The Knee Made Easy

Charalambos Panayiotou Charalambous

The Knee Made Easy

Springer

Charalambos Panayiotou Charalambous
Blackpool Teaching Hospitals
NHS Foundation Trust
Blackpool
Lancashire
UK

ISBN 978-3-030-54505-5 ISBN 978-3-030-54506-2 (eBook)
https://doi.org/10.1007/978-3-030-54506-2

This Springer imprint is published by the registered company Springer Nature Switzerland AG
The registered company address is: Gewerbestrasse 11, 6330 Cham, Switzerland

I dedicate this book to my parents and to all my special teachers and trainers.

Preface

This book aims to provide the reader with a basic understanding of commonly encountered knee conditions and guide as to how these may be managed. It is directed to a wide audience ranging from undergraduate students to those in post-graduate training or in full practice. I hope that not only medical professionals (medical students, general practitioners, orthopaedic surgeons) but also allied health professionals (physiotherapists) find this book of use. It aims to not only transmit knowledge for day-to-day clinical practice but also prepare those with upcoming exams (undergraduate medical, MRCS, FRCS (Orth)).

This book tries to present information in an easily read, succinct way, and break down a vast complex subject into smaller, manageable sections. In particular, this book attempts to unpick and explain those concepts of knee surgery that may be challenging to understand. An attempt is made not only to provide knowledge and information, but also stimulate lateral thinking.

I would like to thank Vignesh Iyyadurai, Project coordinator for Springer Nature, for his support in seeing through the project to its completion. Gratitude is paid to colleagues for their constructive feedback in preparation of this book, particularly Dr. Wael Mati, Consultant Radiologist at Blackpool Victoria Hospital.

My special thanks to Chrysanthos Therapontos for demonstrating through illustrations many of the book's concepts and Tariq Kwaees for helping to demonstrate clinical examination techniques.

Blackpool, Lancashire, UK — Charalambos Panayiotou Charalambous

Contents

Chapter 1
Introduction

When setting out to understand and manage disorders of the knee it is essential to recognise the normal structure and function of this joint. Hence, the clinical anatomy of the knee is initially presented along with a description of the healthy knee joint's biomechanics and function.

The first step in the successful management of knee disorders is the acquisition of a thorough clinical history. Such clinical history elicits the presenting symptoms, their onset, progress and severity, but also determines the patient's overall condition, functional demands, personal circumstances and expectations. Although open ended questions are mainly utilised, specific questioning is also vital in getting a better grasp of the presenting problem and in formulating potential diagnoses. A structured approach for obtaining a clinical history for knee complaints is presented in the fifth chapter.

Clinical examination elicits signs that can supplement the clinical history, and prove or disprove the working diagnosis that the clinician is already considering by having listened to the patient's troubles. The sixth chapter guides as how to perform a structured clinical examination with an emphasis on some of the many special tests described in knee assessment. A structured approach may ensure that important signs are not overlooked.

Clinical history and clinical examination help to guide as to the most likely diagnosis, as well as to potential alternative diagnoses. Once the likely origin of the patient's symptoms is determined, one aims to investigate this further, to confirm or dispute the working diagnosis. The seventh chapter gives an overview of the potential radiological and neurophysiological tests that are available in the diagnosis of knee conditions, helping to guide the reader as to what information these may provide. The value of diagnostic local anaesthetic injections and gait analysis is also discussed.

When managing knee conditions, a wide spectrum of potential interventions are available and it is a skill to decide when and how to intervene. The next chapter introduces some of the challenges faced in treating knee disorders and discusses the role of the management ladder for knee conditions. The next two chapters discuss

C. Panayiotou Charalambous, *The Knee Made Easy*,
https://doi.org/10.1007/978-3-030-54506-2_1

the principles and techniques of injection and needling therapy as well as common surgical procedures employed in the management of the troublesome knee.

Physiotherapy has a huge role to play in the management of knee conditions either in isolation or in combination with other interventions. Although a detailed description of physiotherapy modalities utilised in knee conditions is beyond the scope of this book, the subsequent chapter introduces the reader to some physiotherapy principles viewed from a surgeon's perspective.

Patients don't present with a clinical diagnosis but with symptoms such as pain, stiffness, locking, swelling, instability or weakness. Although common symptoms have common causes, a thorough consideration of what could be accounting for such symptoms may ensure that unusual pathologies are not overlooked. Hence, the subsequent chapters describe a structured consideration of potential causes of common presenting knee symptoms, and advice on how they may be investigated and managed.

The rest of the book reverts to the usual approach of describing specific knee conditions rather than symptoms. These chapters present in greater detail common conditions that may be encountered in clinical practise, their pathogenesis, demographics, clinical symptoms and signs, and guide as to the investigation and management for each.

Reaching a clinical diagnosis relies on knowledge but also on the ability to structure the clinical thought process, to stay open minded, to identify what is vital and eliminate the unnecessary, skills that this book aims to encourage and help develop. Similarly, when it comes to clinical management, this book tries to highlight that one solution does not fit all, but the individualities of the patient and their personal circumstances must be carefully considered. Shared decision making between clinician and patient has a vital role in choosing amongst of many management options. Surgery for many knee conditions may be seen as the last resort, one to be approached with careful consideration and caution.

As a Consultant Surgeon in Trauma and Orthopaedics who has done all my undergraduate and postgraduate training in the United Kingdom, the guidance presented in this book originates from personal experiences, the teachings and "wisdoms" of my senior trainers, peers and colleagues, as well as an extensive literature review. Much of what is presented is commonly available knowledge and every attempt has been made to acknowledge and reference its original sources as warranted. Some may not fully agree with what is presented, some may have opposite views, but that is understandable and acceptable given the uncertainty in much of what we do. Nevertheless, I hope the reader will gain and benefit from what is said, and incorporate some of the advice given in their clinical practise.

Chapter 2
Knee Clinical Anatomy

This chapter describes the normal anatomy of the knee considering the bones, ligaments, muscles, tendons, arterial and nerve supply. The clinical relevance of these structures is also described.

2.1 Knee—Anatomical Structures

We may explore the anatomy of the knee [1–83] in layers, starting from the deepest and moving onto the most superficial:

- Bones
- Joint capsule and ligaments
- Muscles and their tendons
- Subcutaneous tissue and skin

When considering the knee, the bones to describe are the:

- Femur
- Tibia
- Patella
- Fibula

The joints these bones form between them are the:

- Tibiofemoral joint
- Patellofemoral (PF) joint
- Proximal tibiofibular joint

C. Panayiotou Charalambous, *The Knee Made Easy*,
https://doi.org/10.1007/978-3-030-54506-2_2

2.1.1 *Femur*

The femur (thigh bone) is the largest bone in the body. It has three main parts:

1. Femoral head and neck—proximal part
2. Diaphysis (shaft)—middle part
3. Femoral condyles—distal part

The femoral head is connected to the shaft of the femur by the femoral neck. In the coronal plane the femoral neck makes an angle of about 125° (120°–140°) with the femoral shaft. In the axial plane the femoral neck usually makes an anterior inclination in relation to the rest of the femur, which is measured in relation to a line passing through the posterior part of the distal femoral condyles (posterior condylar line). This inclination is in most cases anterior (anteversion) and following skeletal maturity it has been shown to be at an angle of about 16° (+/−6°). On occasions, the femoral neck is inclined posteriorly in relation to the rest of the femur and that is known as retroversion.

The distal femur has two bony prominences projecting distally, the medial and lateral condyles. These are separated anteriorly by the trochlea and posteriorly by the femoral intercondylar notch.

The lateral condyle is larger in a mediolateral and anteroposterior direction as compared to the medial condyle. However, the medial condyle is longer, projecting more distally as compared to the lateral condyle.

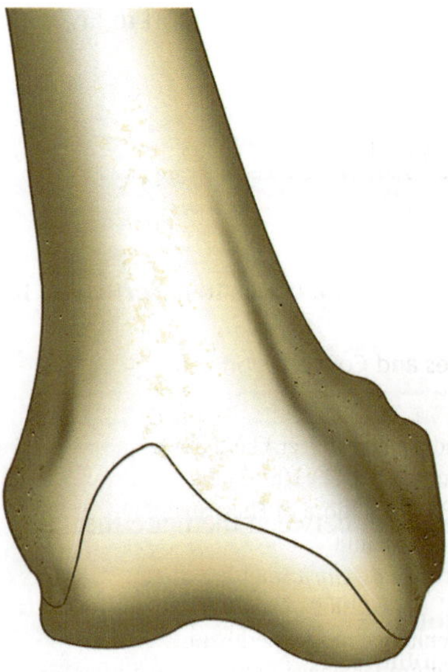

Distal femur showing distal prominence of medial as compared to lateral femoral condyle

The anterior, inferior, and part of the posterior surfaces of the femoral condyles are covered with articular cartilage and articulate with the tibia at the tibiofemoral articulation.

The trochlea is a "U" shaped groove on the anterior part of the distal femur between the two condyles. It has lateral and medial facets covered by articular cartilage and articulates with the patella at the patellofemoral articulation. The lateral facet is larger and extends more proximally than the medial facet. The lateral facet has a relatively steep angle. The cartilage covering the trochlea is much thinner than on the patella, being about 2–3 mm thick.

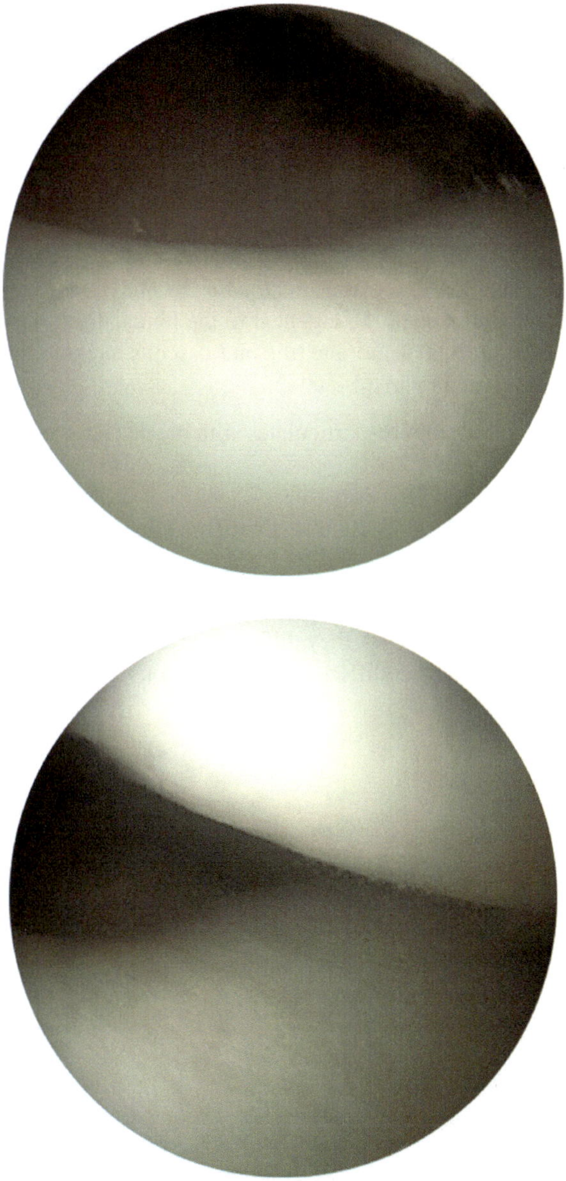

Arthroscopic appearance of the patellofemoral joint, with U shaped trochlea

On the medial aspect of the medial femoral condyle there are two prominences:

1. The medial epicondyle
2. The adductor tubercle

On the lateral aspect of the lateral femoral condyle there is one similar prominence:

1. The lateral epicondyle

A line joining the posterior part of the distal femoral condyles (posterior condylar line) is in about 3° of internal rotation in relation to a line joining the medial and lateral epicondyles (anatomical transepicondylar line) [6].

2.1.2 Tibia

The lower leg has two bones, the tibia and the fibula. The tibia is larger of the 2 and is located on the medial side of the leg, next to the fibula. The tibia is connected to the fibula by a thick fibrous membrane (the interosseous membrane).

The tibia has three main parts:

1. The tibial plateau proximally—articulates with the distal femur at the tibiofemoral joint
2. Diaphysis (shaft)—middle part
3. Tibial plafond—distal part—articulates with the talus at the ankle joint

The tibial plateau has two condyles (medial and lateral) of which the medial is larger in both the anteroposterior and coronal planes. Both condyles are concave in a mediolateral direction. However, they differ in the anteroposterior direction (a difference which along with their difference in dimensions allows their distinction on plain radiographs):

- Medial condyle—concave
- Lateral condyle—convex

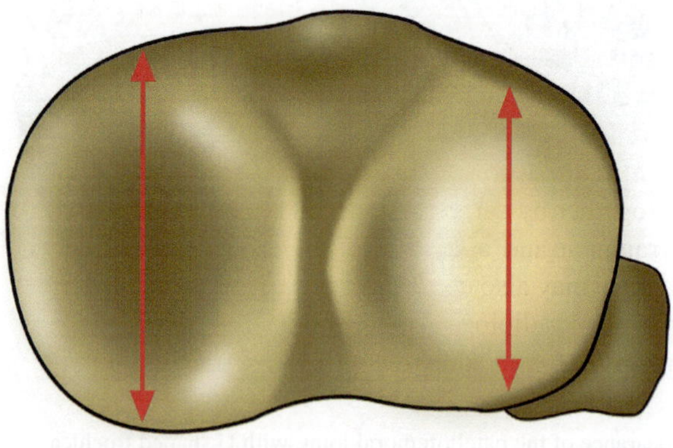

The medial tibial condyle is larger than the lateral

The medial and lateral tibial condyles are separated by the intercondylar area which has two tubercles projecting into the joint (the medial and lateral tibial spines). The upper surface of the condyles is covered with articular cartilage and articulates with the distal femur at the tibiofemoral articulation. The outer part of the lateral condyle articulates with the head of the fibula at the proximal tibiofibular articulation.

The tibial tubercle is a bony prominence located in the midline of the anterior aspect of the tibia, distal to the condyles.

The inter-condylar fossa is located on the posterior aspect of the tibia, between the two condyles.

The lateral condyle has a prominence on its anterolateral aspect (Gerdy's tubercle).

The diaphysis of the tibia is triangular with an anterior, medial and lateral border which form the boundaries of three surfaces—medial, lateral and posterior surfaces. The anterior border (tibial crest/shin) is the most prominent border and is easily palpable.

2.1.3 Patella

The patella (kneecap) is the largest sesamoid bone (a bone located in a tendon separate from the rest of the skeleton) in the body, and is located at the anterior aspect of the knee.

It is triangular in shape with rounded borders, and with its apex pointing inferiorly. Its anterior surface is flat, whilst its posterior surface consists of two condyles (facets) separated by a vertical ridge:

1. Medial facet
2. Lateral facet

The patellar facets are covered with articular cartilage and articulate with the trochlea of the femur at the patellofemoral articulation. The articular cartilage of the patella is very thick (as high as 7 mm), due to the huge forces acting upon the patellofemoral articulation.

In early life the patella is made of cartilage (hence not visible on plain radiographs of the knee). Ossification of the patella begins at the age of about 3–6 years. Usually this occurs from two centres of ossification which eventually unite. However, failure of these to unite may lead to two patellar fragments (bipartite patella) joined together by cartilage rather than bone. In such cases there is usually a large main fragment and a smaller superolateral fragment. Tripartite and even multipartite patellae may also occur. Such developmental variants may be identified for the first time upon radiological imaging of the knee following an injury, where they may be mistaken for an acute fracture.

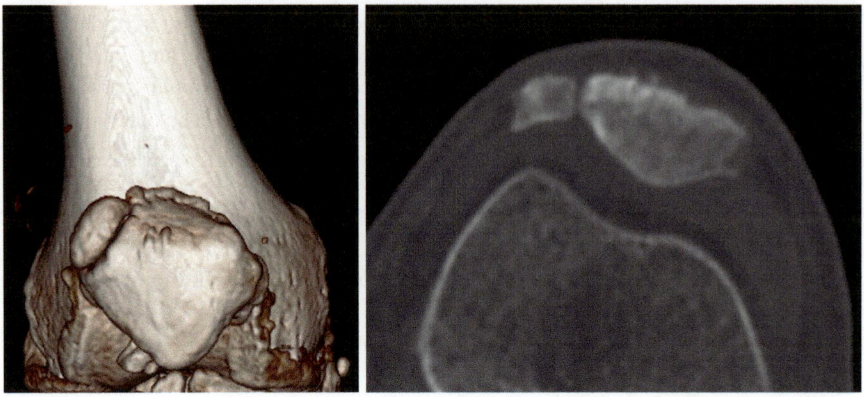

Bipartite patella CT

2.1.4 Fibula

The fibula is the smaller of the two bones of the lower leg. It is located on the posterolateral side of the leg, next to the tibia. The fibula is connected to the tibia by a thick fibrous membrane (interosseous membrane). It articulates with the tibia proximally, at the proximal tibiofibular articulation, and distally at the distal tibiofibular articulation (as part of the ankle joint). The fibula has four main parts:

1. Head—proximal part
2. Neck—between head and shaft
3. Shaft—middle part
4. Lateral malleolus—distal part

The fibular head has an articular facet that faces upwards and medially and which articulates with the lateral condyle of the tibia. The styloid process is a prominence that extends upwards from the posterior part of the fibular head.

2.1.5 Fabella

The fabella is a small sesamoid bone found in 10% to 30% of knees, with evidence that its incidence may be increasing [25, 26]. It is located on the anterior surface of the lateral head of the gastrocnemius muscle, behind the lateral condyle of the femur. The fabella thus articulates with the lateral condyle of the femur.

The fabella may be bony or cartilaginous. It may be a single entity or composed of two or more parts (bi- or tripartite) and hence may be mistaken for loose bodies on radiological imaging.

It is closely related to the common peroneal nerve.

2.2 Knee Joint

The knee is the joint between the distal end of the femur, the proximal end of the tibia, and the posterior surface of the patella. It consists of two articulations:

1. The tibiofemoral articulation—between the medial and lateral condyles of the distal femur and the medial and lateral condyles of the proximal tibia
2. PF articulation—between the patella and femoral trochlea

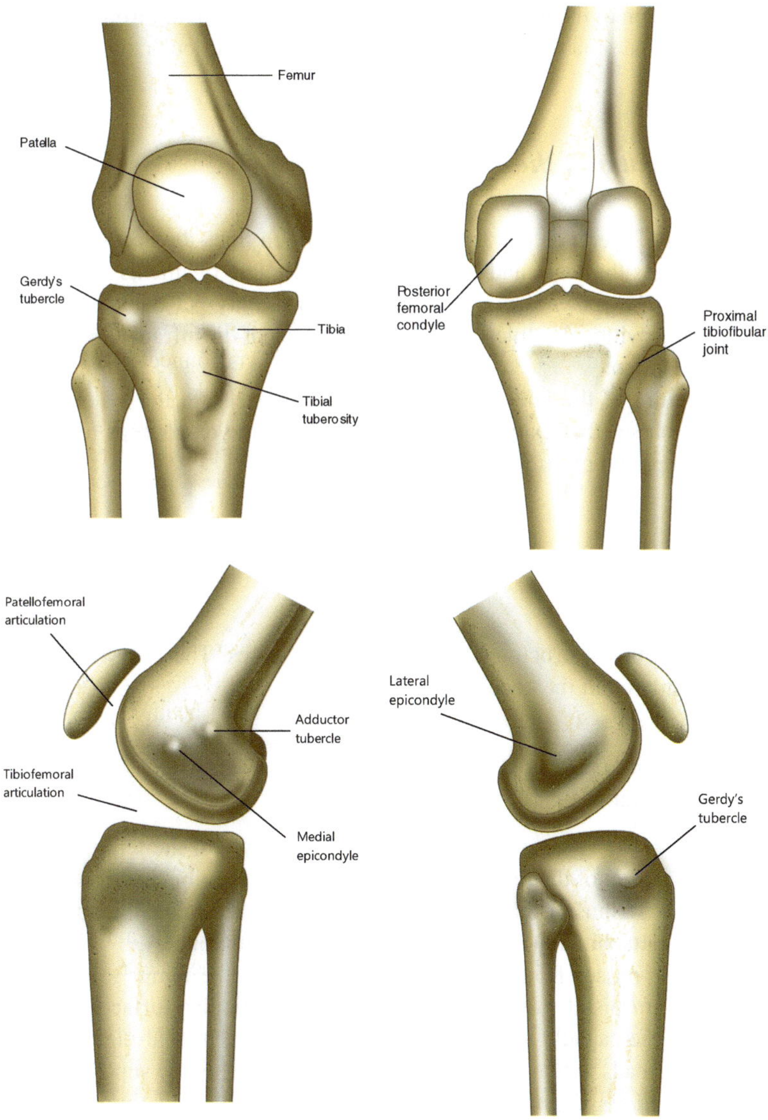

Bones of the knee: anterior and posterior view, side view medial and lateral

2.2.1 Capsule of the Knee Joint

The capsule of the knee joint attaches posteriorly along the superior margins of the femoral condyles and the intercondylar fossa. Anteriorly, it covers the deep surface of the patellar retinaculae up to the superior border of the patella. There is no capsule above the patella, allowing the suprapatellar bursa to communicate with the joint. Medially it extends to the articular margin of the femur and laterally to just proximal to the groove for the popliteus tendon. Distally, the capsule has a short extension, attaching anteriorly at less than 6 mm from the articular tibial border, and posteriorly to the distal margin of the tibial inter-condylar fossa, up to 14 mm from the joint line. On the sides of the tibia the capsule attaches close to the articular surface [27, 28].

2.2.2 Synovium of the Knee Joint

The synovium of the knee is a thin membrane which lines the deep surface of the capsule. It covers the front and the sides of the cruciate ligaments which are thus intracapsular but extrasynovial (within the capsule cavity but outside the synovial cavity). The synovium also lines the posterior surface of the infrapatellar fat pad and the popliteal tendon.

The synovium of the knee joint may be continuous with the synovium of the suprapatellar bursa (that extends proximally deep to the quadriceps tendon, up to about a hand breadth proximal to the patella).

2.2.3 Ligaments

Ligaments are fibrous structures that connect two bones. The following ligaments are to be considered in the knee region:

Medial Collateral Ligament (MCL)
This has three components:

1. *Superficial MCL*—passes from the medial epicondyle of the femur to insert on the medial aspect of the proximal tibia. It inserts on the tibia deep to the tendons of the pes anserinus. This insertion is about 6–8 cm distal to the joint line, and has a broad attachment (2–4 mm wide and 12–18 mm long).
2. *Deep MCL*—passes from the medial epicondyle of the femur to the proximal tibia, 2–3 mm distal to the margin of the tibial articular surface. It is closely attached to the capsule and to the outer border of the medial meniscus. Valgus injury often leads to tear of the deep MCL before tearing the superficial MCL.
3. *Posterior oblique ligament (POL)*—this is a thickening of the posteromedial capsule. Passes from the adductor tubercle and attaches to the posterior surface of the tibia.

Lateral collateral ligament (LCL)—passes from the distal femur (posterior and proximal to the lateral femoral epicondyle) to insert distally onto the anterolateral aspect of the fibular head.

Popliteofibular ligament (arcuate ligament)—passes from the musculotendinous junction of popliteus and inserts onto the posterosuperior medial part of the styloid process of the fibula.

Fabellofibular ligament—passes from the fabella and inserts onto the tip of the styloid process of the fibula.

Anterolateral ligament—this is located deep to the iliotibial band (ITB). It passes from the distal femur (just posterior and proximal to the lateral epicondyle) to insert onto the proximal tibia (about 4–10 mm below the tibial joint line, about 2 cm posterior to Gerdy's tubercle, halfway between Gerdy's tubercle and the fibular head).

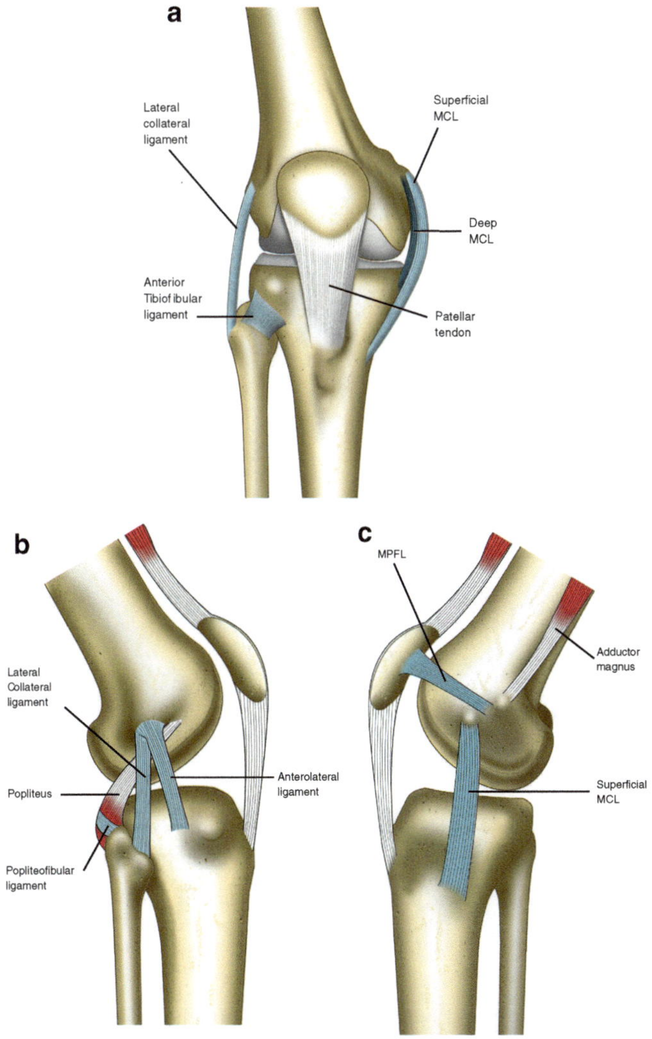

Extra-aricular ligaments of the knee, (**a**) anterior (**b**) lateral (**c**) medial view

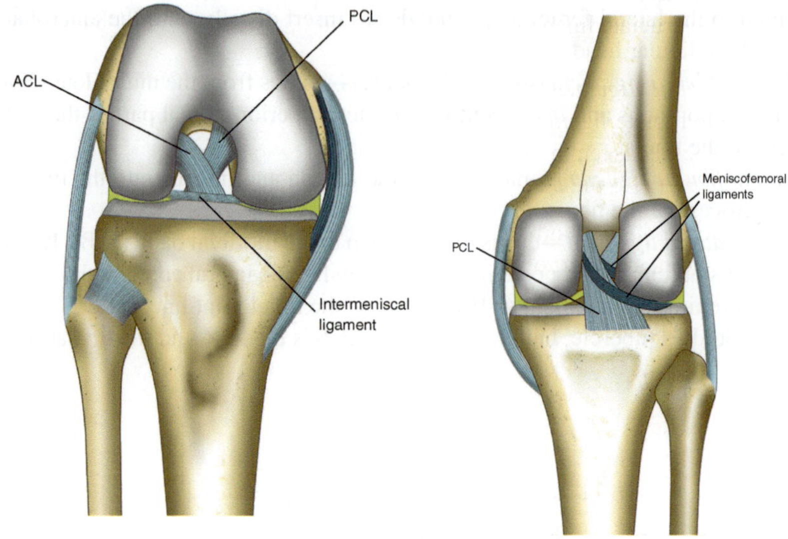

Anterior and posterior views of the cruciate ligaments

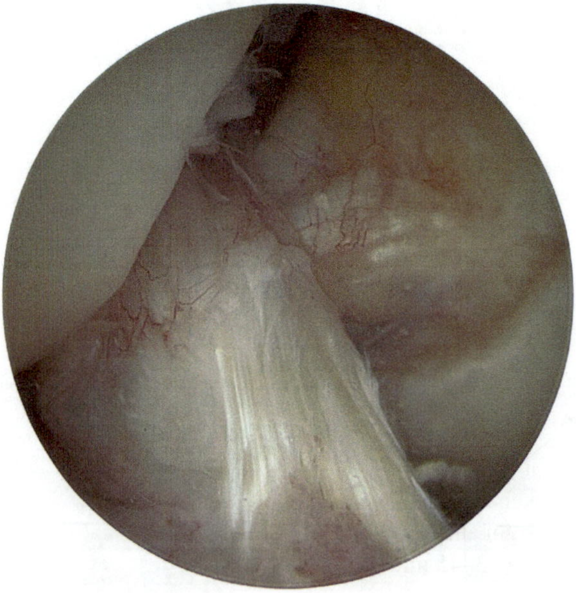

Arthroscopic view of the anterior and posterior cruciate ligaments

Cruciate Ligaments
There are two cruciate ligaments, the anterior and posterior cruciate ligament:

Anterior Cruciate Ligament (ACL)
The anterior cruciate ligament passes from the inferior, inner surface of the lateral condyle of the distal femur and inserts onto the anterior part of the tibial articular surface, just lateral to the medial tibial spine. It consists of two bundles:

1. Anteromedial (AM) bundle—passes from the proximal part of its femoral origin, to the anteromedial part of its tibial insertion
2. Posterolateral (PL) band—passes from the distal part of its femoral origin, to the posterolateral part of its tibial insertion

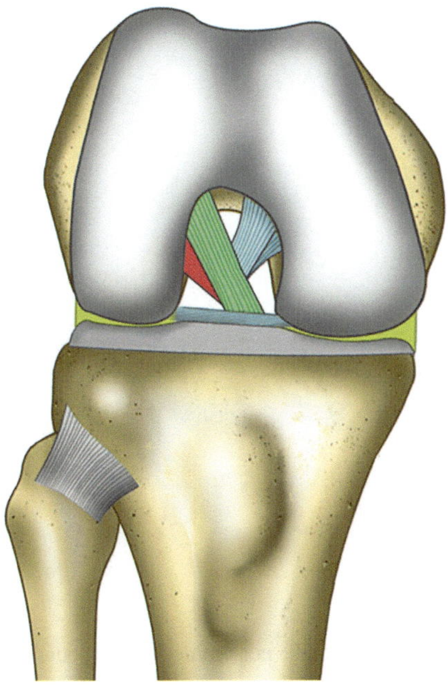

The ACL has an anteromedial bundle (green) and a posterolateral bundle (red)

The mean width of the ACL is about 8 mm (range 5–14 mm), with the AM bundle being thicker than the PL bundle. The middle part of the ACL is narrower than its femoral origin and tibial insertion. The intra-articular length of the ACL is about 32 mm (range 23–45 mm).

Posterior Cruciate Ligament (PCL)

The PCL passes from the medial side of the roof of the inter-condylar notch of the femur (anteroinferior portion of the lateral aspect of the medial femoral condyle) and inserts to the superior aspect of the posterior part of the tibia, in the midline, extending about 12–17 mm distal to the tibial plateau. The PCL consists of two bundles:

1. Anterolateral (AL) bundle—passes from the roof of the notch
2. Posteromedial (PM) bundle—originates mainly from the medial side wall of the notch

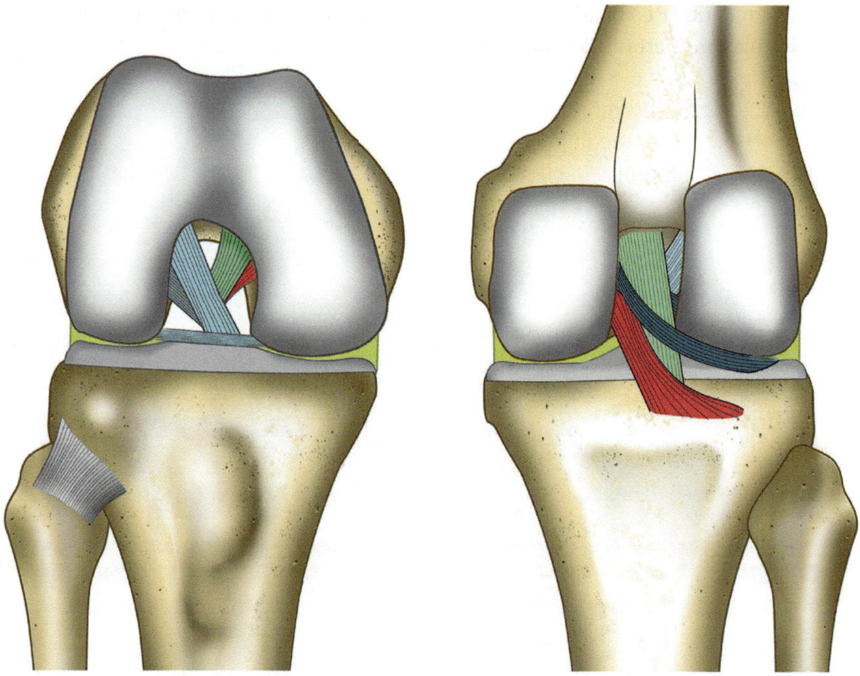

The PCL has an anterolateral (green) and a posteromedial (red) bundle

The fibres of the AL bundle of the PCL insert anteriorly to the fibres of the PM bundle on the tibia.

The femoral origin and tibial insertion of the PCL are much wider than its midsubstance (femoral origin is fan shaped and about 1.7 times wider than the tibial insertion). The length of the PCL is about 29–38 mm, whilst its average cross-sectional area is about 11–13 mm [16, 17]. The AL bundle is thicker and stronger as compared to the PM bundle.

Given the close insertion of the PCL to the tibial joint surface, part of the PCL tibial insertion may be detached during resection of the tibial plateau in total knee replacement arthroplasty, even when implants designed to preserve the PCL are utilised. In line with this, Matziolis G et al. [35] showed that with a flat tibial resection (of 0° slope) about 45 ± 30% of the tibial PCL attachment was removed, whilst with a more oblique resection (slope of 7°), about 70 ± 25% of the tibial PCL attachment was removed. Tibial resection led to complete PCL removal in 20% of male patients and 24% of female patients. Hence, they recommended sparing the tibial insertion, by preserving the posterior tibial cortical bone in the area of attachment of the PCL, rather than resecting the tibial plateau completely.

Medial patellofemoral ligament (MPFL)—Passes from the medial aspect of the distal femur (about 9.5 mm (range 4–22) distal and anterior to the adductor tubercle and proximal and posterior to the medial epicondyle) and inserts with a broad insertion onto the medial edge of the patella (upper two thirds, although in some cases it may extend along the whole medial margin of the patella). The patellar insertion is much wider (about 28 mm (range 16–39)) than the femoral origin. It lies deep to the distal part of vastus medialis. It is a thin but strong structure. The length of the MPFL is about 56 mm.

Medial patellotibial ligament—originates from the anteromedial tibia (about 14 mm distal to the joint line) and inserts onto the inferomedial border of the patella.

Medial patellomeniscal ligament—originates from the inferomedial border of the patella, proximal to the medial patellotibial ligament, and inserts onto the medial meniscus.

Lateral patellofemoral ligament—originates from the lateral femoral epicondyle and inserts onto the lateral border of the patella at its widest part.

Lateral patellomeniscal ligament—connects the inferolateral part of the patella to the anterolateral part of the lateral meniscus.

Lateral patellotibial ligament—this is part of the quadriceps aponeurosis that inserts onto the patella and patellar tendon and onto the proximal tibia between the tibial tuberosity and Gerdy's tubercle [7].

Meniscofemoral ligaments (Humphrey and Wrisberg ligaments)—pass from the posterior horn of the lateral meniscus to the medial femoral condyle, near the origin of the PCL. About 50% of knees have both of these ligaments, but almost all knees have at least one. Gupte CM et al. [33] in an anatomical study of 78 specimens, showed that 93% contained at least one meniscofemoral ligament. The anterior meniscofemoral ligament (aMFL) of Humphrey was seen in 74%, and the posterior meniscofemoral ligament (pMFL) of Wrisberg in 69%. In 50% of the specimens both ligaments were present, and these patients were younger that those with one ligament or none. The authors suggested that the higher incidence of meniscofemoral ligaments in younger cases may be due to their degeneration with age.

2.2.4 Menisci

The menisci are bands of fibrocartilage located between the femoral and tibial condyles [44–47]. There are two menisci:

1. Medial meniscus—located between the medial femoral condyle and medial tibial condyle
2. Lateral meniscus—located between the lateral femoral condyle and lateral tibial condyle

They are C shaped when viewed from above and wedge shaped when viewed in section. The medial meniscus is narrower and larger than the lateral meniscus. The lateral meniscus covers 75–90% of the lateral tibial condyle and the medial meniscus 50–75% of the medial tibial condyle.

They consist of three parts:

1. Anterior horn
2. Body
3. Posterior horn

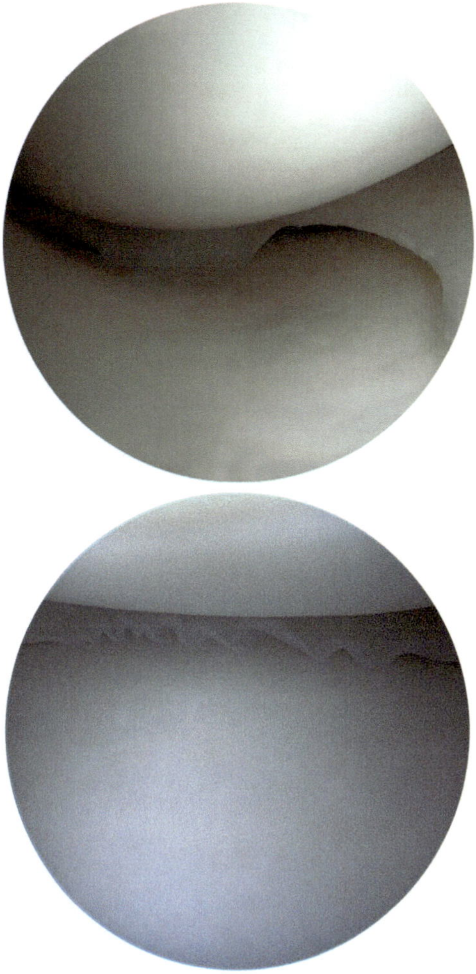

Arthroscopic views of the medial meniscus. Note: the wavy appearance suggestive of an intact medial meniscus

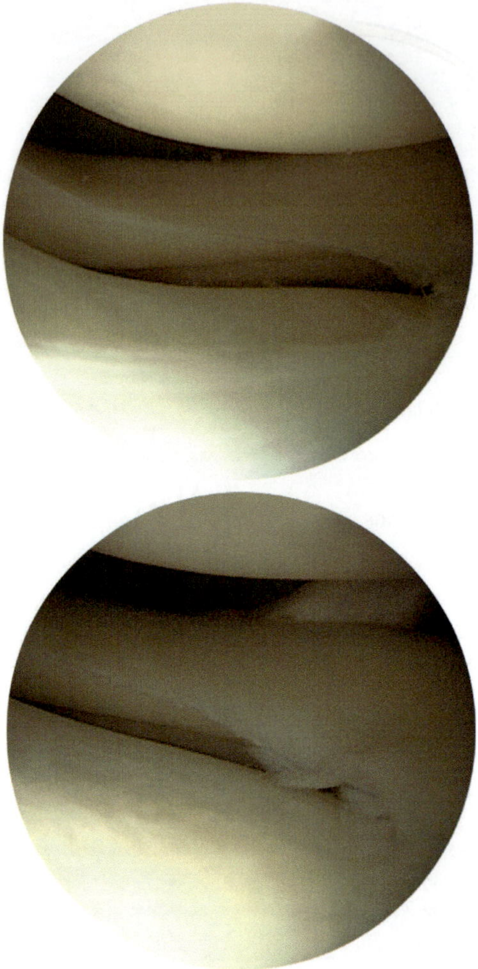

Arthroscopic views of the lateral meniscus, with the popliteus tendon crossing behind it

The anterior and posterior horns are attached to the intercondylar eminence of the tibia. The outer borders of the menisci are attached to the joint capsule and tibia. The attachment of the lateral meniscus to the tibia is interrupted at the junction of its anterior 2/3 s and posterior 1/3 by the popliteus hiatus.

A transverse intermeniscal ligament connects the anterior horn of the medial meniscus to the lateral meniscus.

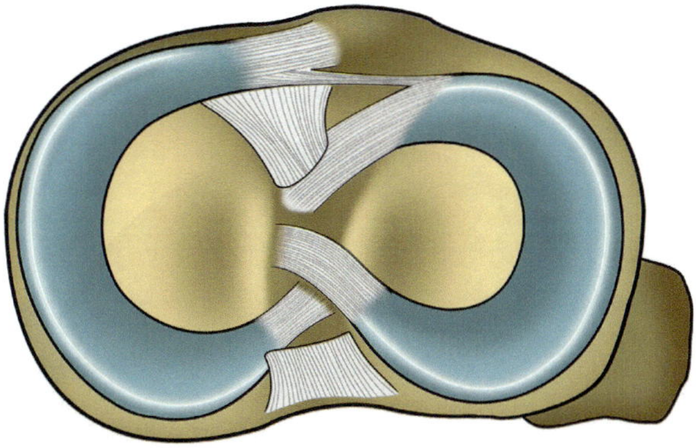

Top view of the medial and lateral menisci

In adults, the meniscus has good blood supply only at its peripheral outer part (about outer 1/3rd).

The meniscus may thus be described into three zones according to its vascularity:

1. Outer zone—red—rich in blood vessels
2. Inner zone—white—avascular
3. Intermediate zone—red-white, intermediate between the outer and inner zones

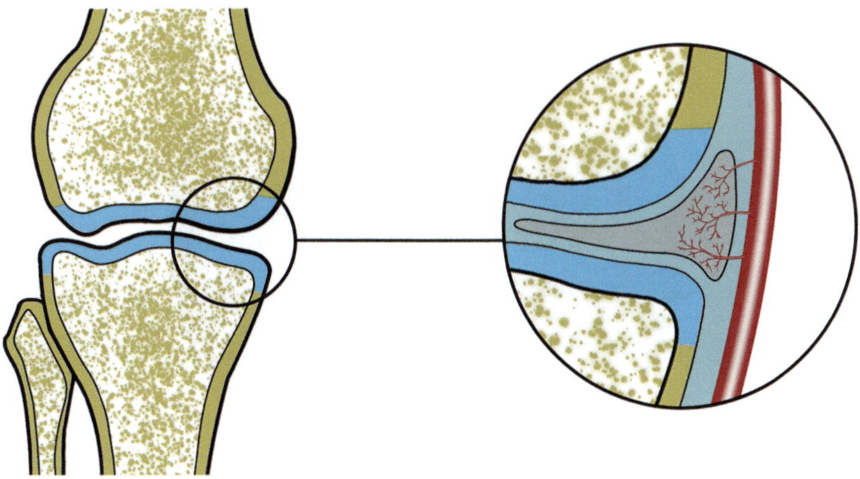

Meniscal blood supply

2.2.5 *Fat pads of the Knee*

These are localised collections of fat located in the knee joint [48–52]. A typical fat pad is macroscopically yellow and lobular in appearance. Three fat pads are considered in the knee joint:

- Suprapatellar
- Prefemoral
- Infrapatellar

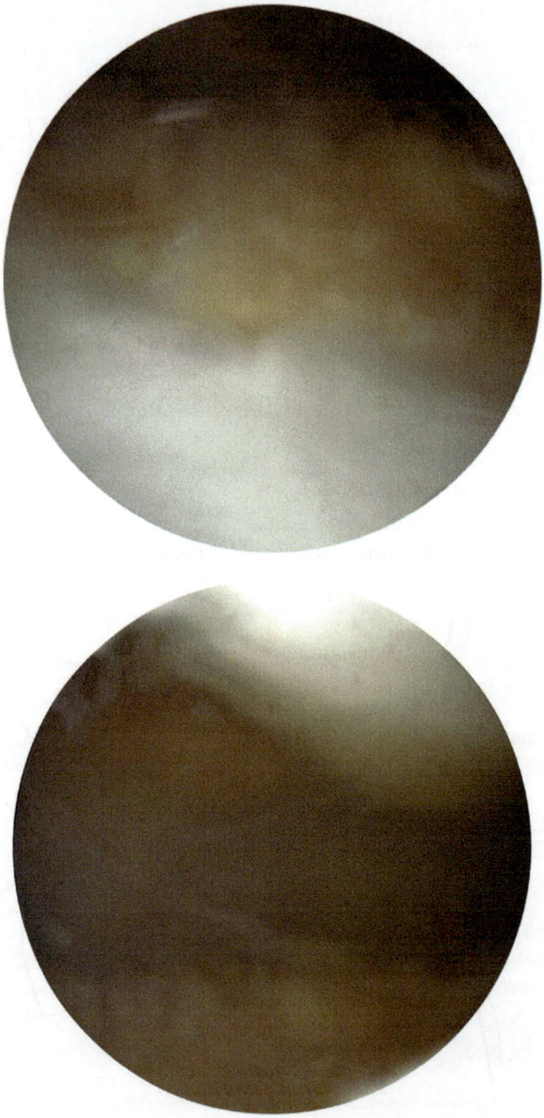

Arthroscopic view of prefemoral and suprapatellar fat pads

Suprapatellar fat pad—located behind the distal part of the quadriceps and superior pole of the patella, anterior to the suprapatellar bursa. It is triangular in shape.

Prefemoral fat pad—located anterior to the distal part of the femur, behind the suprapatellar bursa.

Infrapatellar fat pad—located between the:

- Inferior pole of the patella superiorly
- Anterior part of the tibial plateau inferiorly
- Patellar tendon anteriorly
- Femoral condyles, intercondylar notch, and meniscal horns posteriorly

The infrapatellar fat pad:

- Has a central body, a medial and a lateral extension and in some cases a superior tag
- Has a superior vertical cleft and an inferior horizontal cleft
- The horizontal cleft is located anterior to the tibial insertion of the ACL and below the ligamentum mucosum (which forms the roof of the cleft)
- Is connected to the intercondylar notch by the ligamentum mucosum
- Is extrasynovial, with its deep surface and clefts lined by synovium
- Is innervated mainly by the posterior tibial nerve
- Has a rich blood supply with superficial and deep anastomotic plexuses
- Is broken down only in severe malnutrition

Disorders may arise in the clefts such as ganglion cysts, loose bodies, and nodular synovitis.

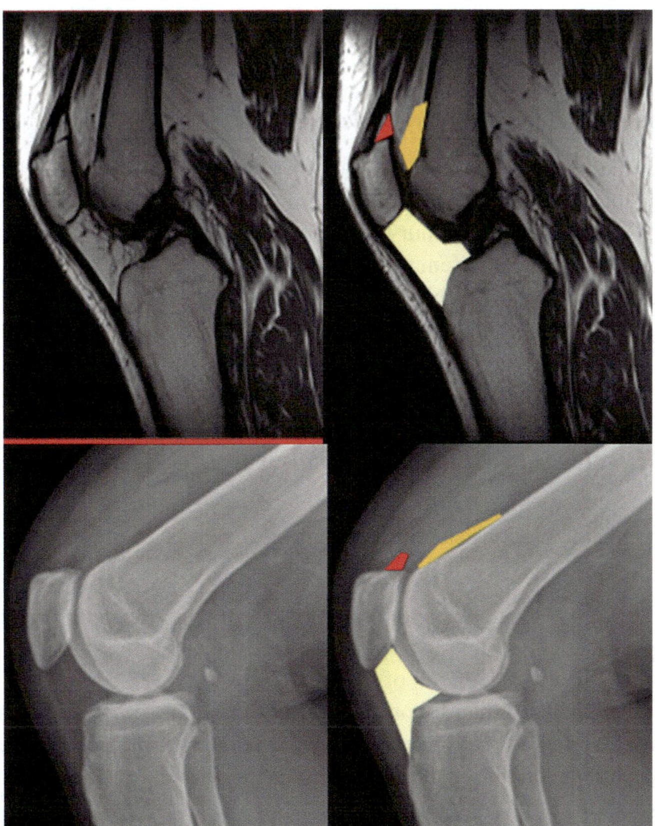

Fat pads (infrapatellar (yellow), suprapatellar (red), prefemoral (orange)

2.3 Proximal Tibiofibular Articulation

The proximal tibiofibular articulation [10] is the joint between the lateral condyle of the tibia and the head of the fibula.

The articular facets of the fibular head and the lateral tibial condyle vary in size, form, and inclination. Based on the morphology of the articular surfaces, multiple types of proximal tibiofibular articulation have been described. For simplicity the following two main types may be considered depending on the joint's axis:

1. Horizontal—circular in shape and located behind a projection of the lateral edge of the tibia
2. Oblique—has a smaller articular surface

The proximal tibiofibular joint is a synovial joint lined with hyaline cartilage. A capsule surrounds the joint and is attached just beyond the joint's articular surfaces. The capsule is lined with synovium and communicates with the knee joint via a subpopliteal recess in a substantial proportion of cases. Anterior and posterior proximal tibiofibular ligaments reinforce the capsule and provide stability.

2.4 Muscles

The muscles around the knee may be described as:

1. Muscles that connect the pelvis to the tibia/fibula
2. Muscles that connect the pelvis to the femur
3. Muscles that connect the femur to the tibia/fibula
4. Muscles that connect the femur to the foot
5. Muscles that connect the tibia/femur to the foot

These are described below [27–30].

2.4.1 Muscles that Connect the Pelvis to the Tibia/Fibula

Quadriceps femoris—consists of four muscles and is located on the front of the thigh:

1 Rectus femoris—located in the middle of the thigh, covering most of the other three quadriceps muscles. It originates from the anteroinferior iliac spine and inserts onto the central tendon of the quadriceps

3. Vastus lateralis—originates from the anterolateral part of the femur and lateral intermuscular septum from the level of the greater trochanter and extends distally. It is orientated obliquely inwards, at an angle of about 40° in relation to the long axis of the femur
4. Vastus medialis—originates from the anteromedial part of the femur and medial intermuscular septum. It runs obliquely outwards at an angle of about 50° in rela-

tion to the long axis of the femur. The vastus medialis obliquus is a part of vastus medialis that originates from the adductor tubercle and distal part of the medial intermuscular septum and runs more obliquely at an angle of about 65° in relation to the long axis of the femur

5. Vastus intermedius—located between vastus lateralis and vastus medialis anterior to the femur and behind rectus femoris (from which it is separated by a bursa). It originates from the anterior surface of the femoral shaft and inserts onto the superior pole of the patella forming the deep layer of the quadriceps tendon

The quadriceps tendon is a trilaminar structure with contributions from the four components of the quadriceps. The most superficial part of this tendon is the rectus femoris, the middle is the vastus lateralis and vastus medialis, and the deep is vastus intermedius. This inserts onto the proximal pole of the patella and gives rise to an aponeurosis that passes over the anterior surface of the patella (to which it is firmly attached) and then gives rise to the patellar tendon. The patellar tendon passes between the inferior pole of the patella and the tibial tuberosity. The aponeurosis also contributes to the lateral and medial patellar retinaculum. Quadriceps is innervated by the femoral nerve (L2, L3, L4).

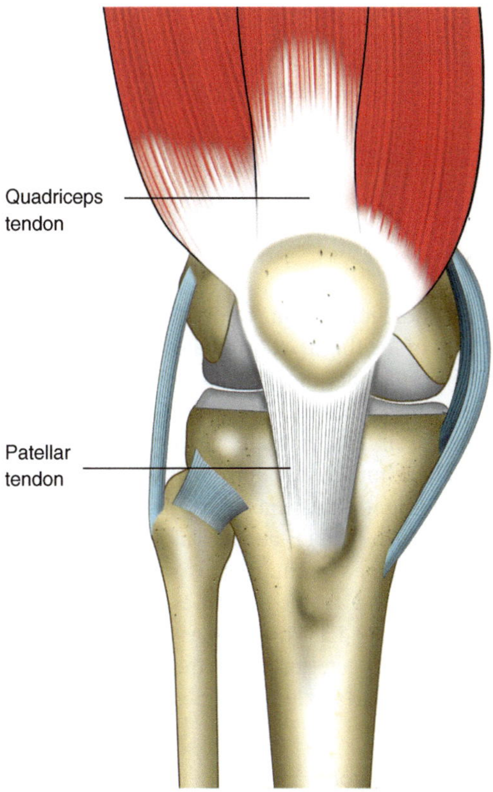

Anterior view of the knee

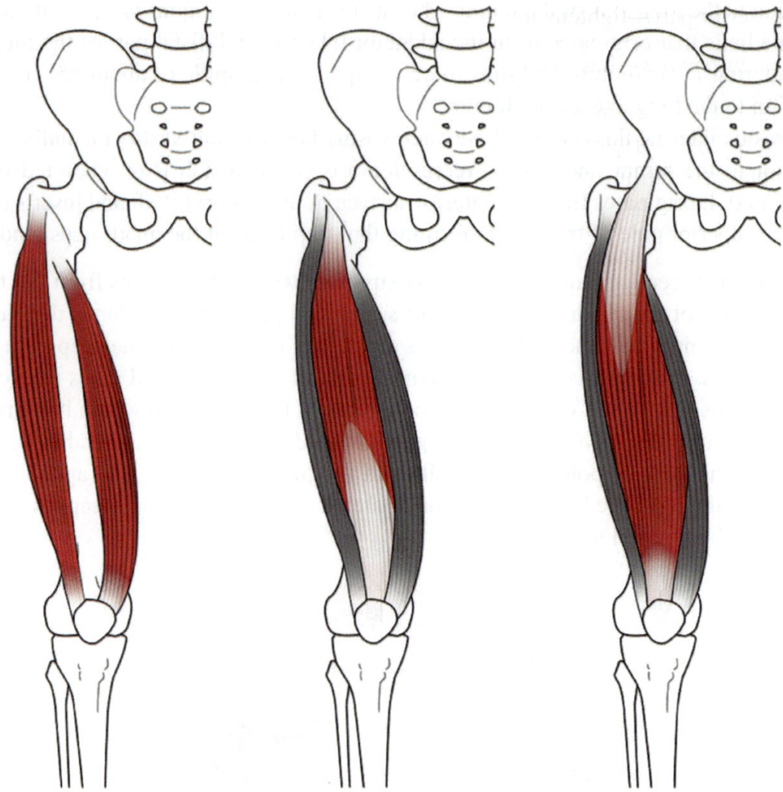

Components of the Quadriceps

ITB [42, 43]—this is a thick, longitudinal, thickening of the fascia lata (the fascia that surrounds the muscles of the thigh). It originates from the anterolateral tubercle of the iliac crest and inserts onto the Gerdy's tubercle of the proximal tibia. Proximally, at the level of the hip, the ITB consists of superficial and deep layers which enclose the tensor fascia latae muscle and which merge into a single layer distal to the tensor fascia latae muscle about the level of the greater trochanter. The ITB receives the tendon of gluteus maximus on its posterior margin.

As it passes vertically distally, the ITB attaches along the length of the thigh to the femur by the lateral intermuscular septum. It is also attached to the distal femur and lateral epicondyle by strong fibrous bands. At the level of the knee the ITB lies in the superficial layer of soft tissues and has connections anteriorly to the quadriceps tendon, patella, patellar tendon, and posteriorly onto the biceps femoris and fibular head.

It may be described in three parts in an anteroposterior direction which tighten in different positions of the knee:

1. Anterior part—tightens in flexion
2. Central part—tightens in mid-flexion

3. Posterior part—tightens in extension

Biceps femoris—has two heads:

1. Long head—originates from the ischial tuberosity
2. Short head—originates from the lateral side of the linea aspera and the lateral supracondylar line of the femur

The two heads form a common tendon which inserts onto the head of the fibula. The long head is innervated by the tibial part of the sciatic nerve and the short head by the common peroneal nerve.

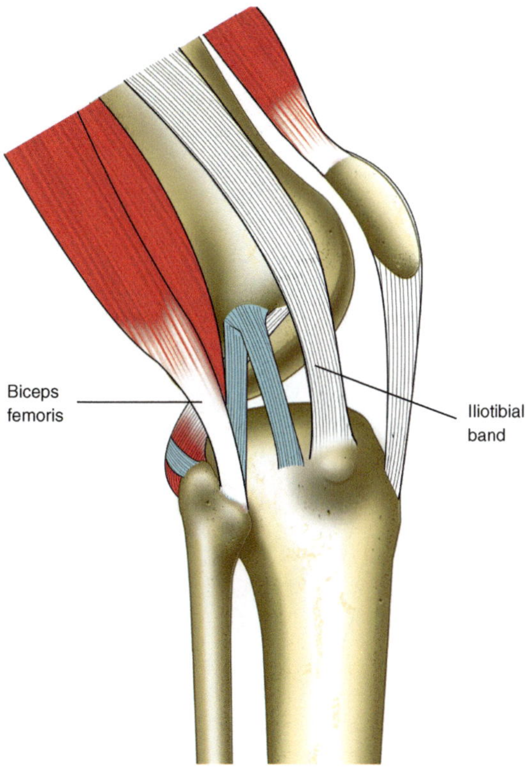

Lateral view of the knee

Semimembranosus [9]—Originates from the ischial tuberosity (with a membranous tendon hence its name) and inserts onto the proximal medial tibia. It is located at the posterior and medial side of the thigh. It has two main attachments:

1. Direct arm—broad attachment to an osseous prominence on the proximal, posterior part of the medial tibial plateau, about 1 cm distal to the joint line
2. Anterior arm—attaches to the proximal tibia, deep to the proximal attachment of the superficial MCL

It is innervated by the tibial branch of the sciatic nerve.

Sartorius—originates from the anterior superior iliac spine and passes obliquely across the anterior thigh to attach to the superomedial surface of the tibia as part of pes anserinus. It consists of a long thin muscle. It is innervated by the femoral nerve.

Gracilis—originates from the symphysis pubis and pubic arch. It runs vertically distally along the thigh, and gives rise to a rounded tendon that passes behind the medial condyle of the femur, curves around the medial condyle of the tibia and inserts onto the upper part of the medial surface of the body of the tibia, below the condyle. At its insertion onto the tibia the gracilis tendon is located just proximal to the tendon of semitendinosus, and is covered by the tendon of the sartorius muscle (as part of pes anserinus). It is innervated by the obturator nerve.

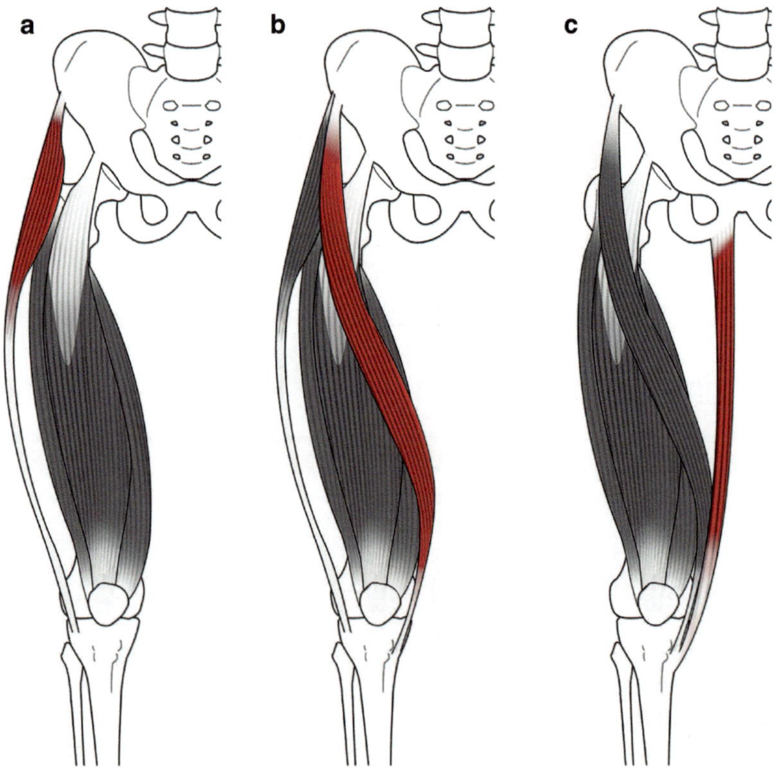

(**a**) Iliotibial band (**b**) Sartorius (**c**) Gracilis

Semitendinosus—originates from the lower part of the ischial tuberosity and from the muscle of the long head of the biceps femoris. It has a long thin muscle which gives rise to a tubular tendon that curves around the medial condyle of the tibia, crosses the medial collateral ligament and inserts at the upper part of the medial surface of the tibia, deep to the insertion of sartorius, and inferior to the insertion of the gracilis tendon (as part of pes anserinus). It is innervated by the tibial part of the sciatic nerve.

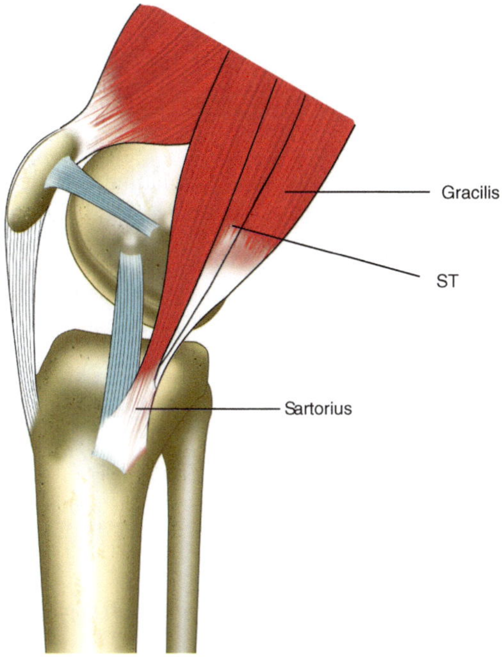

Medial view of the knee

2.4.2 *Muscles that Connect the Pelvis to the Femur*

Adductor Magnus—this is a large muscle which is triangular in shape and is located on the medial side of the thigh.

It consists of two parts:

1. Pubofemoral (adductor part)—originates from the pubic ramus and the ramus of the ischium. It inserts onto the rough line of the femur passing from the greater trochanter to the linea aspera, and onto the linea aspera. It is innervated by the posterior division of the obturator nerve
2. Ischiocondylar part—originates from the ischial tuberosity. It forms a thick muscle that gives rise to a tubular tendon which attaches to the adductor tubercle of the medial femoral condyle. It is innervated by the sciatic nerve

There are several gaps in the tendinous attachment of adductor magnus onto the femur, the lowest one of which is the adductor hiatus. The femoral vessels pass through the adductor hiatus to reach the popliteal fossa.

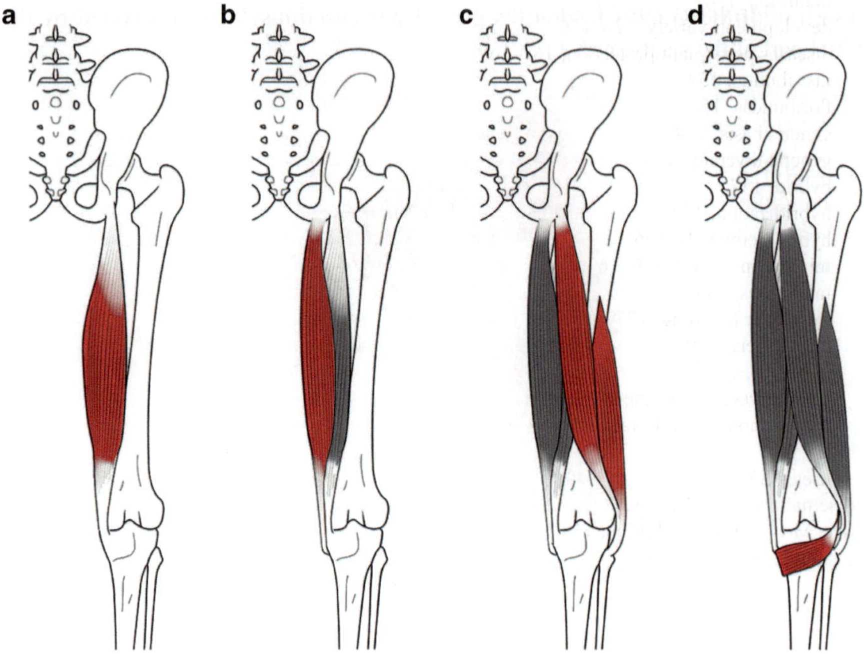

(**a**) Semimembranosus (**b**) Semitendonosus (**c**) Biceps femoris (**d**) Popliteus

2.4.3 Muscles that Connect the Femur to the Tibia

Popliteus—originates from the posterior surface of the tibia, above the soleal line, and passes upwards and laterally giving rise to a tubular tendon that inserts onto the lateral surface of the lateral condyle of the femur. Its tendon separates the lateral meniscus from the lateral collateral ligament. It is innervated by the tibial nerve (L5 and S1).

2.4.4 Muscles that Connect the Femur to the Foot

Gastrocnemius—this is located in the posterior part of the lower leg. It has two muscular heads:

1. Lateral head—originates from the posterior part of the lateral condyle of the femur
2. Medial head—originates from the posterior part of the medial condyle of the femur

The two heads of gastrocnemius and soleus give rise to a common tendon distally (Achilles tendon) which attaches onto the calcaneum. It is innervated by the tibial nerve.

Soleus—located deep to the gastrocnemius. Originates from the posterior surface of the head and upper shaft of the fibula, and the medial border of the tibia. It joins the gastrocnemius aponeurosis to form the Achilles tendon that attaches onto the calcaneum. It is innervated by the tibial nerve.

Soleus has been shown to translate the tibia posteriorly in relation to the femur and hence acts as an agonist to the ACL. In contrast, gastrocnemius tends to translate the tibia anteriorly hence acting as an antagonist to the ACL [83].

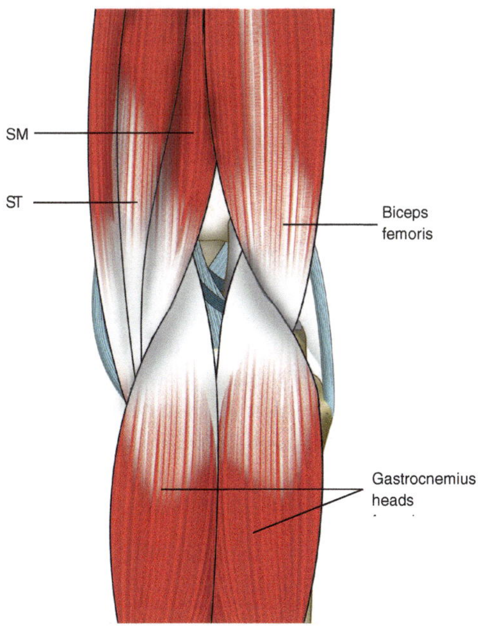

Posterior view of the knee showing gastrocnemius femoral origin

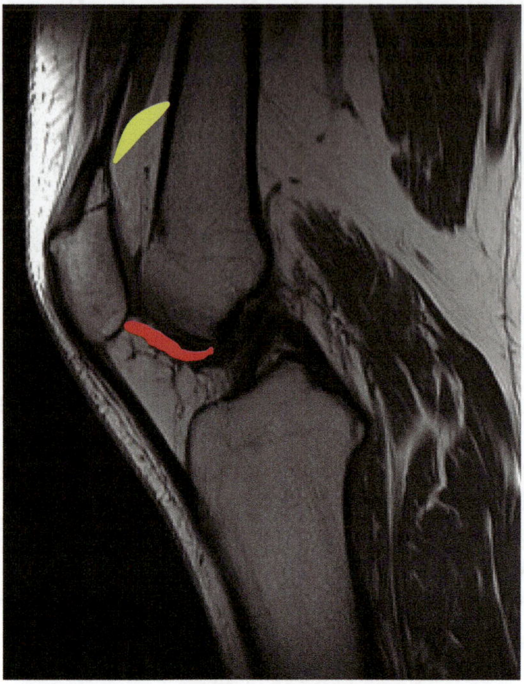

Plicae–infrapatellar (red) suprapatellar (yellow)

2.5 Synovial Folds (Plicae)

Knee plicae are membrane like structures found in the knee [51–54]. They are the remnants of embryonic synovial structures that divide the knee into three separate compartments during development. As these synovial folds break down, a single knee joint evolves. In some cases however these may disappear only partially or not at all, and are thus encountered in the fully developed knee. They are usually incidental, non-symptomatic findings, but may become diseased and contribute to a troublesome knee. They are described as:

1. *Suprapatellar plica*—separates the suprapatellar bursa from the main knee joint cavity
2. *Infrapatellar plica*—located in front of the ACL, passes from the intercondylar notch to the infrapatellar fat pad, at the tip of the patella
3. *Medial patellar plica*—located medial to the medial facet of the patella, and passes longitudinally along the capsule of the knee joint

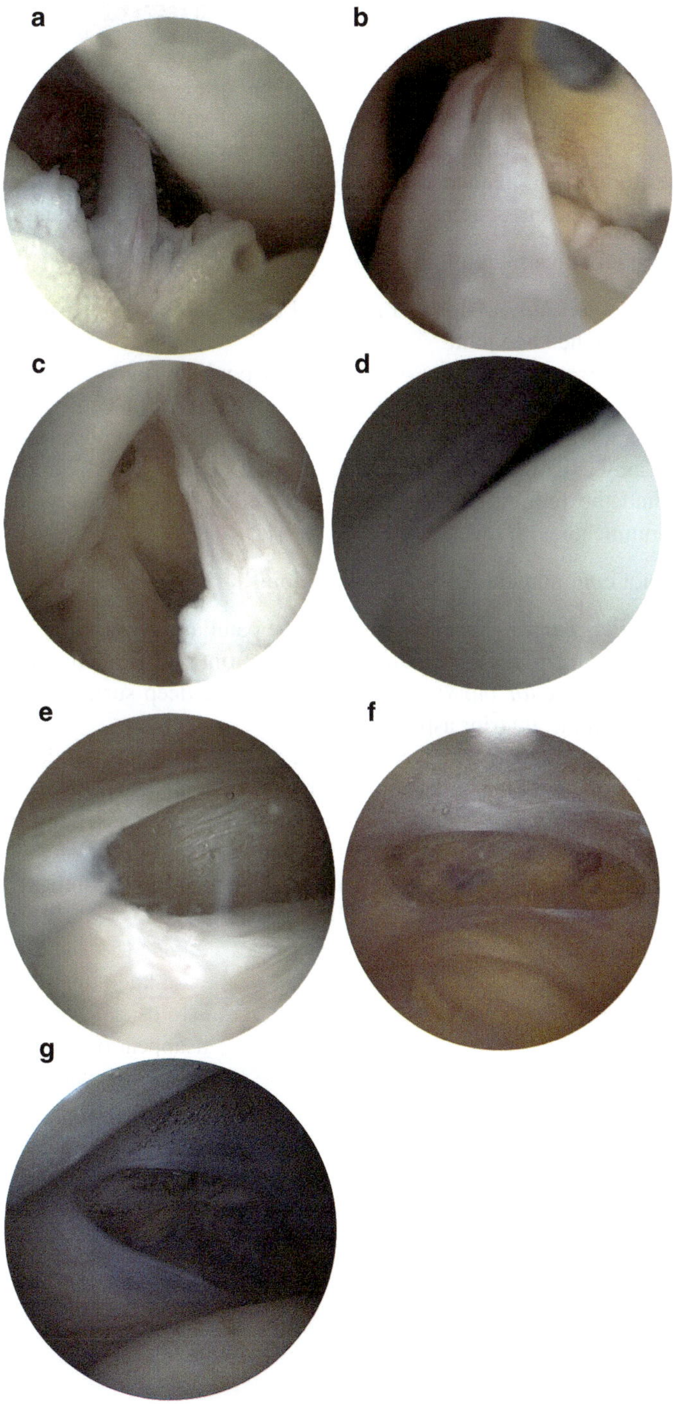

Infrapatellar plica (**a**–**c**), medial plica (**d**, **e**), suprapatellar plica (**f**, **g**)

2.6 Bursae

Several bursae are found in the knee region [58–65]. These are cyst like synovial sacs that facilitate smooth motion between layers of soft tissue (muscles, tendons, ligaments), or between soft-tissue and bone, improving gliding and reducing friction. Their clinical significance is that they may become inflamed or thickened causing pain. The bursae encountered around the knee include the following:

- Bursae communicating with the knee joint
  - *Suprapatellar bursa*—located proximal to the patella and is usually in continuity with the knee joint
  - *Semimembranosus bursa* (also known as popliteal bursa or Baker's cyst)-located just proximal to the attachment of the direct arm of the semimembranosus tendon on the tibia. A defect in the capsule of the posterior part of the knee may exist between the attachment of the direct arm of semimembranosus and the femoral attachment of the medial head of gastrocnemius, and communicate with this bursa
- Bursae not communicating with the knee joint
  - *Prepatellar bursa*—located in front of the patella
  - *Superficial infrapatellar bursa*—located in front of the patellar tendon
  - *Deep infrapatellar bursa*—located between the deep surface of the patellar tendon and the anterior aspect of the tibia
  - *Pes-anserinus bursa*—located between the pes-anserinus tendons' insertion onto the tibia and the underlying insertion of the medial collateral ligament
  - *Biceps femoris bursa*—located between the biceps femoris tendon and the LCL
  - *ITB bursa*—located between the ITB and the lateral part of the femur (its existence has been questioned by more recent anatomical studies)

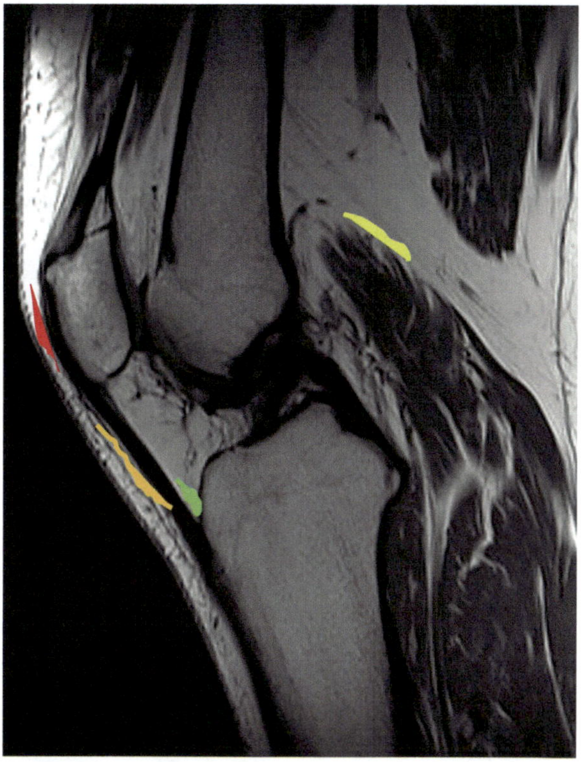

Bursae location - (prepatellar – red, superficial infrapatellar – orange, deep infrapatellar bursa – green, semimembranosus bursa – yellow)

2.7 Anatomy Overview

Consider the axial skeleton as consisting of the vertebral column which articulates via the sacrum to the pelvis. The lower limb is connected to the axial skeleton via:

- The head of the femur which articulates with the pelvis at the hip joint
- Muscles and ligaments that pass between the pelvis and the femur

2.7.1 Orientation of the Knee Bones in Space

Coronal Plane
The femoral head is connected to the shaft of the femur by the femoral neck. In the coronal plane the femoral neck makes an angle of about 125° (120°–140°) with the femoral shaft.

Looking at the knee in the coronal plane the long axis of the femur and the long axis of the tibia, as well as the axes of their articulating surfaces at the tibiofemoral articulation are described below. The long axis is referred to as the anatomical axis.

- Anatomical axis of the femur—line connecting the centre of the femoral shaft in the subtrochanteric area and the centre of the femoral trochlea. This lies about 9° inclination (proximal lateral to distal medial) in relation to the vertical (a line passing vertically down from the symphysis pubis of the pelvis
- Anatomical axis of the tibia—line connecting the centre of the tibial plateau to the centre of the tibial plafond. This lies about 3° inclination (proximal lateral to distal medial) in relation to the vertical (a line passing vertically down from the symphysis pubis of the pelvis)

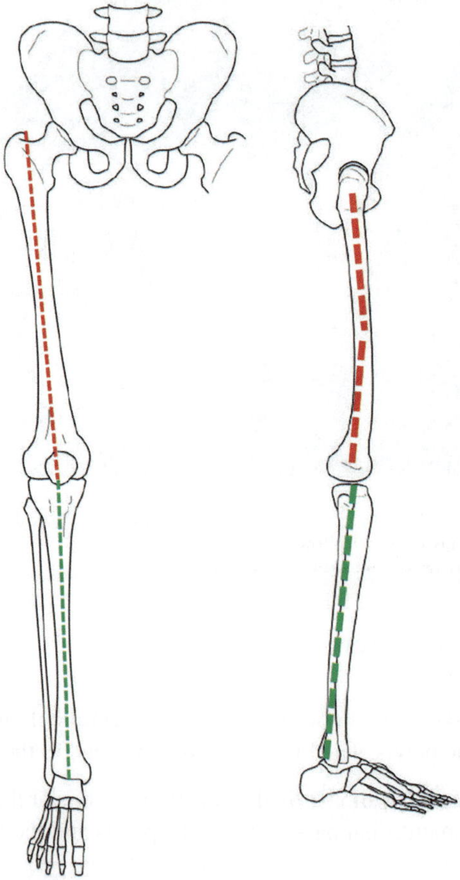

Anatomical axis of the femur (red line) and tibia (green line) in the coronal plane and sagittal plane

- Distal femoral articular axis—line connecting the most distal points of the medial and lateral femoral condyles
- Proximal tibial articular axis—line connecting the most proximal points of the medial and lateral tibial plateau condyles
- Angle between femoral anatomical axis—distal femoral articular axis—the angle between the femoral anatomical axis and the distal femoral articular axis (about 9° in valgus)

- Angle between proximal tibial articular axis and tibial anatomical axis (about 2–3° varus)
- Anatomical femoro-tibial angle—the angle between the anatomical axis of the femur and the anatomical axis of the tibia—about 6° valgus. This is the angle that is clinically measured when assessing coronal alignment

Sagittal Plane

In the sagittal plane the femur has an anterior bowing.

Hasegawa et al. [18] in Japan evaluated the standing sagittal alignment of the whole axial skeleton and lower limbs in volunteers using radiographs. They showed that:

- The femoral axis (centre of the femoral head to centre of the femoral notch) is in extension in relation to the pelvic axis (centre of the femoral head to the middle of the S1 vertebra endplate), with the pelvic-femoral angle between the two axes being about 197° (95% CI—195°–198°)
- The angle between the femoral axis and tibial axis being in slight extension of about 1.6° (95% CI 0.8°–2.3°)

The patella is located anterior to the distal part of the femur just proximal to the trochlea.

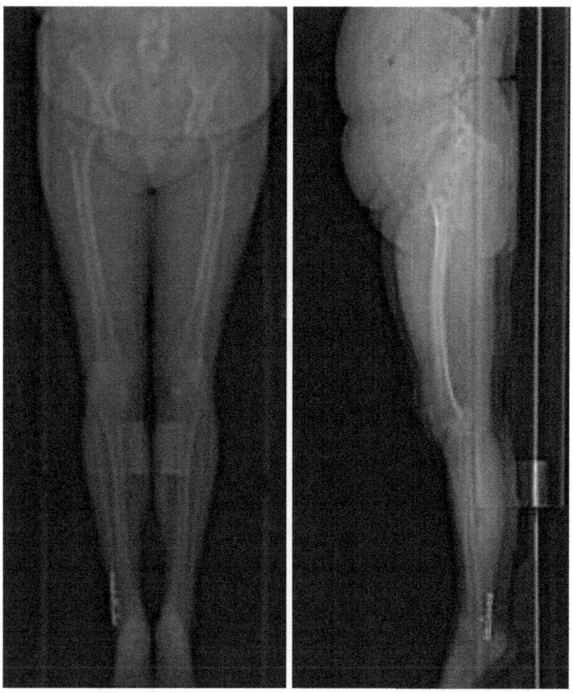

Long leg CT tomogram to assess leg length and alignment

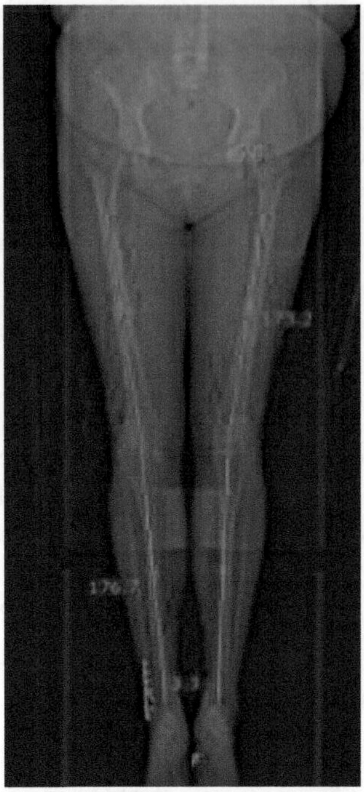

Long leg CT tomogram assessing the angle between the femoral and tibial anatomical axis

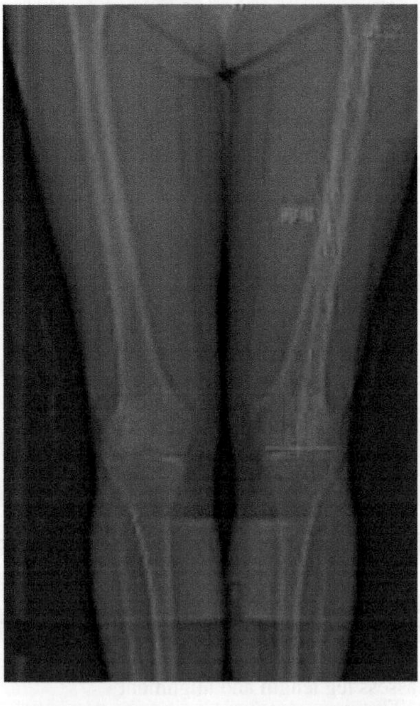

Long leg CT tomogram assessing the angle between the femoral anatomical axis and distal femoral articular line axis

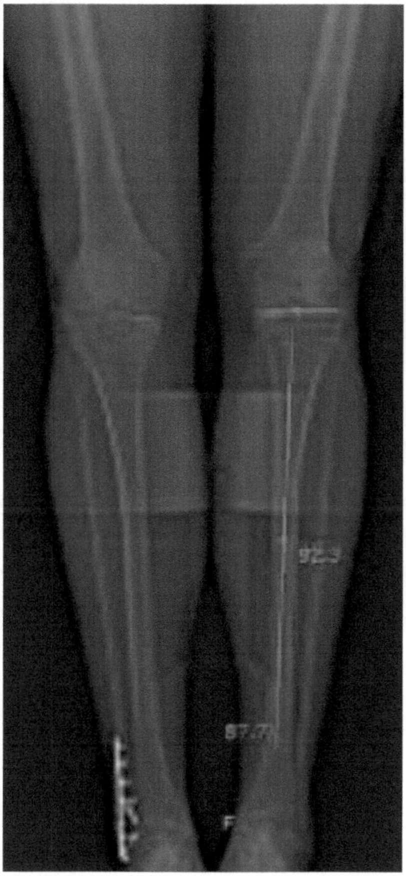

Long leg CT tomogram assessing the angle between the tibial anatomical axis and proximal tibial articular line axis

Axial Alignment

When standing with the feet apart (hip-width) and pointing forwards, the rotation of the distal femur in relation to the pelvis may be described as the:

- Angle between the mediolateral axis of the pelvis (that joins the left and right anterior superior iliac spines) and the posterior condylar line
  - This angle has been shown to be about 11° (+/−7°) internal rotation

The angle between the femoral neck and the mediolateral axis of the pelvis (that joins the left and right anterior superior iliac spines) has been shown to be about 4° (+/−6°) [78].

The posterior condylar line (joining the posterior condyles of the distal femur) is in internal rotation in relation to the axis joining the medial and lateral epicondyles (transepicondylar axis). The posterior condyles may be used as a reference for guiding the rotation of the femoral component in total knee replacement arthroplasty. However, in the presence of a deficient lateral femoral condyle (as in valgus deformity) the internal rotation of the posterior condylar line increases substantially, making it an unreliable reference for the positioning of the femoral component.

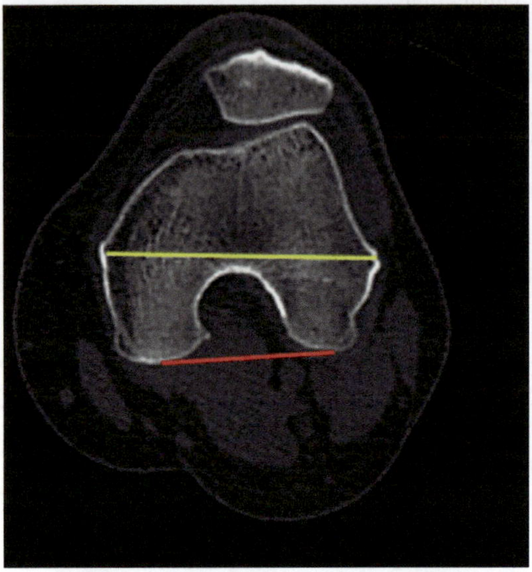

The posterior condylar line (red) is in internal rotation in relation to the trans-epicondylar line (yellow)

2.7.2 *Overview of the Soft Tissue Structures of the Knee*

Taking into account the various structures described above, the following soft tissue areas of the knee may be considered as below.

Anterior Part of the Knee

The quadriceps tendon attaches to the superior pole of the patella. It then gives rise to a thinner aponeurosis that passes over the anterior surface of the patella (to which it is firmly adhered). The quadriceps tendon aponeurosis is continuous and contributes to the medial and lateral patellar retinaculae. Distally the patellar aponeurosis is continuous with the patellar tendon that originates from the inferior pole of the patella and inserts onto the tibial tuberosity [34].

Adductor Canal

This is a triangular space located in the middle third, of the medial part of the thigh. Its boundaries are:

- Laterally—vastus medialis
- Medially—adductor longus and magnus
- Roof—sartorius and sub-sartorial fascia

The adductor hiatus is at the distal end of the adductor canal. It is a gap between the adductor magnus muscle and the femur.

The adductor canal contains the:

- Femoral artery
- Femoral vein
- Saphenous nerve

Medial Part of the Knee—Layers

The soft tissues on the medial and anteromedial part of the knee may be described in three anatomical layers:

- Layer 1—most superficial layer—continuity of the fascia covering the vastus medialis muscle anteriorly and sartorius posteriorly
- Layer 2—intermediate layer—superficial MCL, MPFL, posterior oblique ligament
- Layer 3—deepest layer—deep MCL and capsule

Layers 1 and 2 contribute to the medial patellar retinaculum.

Pes anserinus [55–58]—this is a term used to describe a group of tendons inserting onto the proximal part of the anteromedial tibia. It consists of the tendons of:

1. Sartorius muscles
2. Gracilis
3. Semitendinosus

These are separated from the underlying tibia by a bursa (pes anserinus bursa).

The arrangement of the insertion of the three tendons onto the tibia resembles a goose's foot (pes anserinus in Latin) hence the name.

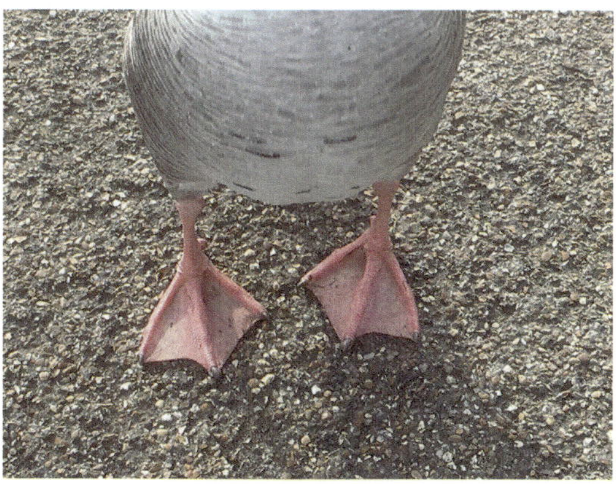

Pes anserinus (goose's foot)

The sartorius tendon fascia is inserted onto the superficial fascial layer of the lower leg. The gracilis and semitendinosus tendons are located on the deep surface of the superficial fascial layer. The sartorius fascia is thus incised to gain access to the semitendinosus and gracilis tendons. An accessory semitendinosus or gracilis are occasionally encountered.

Lateral Part of the Knee—Layers [7]
The soft tissues on the lateral and anterolateral part of the knee may be described in three anatomical layers:

1. Superficial layer—deep fascia—passes over the patella from which it can be separated, laterally it thickens as the ITB
2. Intermediate layer—quadriceps aponeurosis
3. Deep layer—joint capsule—the capsule is thickened forming the lateral patellofemoral ligament and the lateral patellomeniscal ligament

2.7.3 Popliteal Fossa

The popliteal fossa is located on the posterior aspect of the knee. It is diamond-shaped. Its four boundaries are formed by:

1. Biceps femoris laterally
2. Semitendinosus and semimembranosus medially
3. Lateral head of gastrocnemius inferiorly
4. Medial head of gastrocnemius inferiorly

Its floor is formed by the posterior surface of the femur, popliteus muscle, and proximal tibia. Its roof is formed by the thigh fascia.

The popliteal fossa contains the:

- Tibial nerve
- Common peroneal nerve
- Popliteal vessels
- Short saphenous vein
- Lymph nodes
- Semimembranosus bursa

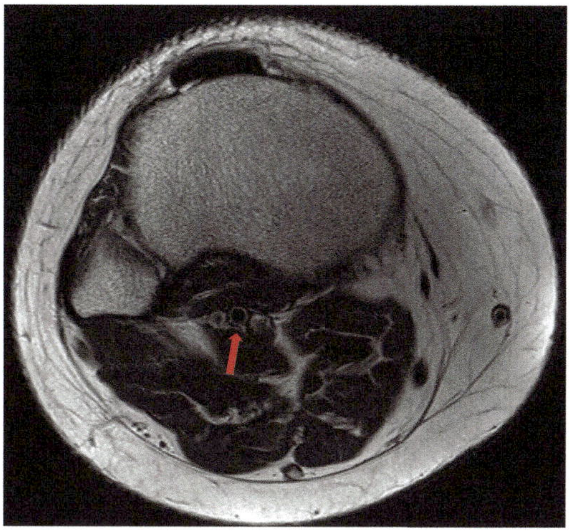

Neurovascular bundle (red arrow) in the popliteal fossa

2.8 Arterial Supply of the Knee and Lower Limb

Consideration of the blood supply of the knee [66–72] is important as its disruption may lead to necrosis of growing or mature bone, or epiphyseal injury with resultant growth disruption in children. Similarly, consideration of the blood supply of the quadriceps is essential, as areas of hypovascularity may predispose to tendon degeneration and tear. The border of two adjacent vascular territories may provide an area of poor perfusion, known as a watershed area. Disruption of perfusion may be due to, amongst others, the aging process, or pathological conditions such as osteonecrosis, or may occur secondary to trauma or surgery.

Femoral Artery

The main artery of the lower limb is the femoral artery. The external iliac artery, one of the terminal branches of the aorta, becomes the femoral artery as it passes under the inguinal ligament at the mid-inguinal point (halfway between the anterior superior iliac spine of the pelvis and the symphysis pubis- where the femoral pulse may be palpated) and enters the anterior aspect of the thigh. It gives rise to the profunda femoris artery, a branch that passes posteriorly and distally, giving branches to the hip joint (femoral neck and head) and to the thigh muscles. The femoral artery also gives rise to the descending genicular (knee) artery, which supplies the knee.

Popliteal Artery

The femoral artery then continues distally to reach the medial part of the thigh, passes through the adductor canal, and reaches the posterior part of the thigh entering the popliteal fossa (located behind the knee), where it becomes the popliteal artery. The popliteal artery pulse can be palpated in the popliteal fossa. The popliteal artery gives rise to genicular branches that supply the knee joint. It passes distally between gastrocnemius and popliteus and just below popliteus it divides into its two terminal branches:

1. Anterior tibial artery
2. Tibio-peroneal trunk—this divides into the:

- Posterior tibial artery
- Peroneal artery

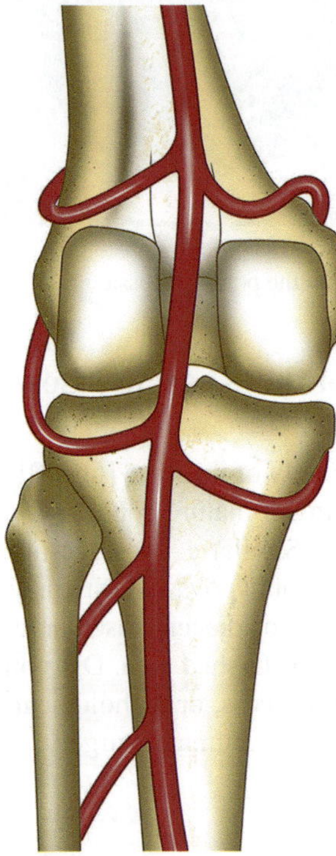

Popliteal artery giving rise to genicular branches

Anterior tibial artery—This passes forwards through the interosseous membrane (between tibia and fibula) to enter the anterior part of the lower leg. It then descends distally between the tibia and fibula. It crosses the anterior part of the ankle to enter the foot where it becomes the dorsalis pedis artery. The dorsalis pedis pulse can be palpated on the dorsum of the foot just lateral to the tendon of extensor hallucis longus. The dorsalis pedis passes inferiorly to enter the sole of the foot and anastomoses with the lateral plantar artery to form the deep plantar arch. It supplies muscles of the anterior part of the lower leg as well as the foot.

Posterior tibial artery—This continues distally, in the posterior compartment of the lower leg, and passes through the tarsal tunnel (located medial to the medial malleolus) along with the tibial nerve to enter the sole of the foot. It then divides into the lateral and medial plantar arteries. Its pulse may be palpated just posterior and inferior to the medial malleolus. It supplies the lateral and posterior parts of the lower leg.

Peroneal artery—This passes distally posterior to the fibula, in the posterior compartment of the lower leg, and supplies muscles of the lateral and posterior part of the lower leg.

Obturator Artery
The obturator artery arises from the internal iliac artery in the pelvis. It passes via the obturator canal to enter the medial thigh, and divides into two branches:

1. Anterior branch—supplies pectineus, obturator externus, adductor muscles and gracilis
2. Posterior branch—supplies the deep gluteal muscles

Gluteal Arteries
The gluteal region is largely supplied by the superior and inferior gluteal arteries. These arteries arise from the internal iliac artery, entering the gluteal region via the greater sciatic foramen.

The superior gluteal artery leaves the foramen above the piriformis muscle, and the inferior gluteal artery below piriformis. The inferior gluteal artery also contributes towards the blood supply of the posterior thigh.

Genicular (Knee) Arteries
These arteries form a network of arteries with multiple smaller branches, plexuses and anastomoses in and around the knee joint that supply the knee. They arise from the popliteal artery and include the:

- Superior lateral genicular artery
- Superior medial genicular artery
- Inferior lateral genicular artery
- Inferior medial genicular artery

A rich intraosseous blood supply exists in the femoral and tibial condyles and patella. Similarly, the deep and superficial soft tissues, ligaments, and outer part of the menisci are richly vascularized.

2.8.1 *Patellar Blood Supply*

The patellar blood supply deserves special consideration- it has two main origins:

1. Arteries penetrating the middle third of the anterior surface of the patella
2. Arteries entering the lower pole of the patella deep to the patellar tendon

This arrangement of patellar arterial supply has several clinical implications including:

- As most blood supply enters the bone distally, there is a potential risk of avascular necrosis of the upper fragment of the patella following a transverse (horizontal) patellar fracture
- Surgery may damage the blood vessels entering the anterior surface of the patella, hence extensive dissection around the patella should be minimised to preserve the prepatellar vascular network
- Excision of the fat pad (as may occur in total knee replacement arthroplasty) may compromise the patellar blood supply

2.8.2 Quadriceps Tendon Blood Supply

The arterial supply to the quadriceps tendon comes from multiple branches which penetrate the tendon and anastomose with an intrasubstance network. These include:

- Descending branches of the lateral circumflex femoral artery
- Medial and lateral superior genicular arteries

Petersen et al. [71] reported that the deep part of the quadriceps tendon has an avascular area which is about 30 mm in length and 15 mm width. Yepes at al [72] localised the hypovascular zone between 1 and 2 cm proximal to the superior pole of the patella, an area which correlates with the location of spontaneous tears of the tendon.

2.9 Veins of the Knee and Lower Limb

Multiple veins exist in the lower leg and knee region. Some of the ones to consider are:

Popliteal vein—located in the popliteal fossa. It arises as the continuation of the posterior tibial vein. It passes through the popliteal fossa and enters the anterior part of the thigh where it becomes the femoral vein. It receives genicular (knee) veins.

Long saphenous vein—this is a subcutaneous vein. It arises on the dorsum of the foot and passes proximally along the medial side of the knee to join the femoral vein in the proximal thigh.

Femoral vein—arises as the continuation of the popliteal vein and passes proximally alongside the femoral artery. It joins the long saphenous vein to become the external iliac vein.

Short saphenous vein—this is a subcutaneous vein. It arises along the posterior lateral part of the ankle and passes proximally along the posterior part of the lower leg, to join the popliteal vein.

2.10 Nerve Supply of the Knee and Lower Limb

The knee region has a rich nerve supply that comes from multiple nerves. Its innervation pattern is variable and the territories of the involved nerves often overlap [73–79].

The lower limb, and hence the knee, are innervated by the lumbar plexus and sacral plexus which arise from the lumbar and sacral nerve roots, and give rise to peripheral nerves as described next.

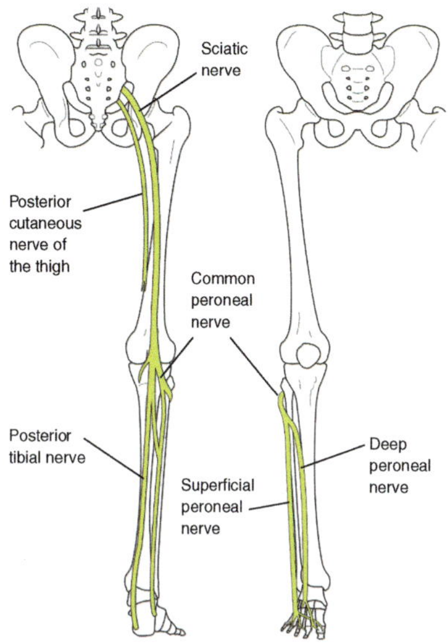

Peripheral nerves of the lower limb

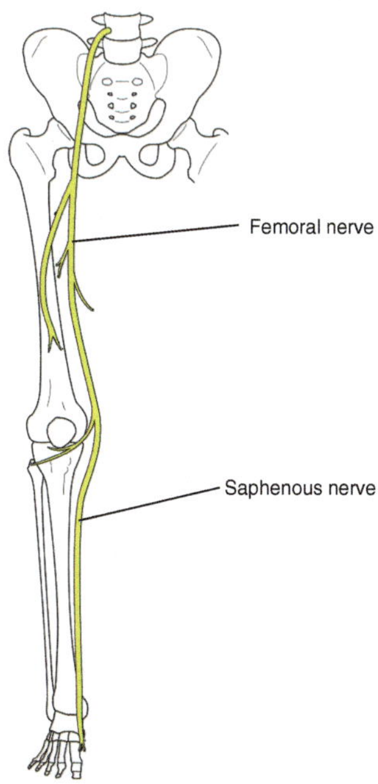

2.10.1 *Sensory Supply of the Knee and Lower Limb*

Sensory supply may be described in terms of:

- Dermatomes—the part of the skin innervated mainly by a specific spinal nerve root
- Peripheral nerve sensory territory—the part of the skin supplied by a specific peripheral nerve that may have contributions from nerve fibres originating in multiple nerve roots

Recognising the difference between root dermatomes/myotomes and peripheral nerve regions is important in looking for the relevant signs and fitting a pattern to clinical findings. The spinal roots may be likened to the central cables that pass from the street to a building. Once they reach the mains, these then feed multiple peripheral wires that light each room. When the light goes off, by examining which bulbs are involved one may recognise whether it is a peripheral wire or a more central cable supply problem.

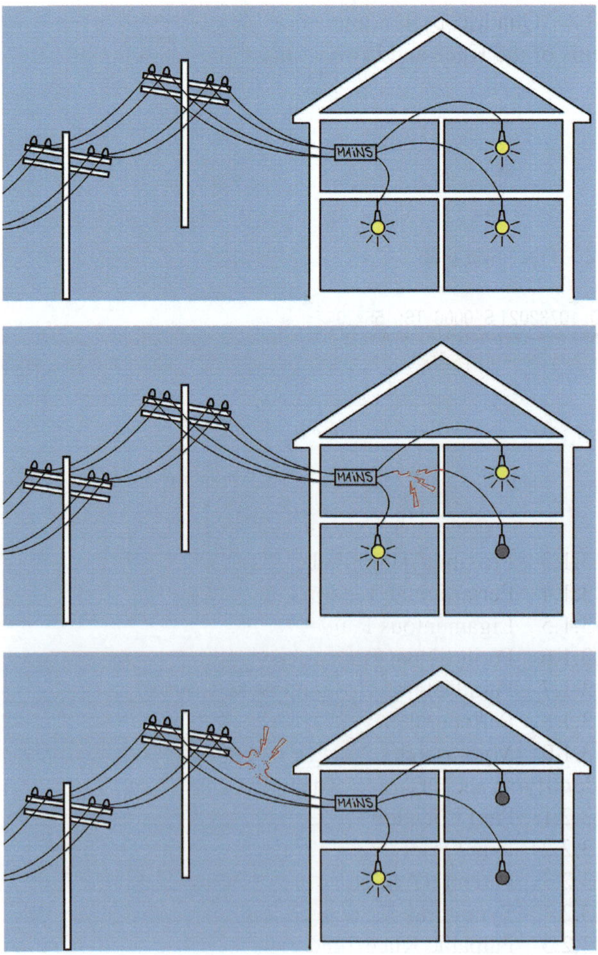

2.10.2 *Motor Supply of the Knee and Lower Limb*

Motor supply may be described in terms of:

- Myotomes—those muscles innervated primarily by a specific spinal nerve root
- Peripheral nerve motor territory—those muscles innervated by a specific peripheral nerve

2.10.3 *Nerves of the Knee and Lower Limb*

The sensory cutaneous supply of the lower limb in terms of dermatomes and peripheral nerves is shown below.

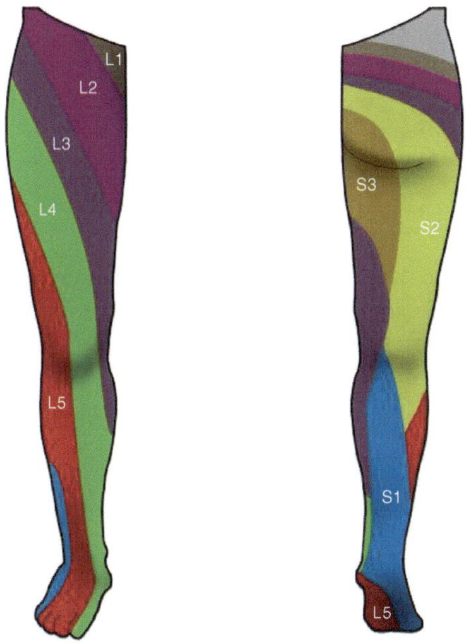

Dermatomes of the lower limb

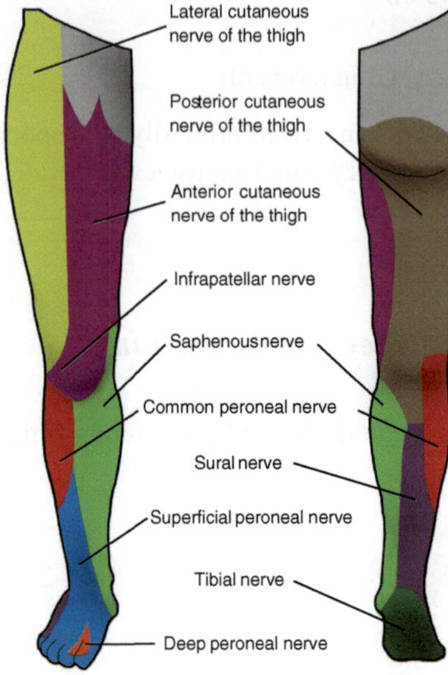

Perpheral nerve distribution of the lower limb

There is often overlap in the exact territories of the dermatomal supply of the lower limb. However, there are some areas more likely to be innervated by a sole nerve root, and these may be tested when examining the lower dermatomes –

- L1—Ilioinguinal area
- L2—Anterior part of the mid-thigh
- L3—Medial part of the knee
- L4—Medial malleolus
- L5—First dorsal web space
- S1—Lateral border of foot
- S2—Posterior middle part of the thigh

The following peripheral nerves may be considered in the innervation of the knee and lower limb:

Lumbar Plexus

The lumbar plexus is found in the lumbar region, within psoas major muscle and anterior to the transverse processes of the lumbar vertebrae. It is formed by the anterior rami of the lumbar spinal nerves L1, L2, L3 and L4 and from the thoracic spinal nerve T12. The anterior rami of L1-L4 spinal roots divide into several cords which then combine to give rise to the six major peripheral nerves of the lumbar plexus. These nerves pass to the lower limb:

1. Iliohypogastric
2. Ilioinguinal
3. Genitofemoral

4. Lateral cutaneous nerve of the thigh
5. Obturator
6. Femoral

Sacral Plexus

This plexus is found on the surface of the posterior wall of the pelvis. It is formed by the anterior rami of the sacral spinal nerves S1, S2, S3 and S4 with contributions from the lumbar spinal nerves L4 and L5 (lumbosacral trunk). These divide into several cords which combine to give rise to several peripheral nerves. These supply pelvic structures as well as the lower limb and include:

- Superior Gluteal
- Inferior Gluteal
- Pudendal
- Posterior cutaneous nerve of the thigh
- Sciatic

Sciatic Nerve

This leaves the pelvis through the greater sciatic foremen, deep to piriformis and gluteus maximus, and enters the posterior part of the thigh. It reaches the proximal part of the popliteal fossa and divides into the:

1. Tibial nerve
2. Common peroneal nerve

   It innervates:

- Hamstrings
- Semitendinosus
- Semimembranosus
- Biceps femoris
- Adductor magnus ischial head
- Articular branches to the hip

Common Peroneal Nerve

This is the lateral division of the sciatic nerve composed of the posterior divisions of L4, 5, S1, 2. It passes from the posterolateral side of the knee curving forwards deep to the biceps femoris tendon, posterior to the fibular head and then curves round the fibular neck. It passes deep to the peroneus longus muscle and divides into:

1. Superficial peroneal nerve
2. Deep peroneal nerve

   The common peroneal nerve also gives rise to:

1. Nerve to the short head of biceps femoris
2. Articular branches to the knee joint and proximal tibiofibular joint
3. Lateral cutaneous nerve of the calf—innervates the skin over the upper lateral leg
4. Lateral sural cutaneous nerve—this joins the medial sural cutaneous branch of the tibial nerve to form the sural nerve. The sural nerve innervates the skin over the lower posterolateral leg

It is of note that in 10% of cases the common peroneal nerve bifurcates more proximally, which must be considered in surgical approaches to the posterolateral part of the knee.

Deep Peroneal Nerve (L4,L5,S1,S2)
This passes distally alongside the anterior tibial vessels, over the interosseous membrane and into the anterior compartment of the leg. It crosses the ankle and enters the dorsum of the foot. It innervates the anterior compartment of the lower leg:

- Tibialis anterior
- Extensor digitorum
- Extensor hallucis longus
- Peroneus tertius

It also gives a cutaneous supply to the dorsum of the foot in the area between the first and second toes.

Superficial Peroneal Nerve (L5,S1,S2)
This innervates the lateral compartment of the lower leg:

- Peroneus longus
- Peroneus brevis

It also provides sensory innervation to the anterolateral part of the lower leg, and the dorsum of the foot (apart from the area between the first and second toes, which is supplied by the deep peroneal nerve).

Saphenous Nerve (L3-L4)
This is a pure sensory nerve. It arises from the femoral nerve in the femoral triangle distal to the inguinal ligament. It passes distally along the thigh, together with the femoral artery and vein, deep to the sartorius muscle. It then traverses the adductor canal. It leaves the adductor canal and becomes subcutaneous by piercing the fascia between vastus medialis and adductor magnus about 10 cm proximal to the medial femoral epicondyle. It descends between the sartorius and gracilis muscles and continues along the medial side of the leg, running along with the saphenous vein. At the ankle, it divides into an anterior and posterior branch which terminate anterior and posterior to the medial malleolus respectively. Proximal to the knee, the saphenous nerve gives rise to a large branch—the infrapatellar nerve (IPN).

The saphenous nerve supplies the:

- Anterior surface of the patella

- Anterior/medial surface of the lower leg
- Medial aspect of the ankle (medial malleolus) and proximal foot

Infrapatellar Nerve

This is a pure sensory nerve. It arises from the saphenous nerve and passes laterally to innervate skin on the anterior part of the knee.

The relationship of the IPN to the sartorius muscle is highly variable. The IPN may emerge from the anterior or posterior border of sartorius or may penetrate the sartorius muscle belly in the distal thigh or the sartorius tendon close to its pes anserinus insertion [79, 80].

Similarly, the relationship of the IPN to the patellar tendon is variable [81]:

1. In most cases it crosses the tibiofemoral joint line medial to the patellar tendon
2. In about 1/3rd of cases it crosses the patellar tendon proximal to the tibiofemoral joint line

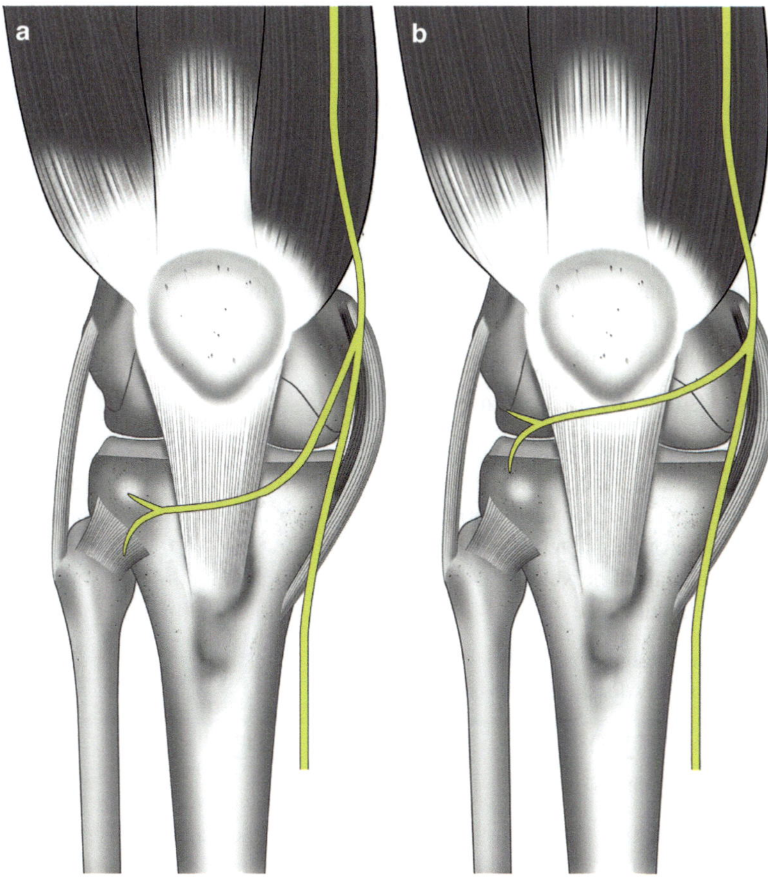

Infrapatellar nerve main patterns in relation to the tibiofemoral joint line and patellar tendon

Kerver et al. [81] showed that the IPN may consist of 1–3 branches. In their study the mean vertical distance of a line passing between the apex of the patella and the uppermost infrapatellar branch (as it passes from medially to laterally) was 70 mm (35–87 mm).

Ackmann et al. [80] compared in a cadaveric study three skin incisions used in total knee replacement arthroplasty, with regards to their rates of injuring the IPN. Their reported rates of injury were:

- Medial parapatellar incision—53%
- Midline incision—47%
- Lateral parapatellar incision—30%

Tibial Nerve

The tibial nerve originates from the sciatic nerve (L4-S3 spinal nerve roots) in the distal, posterior part of the thigh. It passes through the middle of the popliteal fossa and then passes deep to gastrocnemius and under the tendinous arch of the soleus muscle. It continues in the posterior compartment of the leg, on the posterior surface of the tibialis posterior, to reach the distal leg. It then continues deep to the flexor retinaculum, through the tarsal tunnel, posterior to the medial malleolus along with the posterior tibial artery and vein. Just distal to the tarsal tunnel, the tibial nerve gives its two terminal branches, the medial and lateral plantar nerves. It innervates several muscles of the lower leg and foot (via the medial and lateral plantar nerves) as well as giving a sensory supply to the lower leg and foot.

Motor supply by the tibial nerve:

- Gastrocnemius, popliteus, soleus, tIbialis posterior, flexor digitorum longus, flexor hallucis longus
- Small muscles of the foot

Sensory supply by the tibial nerve:

- Articular branches to the knee
- Medial sural cutaneous nerve—joins the lateral sural cutaneous branch of the common peroneal nerve to form the sural nerve that provides sensation to the lateral side of the posterior part of the leg
- Medial calcaneal nerve
- Medial plantar nerve
  - Plantar medial 3 ½ digits
  - Medial 3 ½ dorsal nail beds
- Lateral plantar nerve
  - Lateral plantar surface

  - Lateral 1 ½ toes
  - Lateral 1 ½ dorsal nail beds

2.10.4 Cutaneous Sensory Supply of the Knee

The main peripheral nerves involved in the cutaneous nerve supply of the knee are the:

- Anterior knee—femoral nerve—anterior cutaneous nerve of the thigh
- Anteromedial part
  - Saphenous nerve

    Infrapatellar nerve

  - Obturator nerve—in less than 40% of cases
- Lateral knee
  - Lateral cutaneous nerve of the thigh, femoral nerve
  - Common peroneal nerve
- Posterior—Posterior cutaneous nerve of the thigh
- Posteromedial part—Saphenous nerve
- Posterolateral part—Common peroneal nerve

2.10.5 Deep Sensory Supply of the Knee

Extensive nerve supply of the ligaments, capsule, and synovium is provided by nerves which also innervate the muscles that act on the joint.

Hence, the following nerves contribute to deep knee innervation:

- Femoral—saphenous
- Obturator
- Tibial
- Common peroneal

Their innervation areas include:

- Saphenous nerve: suprapatellar recess, patella, anteromedial and anterolateral joint capsule
- Tibial nerve—joint capsule, infrapatellar fat pad, proximal tibiofibular joint
- Common peroneal nerve—anterolateral capsule, infrapatellar fat pad, tibiofibular joint

- Obturator nerve—superior part of the posteromedial capsule, anteromedial capsule
- Posterior capsule—mainly by the posterior division of the obturator nerve and tibial nerve, and less frequently by the common peroneal and sciatic nerves

Sakamoto et al. [14] showed in a cadaveric study that the femoral nerve supplied branches to the anteromedial aspect of the hip and knee joints, which were derived from the same bundle of the femoral nerve. They concluded that dichotomizing peripheral sensory nerves innervate the hip and knee joints and this could explain the referral of hip pain to the knee.

References

1. Churchill Livingstone Last's Anatomy: Regional and Applied, 12th ed. Sinnatamby CS, editor. Churchill Livingstone, 2011.
2. Flandry F, Hommel G. Normal anatomy and biomechanics of the knee. Sports Med Arthrosc Rev. 2011;19(2):82–92.
3. LaPrade MD, Kennedy MI, Wijdicks CA, LaPrade RF. Anatomy and biomechanics of the medial side of the knee and their surgical implications. Sports Med Arthrosc Rev. 2015;23(2):63–70.
4. James EW, LaPrade CM, LaPrade RF. Anatomy and biomechanics of the lateral side of the knee and surgical implications. Sports Med Arthrosc Rev. 2015;23(1):2–9.
5. Flores DV, Mejía Gómez C, Pathria MN. Layered approach to the anterior knee: normal anatomy and disorders associated with anterior knee pain. Radiographics. 2018;38(7):2069–101.
6. Lyras DN, Loucks C, Greenhow R. Analysis of the geometry of the distal femur and proximal tibia in the osteoarthritic knee: a 3D reconstruction CT scan based study of 449 cases. Arch Bone Jt Surg. 2016;4(2):116–21.
7. Merican AM, Amis AA. Anatomy of the lateral retinaculum of the knee. J Bone Joint Surg Br. 2008;90(4):527–34.
8. Terry GC, LaPrade RF. The posterolateral aspect of the knee. Anatomy and surgical approach. Am J Sports Med. 1996;24(6):732–9.
9. LaPrade RF, Morgan PM, Wentorf FA, Johansen S, Engebretsen L. The anatomy of the posterior aspect of the knee. An anatomic study. J Bone Joint Surg Am. 2007;89(4):758–64.
10. Ogden JA. The anatomy and function of the proximal tibiofibular joint. Clin Orthop Relat Res. 1974;101:186–91.
11. Brockmeyer M, Orth P, Höfer D, Seil R, Paulsen F, Menger MD, Kohn D, Tschernig T. The anatomy of the anterolateral structures of the knee—a histologic and macroscopic approach. Knee. 2019;26(3):636–46.
12. Ariel de Lima D, Helito CP, Lacerda de Lima L, de Castro SD, Costa Cavalcante ML, Dias Leite JA. Anatomy of the anterolateral ligament of the knee: a systematic review. Arthroscopy. 2019;35(2):670–81.
13. Manning BT, Frank RM, Wetters NG, Bach BR, Rosenberg AG, Levine BR. Surgical anatomy of the knee a review of common open approaches. Bull Hosp Jt Dis (2013). 2016;74(3):219–28.
14. Sakamoto J, Manabe Y, Oyamada J, Kataoka H, Nakano J, Saiki K, Okamoto K, Tsurumoto T, Okita M. Anatomical study of the articular branches innervated the hip and knee joint with reference to mechanism of referral pain in hip joint disease patients. Clin Anat. 2018;31(5):705–9. https://doi.org/10.1002/ca.23077. Epub 2018 Apr 16. PMID: 29577432.
15. Saavedra MÁ, Navarro-Zarza JE, Villaseñor-Ovies P, Canoso JJ, Vargas A, Chiapas-Gasca K, Hernández-Díaz C, Kalish RA. Clinical anatomy of the knee. Reumatol Clin. 2012–2013;8(Suppl 2):39–45.

16. Waligora AC, Johanson NA, Hirsch BE. Clinical anatomy of the quadriceps femoris and extensor apparatus of the knee. Clin Orthop Relat Res. 2009;467(12):3297–306.
17. Bowman KF Jr, Sekiya JK. Anatomy and biomechanics of the posterior cruciate ligament, medial and lateral sides of the knee. Sports Med Arthrosc Rev. 2010;18(4):222–9.
18. Hasegawa K, Okamoto M, Hatsushikano S, Shimoda H, Ono M, Homma T, Watanabe K. Standing sagittal alignment of the whole axial skeleton with reference to the gravity line in humans. J Anat. 2017;230(5):619–30.
19. Terry GC, LaPrade RF. The biceps femoris muscle complex at the knee. Its anatomy and injury patterns associated with acute anterolateral-anteromedial rotatory instability. Am J Sports Med. 1996;24(1):2–8.
20. Amis AA, Gupte CM, Bull AM, Edwards A. Anatomy of the posterior cruciate ligament and the meniscofemoral ligaments. Knee Surg Sports Traumatol Arthrosc. 2006;14(3):257–63.
21. Tecklenburg K, Dejour D, Hoser C, Fink C. Bony and cartilaginous anatomy of the patellofemoral joint. Knee Surg Sports Traumatol Arthrosc. 2006;14(3):235–40.
22. Stäubli HU, Dürrenmatt U, Porcellini B, Rauschning W. Anatomy and surface geometry of the patellofemoral joint in the axial plane. J Bone Joint Surg Br. 1999;81(3):452–8.
23. Amis AA. Current concepts on anatomy and biomechanics of patellar stability. Sports Med Arthrosc Rev. 2007;15(2):48–56.
24. Werner S, Durkan M, Jones J, Quilici S, Crawford D. Symptomatic bipartite patella: three subtypes, three representative cases. J Knee Surg. 2013;26(Suppl 1):S72–6.
25. Dalip D, Iwanaga J, Oskouian RJ, Tubbs RS. A comprehensive review of the fabella bone. Cureus. 2018;10(6):e2736. https://doi.org/10.7759/cureus.2736.
26. Berthaume MA, Di Federico E, Bull AMJ. Fabella prevalence rate increases over 150 years, and rates of other sesamoid bones remain constant: a systematic review. J Anat. 2019;235(1):67–79.
27. DeCoster TA, Crawford MK, Kraut MA. Safe extracapsular placement of proximal tibia transfixation pins. J Orthop Trauma. 2004;18(8 Suppl):S43–7.
28. Lowery K, Dearden P, Sherman K, Mahadevan V, Sharma H. Cadaveric analysis of capsular attachments of the distal femur related to pin and wire placement. Injury. 2015;46(6):970–4.
29. Robinson JR, Bull AM, Amis AA. Structural properties of the medial collateral ligament complex of the human knee. J Biomech. 2005;38(5):1067–74.
30. Amis AA, Firer P, Mountney J, Senavongse W, Thomas NP. Anatomy and biomechanics of the medial patellofemoral ligament. Knee. 2003;10(3):215–20.
31. Edwards A, Bull AM, Amis AA. The attachments of the anteromedial and posterolateral fibre bundles of the anterior cruciate ligament. Part 2: femoral attachment. Knee Surg Sports Traumatol Arthrosc. 2008;16(1):29–36.
32. Edwards A, Bull AM, Amis AA. The attachments of the anteromedial and posterolateral fibre bundles of the anterior cruciate ligament: Part 1: tibial attachment. Knee Surg Sports Traumatol Arthrosc. 2007;15(12):1414–21.
33. Gupte CM, Smith A, McDermott ID, Bull AM, Thomas RD, Amis AA. Meniscofemoral ligaments revisited. Anatomical study, age correlation and clinical implications. J Bone Joint Surg Br. 2002;84(6):846–51.
34. Basso O, Johnson DP, Amis AA. The anatomy of the patellar tendon. Knee Surg Sports Traumatol Arthrosc. 2001;9(1):2–5.
35. Matziolis G, Mehlhorn S, Schattat N, Diederichs G, Hube R, Perka C, Matziolis D. How much of the PCL is really preserved during the tibial cut? Knee Surg Sports Traumatol Arthrosc. 2012;20(6):1083–6.
36. Hinckel BB, Lipinski L, Arendt EA. Concepts of the distal medial patellar restraints: medial patellotibial ligament and medial patellomeniscal ligament. Sports Med Arthrosc Rev. 2019;27(4):143–9.
37. Hinckel BB, Gobbi RG, Demange MK, Pereira CAM, Pécora JR, Natalino RJM, Miyahira L, Kubota BS, Camanho GL. Medial patellofemoral ligament, medial patellotibial ligament, and medial patellomeniscal ligament: anatomic, histologic, radiographic, and biomechanical study. Arthroscopy. 2017;33(10):1862–73.
38. Tanaka MJ. The anatomy of the medial patellofemoral complex. Sports Med Arthrosc Rev. 2017;25(2):e8–e11.

39. Trinh TQ, Ferrel JR, Bentley JC, Steensen RN. The anatomy of the medial patellofemoral ligament. Orthopedics. 2017;40(4):e583–8.
40. DeFroda SF, Shah KN, Lemme N, Koruprolu S, Ware KJ, Owens BD. Biomechanical properties of the lateral patellofemoral ligament: a cadaveric analysis. Orthopedics. 2018;41(6):e797–801.
41. Capkin S, Zeybek G, Ergur I, Kosay C, Kiray A. An anatomic study of the lateral patellofemoral ligament. Acta Orthop Traumatol Turc. 2017;51(1):73–6.
42. Fairclough J, Hayashi K, Toumi H, Lyons K, Bydder G, Phillips N, Best TM, Benjamin M. The functional anatomy of the iliotibial band during flexion and extension of the knee: implications for understanding iliotibial band syndrome. J Anat. 2006;208(3):309–16.
43. Godin JA, Chahla J, Moatshe G, Kruckeberg BM, Muckenhirn KJ, Vap AR, Geeslin AG, LaPrade RF. A Comprehensive reanalysis of the distal iliotibial band: quantitative anatomy, radiographic markers, and biomechanical properties. Am J Sports Med. 2017;45(11):2595–603.
44. Fox AJ, Wanivenhaus F, Burge AJ, Warren RF, Rodeo SA. The human meniscus: a review of anatomy, function, injury, and advances in treatment. Clin Anat. 2015;28(2):269–87.
45. Bryceland JK, Powell AJ, Nunn T. Knee Menisci. Cartilage. 2017;8(2):99–104.
46. Gray JC. Neural and vascular anatomy of the menisci of the human knee. J Orthop Sports Phys Ther. 1999;29(1):23–30.
47. Assimakopoulos AP, Katonis PG, Agapitos MV, Exarchou EI. The innervation of the human meniscus. Clin Orthop Relat Res. 1992;275:232–6.
48. Macchi V, Stocco E, Stecco C, Belluzzi E, Favero M, Porzionato A, De Caro R. The infrapatellar fat pad and the synovial membrane: an anatomo-functional unit. J Anat. 2018;233(2):146–54.
49. Mace J, Bhatti W, Anand S. Infrapatellar fat pad syndrome: a review of anatomy, function, treatment and dynamics. Acta Orthop Belg. 2016;82(1):94–101.
50. Roth C, Jacobson J, Jamadar D, Caoili E, Morag Y, Housner J. Quadriceps fat pad signal intensity and enlargement on MRI: prevalence and associated findings. AJR Am J Roentgenol. 2004;182(6):1383–7.
51. Patel SJ, Kaplan PA, Dussault RG, Kahler DM. Anatomy and clinical significance of the horizontal cleft in the infrapatellar fat pad of the knee: MR imaging. AJR Am J Roentgenol. 1998;170(6):1551–5.
52. Kim SJ, Min BH, Kim HK. Arthroscopic anatomy of the infrapatellar plica. Arthroscopy. 1996;12(5):561–4.
53. Kent M, Khanduja V. Synovial plicae around the knee. Knee. 2010;17(2):97–102.
54. Dupont JY. Synovial plicae of the knee. Controversies and review. Clin Sports Med. 1997;16(1):87–122.
55. Olewnik Ł, Gonera B, Podgórski M, Polguj M, Jezierski H, Topol M. A proposal for a new classification of pes anserinus morphology. Knee Surg Sports Traumatol Arthrosc. 2019;27(9):2984–93.
56. Charalambous CP, Kwaees TA. Anatomical considerations in hamstring tendon harvesting for anterior cruciate ligament reconstruction. Muscles Ligaments Tendons J. 2013;2(4):253–7.
57. Reina N, Abbo O, Gomez-Brouchet A, Chiron P, Moscovici J, Laffosse JM. Anatomy of the bands of the hamstring tendon: how can we improve harvest quality? Knee. 2013;20(2):90–5.
58. Mochizuki T, Akita K, Muneta T, Sato T. Pes anserinus: layered supportive structure on the medial side of the knee. Clin Anat. 2004;17(1):50–4.
59. Hennigan SP, Schneck CD, Mesgarzadeh M, Clancy M. The semimembranosus-tibial collateral ligament bursa. Anatomical study and magnetic resonance imaging. J Bone Joint Surg Am. 1994;76(9):1322–7.
60. Nakamura T, Suzuki D, Murakami G, Cho BH, Fujimiya M, Kozuka N. Human fetal anatomy of the posterior semimembranosus complex at the knee with special reference to the gastrocnemio-semimembranosus bursa. Knee. 2011;18(4):271–7.
61. Rauschning W, Lindgren PG. The clinical significance of the valve mechanism in communicating popliteal cysts. Arch Orthop Trauma Surg. 1979;95(4):251–6.
62. Rauschning W. Anatomy and function of the communication between knee joint and popliteal bursae. Ann Rheum Dis. 1980;39(4):354–8.

63. Rauschning W, Lindgren PG. Popliteal cysts (Baker's cysts) in adults. I. Clinical and roentgenological results of operative excision. Acta Orthop Scand. 1979;50(5):583–91.
64. Herman AM, Marzo JM. Popliteal cysts: a current review. Orthopedics. 2014;37(8):e678–84.
65. Steinbach LS, Stevens KJ. Imaging of cysts and bursae about the knee. Radiol Clin N Am. 2013;51(3):433–54.
66. Shim SS, Leung G. Blood supply of the knee joint. A microangiographic study in children and adults. Clin Orthop Relat Res. 1986;208:119–25.
67. Barner KL, Mayer CM, Orth C, Tran QV, Olinger AB, Wright BW. Mapping the genicular arteries to provide a caution zone during knee surgery. Clin Anat. 2019; https://doi.org/10.1002/ca.23535.
68. Hirtler L, Lübbers A, Rath C. Vascular coverage of the anterior knee region—an anatomical study. J Anat. 2019;235(2):289–98.
69. Wang D, Shen Z, Jiang D, Li X, Fang X, Leng H, Zhang W. Qualitative and quantitative analysis of patellar vascular anatomy by novel three-dimensional micro-computed-tomography: Implications for total knee arthroplasty. Knee. 2019;26(6):1330–7.
70. Reipond L, Trompeter A, Szarko M. Neurovascular anatomy around the knee: Relevance of the dangers of self-drilling external fixator pin tips. SICOT J. 2019;5:9. https://doi.org/10.1051/sicotj/2019006.
71. Petersen W, Stein V, Tillmann B. Blood supply of the quadriceps tendon. Unfallchirurg. 1999;102(7):543–7.
72. Yepes H, Tang M, Morris SF, Stanish WD. Relationship between hypovascular zones and patterns of ruptures of the quadriceps tendon. J Bone Joint Surg Am. 2008;90(10):2135–41.
73. Tran J, Peng PWH, Gofeld M, Chan V, Agur AMR. Anatomical study of the innervation of posterior knee joint capsule: implication for image-guided intervention. Reg Anesth Pain Med. 2019;44(2):234–8.
74. Tran J, Peng PWH, Lam K, Baig E, Agur AMR, Gofeld M. Anatomical study of the innervation of anterior knee joint capsule: implication for image-guided intervention. Reg Anesth Pain Med. 2018;43(4):407–14.
75. Deutsch A, Wyzykowski RJ, Victoroff BN. Evaluation of the anatomy of the common peroneal nerve. Defining nerve-at-risk in arthroscopically assisted lateral meniscus repair. Am J Sports Med. 1999;27(1):10–5.
76. Kim SY, Le PU, Kosharskyy B, Kaye AD, Shaparin N, Downie SA. Is genicular nerve radiofrequency ablation safe? A literature review and anatomical study. Pain Physician. 2016;19(5):E697–705.
77. Patterson DC, Cirino CM, Gladstone JN. No safe zone: the anatomy of the saphenous nerve and its posteromedial branches. Knee. 2019;26(3):660–5.
78. Uemura K, Atkins PR, Fiorentino NM, Anderson AE. Hip rotation during standing and dynamic activities and the compensatory effect of femoral anteversion: an in-vivo analysis of asymptomatic young adults using three-dimensional computed tomography models and dual fluoroscopy. Gait Posture. 2018;61:276–81.
79. Henry BM, Tomaszewski KA, Pękala PA, Ramakrishnan PK, Taterra D, Saganiak K, Mizia E, Walocha JA. The variable emergence of the infrapatellar branch of the saphenous nerve. J Knee Surg. 2017;30(6):585–93.
80. Ackmann T, Von Düring M, Teske W, Ackermann O, Muller P, Von Schulze Pellengahr C. Anatomy of the infrapatellar branch in relation to skin incisions and as the basis to treat neuropathic pain by cryodenervation. Pain Physician. 2014;17(3):E339–48.
81. Mochida H, Kikuchi S. Injury to infrapatellar branch of saphenous nerve in arthroscopic knee surgery. Clin Orthop Relat Res. 1995;320:88–94.
82. Kerver AL, Leliveld MS, den Hartog D, Verhofstad MH, Kleinrensink GJ. The surgical anatomy of the infrapatellar branch of the saphenous nerve in relation to incisions for anteromedial knee surgery. J Bone Joint Surg Am. 2013;95(23):2119–25.
83. Elias JJ, Faust AF, Chu YH, Chao EY, Cosgarea AJ. The soleus muscle acts as an agonist for the anterior cruciate ligament. An in vitro experimental study. Am J Sports Med. 2003;31(2):241–6.

Chapter 3
Knee Biomechanics: Tibiofemoral Articulation

This chapter describes the direction and components of knee motion as well as the muscles acting upon the tibiofemoral articulation. In addition, it explores the forces acting on the tibiofemoral joint and describes the various structures contributing to its stability.

3.1 Knee Flexion/Extension at the Tibiofemoral Joint [1–16]

In relation to the tibia, the femur rolls (equivalent to a car wheel rolling down the road), slides (equivalent to a wheel sliding on an icy surface), and rotates (equivalent to a wheel spinning without moving).

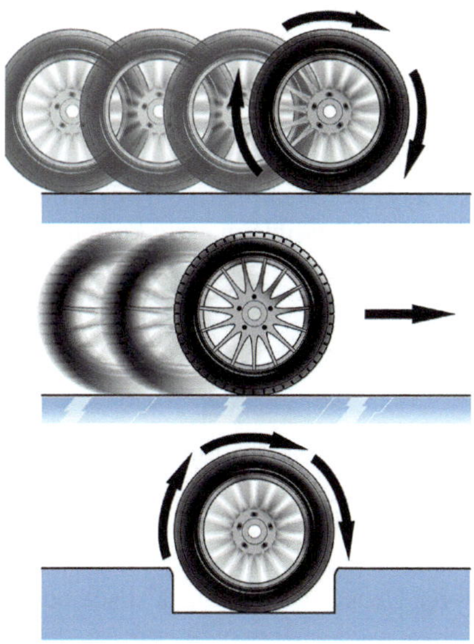

Wheel rolling, sliding, spinning is analogous to femoral condyle motion during knee flexion/extension

C. Panayiotou Charalambous, *The Knee Made Easy*,
https://doi.org/10.1007/978-3-030-54506-2_3

It has been shown that the medial and lateral femoral condyles exhibit different patterns of motion (which is related to their distinct anatomical features- the medial femoral condyle being longer):

- The lateral femoral condyle rolls posteriorly and slides in relation to the tibia as the knee flexes.
- The medial femoral condyle rotates but does not roll back or slide with flexion up to 110°. Minor posterior movement of the medial femoral condyle may occur with higher degrees of flexion (but which is much less that that seen in the lateral femoral condyle).

  Hence, posterior "roll-back" occurs laterally but not medially
- The contact point between the femoral condyles and the tibia moves posteriorly as the knee flexes. The femoral condyles are not fully circular, hence the position of the contact point does not parallel the position of the femoral condyles (the contact point may thus move posteriorly without the medial femoral condyle doing so).

3.2 Initiation of Knee Extension (Screw Home Mechanism)

At terminal extension, the knee joint is slightly hyperextended and stabilized with the tightening of the cruciate and collateral ligaments. As the length of the medial femoral condyle is longer than the length of the lateral condyle, when the foot is free (open chain motion) the tibia rotates externally about 15° on the femur during the last 20° of extension, and the tibial tuberosity is seen moving laterally. This is called the screw-home motion. When the foot is fixed on the ground (closed chain motion) the same effect is achieved by internal rotation of the femur in relation to the tibia.

Reversal of the screw home mechanism occurs during knee flexion from extension [11–13]. It is of note that such motion is not obligatory (simply related to anatomical factors) but also may also be influenced by dynamic factors as some passive internal/external rotation is still possible in early knee flexion.

3.3 Range of Motion at the Knee

Range of motion may be described as the range of motion that can occur in a particular direction (*anatomical range of motion*). However, it is important to recognise that in real life a great variation may exist in the amount of motion that can be achieved between individuals with healthy knees, due to anatomical (bony and soft tissue) and other factors. Hence, comparing a diseased knee with the opposite healthy knee of the same individual may provide more meaningful information, rather than simply comparing it to the general population.

Range of motion may also be described in terms of *functional range of motion.* This is defined as the minimum range of motion necessary to perform activities of daily living in a comfortable and effective fashion, and it is often much less than the anatomical range of motion:

Hence, although attaining full motion is a reasonable goal of knee interventions, it should be recognised that a smaller range of motion is required to perform many of the daily activities of life and achieve efficient function. It should be remembered however, that the functional range will depend on the individual with their specific circumstances and functional demands. Certain individuals may need much greater levels of mobility than the average "norm" due to occupational, religious (such as sitting with legs crossed, kneeling for praying) or recreational (sports) reasons [13–16].

Anatomical motion at the tibiofemoral joint may be described in three planes—sagittal, axial and frontal, and some of the values reported in western populations include:

Sagittal plane

- 10° hyperextension to 134° flexion, actively [13]
- 15° hyperextension to 145° flexion passively [14]

Axial (Transverse) Plane

In full extension—motion is not usually possible, because of interlocking of the femoral and tibial condyles.

At 90° of flexion:

- External rotation—45°
- Internal rotation—30°

Frontal Plane

In full extension—motion is not usually possible, because of interlocking of the femoral and tibial condyles.

At up to 30° of flexion

- Slight abduction/adduction possible

Functional Range of Motion

Most daily activities require much less motion than is potentially possible at the tibiofemoral articulation.

Rowe PJ et al [14] examined how much knee motion is sufficient for normal daily life in 20 normal subjects (mean age = 67 years), in a western setting, using flexible electrogoniometry during several functional activities. They evaluated normal gait, walking on slopes, stair negotiation, using standard and low chairs, and using a bath. They showed that:

- Normal gait and slopes require less than 90° of knee flexion
- Ascending/descending stairs (with 165 mm riser, 280 mm tread) and sitting down or sit to stand from a chair (380 or 460 mm high) require 90–120° of flexion
- Bath use requires about 135° of knee flexion
  - Getting in—from standing alongside bath, stepping in and sitting down (590 mm high)
  - Getting out—from sitting to standing up, stepping out, standing alongside bath

They concluded that achievement of 110° of flexion is a suitable goal for the rehabilitation of the injured or operated knee.

However, some individuals may require much more motion than the average minimum. In Asia and the Middle East many activities are performed while squatting, kneeling, or sitting cross-legged. These positions demand a greater range of motion than that typically required in Western populations. Similarly, deep kneeling is needed for prayer amongst Muslims and in Japan for traditional ceremonies.

- Hemmerich et al [15] showed that a mean maximum knee flexion of about 157° was required for squatting with heels up. Zhou et al [16] evaluated the kinematics of lower limbs of healthy Chinese people sitting cross-legged showing that about 132° of knee flexion was necessary.

3.4 Muscles Bringing about Motion

Muscles attach via their tendons to bones. Upon contraction they exert forces in a direction influenced by the site of muscle origin, muscle fibre orientation and site of tendon insertion [9, 10]. Through contraction a muscle may:

- Move a body segment in line with the direction of its pull
  - In leg extension the quadriceps contracts, moving the tibia forwards in relation to the femur
- Slow down a body segment motion occurring in a direction opposite to its pull
  - In flexing the knee from a fully extended position, quadriceps contracts opposing the effect of gravity and preventing an uncontrolled leg drop
- Oppose a muscle acting in an opposite direction, to stabilise a body segment in a particular position—hamstrings contract opposing the quadriceps in the anterior cruciate ligament (ACL) deficient knee—this limits anterior translation of the tibia and hence improves the stability of the tibiofemoral joint.
- Stabilise a body segment so that it rotates rather than translate under the action of another muscle. This is equivalent to a force acting on a wheel. If the force is unopposed it will cause the wheel to rotate but also translate in the direction

of the applied force. However, if an opposite force is applied to the wheel at the same time, it can stabilise the wheel so that it simply rotates rather than translate. This force may be applied in an opposite direction to the distracting force, causing the wheel to translate, or in any other direction (such as perpendicular to the distracting force). Quadriceps contracts opposing the action of hamstring tendons during knee flexion and limiting distraction of the tibiofemoral articulation.

By recognising the anatomical origin and insertion of muscles in relation to the joints across which they act, one may determine the movement they can achieve upon contraction. This can form the basis of assessing the strength of these muscles and formulating a diagnosis when knee motion or knee stability is impaired.

In considering knee motion, it is important to appreciate that although a muscle may be described as having a major function:

- Different parts of the muscle may have different effects with regards to moving or stabilising a body segment (such as the different heads of quadriceps)
- A muscle can exert different effects depending on leg position (hamstring muscles in internal versus external rotation of the lower leg).

The above may help explain at least partly:

- The variability that may be observed in the detrimental effect of muscle dysfunction between individuals
- The variability in strength improvement achieved by exercises targeting specific muscles between individuals

The quadriceps and hamstring have been shown to work in a coordinated way in bringing about motion during functional activities of the knee.

Quadriceps
- All four heads—extend the knee
- Rectus femoris—flexes the hip

Hamstrings (semimembranosus, semitendinosus and biceps femoris)—these act upon two joints—the hip and knee and are thus bi-articular muscles. Their individual actions are described below:

Semitendinosus
- Extends the hip when the trunk is fixed
- Flexes the knee and internally rotates the lower leg when the knee is flexed

Semimembranosus
- Extends the hip
- Flexes the knee and internally rotates the lower leg when the knee is flexed

Long head of biceps femoris
- Extends the hip
- Flexes the knee

- Externally rotates the lower leg with the knee in flexion

Gracilis
- Adducts, internally rotates and flexes the hip
- Flexes the knee

Adductor Magnus
- Extends and adducts the hip
- The part attached to the linea aspera acts as an external rotator of the femur
- The part attached to the adductor tubercle acts as an internal rotator of the femur

Sartorius
- Flexes and externally rotates the femur at the hip
- Flexes the knee and internally rotates the lower leg

Iliotibial Band (ITB)
- Extends, abducts, and laterally rotates the hip
- Contributes to the lateral stability of the knee, resisting varus stress and internal rotation of the tibia on the femur

Popliteus
Popliteus has the following functions:
- When the foot is in contact with the ground (closed chain)—rotates the femur externally on the tibia at the beginning of knee flexion unlocking the knee
- When the foot is not in contact with the ground (open chain)—rotates the tibia internally on the femur at the beginning of knee flexion
- Contributes to knee flexion
- Popliteus is attached to the lateral meniscus and draws it posteriorly during knee flexion to avoid crushing it between the tibia and femur

3.4.1 Muscles Controlling Tibiofemoral Joint Motion

Several muscles bring about motion at the tibiofemoral joint as below:

Extension
- Quadriceps

Flexion
- Hamstrings
  - Semimembranosus
  - Semitendinosus
  - Biceps femoris
- Gracilis
- Sartorius
- Popliteus

Internal rotation
- Semimembranosus
- Semitendinosus
- Sartorius
- Gracilis

External rotation
- Biceps femoris

3.5 GAIT

Having considered motion at the knee, it is important to relate this motion to the overall gait cycle [10, 17].

Normal gait is divided into two phases:

1. Stance phase
   a. Heel strike
   b. Foot flat
   c. Heel off
   d. Toe off
2. Swing phase
   a. Hip extension
   b. Knee flexion
   c. Ankle dorsiflexion
   d. Hip flexion

Motion of the knee during the gait cycle may be summarised as below:

- The knee extends twice during each step
  - At the end of the swing phase
  - Late in stance phase
- The knee shows its largest flexion during the swing phase
  - Soon after toe off (for foot clearance off the ground to occur)
  - Before heel strike
- The tibia rotates internally with flexion and externally with extension

Looking at knee flexion/extension in each gait phase:

Stance
- Heel strike to foot flat—knee flexion
- Foot flat to heel off—knee flexion is completed and extension begins
- Heel off to toe off—extension completed and knee begins to flex again

Swing
- Maximum knee flexion is reached soon after toe off
- Maximum extension is shown just before heel strike

Quadriceps and hamstrings contract and relax during the gait cycle to achieve the desired knee motion:

- Quadriceps contraction is high at mid-stance
- It then progressively declines as the knee extends. Once the trunk moves anterior to the knee, extension stability is provided passively, hence the quadriceps relaxes.
- At the end of stance the knee begins to flex. There is no quadriceps contraction at this time, as the body lies anterior to the knee providing stability.
- As swing progresses quadriceps contracts to extend the knee, to oppose gravity, decelerate the leg and stabilize the knee just before heel strike.
- Co-contraction of the hamstrings towards the end of the swing phase limits knee hyperextension.
- Between heel strike and flat foot the knee flexes as the hamstrings contract.
- The hamstrings contract at toe off to flex the knee, allowing foot clearance during swing.

3.6 Forces Transmitted by the Tibiofemoral Joint

The knee is a weight bearing joint, with huge amounts of forces transmitted through the tibiofemoral joint [18–27].

The forces transmitted across the knee joint are the result of:

- Transmitted weight—weight of body and upper leg
- Ground reaction force (GRF)—opposing force exerted by the ground upon weightbearing
- Forces generated by the surrounding muscles which contract in order to maintain position of the limb in space, move the bones in relation to each other, and also achieve joint stability
- Forces in surrounding soft tissues (such as ligament tension)
- Friction force between the articular surfaces
- Compressive and shear forces exerted by the muscles acting across the joint
- Acceleration forces of the foot and tibia

3.6.1 Forces Acting on the Tibiofemoral Joint

Analysis of the forces acting on the tibiofemoral joint has suggested that huge forces are transmitted during normal daily activities [12–14] with most resultant forces being in the region of 2.2–3.5 times the Body Weight (BW). Forces associated with some activities are as below:

- Stair descending 3.5 BW
- Stair ascending 3.2 BW
- Level walking 2.6 BW
- Downhill walking (19% gradient)-8 BW
- One legged stance 2.6 BW
- Knee bending 2.5 BW
- Standing up 2.5 BW
- Sitting down 2.3 BW
- 2-legged stance 1.1 BW
- Ergometer cycling—1.2 BW (hence cycling is considered as a low demand activity for the knee joint)

The knee has two peak forces during normal gait:

1. Quadriceps contraction just after heel strike as the weightbearing leg accepts weight
2. When the forefoot is pushing off the ground, propulsing the body forwards

3.7 Tibiofemoral Joint Loading [28–36]

Tibiofemoral joint loading in both the static and dynamic states is considered. The mechanical axis and adduction moment are described next. The mechanical axis represents the line of transmission of the body weight to the ground via the lower limb, whereas the adduction moment represents the action of the GRF (the force which opposes the body weight upon contact with the ground) on the knee.

3.8 Weightbearing—Mechanical Axis

In evaluating tibiofemoral loading, the weightbearing axis of the whole lower limb and its influence upon the knee is considered. This is a static assessment of the weightbearing limb and gives an indication as to how the body weight is transmitted through the lower limb and knee to the floor, in double leg stance.

When standing still, the body and lower limbs may be considered analogous to a table with legs. The weight of the table (excluding the weight of its legs) passes onto the legs at the point of contact with that table's flat surface, and through them to the floor. In the case of the lower limbs, this connection is at the hip joint, whereby the femoral head articulates with the pelvis, and hence with the axial skeleton and the rest of the body. The weightbearing axis may be assessed based on standing long leg films.

The weightbearing axis is represented by a line connecting the centre of the femoral head to the centre of the distal tibial plafond (at the ankle). This normally passes through, or very near to the centre of the knee, and makes an angle of 3°with the vertical axis (an axis that passes from the symphysis pubis vertically towards the ground).

In the normal knee the weightbearing axis passes just medial to the medial spine of the tibia, but moves medially in varus deformities and laterally in valgus deformities.

In relation to weightbearing, the mechanical axis of the femur and the mechanical axis of the tibia may also be described as the axis of weight transmission across these bones:

- Mechanical axis femur—line connecting the centre of the femoral head to the centre of the distal femur (centre of knee)
- Mechanical axis of the tibia—line connecting the centre of the tibial plateau (knee) to the centre of the distal tibial plafond
- Angle between femoral mechanical axis—distal femoral articular axis—the angle between the femoral mechanical axis and the distal femoral articular axis (about 3° in valgus)
- Angle between proximal tibial articular axis and tibial mechanical (or anatomical) axis (about 3° varus)

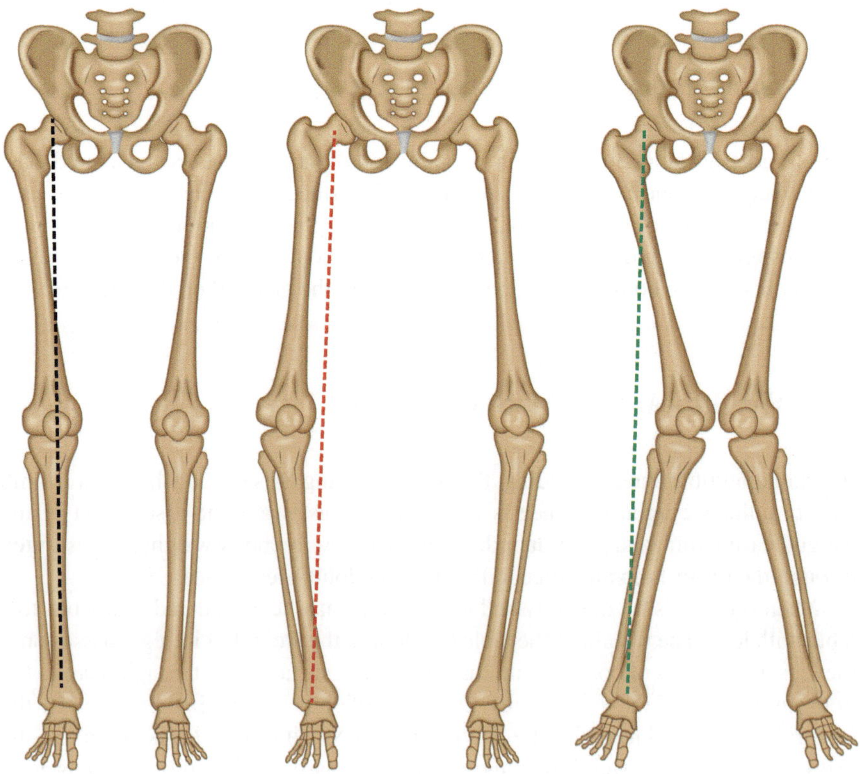

Weight bearing axis of knee with neutral, varus and valgus alignment

The mechanical axis of the femur and tibia, when combined, form the mechanical axis of the lower limb. In normal limb alignment, this mechanical axis of the lower limb coincides with the weightbearing axis of the whole lower limb. However, in the presence of deformity there may be deviation between the mechanical and weightbearing axes.

- The angle between the mechanical axis of the femur and the mechanical axis of the tibia is known as the mechanical femoro-tibial angle (MFTA) (normally 180°).

Describing the mechanical axis of the femur and tibia in isolation, is vital in arthroplasty surgery in the planning of the orientation of the replaced articular surfaces. In the absence of an anatomical deformity of the femur and tibia, the joint orientation may be planned in relation to the anatomical axis of the femur and tibia. However, in the presence of anatomical deformity such reliance on anatomical axes becomes difficult. Aligning the joint orientation in relation to the desired mechanical axis can give the desired outcome.

It is of note that the weightbearing axis does not fully reflect the magnitude of knee loading under dynamic conditions, and may only predict about 50% of peak forces applied. Other forces such as muscle co-contraction and ligamentous strain, as well as the GRF play a role in knee loading.

Similarly, the weightbearing axis may not fully predict the force distribution across the knee. Johnson F. et al [33] compared the static weightbearing axis with loading of the tibial plateau as measured dynamically by gait analysis. They found that in about 70% of cases with valgus deformities, the load remained medial. This suggested that the knee is loaded more medially than a static weightbearing axis would predict. Hence, they suggested that examination of a radiograph of a static knee cannot provide a full estimate of the distribution of load.

Johnson F. et al [33] also determined the varus/valgus tibiofemoral angles at which the entire load would be carried by the medial or lateral compartment respectively:

- Varus 4°—load entirely carried by the medial compartment
- Valgus 15°—load entirely carried by the lateral compartment

Hence, for low tibiofemoral valgus angulation, the load is predominantly medial. With a varus deformity the load on the medial plateau is almost 100%.

The above lack of correlation between the static mechanical axis and the dynamic weight bearing axis may be due to differences in the forces acting upon the knee during static and dynamic conditions:

- In the static neutral knee the GRF passes through the centre of the knee, and no horizontal forces exist.
- In the static varus knee the GRF passes medially to the centre of the knee, and the load on the medial compartment is correspondingly greater.
- However, during dynamic loading of the knee (in the stance phase of gait) there is an additional horizontal component to the GRF, which shifts its force vector more medially.

The mechanical axis is used to guide how realignment procedures are performed, to shift weight away from an overloaded compartment.

- In osteotomy of the varus knee (opening wedge, closing wedge) the varus deformity is corrected. This shifts the mechanical axis laterally. The mechanical axis is often moved to a point located about 62% of the medial to lateral width of the tibial plateau from the medial tibial edge—passing close to the lateral spine (known as the Fujisawa point). However, this is not absolute and the exact shift may vary according to individual characteristics [31, 35].

However, such static shifts in the weightbearing axis, may not fully represent equivalent shifts in compartmental pressures upon dynamic loading. Tension in ligaments may influence compartmental forces and contact pressures, even when the mechanical axis is well re-aligned. Agneskirchner et al [36] showed that:

- An opening wedge high tibial osteotomy (HTO) without release of the medial collateral ligament (MCL) results in a significant increase of pressure in the medial compartment of the tibiofemoral joint, despite the fact that the mechanical axis has been shifted into valgus.
- Only after a complete release of the MCL there was a significant decrease of pressure of the medial joint compartment observed after opening wedge HTO.

3.9 Knee Adduction Moment

In evaluating force transmission through the lower limb and knee under dynamic conditions, the knee adduction moment is considered:

- The force exerted by the lower limb on the ground is due to the body and limb weight and is applied at the point of contact between the foot and the ground.
- The ground exerts an equal and opposite force which originates at the point of contact with the foot and passes upwards through the centre of body mass (usually located at the level of the S2 vertebra). This GRF may be viewed in the coronal and sagittal planes.

3.9.1 Relation of the GRF to the Knee in the Coronal Plane

When standing still, the legs are usually positioned apart. However, when walking the hip and tibia are adducted. Hence, during the stance phase of gait the leg makes contact with the ground with the leg in an adducted position. This is visible when looking at an individual from the front and can be more obvious when ascending or descending stairs. This means that the point at which the foot makes contact with the ground is medial to the knee.

As a result, the GRF vector (upward vector) which passes from:

- The center of pressure of the foot to
- The center of mass of the body

acts medial to the knee.

Given its orientation and position, this force causes an adduction (varus) moment at the knee joint (pulling the tibia in further adduction in relation to the femur). This compresses the medial compartment more than the lateral compartment, and hence most of the force goes through the medial compartment.

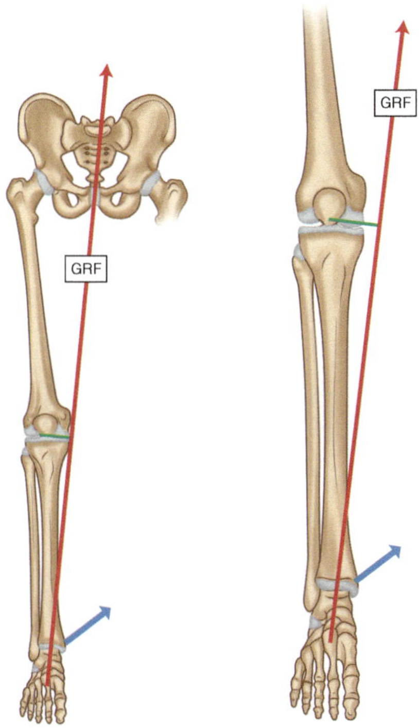

Adduction moment due to GRF

This resultant adduction moment leads to compression of the medial compartment and unloading of the lateral compartment, which is resisted by the lateral ligamentous structures and iliotibial band. Hence, medial compartment loading is determined mainly by the GRF. In contrast, the force transmitted by the lateral compartment is mainly due to muscle and ligament action. This could explain the predisposition of the medial compartment to degenerative changes and osteoarthritis.

The adduction moment = force multiplied by the distance from the point of action (from the knee)

- The more medial the GRF passes in relation to the knee, the greater the adduction moment.

Understanding the adduction moment can help determine some of the factors influencing its magnitude. The orientation and position of the GRF in relation to the centre of the knee, and its size, influences the magnitude of the adduction moment.

- The location of the centre of mass relative to the centre of contact of the foot with the ground influences the orientation of the GRF. Weak hip abductors may lead to a shift in the centre of mass away from the weightbearing leg increasing the adduction moment
- The alignment of the knee influences the position of the GRF in relation to the knee (increased in varus deformity)
- The larger the GRF, the greater the magnitude of the adduction moment. The size of the GRF is influenced by body weight—as body weight increases, GRF and thus the adduction moment increase.

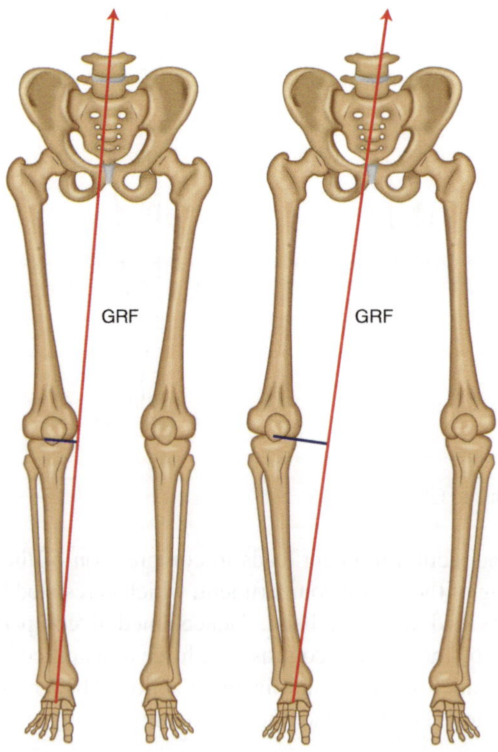

Varus alignment moves the GRF medially in relation to the knee, increasing the adduction moment

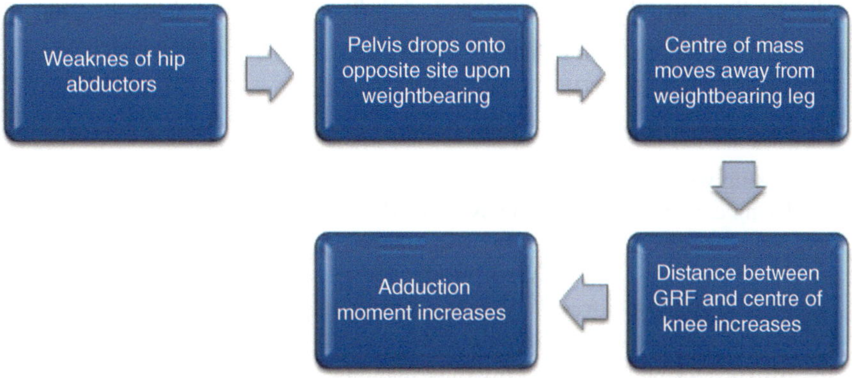

Weakness of the hip abductors may lead to an increase in the adduction moment acting on the knee

The adduction moment is clinically important as it has been related to the severity of medial compartment arthritis, severity of symptoms of medial compartment arthritis, and rate of arthritis progression.

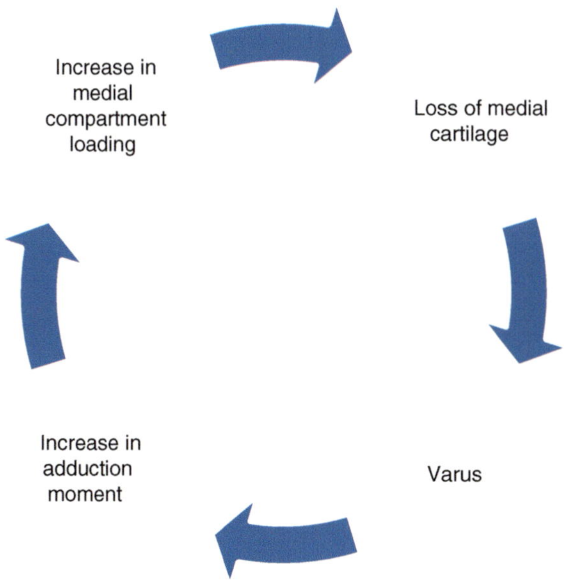

Articular cartilage degeneration leads to an increase in the adduction moment, which leads to further cartilage degeneration

In addition, recognition of the adduction moment helps to consider interventions to minimise tibiofemoral joint loading, and improve clinical symptoms caused by arthritis. The knee adduction moment may be decreased by:

- Moving laterally the point of contact of the foot with the ground by using a lateral wedge orthosis

- Improving limb alignment—reducing varus by:
  - Medial compartment unloading knee brace
  - Re-alignment surgery-osteotomy
- Reducing the size of the GRF by:
  - Losing weight
  - Using cane or other walking assisting devices
- Altering certain gait parameters
  - Moving the trunk over the standing limb shifts the centre of mass towards the standing leg, reducing the adduction moment
  - Moving the centre of foot pressure laterally by walking with the foot externally rotated

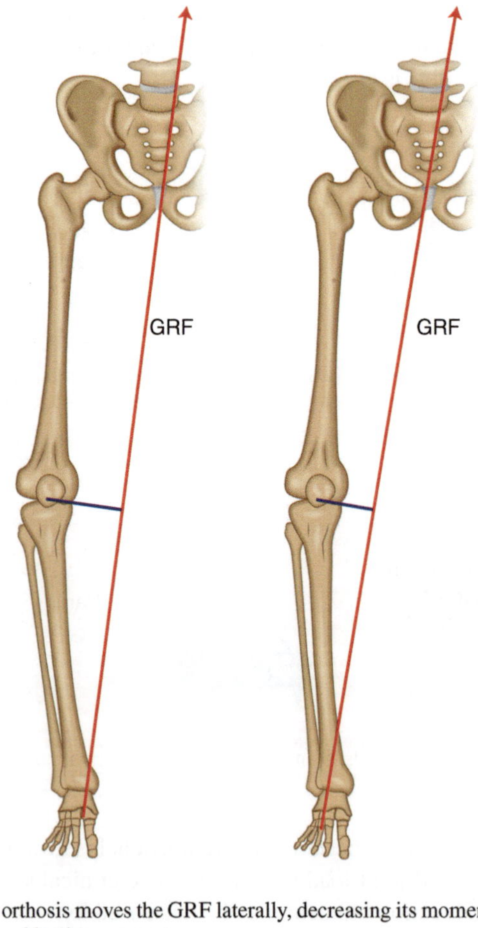

A foot lateral wedge orthosis moves the GRF laterally, decreasing its moment arm on the knee, and hence decreasing the adduction moment

3.10 Menisci and Loading of the Knee

In considering the biomechanics of the tibiofemoral articulation it is essential to consider the activity of the medial and lateral menisci. They have important functions [37, 38] including:

- Distribute knee load, reducing localised stress on the articular surface
- Transmit weight—load sharing
- Enhance lubrication
- Improve stability

The medial and lateral menisci may transmit 50% and 70% of their compartment's load in extension, and 85% and 90% in flexion, respectively.

When a force is applied on a surface the stress created depends on the area over which that force is applied:

- Stress = force/area over which the force is exerted

The greater the area over which the force is applied the smaller the stress created.

- The contact area between two conforming surfaces (convex on concave) is larger than the contact area between two non-conforming surfaces (convex on flat or convex on convex).

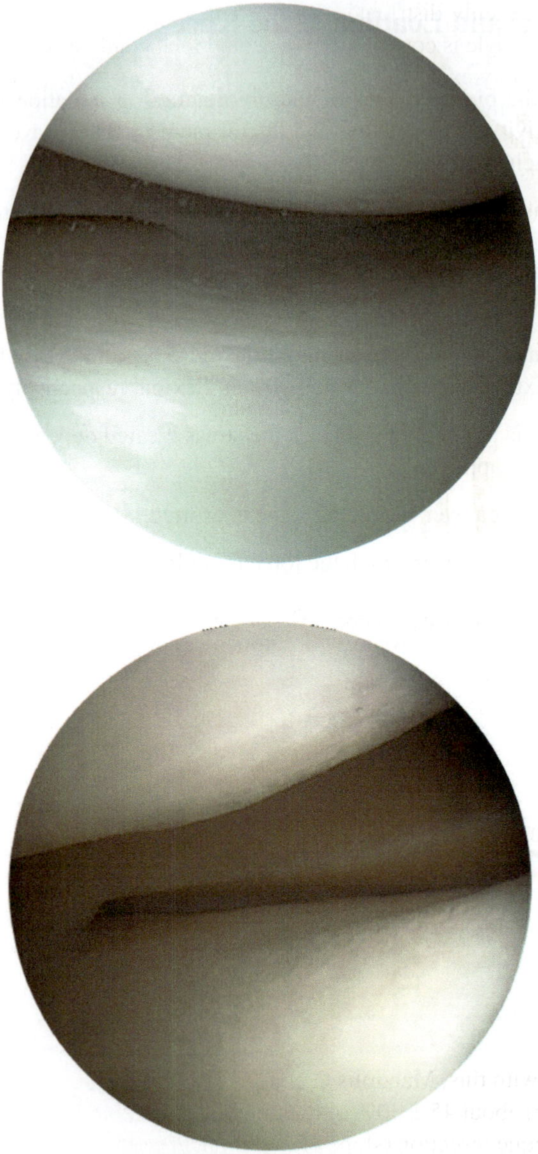

Arthroscopic view of the medial and lateral compartments showing the different geometry between the medial and lateral tibial plateau

Hence, when two articular surfaces come in contact and a force is transmitted across them, the localised stress created will depend on the area of contact between the two articulating surfaces. Localised high levels of stress can have detrimental effects upon the articular cartilage, predisposing to early degeneration. The femoral and the tibial articular surfaces are not fully conforming, hence at any point the load application is not evenly distributed across the whole of the articular surfaces. The medial femoral condyle is convex but the medial tibial condyle is concave, thus some element of conformity exists. In contrast, both the lateral femoral condyle and lateral tibial condyle are convex which increases their point loading. The menisci between the condyles help to increase the surface area of contact and in this way reduce the point peak stresses. This is equivalent to someone sitting on a hard rock. A painful bum due to localised pressure by the rock may be relieved by using a soft cushion to sit on.

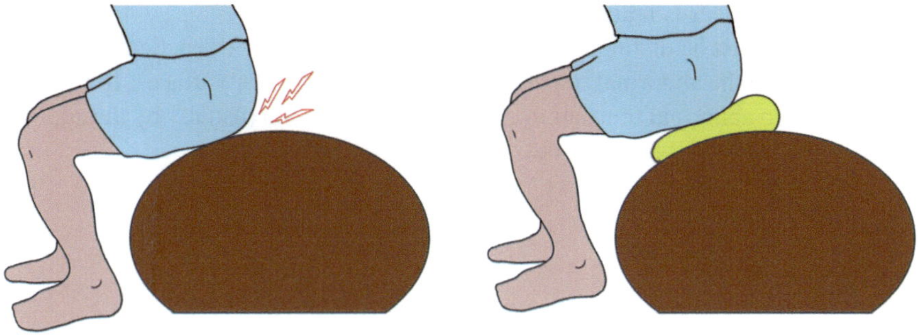

The meniscus acts like a cushion to reduce stresses, analogous to using a cushion when seating on a rock

The femur transmits force to the tibia at the point of contact between the two. If there is a large contact area the force is distributed across this, and hence no point of articular cartilage is subjected to a high stress. In contrast, if the contact area is small the localised force is larger, and hence the stress upon the articular cartilage is higher.

Following meniscectomy the contact area decreases, and hence contact pressures increase:

- Post medial meniscectomy contact pressures may increase by 100% whereas following lateral meniscectomy contact pressures may increase by 200–350% [39]

3.11 Forces with Aquatic Exercises [25–27]

Aquatic exercises are used in knee rehabilitation to allow mobilisation and strengthening whilst keeping loading of the knee joint to a minimum. Buoyancy reduces the load upon the knee as compared to exercises done out of water.

Kutzner et al [27] showed that the joint forces were reduced by 36–55% during weightbearing and dynamic exercises. However, consideration must also be made to drag forces in the water that oppose the muscle action. The same authors showed that during non-weight bearing aquatic activities high velocities increase the joint forces by about 60%, a factor to be considered when planning an aquatic exercise program.

3.12 Tibiofemoral Joint Stability

Tibiofemoral joint stability refers to the ability of a joint to maintain the normal relation of its articulating surfaces to avoid troublesome clinical symptoms.

Instability of a joint describes an abnormal translation of one articular surface in relation to the other. This can vary from dislocation where there is complete loss of contact between the articular surfaces, to subluxation where some contact between the articular surfaces is maintained.

Instability must be distinguished from laxity. In instability the patient has symptoms, related to the abnormal translation between the articular surfaces. In contrast, laxity refers to abnormal translation evident on examination (usually by the application of a force by the examiner) but which is not symptomatic.

3.12.1 Joint Stability

In considering stability of a joint one may look at static and dynamic stabilisers [40–75].

Static stabilisers: those factors that are constant in shape and size, parameters that cannot be altered according to the need of stability. These include:

- Shape of the articular surfaces
  - Conforming surfaces—ball in a cup
  - Non-conforming surfaces—flat on flat surface, ball on a flat surface
- Negative intra-articular pressure providing a suction force of one articular surface on the other
- Ligaments, menisci

Ligaments are fibrous structures that connect two bones. Ligaments are static stabilisers as they cannot actively change their shape or size to limit motion. Instead, when a force is applied, all they can do is stretch from a resting lax state to a taut state. Ligaments may provide stability in two ways:

1. Check-rein effect—the ligament allows motion between two bones in a direction along the line of the ligament, until it stretches to its maximum length at which no further movement is allowed
2. Buttress effect—the ligament acts like a fence, limiting motion in a direction perpendicular to the ligament

At the knee, ligaments function in a check rein mechanism.

The mode by which a ligament exerts its effect may be influenced by the way in which a ligament is attached to bone (its origin and insertion). These functions may be explained by the analogy of the rope used to anchor a boat onto the dock cleat [76]:

- A rope passing from the cleat to the boat will allow some movement up to the point it becomes taut. However, such a rope may not stop the boat from moving sideways at an angle and colliding with neighbour boats!
- A rope passing on either side of the boat and also round its back may stop it from drifting into the open sea but in addition limit the extent to which it can slide side to side.

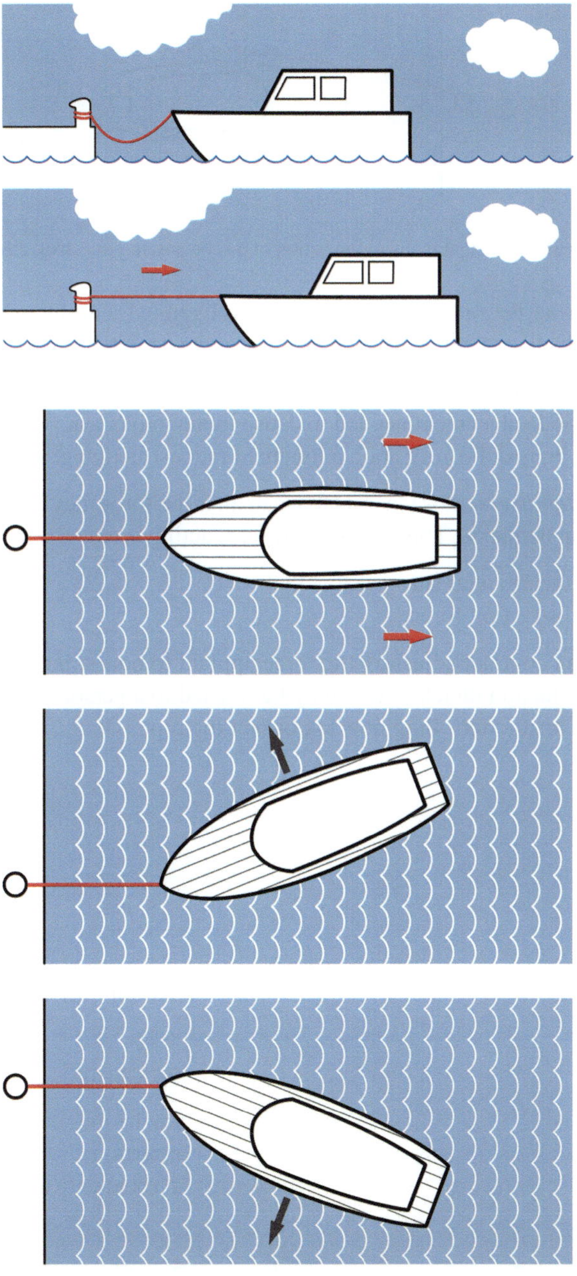

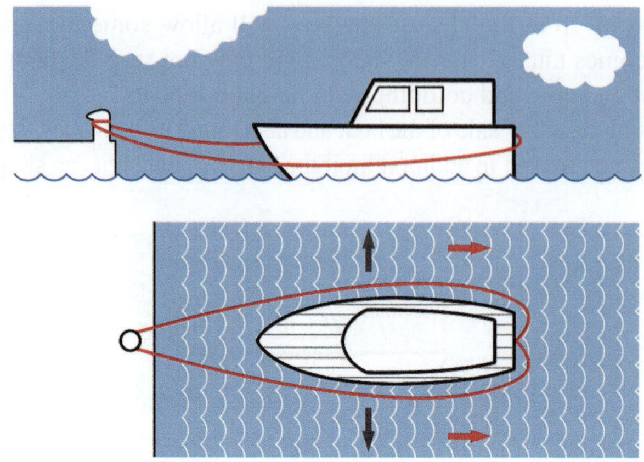

The action of ligaments is analogous to the action of a rope passing to a dock cleat

In considering the origin and insertion of a ligament and the axis along which joint motion/displacement occurs the following can be determined:

- Direction of displacement resisted by the ligament
- Direction of displacement needed to cause ligamentous tear
- Effect of a bony deformity upon a ligament reconstruction graft

Dynamic stabilisers: those factors that can alter the force they exert across a joint as the situation demands. This refers to muscles acting across a joint in order to:

1. Compress the articular surfaces together
2. Oppose a distracting force

Muscles can contract adjusting the force applied to bones, hence adjusting joint stability as a situation dictates. This may be likened to a person pulling on the rope anchoring the boat (controlling how lax or taut the rope is).

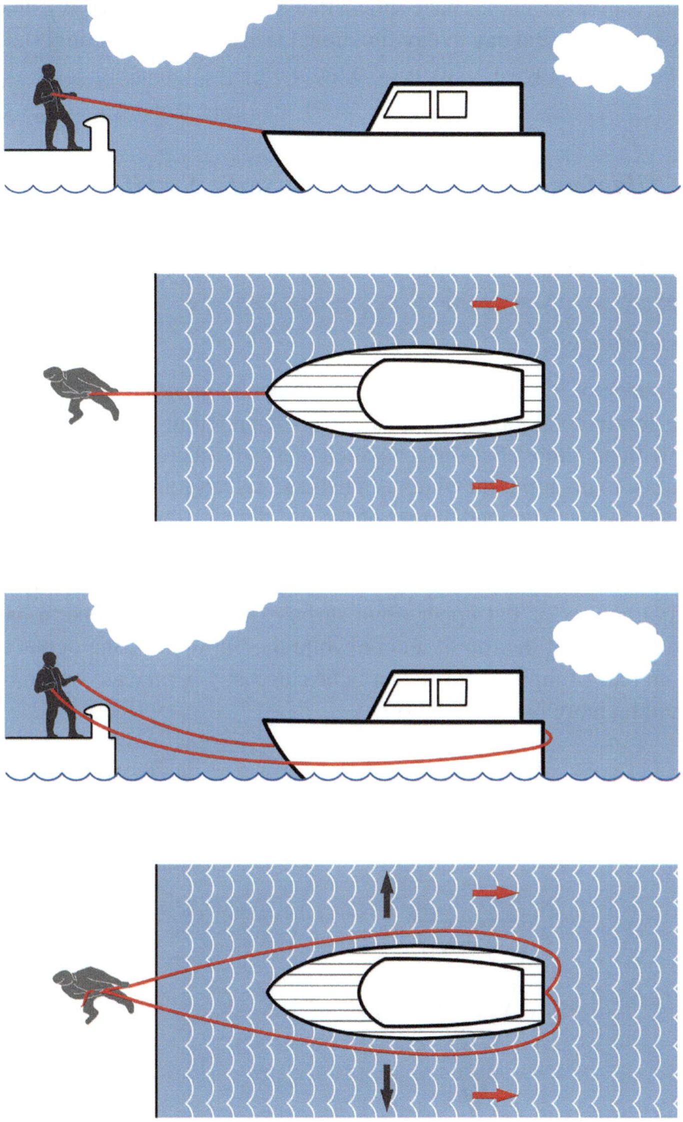

Muscles are considered the main stabilisers of joints. This would explain why joints whose main ligaments are torn can continue to be stable allowing return to normal activities. In addition, by strengthening certain muscles a greater stabilising force may be exerted across a joint. Similarly, by getting muscles to work in a more balanced and coordinated way joint stability may be improved.

Electromyographic studies have shown that a coordinated quadriceps/hamstrings activity occurs in normal day to day functional tasks (such as walking, stair ascending/descending) and such activity is even more important in ligamentous deficiency.

3.12.2 *Tibiofemoral Joint Stability – Static Stabilizers*

If we examine the potential stabilisers described above, for the tibiofemoral joint we can see that:

1. *Bone morphology*

    - The shape of the femur and tibia do not confer substantial inherent stability. The tibiofemoral joint involves a curved distal femur (part of a ball) articulating with an almost flat surface which makes it inherently unstable. This is in contrast to the hip joint which is a ball and socket joint, but the acetabulum is a deep socket. The medial part of the tibiofemoral joint involves articulating of the convex distal femur with a concave tibial surface, whereas the lateral part of the tibiofemoral joint involves articulating of the convex distal femur with a convex or flat upper tibial surface. This is almost like a ball of ice-cream sitting at the top of a cone while the hip joint is analogous to an ice-cream ball sitting in a plastic cup; one can easily appreciate which of the two would be more likely to slip off.

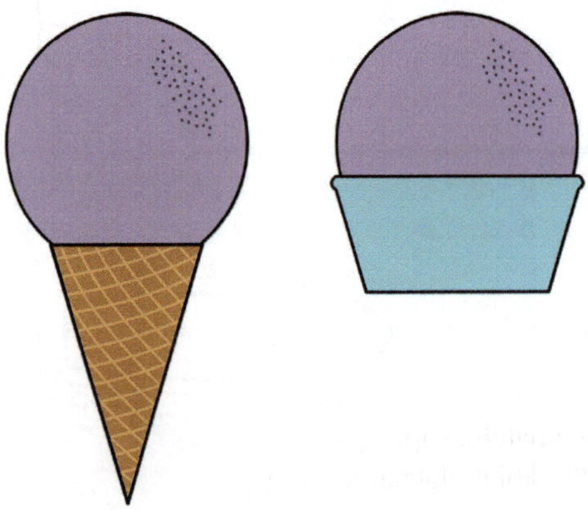

The knee articulation is almost like a ball of ice-cream sitting at the top of a cone while the hip joint is analogous to an ice-cream ball sitting in a plastic cup

- It has been shown that:
  - Depth of the medial tibial plateau—as it increases, tibiofemoral stability increases
  - Sphericity of the medial femoral condyle—as it increases, tibiofemoral stability decreases

- Tibial slope—the upper part of the tibia has a slope when looking at it from the side (anterior part being higher than the posterior part creating a posteriorly directed slope). It is quantified by measuring the angle between a line perpendicular to the middle part of the tibial diaphysis and a line representing the posterior inclination of the tibial plateau. It is usually about 10°. Hence, there is a tendency for the femur to slide down this slope, in a posterior and inferior direction.
- Shape of the femoral notch—a pyramidal shape notch may confer more stability than a dome shaped notch.
- Medial tibial spine volume—as it increases, tibiofemoral stability increases.

It is recognised that:

- There is substantial variation in the magnitude of tibial slope between individuals.
- There is variation in the slope between the knees of a particular individual.
- The medial and lateral tibial slopes may differ within an individual.
- In the intact knee, application of a compressive force to the knee (during weightbearing) produces an anteriorly directed shear force on the tibia which leads to anterior shift of the tibia in relation to the femur. This shift is resisted by an intact ACL. The magnitude of this anterior directed force may be influenced by the surrounding bone morphology.
- The above may explain the predisposition of some individuals to ACL tear (as their bone geometry may confer increased strain on the ACL).
- Furthermore, it may explain the ability of some individuals to cope with a torn ACL without much instability, whereas others cannot. It may be that in some cases the bone morphology helps compensate for the lost ACL.

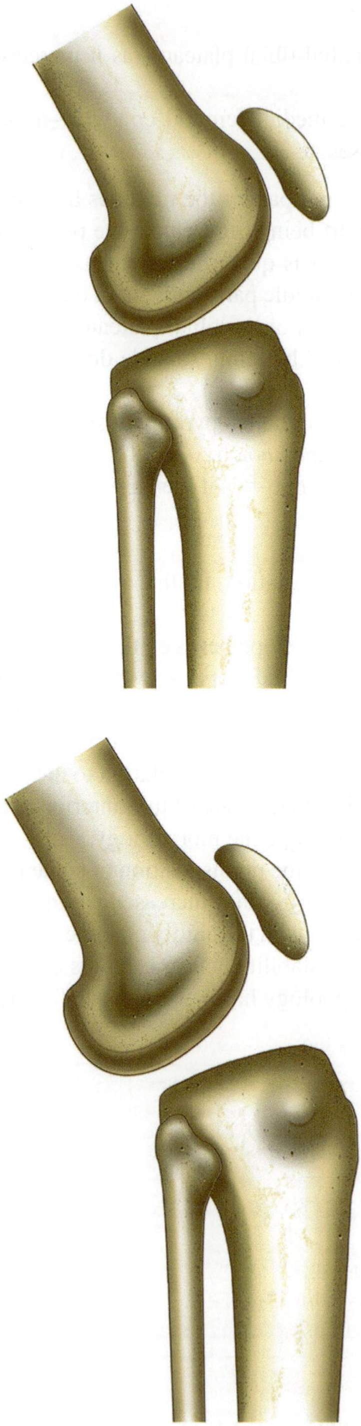

As the posterior slope increases the femur tends to roll backwards on the tibia increasing the strain on the ACL

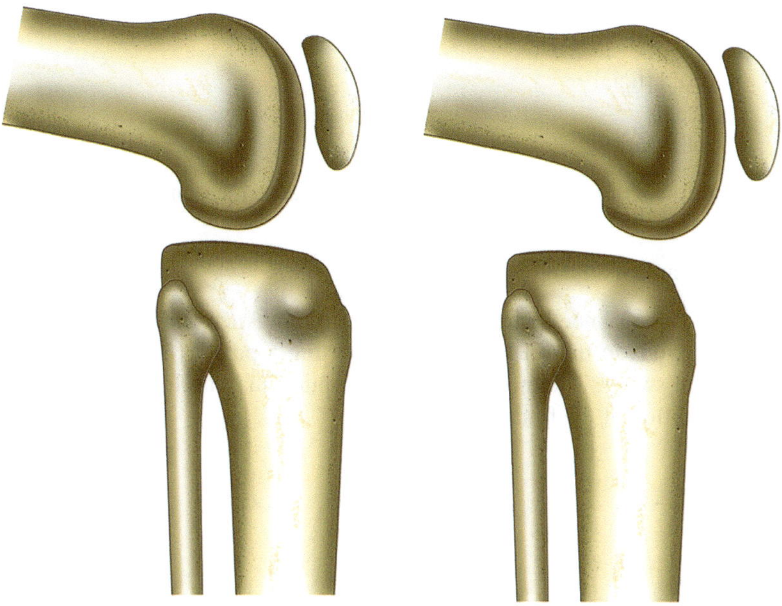

As the posterior slope decreases or reverses the femur tends to roll anteriorly in relation to the tibia, increasing the strain on the PCL

2. Menisci

   - The menisci improve the conformity of the articular surfaces, especially in the lateral compartment, almost like a cushion between two uneven surfaces.
   - The posterior meniscal horns also limit the effective posterior translation of the femur on the tibia (equivalent to anterior translation of the tibia in relation to the femur), by acting as wedges between the two.
   - The menisci also insert onto the tibia and are connected to the femur via ligamentous structures. As they are connected to both bones, they can contribute to knee stability, acting as check reins.

3. Intra-articular pressure

   - There is a suction effect of the negative intra-articular pressure found in the tibiofemoral joint, but this is a minor contributor to joint stability.

4. Patellar tendon

   - The patellar tendon may act as a passive knee stabiliser in an anterior and posterior direction. It may limit the anterior translation of the tibia by exerting a buttress effect and posterior translation of the tibia on the femur due to a check rein effect.

5. Knee capsule

   - The tibiofemoral joint capsule is thin and loose fitting, especially at its superior part. However, the joint capsule is reinforced by ligaments which contribute to stability:

- The medial collateral ligament resists lateral translation of the tibia in relation to the femur and has three components:
  - Superficial
  - Deep
  - Oblique
- The posterior part of the capsule resists anterior translation of the tibia on the femur

6. Knee ligaments

- The role of knee ligaments in supporting the knee and providing stability is analogous to that of two ropes supporting a person sitting on the seat of a frame swing. The mode of ACL disruption may be likened to the mode of disruption of the frame swing.

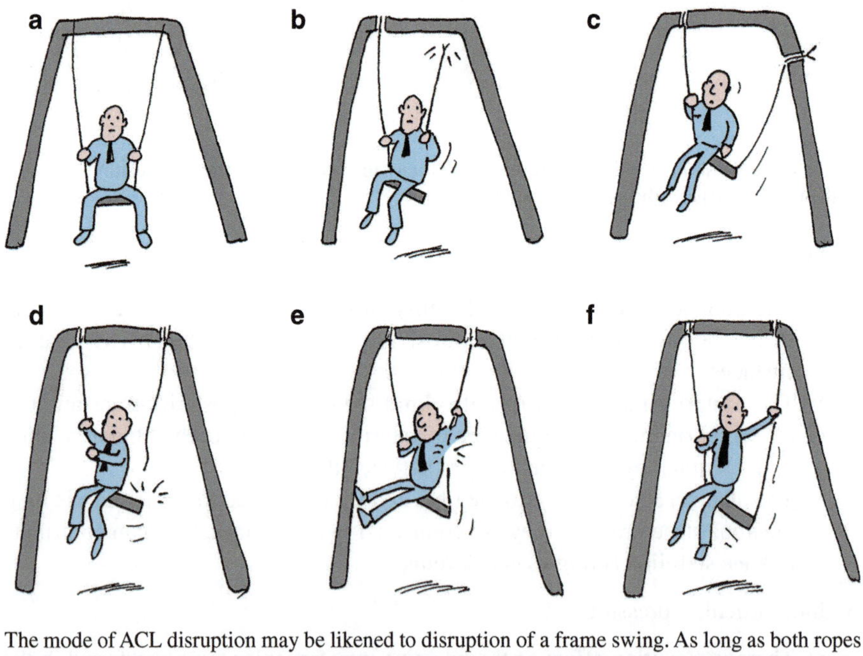

The mode of ACL disruption may be likened to disruption of a frame swing. As long as both ropes are taut and balanced one can happily swing along (**a**). However, one cannot swing happily if one rope: Pulls off the swing frame and floats in free space (analogous to a bony avulsion of the ACL from its femoral origin) (**b**). Pulls off and reattaches lower down the frame (analogous to an avulsion of the ACL from its femoral origin and healing onto the PCL) (**c**). Pulls off the swing seat (analogous to an avulsion of the ACL from its tibial insertion) (**d**). Snaps halfway down its length (analogous to a mid-substance ACL tear) (**e**). Stretches out (analogous to the ACL stretching and lengthening, which thus becomes lax—this may be observed in tibial spine avulsion in children whereby although the avulsed fragment heals in a satisfactory position the stretched ACL may account for continued instability) **(f)**

In considering the contribution of ligaments to joint stability it is important to consider primary and secondary ligamentous restraints:

- Primary restraint—a structure that is the main opposing force to a particular translation or angulation
- Secondary restraint—a structure that contributes to a lesser extent in providing an opposing force to a particular translation or angulation, but becomes translation when the primary restraint is dysfunctional

The following describe the various ligamentous restraints to tibiofemoral instability in various directions:

Anterior laxity (translation of the tibia)
- Primary restraint: ACL
- Secondary restraint: MCL

Posterior laxity (translation of the tibia)
- Primary restraint: PCL. The AL band of the PCL is the primary restraint to posterior tibial translation from 30 to 120° knee flexion with the PM band becoming the main restraint in deeper flexion.
- Secondary restraint: PLC, meniscofemoral ligaments

Valgus laxity
- Primary restraint:
  - Superficial MCL—throughout knee flexion, more apparent at 30° of flexion
  - Posteromedial capsule—in extension
- Secondary restraints:
  - ACL, PCL, posterior capsule
  - Deep MCL

Varus laxity
- Primary restraint: LCL, PLC
- Secondary restraints: ACL with the knee in extension

External Rotation of the Tibia
- Primary restraint—PLC—the lateral structures pass posteriorly as they pass from proximal to distal, hence they slacken with tibial internal rotation and become tight with tibial external rotation. Their ability to resist tibial external rotation is greatest at 30° of knee flexion. They exert a smaller effect at 90° of flexion.
  - Popliteo-fibular ligament is the primary restraint to tibial external rotation at all angles of flexion
- Secondary restraints—PCL (at 90° flexion), MCL, ACL

Role of Individual Ligaments to Tibiofemoral Stability
The function of the main knee ligaments contributing to tibiofemoral stability may thus be described as below:

ACL—primary restraint to anterior translation of the tibia on the femur.

It has been suggested (but not uniformly accepted) that:

- The AM band is the primary restraint to anterior tibial translation at 90° of flexion
- The PL band is the primary restraint at 20° of flexion

Hence:

- Dividing the AM band has a greater effect on the anterior drawer test
- Dividing the PL band has a greater effect on the Lachman test

The ACL also resists internal rotation of the tibia on the femur and varus with the knee in extension.

The ACL may thus be disrupted by:

- Hyperextension of the knee
- Internal rotation of the tibia on the femur

PCL—primary restraint to posterior translation of the tibia on the femur

- The AL band is slack when the knee is extended and tightens when the knee flexes. It is the primary restraint to posterior tibial translation between 30 and 120° knee flexion
- The PM band is tight in extension, slackens when the knee flexes, and becomes tight with hyperflexion. It is the main restraint to posterior tibial translation in deeper flexion.

Hence, with the knee in extension the PCL does not contribute to stability and this may account for the lack of instability symptoms in many patients with a torn PCL.

The PCL also resists external rotation of the tibia on the femur.

The PCL may thus be disrupted by:

- Posterior translation of the tibia in relation to the femur with the knee in flexion—such as due to direct blow on the anterior part of the tibia forcing it backwards
- External rotation of the tibia on the femur

Medial collateral ligament—resists valgus angulation and external rotation of the tibia in relation to the femur. It is thus disrupted by:

- Forcing the tibia in a lateral direction in relation to the femur
- Externally rotating the tibia in relation to the femur

The deep part of the MCL often gets disrupted prior to the superficial-MCL upon valgus loading.

Lateral collateral ligament—resists varus angulation and external rotation of the tibia in relation to the femur. The lateral ligament is the primary restraint to varus at 5–25° of knee flexion. It may thus be disrupted by:

- Forcing the tibia in a medial direction in relation to the femur
- Externally rotating the tibia on the femur

- *Meniscofemoral ligaments*—act as secondary restraints to posterior translation of the tibia in relation to the femur. They may remain intact when the PCL tears, and may help in the healing of the PCL by acting as an internal splint for a torn PCL.

3.12.3 Dynamic Tibiofemoral Joint Stabilisers

Most of the stability of the tibiofemoral joint is brought about by contraction of the muscles which cross the knee. These work to stabilise the tibia on the femur. As they exert their force in an opposite direction they may balance out and provide stability. They thus form force couples:

Sagittal force couple:
- Anterior—Quadriceps
- Posterior—Hamstrings

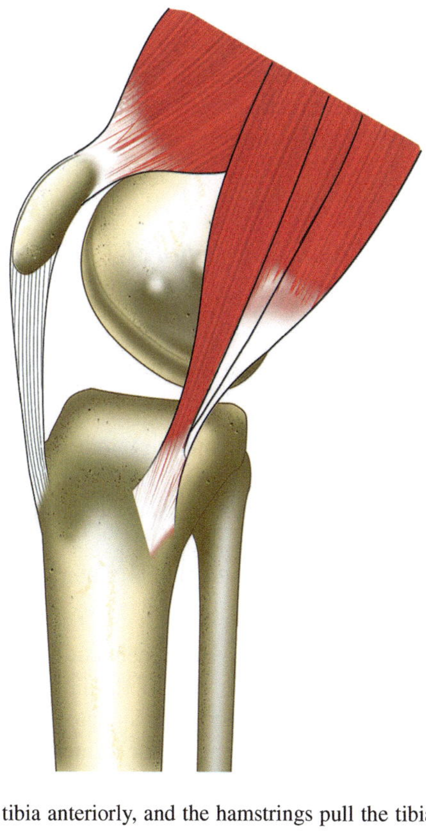

The quadriceps pulls the tibia anteriorly, and the hamstrings pull the tibia posteriorly, forming a force couple

Coronal force couple:
- Medial stabilisers—semimembranosus, pes anserinus, vastus medialis
- Lateral stabilisers—biceps femoris, iliotibial band, vastus lateralis

3.12.3.1 Sagittal Quadriceps/Hamstring Force Couple

- Quadriceps pulls the tibia anteriorly
- Hamstrings pull the tibia posteriorly

Acting together they stop the tibia sliding backwards or forwards in relation to the femur. However, if one of these muscles is weak, the tibia may be pulled forwards or backwards by the remaining intact muscle. A similar imbalance may occur if one of the couple is abnormally overactive.

Hamstring/Quadriceps coordination is of particular importance in the presence of ligament disruption to compensate for the lost ligament rather than aggravating the effects of its loss. This is important in the ACL deficient knee, whereby the hamstrings act as agonists of the ACL and compensate for its disruption, whereas the quadriceps acts as antagonist.

- Hamstring/Quadriceps coordination is also vital to minimise the strain on intact ligaments and hence reduce the risk of their disruption. Similarly, muscle coordination following ligament reconstruction helps to prevent undue strain on the graft reducing the risk of graft failure.

3.12.4 Core Control and Tibiofemoral Joint Stability [75, 77–87]

In considering knee stability it is vital to recognise that we do not simply have a tibia that moves on the femur. Instead:

- The tibia articulates with the femur, and the femur articulates with the pelvis at the hip joint.
- The pelvis articulates with the lumbosacral spine (part of the axial skeleton) at the sacroiliac articulation.
- The axial skeleton has various components that exhibit mobility relative to each other.

Hence, in order to allow coordinated movements of the knee, there is a need for well controlled and coordinated movements of the femur on the pelvis, and well controlled, coordinated movements of the axial skeleton. In this way the axial skeleton can provide a stable platform for the femur to move upon, and the femur can provide a stable platform for the tibia to move in relation to.

Control and coordination of the femur on the pelvis is provided by the various muscles passing from the pelvis to the femur as described above. Control and coordination of the axial skeleton is provided by the core muscles.

The core has been described as a "box" with the:

- Abdominal muscles at the front
- Para-spinal muscles, thoraco-lumbar fascia and glutae at the back
- Diaphragm forms the roof
- Pelvic floor, hip joint muscles (hip adductors, gluteus medius, ilio-psoas hip extensors) form the floor

The core muscles provide a corset that helps to stabilise the vertebral column both at rest and during limb movements (similar to a belt worn by weight lifters to get more stability during weight lifting). Contraction of the diaphragm increases the intra-abdominal pressure which also helps to stabilise the lumbar spine.

The core provides a stable platform for the lower spine and lower limbs to work. A stable core allows strong coordinated motion of the lower limbs. A weak core cannot provide the stability needed for limb motion to occur in a coordinated way as to exert sufficient power to achieve its goals. A weak core is an analogous to a weight lifter trying to lift a heavy weight bar which has substantial weight imbalance between its two ends.

Hence, in improving stability of the tibiofemoral joint, there is a need to address not only those muscles that pass between the femur and tibia but also the muscles that give pelvic and core stability. This is achieved by improving muscle strength but also muscle endurance. Individuals may be taught to recruit muscles (that have been inactive) either in isolation or as part of a group of muscles. Once a muscle is awakened and recruited further training can enhance its function.

Central to core activity is proprioception, the ability to subconsciously sense joint position and the movement of body segments (Proprioception is discussed more extensively in the Physiotherapy chapter).

3.12.5 Hip Muscles

The hip muscles need special consideration as, like the core, their adequate function may help improve functional stability of the knee. The muscles of the hip may control the position of the femur, limiting knee postures or force distribution that could predispose to instability. The hip muscles to consider are:

- Hip extensors
- Hip abductors
- Hip external rotators

Weakness of these may lead to dynamic valgus of the knee, increasing the strain on the ACL and predisposing to ACL tear when landing from a jump.

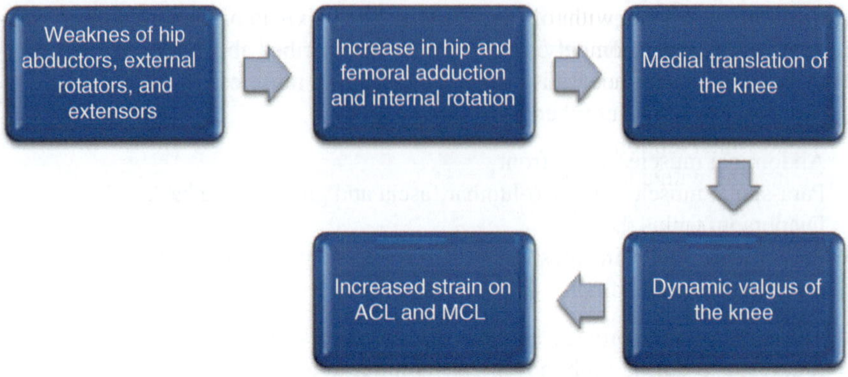

Hip weakness may lead to dynamic valgus upon landing and increased strain on the ACL and MCL

Similarly, weakness of sagittal muscles may predispose to ACL tear. When landing from a jump, the hip and knee are in flexion and the GRF passes posterior to the knee. This creates a flexion moment on the knee which is opposed by contraction of the quadriceps. This contraction of the quadriceps pulls the tibia anteriorly in relation to the femur which increases the strain on the ACL and may increase the risk of ACL tear. Weak hip extensors (gluteus maximus, hamstrings), may be compensated by a posterior lean of the trunk. However, this may increase the flexion moment of the knee, leading to higher quadriceps activation and higher strain on the ACL. Females show less knee, hip, and trunk flexion during gait and landing compared to males and also have an increased risk of ACL tear.

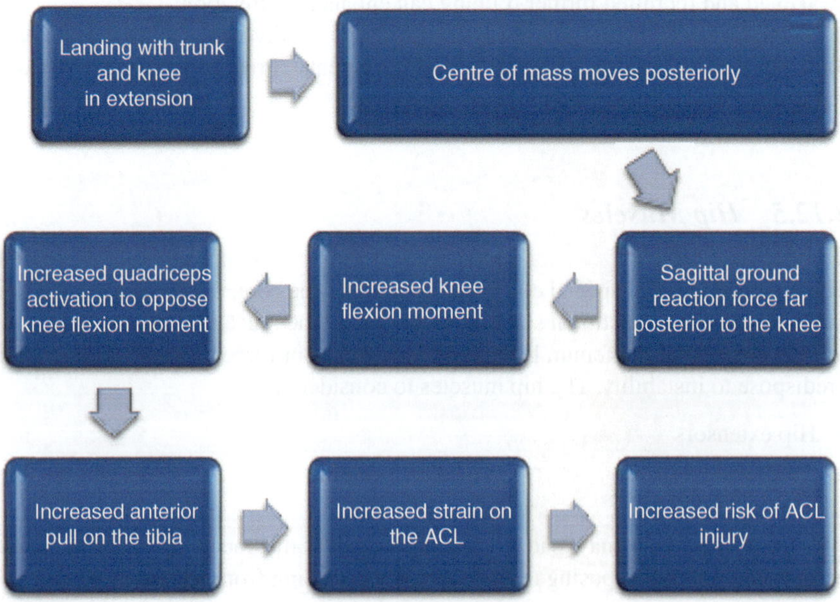

Landing with trunk and knee in extension may lead to an increased strain on the ACL

In contrast, landing with the trunk flexed moves the centre of mass anteriorly and reduces the flexion moment on the knee, and hence the quadriceps activation and ACL strain. Greater knee flexion may also increase hamstring activation which may reduce anterior tibial shear force on the ACL [75].

Hence, intervention programs designed to reduce the risk of ACL tear promote jump landing with a less erect posture:

- Increased trunk, hip and knee flexion
- Hips abducted, less knee valgus

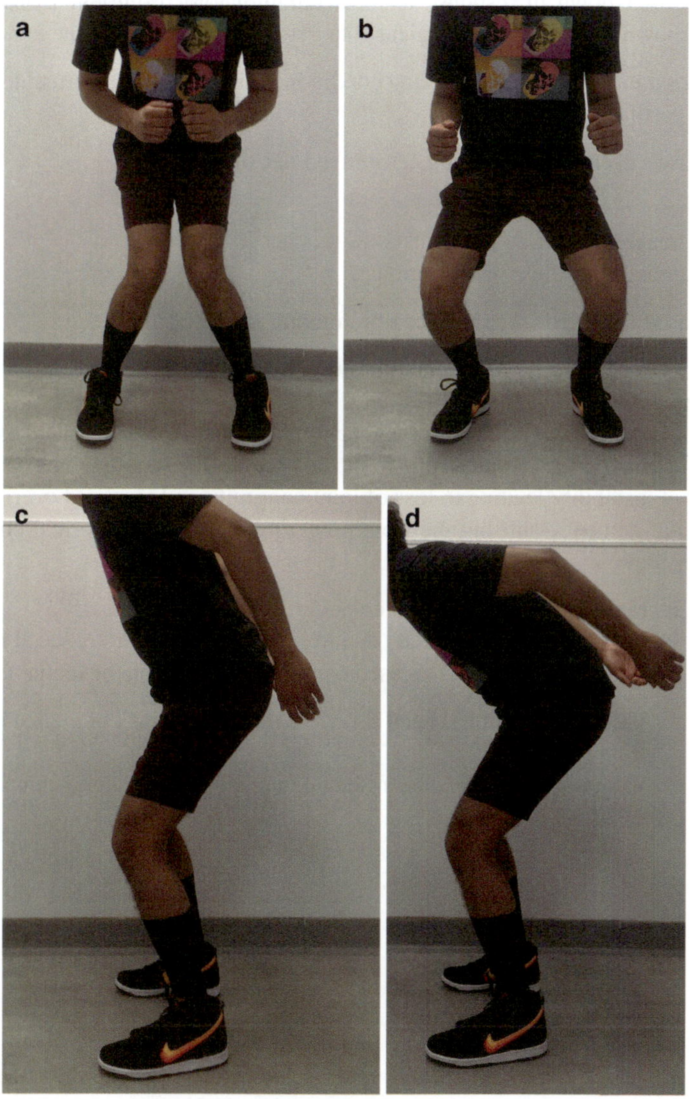

Landing with the hips in adduction (**a**) and the trunk extended (**c**) increases ACL strain. Landing with the hips in abduction (**b**) and the trunk flexed (**d**) reduces ACL strain

3.13 Biomechanics of Tibiofemoral Degeneration [88–97]

Degeneration of articular cartilage and subsequent development of osteoarthritis may be influenced by both biological and biomechanical factors.

Biological factors, include:
The ability of articular cartilage to:

- Adapt to increased or repeated loading
- Regenerate following an insult
- Resist breakdown in response to local inflammatory reactions—synovitis has been shown to precede radiological changes of osteoarthritis of the knee

Biomechanical factors include any condition which leads to abnormal loading of articular cartilage such as:

1. Increased overall forces acting across the knee due to:
   - Rise in body weight
   - Increased adduction moment
   - Increased muscle co-contraction
2. Increased localised forces on the tibiofemoral joint due to:
   - Loss of conformity of articulating surfaces –secondary to post-traumatic fracture deformity, malunion
   - Loss of meniscal protection (degenerate or traumatic tear, surgical excision)
   - Joint incongruity (such as due to intra-articular fracture malunion)
   - Joint instability leading to loss of joint congruity and localised overloading
   - Malalignment—shifting the weight bearing axis from its normal position—this may:
     - Increase local loading of articular cartilage (contact stress)
     - Predispose to meniscal tear (due to increased loads and reduced meniscal mobility secondary to increased compression between the femur and tibia):

       Varus alignment has been shown to increase the risk of medial meniscal tears by two fold
       Valgus alignment has been shown to predispose to lateral meniscal tears

3.13.1 *Primary Medial Compartment OA with Intact ACL*

The following may be considered in the development of medial compartment OA in the ACL intact knee:

- Due to the adduction moment, most of the load on weightbearing goes through the medial compartment of the knee, hence this is more prone to developing degeneration.
- OA begins with the knee in extension giving rise to tibial anteromedial arthritis because:
  - The knee is mainly in extension during weightbearing
  - The relation of the tibia to the femur is maintained in the knee with an intact ACL, hence the anterior part of the tibial plateau is loaded more than the posterior tibial plateau.
- As the articular cartilage is worn and lost, a varus deformity develops, increasing the adduction moment further.
- The MCL does not shorten, because each time the knee flexes, the femur roles back onto normal, intact, and thus thick, tibial cartilage, stretching the MCL out to length.
- With disease progression, the ACL degenerates and becomes dysfunctional.
- With ACL dysfunction, the tibia translates anteriorly in relation to the femur. This leads to increased loading of the posterior part of the tibia and as a result arthritis progresses posteriorly on the tibia.
- The MCL can no longer be stretched out to normal length during knee flexion (i.e. the MCL is shorter in both extension and flexion) hence the MCL contracts.
- Eventually OA moves to the lateral compartment.

In such circumstances:

- If OA is limited to the anteromedial part of the tibial plateau, unicompartmental knee replacement arthroplasty may be an appropriate surgical management option.
- As arthritis progresses to involve the posteromedial or lateral compartment, total knee replacement arthroplasty may be more appropriate.

ACL degeneration has been shown to be highly prevalent in knees with cartilage defects, and may be involved in the pathogenesis of knee OA [91].

a
b
c

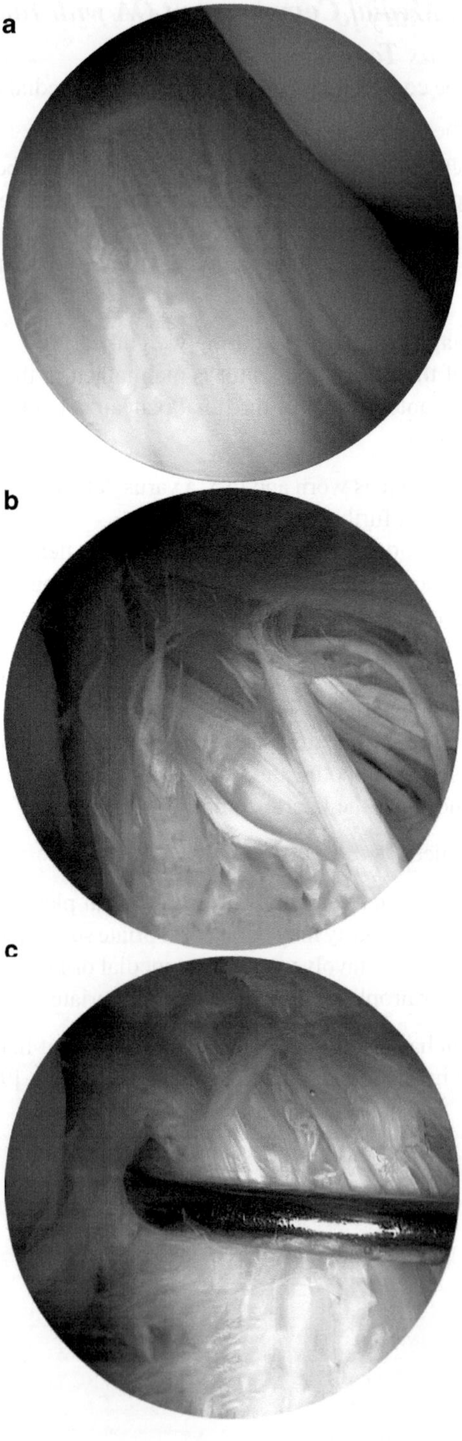

Arthroscopic view of non-degenerate **(a)** and degenerate **(b, (c)** ACL

3.13.2 OA Secondary to ACL Deficiency (Due to Previous Tear)

The following may be considered in the development of medial compartment OA in the ACL deficient knee:

- The tibia translates anteriorly in relation to the femur leading to posterior tibiofemoral contact in extension, which leads to increased loading of the posterior part of the tibial plateau.
- Hence, in ACL deficiency, arthritis in the medial compartment begins posteromedially.
- In these circumstances, the length of the MCL is maintained, and the lateral compartment is often preserved.

The above may influence the choice of surgical management options:

- If instability is the main symptom—ACL reconstruction may be performed followed by medial compartment unicompartmental knee replacement arthroplasty (if there is persistent pain).
- If both pain and instability are troublesome—combined ACL reconstruction + medial compartment unicompartmental knee replacement arthroplasty is an option. Outcomes of such combined procedures have been shown to be similar to those of medial compartment unicompartmental knee replacement arthroplasty in the presence of an intact ACL.

3.13.3 OA Associated with PCL Deficiency

Chronic PCL deficiency has been related to increased risk of knee OA, mainly of the medial compartment and patellofemoral (PF) compartment

- Cadaveric studies have shown that sectioning the PCL increases the contact pressures in the medial and PF compartments, hence the predisposition of these to degeneration.

3.13.4 Primary Lateral Compartment OA

The following may be considered in the development of lateral compartment OA:

In severe valgus deformities, the weightbearing axis passes through the lateral compartment with the GRF causing a valgus moment. Hence, severe valgus deformities are associated with lateral compartment arthritis.

However, in mild valgus knee alignment the adduction moment passes medial to the knee. Despite this, even mild-valgus alignment increases the risk of lateral compartment arthritis suggesting that other biomechanical factors may have a role to play. Such factors may include:

- Increased muscle co-contraction which raises contact pressures.
- Sensitivity of the lateral compartment to changes in loading, due to less conformity of its articulating surfaces.
- Increased risk of lateral meniscal degeneration with valgus alignment, and the greater sensitivity of the lateral compartment to loss of the lateral meniscus (due to less conformity of its articulating surfaces). Lateral meniscal degeneration may be due to increased local loading and reduced meniscal mobility secondary to increased compressive forces.

Felson et al [96] and Hayashi et al [97] reported that:

- Valgus of about 1–3° was associated with an increased risk of lateral OA progression.
- Valgus greater than 3° was associated with articular cartilage damage on MRI in knees without OA. There was a strong relation of valgus with progressive lateral meniscal damage.

References

1. Flandry F, Hommel G. Normal anatomy and biomechanics of the knee. Sports Med Arthrosc Rev. 2011;19(2):82–92.
2. Winter DA. Biomechanics and motor control of human movement. 2nd ed. New York: John Wiley; 1990.
3. Freeman MA, Pinskerova V. The movement of the normal tibio-femoral joint. J Biomech. 2005;38(2):197–208.
4. Pinskerova V, Johal P, Nakagawa S, Sosna A, Williams A, Gedroyc W, Freeman MA. Does the femur roll-back with flexion? J Bone Joint Surg Br. 2004;86(6):925–31.
5. Nagerl H, Walters J, Frosch KH, Dumont C, Kubein-Meesenburg D, Fanghanel J, Wachowski MM. Knee motion analysis of the non-loaded and loaded knee: a re-look at rolling and sliding. J Physiol Pharmacol. 2009;60(Suppl 8):69–72.
6. Blaha JD, Mancinelli CA, Simons WH, Kish VL, Thyagarajan G. Kinematics of the human knee using an open chain cadaver model. Clin Orthop Relat Res. 2003;(410):25–34.
7. Iwaki H, Pinskerova V, Freeman MA. Tibiofemoral movement 1: the shapes and relative movements of the femur and tibia in the unloaded cadaver knee. J Bone Joint Surg Br. 2000;82(8):1189–95.
8. Nakagawa S, Kadoya Y, Todo S, Kobayashi A, Sakamoto H, Freeman MA, Yamano Y. Tibiofemoral movement 3: full flexion in the living knee studied by MRI. J Bone Joint Surg Br. 2000;82(8):1199–200.
9. Hill PF, Vedi V, Williams A, Iwaki H, Pinskerova V, Freeman MA. Tibiofemoral movement 2: the loaded and unloaded living knee studied by MRI. J Bone Joint Surg Br. 2000;82(8):1196–8.
10. Kim HY, Kim KJ, Yang DS, Jeung SW, Choi HG, Choy WS. Screw-home movement of the tibiofemoral joint during normal gait: three-dimensional analysis. Clin Orthop Surg. 2015;7(3):303–9.
11. Hallén LG, Lindahl O. The "screw-home" movement in the knee-joint. Acta Orthop Scand. 1966;37(1):97–106.
12. Mulholland SJ, Wyss UP. Activities of daily living in non-Western cultures: range of motion requirements for hip and knee joint implants. Int J Rehabil Res. 2001;24(3):191–8.
13. American Academy of Orthopaedic Surgeons. Joint motion: method of measurement and recording. New York: Churchill Livingstone; 1991.

14. Rowe PJ, Myles CM, Walker C, Nutton R. Knee joint kinematics in gait and other functional activities measured using flexible electrogoniometry: how much knee motion is sufficient for normal daily life? Gait Posture. 2000;12(2):143–55.
15. Hemmerich A, Brown H, Smith S, Marthandam SS, Wyss UP. Hip, knee, and ankle kinematics of high range of motion activities of daily living. J Orthop Res. 2006;24(4):770–81.
16. Zhou H, Liu A, Wang D, Zeng X, Wei S, Wang C. Kinematics of lower limbs of healthy Chinese people sitting cross-legged. Prosthetics Orthot Int. 2013;37(5):369–74.
17. Ciccotti MG, Kerlan RK, Perry J, Pink M. An electromyographic analysis of the knee during functional activities. I. The normal profile. Am J Sports Med. 1994;22(5):645–50.
18. Costigan PA, Deluzio KJ, Wyss UP. Knee and hip kinetics during normal stair climbing. Gait Posture. 2002;16(1):31–7.
19. Li G, Rudy TW, Sakane M, Kanamori A, Ma CB, Woo SL. The importance of quadriceps and hamstring muscle loading on knee kinematics and in-situ forces in the ACL. J Biomech. 1999;32(4):395–400.
20. Shelburne KB, Torry MR, Pandy MG. Contributions of muscles, ligaments, and the ground-reaction force to tibiofemoral joint loading during normal gait. J Orthop Res. 2006;24(10):1983–90.
21. Shelburne KB, Torry MR, Pandy MG. Muscle, ligament, and joint-contact forces at the knee during walking. Med Sci Sports Exerc. 2005;37(11):1948–56.
22. Kuster M, Sakurai S, Wood GA. Kinematic and kinetic comparison of downhill and level walking. Clin Biomech (Bristol, Avon). 1995;10(2):79–84.
23. Kutzner I, Heinlein B, Graichen F, Rohlmann A, Halder AM, Beier A, Bergmann G. Loading of the knee joint during ergometer cycling: telemetric in vivo data. J Orthop Sports Phys Ther. 2012;42(12):1032–8.
24. Kutzner I, Heinlein B, Graichen F, Bender A, Rohlmann A, Halder A, Beier A, Bergmann G. Loading of the knee joint during activities of daily living measured in vivo in five subjects. J Biomech. 2010;43(11):2164–73.
25. Ericson MO, Nisell R. Tibiofemoral joint forces during ergometer cycling. Am J Sports Med. 1986;14(4):285–90.
26. Heywood S, McClelland J, Geigle P, Rahmann A, Villalta E, Mentiplay B, Clark R. Force during functional exercises on land and in water in older adults with and without knee osteoarthritis: Implications for rehabilitation. Knee. 2019;26(1):61–72.
27. Kutzner I, Richter A, Gordt K, Dymke J, Damm P, Duda GN, Günzl R, Bergmann G. Does aquatic exercise reduce hip and knee joint loading? In vivo load measurements with instrumented implants. PLoS One. 2017;12(3):e0171972. https://doi.org/10.1371/journal.pone.0171972.
28. Stryker. The measurement and analysis of axial deformity of the knee. Krackow KA: Stryker; 2008. Accesesd on 30/3/2020 at https://www.medschool.lsuhsc.edu/ortho/docs/How%20to%20Measure%20Knee%20Alignment.pdf
29. Cherian JJ, Kapadia BH, Banerjee S, Jauregui JJ, Issa K, Mont MA. Mechanical, Anatomical, and Kinematic Axis in TKA: Concepts and Practical Applications. Curr Rev Musculoskelet Med. 2014;7(2):89–95.
30. Favre J, Jolles BM. Gait analysis of patients with knee osteoarthritis highlights a pathological mechanical pathway and provides a basis for therapeutic interventions. EFORT Open Rev. 2017;1(10):368–74.
31. Amis AA. Biomechanics of high tibial osteotomy. Knee Surg Sports Traumatol Arthrosc. 2013;21(1):197–205.
32. Shelburne KB, Torry MR, Steadman JR, Pandy MG. Effects of foot orthoses and valgus bracing on the knee adduction moment and medial joint load during gait. Clin Biomech (Bristol, Avon). 2008;23(6):814–21.
33. Johnson F, Leitl S, Waugh W. The distribution of load across the knee. A comparison of static and dynamic measurements. J Bone Joint Surg (Br). 1980;62(3):346–9.
34. Davies-Tuck ML, Wluka AE, Wang Y, Teichtahl AJ, Jones G, Ding C, Cicuttini FM. The natural history of cartilage defects in people with knee osteoarthritis. Osteoarthr Cartil. 2008;16(3):337–42.

35. Fujisawa Y, Masuhara K, Shiomi S. The effect of high tibial osteotomy on osteoarthritis of the knee. An arthroscopic study of 54 knee joints. Orthop Clin North Am. 1979;10(3):585–608.
36. Agneskirchner JD, Hurschler C, Wrann CD, Lobenhoffer P. The effects of valgus medial opening wedge high tibial osteotomy on articular cartilage pressure of the knee: a biomechanical study. Arthroscopy. 2007;23(8):852–61.
37. Fox AJ, Wanivenhaus F, Burge AJ, Warren RF, Rodeo SA. The human meniscus: a review of anatomy, function, injury, and advances in treatment. Clin Anat. 2015;28(2):269–87.
38. Bryceland JK, Powell AJ, Nunn T. Knee Menisci. Cartilage. 2017;8(2):99–104.
39. Rao AJ, Erickson BJ, Cvetanovich GL, Yanke AB, Bach BR Jr, Cole BJ. The meniscus-deficient knee: biomechanics, evaluation, and treatment options. Orthop J Sports Med. 2015;3(10):2325967115611386.
40. Pappas E, Zampeli F, Xergia SA, Georgoulis AD. Lessons learned from the last 20 years of ACL-related in vivo-biomechanics research of the knee joint. Knee Surg Sports Traumatol Arthrosc. 2013;21(4):755–66.
41. Dargel J, Gotter M, Mader K, Pennig D, Koebke J, Schmidt-Wiethoff R. Biomechanics of the anterior cruciate ligament and implications for surgical reconstruction. Strategies Trauma Limb Reconstr. 2007;2(1):1–12.
42. Shelburne KB, Pandy MG, Anderson FC, Torry MR. Pattern of anterior cruciate ligament force in normal walking. J Biomech. 2004;37(6):797–805.
43. Rosenberg TD, Rasmussen GL. The function of the anterior cruciate ligament during anterior drawer and Lachman's testing. An in vivo analysis in normal knees. Am J Sports Med. 1984;12(4):318–22.
44. Kittl C, Inderhaug E, Williams A, Amis AA. Biomechanics of the anterolateral structures of the knee. Clin Sports Med. 2018;37(1):21–31.
45. Kittl C, El-Daou H, Athwal KK, Gupte CM, Weiler A, Williams A, Amis AA. The role of the anterolateral structures and the ACL in controlling laxity of the intact and ACL-deficient knee. Am J Sports Med. 2016;44(2):345–54.
46. LaPrade MD, Kennedy MI, Wijdicks CA, LaPrade RF. Anatomy and biomechanics of the medial side of the knee and their surgical implications. Sports Med Arthrosc Rev. 2015;23(2):63–70.
47. Robinson JR, Bull AM, Amis AA. Structural properties of the medial collateral ligament complex of the human knee. J Biomech. 2005;38(5):1067–74.
48. James EW, LaPrade CM, LaPrade RF. Anatomy and biomechanics of the lateral side of the knee and surgical implications. Sports Med Arthrosc Rev. 2015;23(1):2–9.
49. Lasmar RC, Marques de Almeida A, Serbino JW Jr, Mota Albuquerque RF, Hernandez AJ. Importance of the different posterolateral knee static stabilizers: biomechanical study. Clinics (Sao Paulo). 2010;65(4):433–40.
50. Bowman KF Jr, Sekiya JK. Anatomy and biomechanics of the posterior cruciate ligament, medial and lateral sides of the knee. Sports Med Arthrosc Rev. 2010;18(4):222–9.
51. Halewood C, Amis AA. Clinically relevant biomechanics of the knee capsule and ligaments. Knee Surg Sports Traumatol Arthrosc. 2015;23(10):2789–96.
52. Amis AA, Bull AM, Gupte CM, Hijazi I, Race A, Robinson JR. Biomechanics of the PCL and related structures: posterolateral, posteromedial and meniscofemoral ligaments. Knee Surg Sports Traumatol Arthrosc. 2003;11(5):271–81.
53. Amis AA, Firer P, Mountney J, Senavongse W, Thomas NP. Anatomy and biomechanics of the medial patellofemoral ligament. Knee. 2003;10(3):215–20.
54. Gupte CM, Bull AM, Thomas RD, Amis AA. A review of the function and biomechanics of the meniscofemoral ligaments. Arthroscopy. 2003;19(2):161–71.
55. Turnick DR, Vacek PM, DeSarno MJ, Gardner-Morse MG, Tourville TW, Slauterbeck JR, Johnson RJ, Shultz SJ, Beynnon BD. Combined anatomic factors predicting risk of anterior cruciate ligament injury for males and females. Am J Sports Med. 2015;43(4):839–47.
56. Wordeman SC, Quatman CE, Kaeding CC, Hewett TE. In vivo evidence for tibial plateau slope as a risk factor for anterior cruciate ligament injury: a systematic review and meta-analysis. Am J Sports Med. 2012;40(7):1673–81.

57. Grassi A, Signorelli C, Urrizola F, Raggi F, Macchiarola L, Bonanzinga T, Zaffagnini S. Anatomical features of tibia and femur: influence on laxity in the anterior cruciate ligament deficient knee. Knee. 2018;25(4):577–87.
58. Petrigliano FA, Suero EM, Voos JE, Pearle AD, Allen AA. The effect of proximal tibial slope on dynamic stability testing of the posterior cruciate ligament- and posterolateral corner-deficient knee. Am J Sports Med. 2012;40(6):1322–8.
59. Herman B, Litchfield R, Getgood A. Role of osteotomy in posterolateral instability of the knee. J Knee Surg. 2015;28(6):441–9.
60. Novaretti JV, Sheean AJ, Lian J, De Groot J, Musahl V. The role of osteotomy for the treatment of PCL injuries. Curr Rev Musculoskelet Med. 2018;11(2):298–306.
61. Savarese E, Bisicchia S, Romeo R, Amendola A. Role of high tibial osteotomy in chronic injuries of posterior cruciate ligament and posterolateral corner. J Orthop Traumatol. 2011;12(1):1–17.
62. Shelburne KB, Kim HJ, Sterett WI, Pandy MG. Effect of posterior tibial slope on knee biomechanics during functional activity. J Orthop Res. 2011;29(2):223–31.
63. Chen CY, Jiang CC, Jan MH, Lai JS. Role of flexors in knee stability. J Formos Med Assoc. 1995;94(5):255–60.
64. Schipplein OD, Andriacchi TP. Interaction between active and passive knee stabilizers during level walking. J Orthop Res. 1991;9(1):113–9.
65. Shelburne KB, Torry MR, Pandy MG. Effect of muscle compensation on knee instability during ACL-deficient gait. Med Sci Sports Exerc. 2005;37(4):642–8.
66. Liu W, Maitland ME. The effect of hamstring muscle compensation for anterior laxity in the ACL-deficient knee during gait. J Biomech. 2000;33(7):871–9.
67. Liu W, Maitland ME. Influence of anthropometric and mechanical variations on functional instability in the ACL-deficient knee. Ann Biomed Eng. 2003;31(10):1153–61.
68. Torry MR, Decker MJ, Ellis HB, Shelburne KB, Sterett WI, Steadman JR. Mechanisms of compensating for anterior cruciate ligament deficiency during gait. Med Sci Sports Exerc. 2004;36(8):1403–12.
69. Elias JJ, Faust AF, Chu YH, Chao EY, Cosgarea AJ. The soleus muscle acts as an agonist for the anterior cruciate ligament. An in vitro experimental study. Am J Sports Med. 2003;31(2):241–6.
70. Sherbondy PS, Queale WS, McFarland EG, Mizuno Y, Cosgarea AJ. Soleus and gastrocnemius muscle loading decreases anterior tibial translation in anterior cruciate ligament intact and deficient knees. J Knee Surg. 2003;16(3):152–8.
71. Begalle RL, Distefano LJ, Blackburn T, Padua DA. Quadriceps and hamstrings coactivation during common therapeutic exercises. J Athl Train. 2012;47(4):396–405.
72. Noyes FR, Barber-Westin SD, Fleckenstein C, Walsh C, West J. The drop-jump screening test: difference in lower limb control by gender and effect of neuromuscular training in female athletes. Am J Sports Med. 2005;33(2):197–207.
73. Blackburn JT, Padua DA. Sagittal-plane trunk position, landing forces, and quadriceps electromyographic activity. J Athl Train. 2009;44(2):174–9.
74. Bennett DR, Blackburn JT, Boling MC, McGrath M, Walusz H, Padua DA. The relationship between anterior tibial shear force during a jump landing task and quadriceps and hamstring strength. Clin Biomech (Bristol, Avon). 2008;23(9):1165–71.
75. Kwak SD, Ahmad CS, Gardner TR, Grelsamer RP, Henry JH, Blankevoort L, Ateshian GA, Mow VC. Hamstrings and iliotibial band forces affect knee kinematics and contact pattern. J Orthop Res. 2000;18(1):101–8.
76. Charalambous CP. The shoulder made easy. Springer: Cham; 2019.
77. Huxel Bliven KC, Anderson BE. Core stability training for injury prevention. Sports Health. 2013;5(6):514–22.
78. Willson JD, Dougherty CP, Ireland ML, Davis IM. Core stability and its relationship to lower extremity function and injury. J Am Acad Orthop Surg. 2005;13(5):316–25.
79. Kibler WB, Press J, Sciascia A. The role of core stability in athletic function. Sports Med. 2006;36(3):189–98.
80. Brazen DM, Todd MK, Ambegaonkar JP, Wunderlich R, Peterson C. The effect of fatigue on landing biomechanics in single-leg drop landings. Clin J Sport Med. 2010;20(4):286–92.

81. Renström P, Arms SW, Stanwyck TS, Johnson RJ, Pope MH. Strain within the anterior cruciate ligament during hamstring and quadriceps activity. Am J Sports Med. 1986;14(1):83–7.
82. Hogervorst T, Brand RA. Mechanoreceptors in joint function. J Bone Joint Surg Am. 1998;80(9):1365–78.
83. Jerosch J, Prymka M. Proprioception and joint stability. Knee Surg Sports Traumatol Arthrosc. 1996;4(3):171–9.
84. Johansson H, Sjölander P, Sojka P. A sensory role for the cruciate ligaments. Clin Orthop Relat Res. 1991;268:161–78.
85. Johansson H. Role of knee ligaments in proprioception and regulation of muscle stiffness. J Electromyogr Kinesiol. 1991;1(3):158–79.
86. Lattanzio PJ, Petrella RJ. Knee proprioception: a review of mechanisms, measurements, and implications of muscular fatigue. Orthopedics. 1998;21(4):463–70.
87. Jeong HS, Lee SC, Jee H, Song JB, Chang HS, Lee SY. Proprioceptive training and outcomes of patients with knee osteoarthritis: a meta-analysis of randomized controlled trials. J Athl Train. 2019;54(4):418–28.
88. Moschella D, Blasi A, Leardini A, Ensini A, Catani F. Wear patterns on tibial plateau from varus osteoarthritic knees. Clin Biomech (Bristol, Avon). 2006;21(2):152–8.
89. Lohmander LS, Englund PM, Dahl LL, Roos EM. The long-term consequence of anterior cruciate ligament and meniscus injuries: osteoarthritis. Am J Sports Med. 2007;35(10):1756–69.
90. White SH, Ludkowski PF, Goodfellow JW. Anteromedial osteoarthritis of the knee. J Bone Joint Surg Br. 1991;73(4):582–6.
91. Hasegawa A, Otsuki S, Pauli C, Miyaki S, Patil S, Steklov N, Kinoshita M, Koziol J, D'Lima DD, Lotz MK. Anterior cruciate ligament changes in the human knee joint in aging and osteoarthritis. Arthritis Rheum. 2012;64(3):696–704.
92. Harman MK, Markovich GD, Banks SA, Hodge WA. Wear patterns on tibial plateaus from varus and valgus osteoarthritic knees. Clin Orthop Relat Res. 1998;352:149–58.
93. MacDonald P, Miniaci A, Fowler P, Marks P, Finlay B. A biomechanical analysis of joint contact forces in the posterior cruciate deficient knee. Knee Surg Sports Traumatol Arthrosc. 1996;3(4):252–5.
94. Logan M, Williams A, Lavelle J, Gedroyc W, Freeman M. The effect of posterior cruciate ligament deficiency on knee kinematics. Am J Sports Med. 2004;32(8):1915–22.
95. Gill TJ, DeFrate LE, Wang C, Carey CT, Zayontz S, Zarins B. Li G The effect of posterior cruciate ligament reconstruction on patellofemoral contact pressures in the knee joint under simulated muscle loads. Am J Sports Med. 2004;32(1):109–15.
96. Felson DT, Nevitt MC, Yang M, Clancy M, Niu J, Torner JC, Lewis CE, Aliabadi P, Sack B, McCulloch C, Zhang Y. A new approach yields high rates of radiographic progression in knee osteoarthritis. J Rheumatol. 2008;35(10):2047–54.
97. Hayashi D, Englund M, Roemer FW, Niu J, Sharma L, Felson DT, Crema MD, Marra MD, Segal NA, Lewis CE, Nevitt MC, Guermazi A. Knee malalignment is associated with an increased risk for incident and enlarging bone marrow lesions in the more loaded compartments: the MOST study. Osteoarthr Cartil. 2012;20(11):1227–33.

Chapter 4
Knee Biomechanics—Patellofemoral Articulation

This chapter describes the direction and components of patellofemoral (PF) motion, as well as the muscles acting upon the patella to achieve that motion. In addition, it explores the forces acting on the PF joint. Furthermore, it describes the various structures contributing to stability of the patella in relation to the femoral trochlea. The biomechanical factors leading to PF degeneration are also discussed.

The PF articulation is the joint between the posterior surface of the patella and the femoral trochlea. The patella has several biomechanical functions [1–5] including:

- Enhances the function of the quadriceps, facilitating knee extension
- Increases the moment arm of the quadriceps muscle in relation to the centre of rotation of the knee (as it translates the quadriceps tendon more anterior in relation to the centre of the knee)
- Concentrates the pull of the four heads of the quadriceps tendon increasing its effectiveness
- Minimises friction between the quadriceps tendon and the femur

The patella may move in various directions in relation to the femoral trochlea. The main motion is a proximal to distal translation as the knee flexes. In addition the patella exhibits:

- Medial and lateral translation
- Medial and lateral rotation—the inferior pole aims medially and laterally respectively
- Medial or lateral tilt—medial or lateral facet respectively tilts posteriorly towards the trochlea
- Superior or inferior tilt—superior or inferior pole of the patella respectively tilts posteriorly towards the trochlea

C. Panayiotou Charalambous, *The Knee Made Easy*,
https://doi.org/10.1007/978-3-030-54506-2_4

4.1 Patellofemoral Motion

The following may be considered:

- In full knee extension the patella lies proximally to the femoral trochlea and slightly lateral to the midline. It may be normal for the patella to be slightly tilted laterally in extension, but such tilting is usually reducible.
- As the knee flexes the patella moves more centrally, the lateral facet making initial contact followed by the medial facet.
- The patella gains contact with the trochlea at 10–20° of knee flexion and centralises in the inter-condylar groove beyond 30°. The patella also rotates laterally, hence in deep flexion it is mainly the lateral facet that is in contact with the femoral condyle.
- Lin et al. [6] evaluated in vivo patellar motion when the knee was voluntarily extended from 15° flexion to full extension. During knee extension the patella:
  - Extended 8°
  - Tilted laterally 2°
  - Translated laterally 3 mm
  - Translated proximally 10 mm
- At the commencement of flexion, the distal part of the patella makes contact with the proximal part of the femoral trochlea. With deeper flexion the articulating area of the patella moves proximally, and the articulating area of the femur moves more inferiorly and posteriorly. Hence, the contact area between the patella and trochlea increases in deeper flexion.

4.2 Patellar Motion in Relation to the Femur and Tibia

- The patella is located in the quadriceps tendon and thus is not attached to the distal femur. However, the patella is attached (tethered) to the tibia by the patellar tendon. Hence, the patella follows the motion of the tibia, but the femur and patella can move independently to each other.
- When the foot is not supported (open chain motion), the tibia can rotate in relation to the femur. The patella moves along with the tibia relative to the femur.
- During weightbearing when the foot and hence tibia are supported on the ground (closed chain knee motion) internal rotation of the femur may occur in relation to the tibia. This internal rotation of the femur occurs under the patella. This brings the lateral part of the femoral trochlea closer to the lateral facet of the patella. Lateral subluxation of the patella and compression of the lateral patellar facet against the femur during weightbearing activities, may thus be secondary to the femur rotating under the patella, rather than due to the patella primarily translating or tilting laterally in relation to the femur.

4.3 Patellofemoral Joint Forces

The PF joint is subjected to high transmitted forces, which can be several times the body weight (BW). Understanding the PF forces, may help explain how they change in various pathological conditions, and help apply interventions to minimise symptoms due to such force changes.

The PF force is the compression force between the patella and femur. It is the result of the:

- Quadriceps pull force
- Patellar tendon tension (force)

The PF force is influenced by the:

- Strength of the quadriceps contraction—increasing with stronger contraction
- Patellar tendon tension—increasing with increased tension
- Degree of knee flexion—increasing with deeper knee flexion

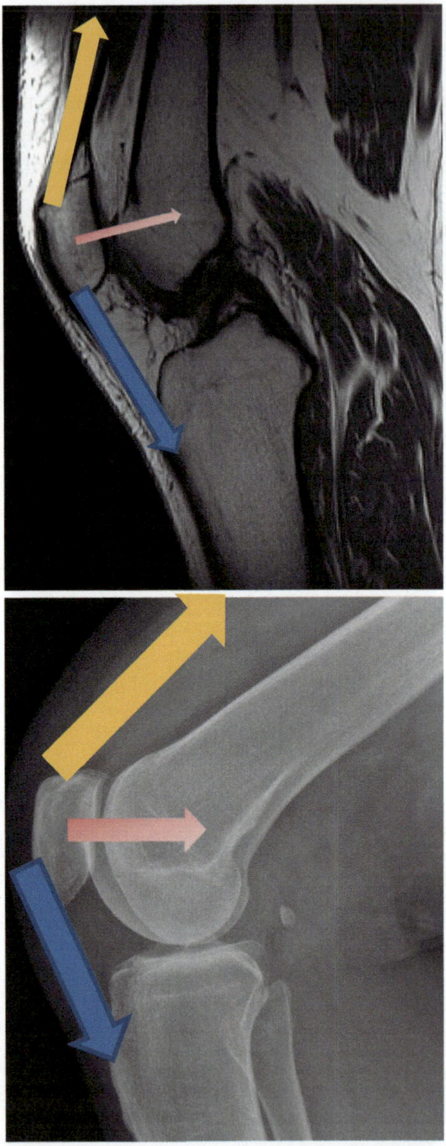

Patellofemoral joint forces (Quadriceps -orange, Patellar tendon—blue, Resultant joint force—red). Joint force is much greater in deeper flexion

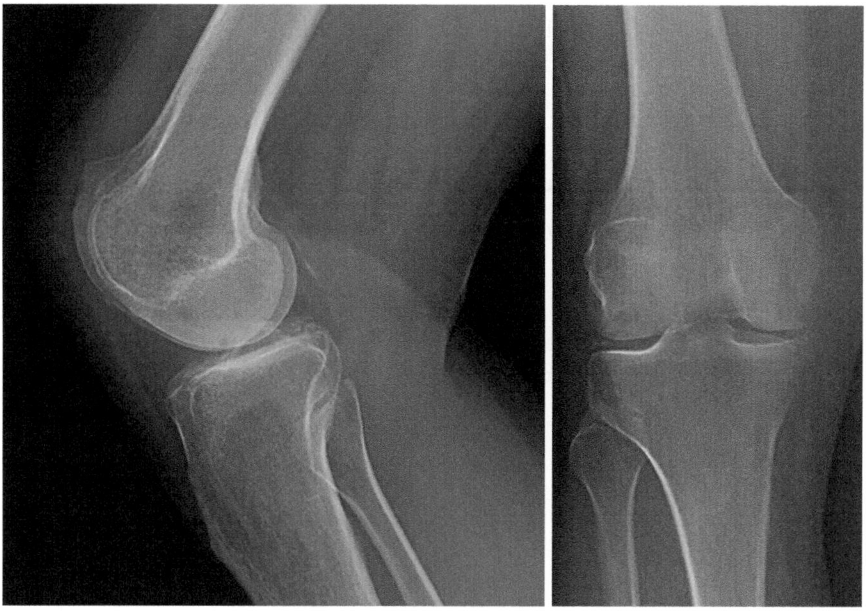

Absent patella (post patellectomy for trauma), which reduces the efficiency of the quadriceps as it brings it closer to the centre of the knee. The patient continues to mobilise and function but with a less efficient quadriceps

To explain this the following may be considered. The attachment of the quadriceps tendon and the patellar tendon to the patella, are like having two strings attached at the two ends of the patella, with one string pulling the patella upwards and one downwards. If both strings are in line, all they achieve is suspending the patella in a vertical orientation, without pressing it against the femoral trochlea. In contrast, if both strings are pulling the patella in a similar direction, backwards towards the trochlea, the force of the patella on the trochlea will rise. Hence, in knee extension PF forces are minimal, whereas in knee flexion they rise. Similarly, the higher the tension of the strings (equivalent to the magnitude of the quadriceps contraction and patella tendon tension) the tighter the pull on the patella against the trochlea, and hence the higher the patellar force between the patella and trochlea.

The magnitude of quadriceps contraction is related to its attempt to oppose knee flexion which is at least partly driven by the action of the ground reaction force (GRF). Knee flexion is also driven by contraction of the hamstrings.

The GRF is generated by the BW coming into contact with the ground. In the sagittal plane, the GRF originates at the point of foot contact with the ground, and passes upwards towards the body's centre of gravity (that is located anterior to the sacrum at about the S2 level). The magnitude and orientation of the GRF may thus help determine the activity in the quadriceps, and hence the size of the PF forces in physiological as well as pathological conditions.

- In full knee extension or hyperextension, the GRF falls in front of the knee, hence there is no need for quadriceps to contract to keep the knee straight. However, as the knee flexes (as in squatting) the GRF falls behind the knee, hence quadriceps contracts to oppose further knee flexion. Knee flexion is brought about by contraction of the hamstrings, which the quadriceps also opposes. The PF force is thus influenced by the degree of knee flexion (higher as knee flexion increases):
  - In full knee extension the PF force is zero as no forces are acting on the PF joint
  - In knee flexion the PFR force increases with deeper knee flexion:
    - 0° BW at 15° of knee flexion
    - 12.9 BW at 135°of knee flexion

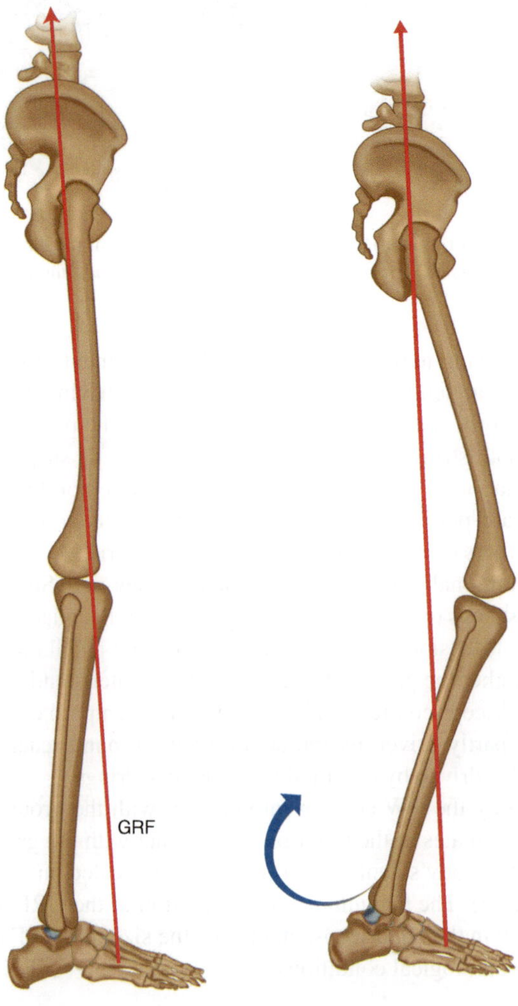

GRF in sagittal plane with the knee in extension and flexion

The PF force may also vary according to the activity performed with some of the values reported in literature being:

- 0.6 BW at level walking
- 7.7 BW at jogging
- 20 BW at jumping

Trepczynski et al. [7] calculated tibiofemoral and PF forces using a musculoskeletal model and reported that:

- Peak PF forces of 2.9–3.4 BW occurred and varied little across activities
- Peak PF forces showed significant variability, ranging from less than 1BW during walking to greater than 3BW during high flexion activities

The PF force is worse on descending than ascending stairs due to the eccentric contraction of quadriceps. The forces on stair descend may be eight times higher compared to level walking [8].

PF force during cycling is less than other activities of daily living (about 1.3 BW) [9]. It has been shown to:

- Increase with work load and decreased saddle height
- Be unrelated to pedalling rates or foot position

Consideration of the PF force in relation to the GRF in the sagittal plane, may also explain the quadriceps activity in certain disorders:

- In the presence of weakness of the extensor muscles of the hip, the individual may move the body (and hence the centre of gravity) backwards in order to achieve hip extension. This moves the GRF vector further away from the knee increasing the force required by quadriceps to oppose this force.
- In fixed flexion deformity the GRF passes behind the knee, increasing the work that must be done by the quadriceps. The greater the flexion deformity the greater is the lever arm of the GRF, and hence the greater the counteractive force needed by quadriceps. As the flexion deformity is fixed, the quadriceps must be constantly active to oppose the flexed posture of the knee upon weightbearing.
- In the presence of a tight quadriceps or tight patellar tendon (as in post-trauma or post-surgical scarring) much stronger quadriceps contractions, and thus higher forces, need to be exerted for motion to occur, increasing the compression force between patella and trochlea.
- In the presence of quadriceps weakness, leaning forwards brings the centre of gravity forwards, and hence the GRF closer to the knee, thus reducing the work required by quadriceps.
- In the presence of a painful PF joint, the patient may try to keep the knee straight when mobilising, such as when descending stairs. `This is done to limit quadriceps contraction, limit the PF forces and thus help improve pain.

4.4 Variation of Patellar Contact Pressures with Knee Flexion

It is also important to recognise that PF contact pressures are influenced by the force applied and also by the area upon which such force is exerted:

- Stress = Force divided by area over which the force is exerted.

Hence, local stress (equivalent to PF contact pressure) is influenced by the area of contact between the patella and trochlea. With knee flexion, as the patella engages with the trochlea, the area of the patella moves proximally and of the trochlea moves posteriorly. Furthermore, the size of the contact area increases. Hence, PF stress increases between 30° and 90° of knee flexion, being highest at 90°. With higher knee flexion angles the contact area increases and contact stress is reduced. Degeneration of the patella often occurs in those areas that correspond to articulation in 40–80° of knee flexion, where contact pressures are high.

4.5 Asymmetrical Loading of the Patella

It is also important to recognise that loading of the PF joint may not be symmetrical but one of the facets may be loaded more than the other:

- Lateral translation or tilting of the patella compresses the lateral facet of the patella on the trochlea
- Medial translation or tilting of the patella compresses the medial facet of the patella on the trochlea

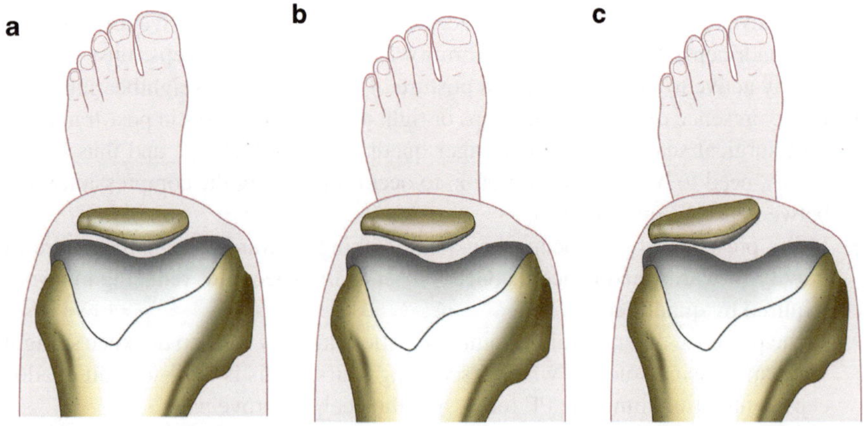

(a) Normal patellar alignment (b) Lateral patellar translation (c) Lateral patellar tilting

As described above, the patella is attached to the tibia via the patellar tendon, hence rotation of the tibia tends to drag the patella along, altering local PF loading:

- External tibial rotation—increases the pressure between the lateral patellar facet and trochlea
- Internal tibial rotation—increases the pressure between the medial patellar facet and trochlea
- External tibial rotation has been related to instability and lateral compression syndrome
- Cadaveric studies have shown that lateralisation to the tibial tubercle increases the lateral PF contact pressures, which are reduced by tubercle medialization.

In contrast, femoral rotation leads to patellar translation in relation to the femur –

- Internal femoral rotation—the lateral trochlear facet presses on the lateral facet of the patella increasing contact pressures
- External femoral rotation—the medial trochlear facet pushes on the medial facet of the patella increasing contact pressures

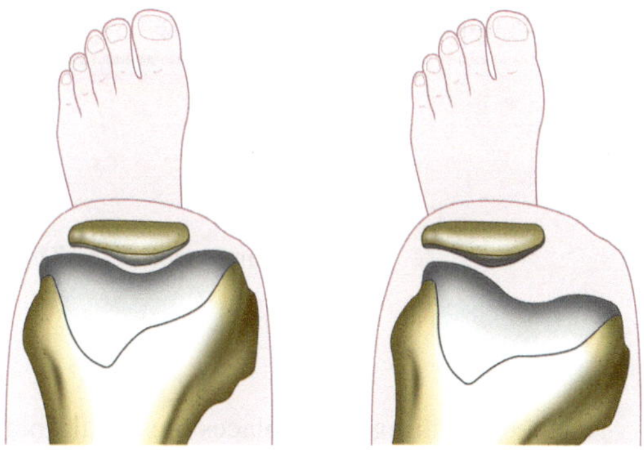

Internal rotation of the femur under the patella

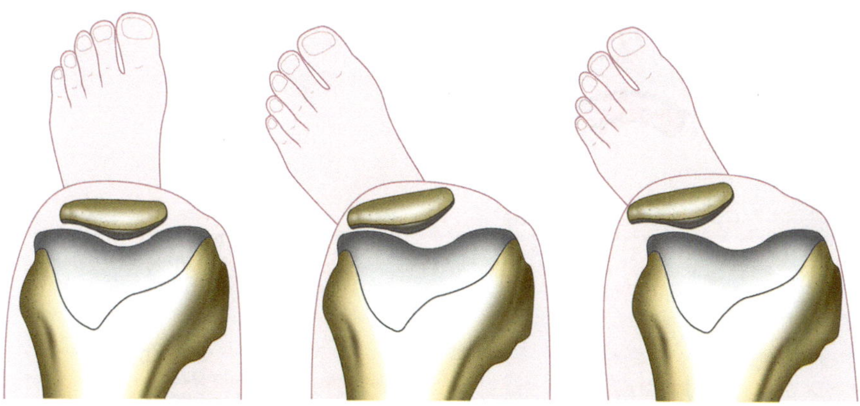

External rotation of the tibia, dragging the patella along

Any conditions which lead to maltracking of the patella in relation to the femur may alter PF forces and thus contact pressures. Such conditions may be structural or functional:

Structural

- Femoral neck anteversion (femoral neck angled more anteriorly than normal). This leads to compensatory internal rotation of the femur in an attempt to minimise the anterior subluxation of the femoral head from the acetabulum, and maintain concentric reduction of the head in the acetabulum
- Femoral shaft internal rotation (idiopathic, post-traumatic)
- Tibial external tibial rotation (idiopathic, post-traumatic)
- Structural knee valgus
- Trochlear dysplasia
- Patella alta/baja
- Structural foot pronation

Functional [10–18]

- Weakness of hip abductors and external rotators—leading to femoral adduction and internal rotation
- Foot pronation due to muscle/ligamentous imbalance—leading to tibial and femoral internal rotation

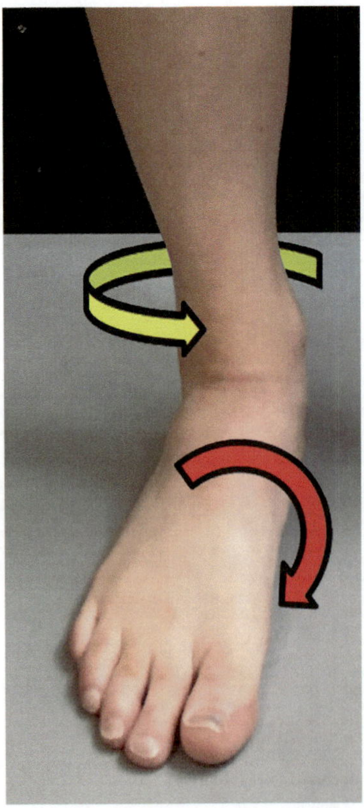

Foot pronation leads to internal tibial rotation

- Dynamic knee valgus
  - Due to:
    - muscle/ligamentous imbalance
    - abnormal bony kinetics—secondary to internal rotation of the femur, tibia or both
  - Dynamic valgus may lead to lateral patella maltracking and hence increased PF pressures.
- Soft tissue factors—muscle imbalance, ligamentous tightness, ligamentous laxity

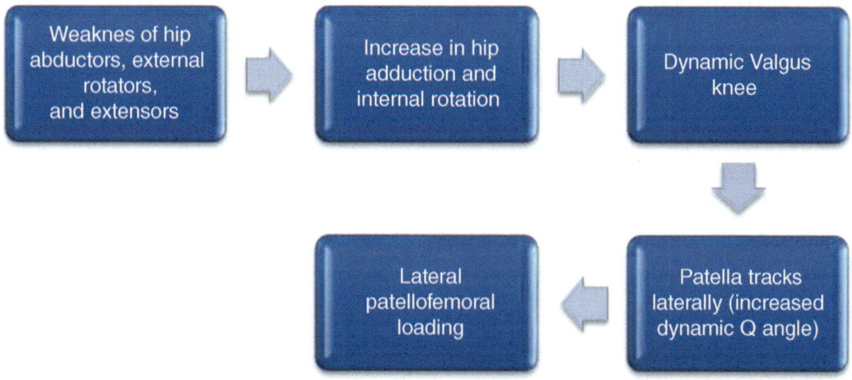

Hip weakness may lead to lateral Patellofemoral joint loading

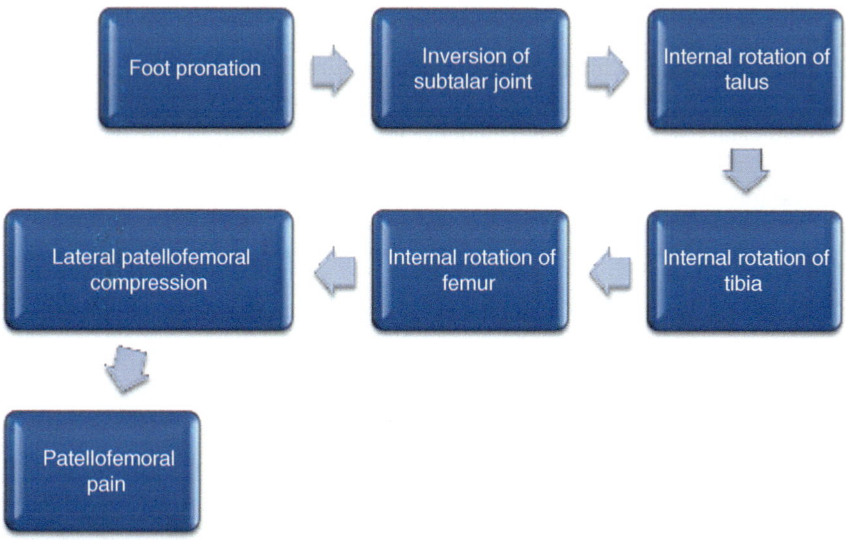

Foot pronation may lead to increased patellofemoral joint loading and pain

Souza RB et al. [19] looked at PF joint kinematics, femoral rotation, and patellar rotation between females with PF pain and pain-free controls using magnetic resonance imaging (MRI). Cases with PF pain showed greater lateral patellar translation at all angles evaluated and greater lateral patella tilt at 0–30° of knee flexion. Similarly, greater internal femoral rotation was observed in the PF pain group. No group differences in patella rotation were found. Hence, the authors concluded that altered PF joint kinematics in females with PF pain is related to excessive internal femoral rotation, as opposed to lateral patellar rotation.

4.6 Patella Alta

Patella alta refers to a condition whereby the patella lies in a much higher than expected position in relation to the femoral trochlea. Hence, during knee flexion the patella takes much longer to engage with the trochlea, as it has to travel from a much more proximal starting position.

Patella alta is associated with a higher risk of anterior knee pain. This may be explained by biomechanical studies [20–23] which have shown that patella alta is associated with higher PF contact pressures during knee flexion:

- Luyckx et al. [21] showed in cadavers that during knee flexion the PF contact force increased with increasing knee flexion, up to a maximum, and was then followed by a decrease. This drop in PF contact pressures coincided with the onset of contact between the quadriceps tendon and the trochlea, which allowed load sharing. In initial flexion patella alta was associated with a lower patellar contact force. However, in high degrees of flexion, patella alta was associated with higher contact forces than those of normal patellar height, as contact of the quadriceps tendon with the trochlea, and hence force sharing, was delayed until deeper flexion. Thus, the maximal PF contact force and contact pressure increased significantly with increasing patellar height. When averaged across all flexion angles, a high riding patellar position was associated with the highest contact pressures.

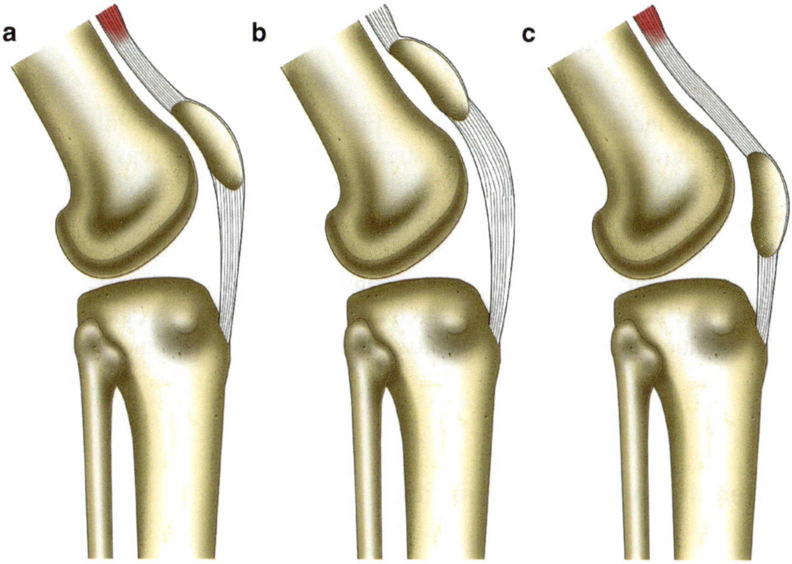

Variations in patellar height (**a**) Normal (**b**) Patella alta (**c**) Patella baja

Patella alta, has been shown to be associated with osteoarthritic changes of the PF joint, and with an increased risk of worsening of these degenerative features over time.

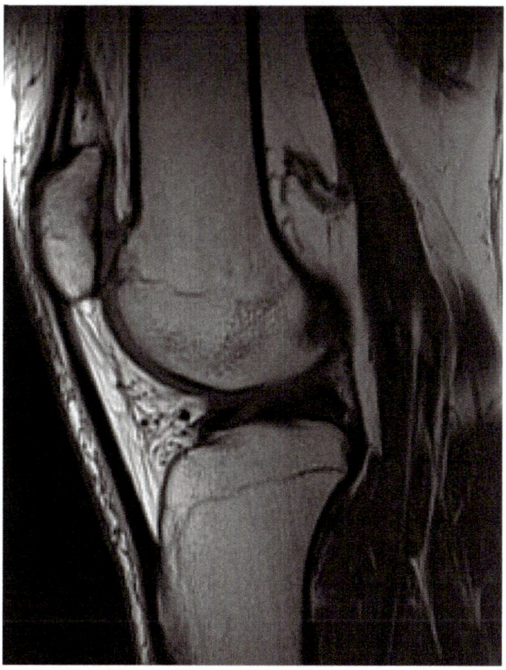

Patella alta

4.7 Downhill Walking Induced Muscle Damage and Delayed Onset Muscle Soreness [24–26]

Downhill walking increases substantially the PF contact forces. Downhill walking has also been shown to be efficient in strengthening the quadriceps. However, intense eccentric contractions, associated with an intense episode of downhill walking may lead to microtrauma due to a high strain of muscle fibers and extracellular matrix. This may lead to muscle inflammation and raised creatinine kinase. Clinically, this presents as anterior quadriceps muscle soreness, weakness, and difficulty mobilising. It appears within 24–48 h and takes several days (about 96 h to settle). Preconditioning with lesser episodes of eccentric exercises may reduce its intensity.

4.8 Patellofemoral Joint Stability

PF joint stability refers to the ability of the joint to maintain the normal relation of its articulating surfaces (patella and trochlea) to avoid troublesome clinical symptoms.

Instability of the PF joint describes an abnormal translation of the patella in relation to the trochlea which causes troublesome symptoms to the patient. This can be:

- Dislocation where there is complete loss of contact between the articular surfaces of the patella and trochlea
- Subluxation where some contact between the patella and trochlea articular surfaces is maintained

PF instability is different from PF laxity. In instability the patient has symptoms, related to the abnormal PF translation. In contrast, laxity refers to abnormal PF translation recognised by the patient or seen on clinical examination but which is not symptomatic.

It is of note that although when describing PF instability we refer to the position of the patella in relation to the trochlea, any abnormal positioning of the patella may be primary due to the patella translating or secondary due to the trochlea translating in relation to the patella.

Patellar instability usually occurs in a lateral direction (this refers to the position of the patella in relation to the femur), and more rarely in a medial direction. For the purposes of this chapter, lateral patellar instability is considered.

4.9 PF Joint Stabilisers

In considering PF stability one may look at static and dynamic stabilisers [27–52].

Static stabilisers: those parameters that are constant in shape and size. These include:

- Shape of the articular surfaces
- Ligaments

Ligaments are fibrous structures that connect two bones. Ligaments cannot actively change their shape or size to limit motion. Instead, upon application of a distracting force, they stretch from a resting lax to a taut state. Ligaments of the PF joint provide:

1. Check-rein effect—the ligament allows translation between two bones in a direction along the line of the ligament, until it stretches to a maximum length at which no further movement is possible.

Dynamic stabilisers: those parameters that can change the force they exert across a joint as the situation demands. Muscles are considered the main stabilisers of joints. This would explain why:

- PF joints the ligaments of which are torn following a dislocation can continue to be stable allowing return to normal activities.
- By muscle strengthening and by getting the muscles to work in a more balanced and coordinated way joint stability may be improved.

The following static and dynamic factors apply to the PF articulation:

4.9.1 Static Factors

4.9.1.1 Bone and Articular Cartilage Morphology

The PF articulation has conforming surfaces which contribute to stability. The trochlea is "U" shaped with concave lateral and medial facets covered by articular cartilage. The articular surface of the patella is "V" shaped, consisting of medial and lateral facets separated by a vertical ridge. Hence, the "V" sits in the "U".

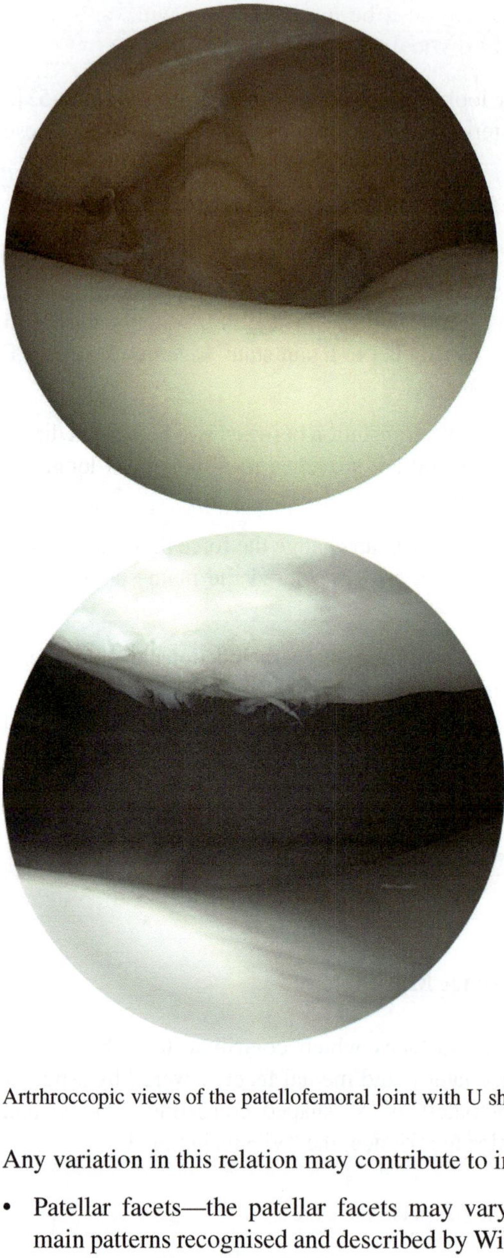

Artrhroccopic views of the patellofemoral joint with U shaped trochlea

Any variation in this relation may contribute to instability.

- Patellar facets—the patellar facets may vary amongst individuals, with three main patterns recognised and described by Wiberg's classification [34], based on a skyline radiograph at 30° flexion:
  - Type I—symmetrical patella—the medial facet has concave shape and has almost the same size as the lateral facet which is also concave
  - Type II- medial facet is smaller than the lateral facet, lateral facet is concave but medial facet is flat or slightly convex—most common (prevalance about 80%)
  - Type III— medial facet is substantially smaller, almost vertical

In addition to the above, the patella may also be flat or concave with no distinct separate facets, patterns which are also encountered in instability.

- Trochlea—The lateral facet of the trochlea is usually larger than the medial and extends more proximally. It improves patellar lateral stability by providing a lateral bony buttress. The trochlear depth may vary amongst individuals being:
  - Normal depth (U shaped)
  - Shallow (less U shaped)
  - Flat
  - Convex
  - Convex with a prominence or bump (this is an extension of the trochlear groove above the level of the anterior femoral cortex. The patella must pass over this bump to enter the trochlea)
- The depth of the trochlea may be assessed on radiological imaging (MRI, Computed Tomography (CT), plain radiographs) by measuring the angle between the lateral and medial trochlear facets (the angle from the highest point of the facets to the lowest point of the trochlear groove). This angle is normally about $138 \pm 6°$. An angle >145° suggests trochlear dysplasia (less depth of the trochlea) and may be related to a tendency for patellar subluxation [37, 45, 46].
- Trochlear dysplasia refers to the trochlea being of abnormal shape which makes it shallower than the average normal. It is seen in <2% of the population but in about 85% of those with patellar instability [37].
- About 96% of those with patellar dislocation may have radiographic evidence of trochlear dysplasia [32].

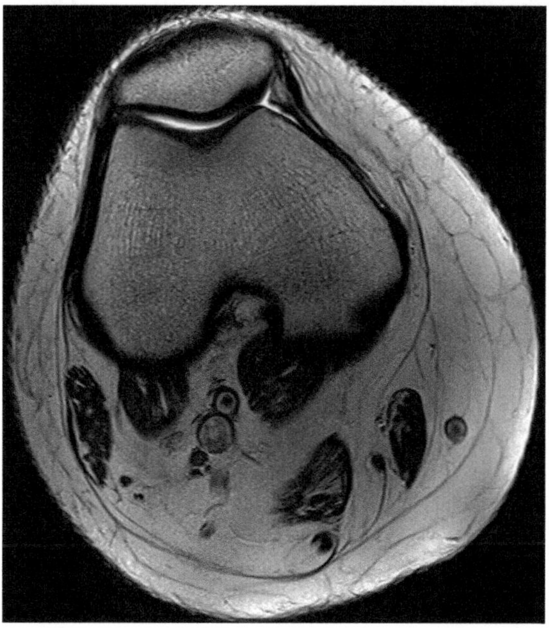

Congruent patellofemoral joint, well formed trochlea

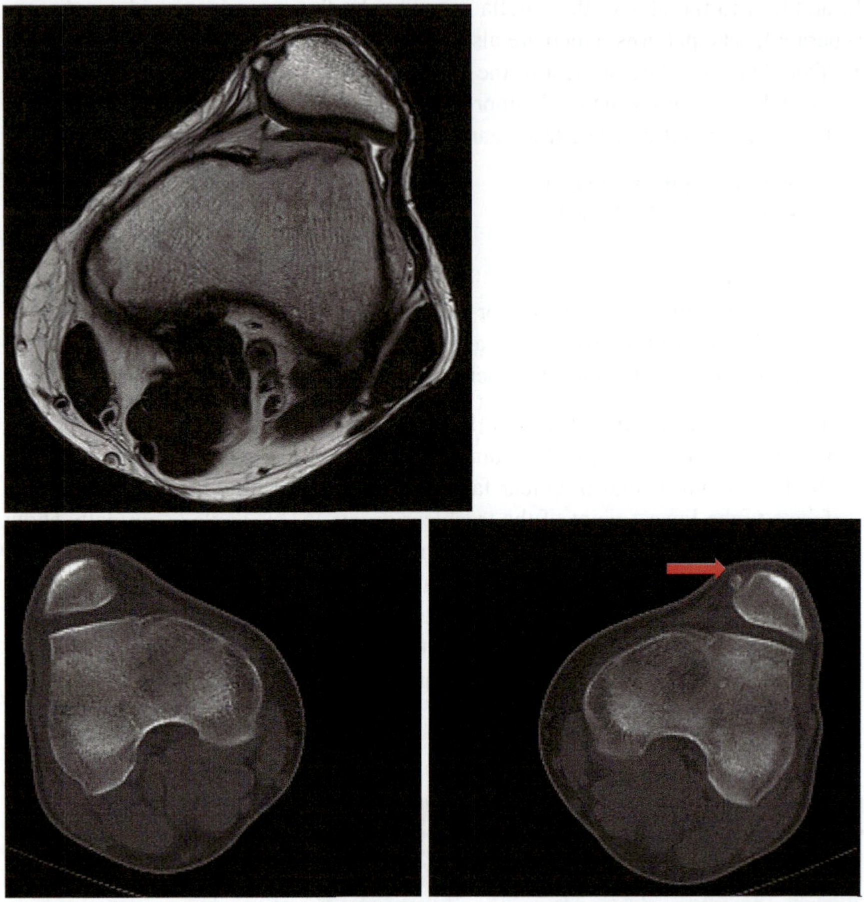

Trochlear dysplasia, lateral subluxation of the patella, and medial ossicle (red arrow) consistent with MPFL avulsion injury

Keshmiri et al. [29] examined what contributes to the trochlea being of abnormal shape and losing its normal depth. They compared the morphology of adult knees with and without trochlear dysplasia on MRI, and reported that no significant differences were seen in the dimensions of the lateral femoral condyle between the two groups. However, the dimensions of the medial femoral condyle (height, width, depth) were significantly smaller in the dysplastic as compared to the control group. They concluded that patients with a dysplastic trochlea have a hypoplastic medial rather than a hypoplastic lateral femoral condyle.

4.9.1.2 Ligaments

The following ligaments provide a static restraint to patellar instability:

- Medial patellofemoral ligament (MPFL)—resists lateral translation of the patella in relation to the trochlea. It is the primary restraint to lateral displacement of the patella. It is tightest at 30° of knee flexion.
- Medial patellomeniscal ligament—resists lateral translation of the patella
- Medial patellotibial ligament—resists lateral translation of the patella
- Medial retinaculum—resists lateral translation of the patella
- Lateral retinaculum—resists medial translation of the patella
- Lateral patellotibial ligament—resists medial translation of the patella
- Lateral patellomeniscal ligament—resists medial translation of the patella

The medial and lateral restraints also act as restraints to anterior translation of the patella in relation to the trochlea—essentially compressing the patella against the trochlea.

4.9.1.3 Tendons

- Quadriceps—resists distal translation of the patella and anterior lifting of the proximal pole of the patella off the femur
- Patellar tendon—resists proximal translation of the patella and anterior lifting of the distal pole of the patella off the femur
- Iliotibial band—resists medial translation of the patella in relation to the trochlea

The tension in these tendons exerts a check-rein effect in addition to any dynamic effect achieved by their muscle contraction:

- If the patellar tendon tears the patella is pulled proximally by the quadriceps tendon attachment—a substantial migration can occur due to active quadriceps muscle contraction.
- If the quadriceps tendon tears the patella springs distally due to its attachment of the patellar tendon. However, such retraction is minimal as there is no active muscle contraction distally.

4.9.1.4 The following describe the various static ligamentous/tendinous restraints to PF instability in various directions:

Lateral Patellar Translation

- Primary restraint
  - MPFL
- Secondary restraints
  - Medial patellotibial ligament
  - Medial patellomeniscal ligament
  - Medial patellar retinaculum

Panagiotopoulos et al. [34] in a cadaveric study showed that the contribution of MPFL to lateral patellar stability was more than 50%. The medial patellomeniscal ligament contributes about 24% whilst the medial patellotibial ligament and medial retinaculum contribute about 13% each.

Medial Patellar Translation

- Lateral patellar retinaculum
- Lateral patellotibial ligament
- Lateral patellomeniscal ligament
- Iliotibial band
- Joint capsule

Proximal Patellar Translation

- Patellar tendon
- Medial and lateral retinaculae

Distal Patellar Translation

- Quadriceps tendon
- Medial and lateral retinaculae

4.9.1.5 Interaction of Static Restraints

A balance in tension between the medial and lateral static stabilisers is essential in maintaining patellar stability. Imbalance between the medial and lateral static restraints may lead to patellar instability such as:

- Tight iliotibial band or lateral patellar retinaculum in relation to the medial restraints—leading to lateral patellar instability
- Lax medial restraints in relation to lateral restraints—leading to lateral patellar instability

- Decreased slope of the lateral facet on the trochlea- leading to lateral patellar instability
- Deficient lateral patellar retinaculum—leading to medial patellar instability

The contribution of static constraints varies according to the position of knee flexion. When the knee is extended the patella lies outside the trochlea and the quadriceps is relaxed or only slightly contracted. Hence, the patella is not under tension and can be easily moved from side to side.

Patellar stability in this knee position relies on:

- The medial and lateral ligamentous/tendinous structures

- At 30° of knee flexion the patella engages with the trochlea. From this stage on, the osseous components (trochlea and patella shape) provide the major contribution to patellar stability. The height and slope of the lateral facet in relation to the medial facet, becomes the primary restraint to lateral patellar translation. Furthermore, in deep knee flexion the angle between the quadriceps force and patellar tendon force decreases which means the patella is pulled more firmly against the trochlea, improving its stability.

4.9.2 Dynamic Factors in PF Stability

Dynamic factors include the muscles of the knee, core, hip, and rest of the lower limb.

4.9.2.1 Knee Muscles

- Quadriceps

The various components of quadriceps act in a balanced and coordinated way to compress the patella against the trochlea improving PF stability. A balance between the quadriceps medial and lateral components is essential to maintain PF congruency. Imbalance between the two may predispose to patellar instability:

- Underactivity of vastus medialis in relation to vastus lateralis may increase tendency of the patella to translate laterally
- Dysfunction of vastus lateralis may increase the tendency of the patella to translate medially

The direction of the resultant force brought about by quadriceps contraction guides the direction of pull on the patella. Hence, the overall line of pull of the quadriceps may influence patellar stability. The resultant force of the quadriceps, under physiological conditions, is in an upward and lateral direction due to the:

- Origin of the quadriceps in relation to its patellar insertion—rectus femoris originates partly from the anterior inferior iliac spine
- Angulation of the femur in the coronal plane, and hence line of action of the quadriceps –femur passes from a proximal lateral to a distal medial direction

In relation to the above, consideration must be paid to the *biomechanical Q angle*. This is the angle between:

- The line representing the resultant force of the quadriceps tendon
- A line drawn from the insertion of the patellar tendon to the centre of the patella

The higher the Q angle, the more lateral the quadriceps pull on the patella, which may predispose to lateral patellar instability.

The *clinical Q angle* has been described as an angle that can be assessed clinically and be used as a surrogate of the biomechanical Q angle. The clinical Q-angle is the angle formed by the intersection of:

- A line drawn from the anterior superior iliac spine (which is easily clinically palpable) to the center of the patella—this line is used as an approximation of the resultant force of the quadriceps on the patella
- A line drawn from the center of the patella to the tibial tubercle—as a representation of the pull of the patellar tendon on the patella

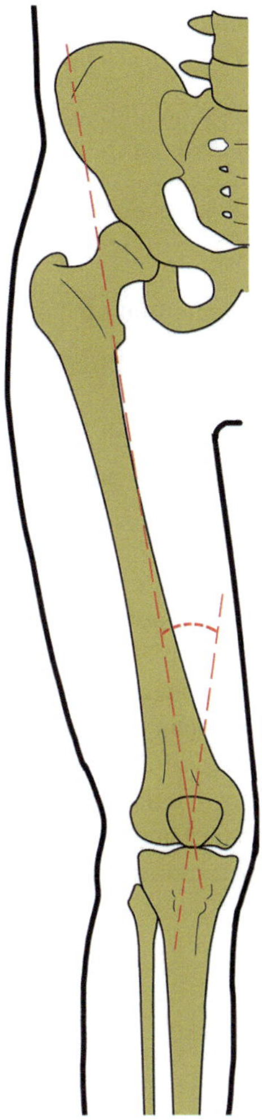

Clinical assessment of the Q angle

The clinical Q angle may be assessed with the knee in slight flexion, to allow the patella to center in the trochlea. The clinical Q angle has been shown to be an underestimation of the biomechanical Q angle.

The clinical Q angle varies in males and females with some of the reported values reported in literature including:

- Males—8°-14°
- Females—11°-20°

The Q angle, and hence lateral pull on the patella may be increased by the following:

- Wider pelvic anatomy (associated with female sex)
- Weak external rotators or abductors of the hip—which leads to:
  - Functional adduction and internal rotation of the femur
- Hip anteversion which leads to:
  - Compensatory femoral internal rotation
- Structural femoral adduction or internal rotation
- Valgus deformity of the knee
- Genu recurvatum—knee hyperextension
- Foot pronation (pes planus or flat feet)- pronation of the foot leading to increased knee valgus

4.9.2.2 Muscles of the Core, Hip, Foot and Ankle

As described above for PF loading, adequate strength and coordination of the core and hip muscles is essential to maintain normal positioning of the femur in relation to the patella and tibia. Dysfunction of these may predispose to patellar instability. Similarly, foot position may affect patellar positioning and can be influenced by the activity of muscles acting on the foot and ankle.

- Proprioception plays an important role in the functioning of the muscles involved in PF stability.

4.10 Lateral PF Instability

Lateral patellar instability (subluxation/dislocation) usually occurs when the knee is at about 20–30° of knee flexion (either with the knee flexing or extending). Several factors may account for this:

- In normal knee motion, at about 20° of knee flexion the patella shifts and tilts laterally, suggesting that the main force vector on the patella (brought about by the quadriceps muscle contraction and static restraints) is in a lateral direction.
- In early knee flexion, the tibia is in external rotation, the femur is internally rotated and the knee is in valgus which further predispose to lateral patellar translation.

With higher knee flexion, the patella is less likely to dislocate, as it engages deeper in the trochlea. Farahmand et al. [53] assessed the patellar lateral force-displacement behaviour in normal human cadavers at various flexion angles. A 5 mm lateral patellar displacement required a constant displacing force (consistent with a constant lateral instability) up to 60° knee flexion. Following this, the displacing force magnitude increased. Nevertheless, lateral patellar dislocation may also occur in deeper flexion if there is substantial trochlear bony deficiency or other bony abnormality.

In evaluating lateral PF instability there is a need to consider conditions which lead to lateral maltracking of the patella in relation to the femur predisposing it to lateral instability. These may primarily involve the:

- Core
- Hip
- Knee
- Lower leg, ankle, foot

Such conditions may be structural or functional:

Structural
- Femoral neck anteversion
- Femoral internal rotation
- Tibial external tibial rotation
- Structural knee valgus
- Trochlear dysplasia
- Lateralization of the tibial tubercle
- Patella alta
- Structural foot pronation

Patella Alta—as described above, patella alta refers to a condition whereby the patella at rest lies in a much higher than expected position [47, 48]. Hence, during knee flexion, the patella takes much longer to engage with the trochlea, as it has to travel from a much more proximal starting position. Clinically, patella alta is related to a higher risk of lateral patellar instability [49]. This may be explained by the delayed engagement with the trochlea, hence relying for a greater part of the knee flexion cycle on soft tissue restraints for stability. As the patella spends more time outside the groove, there is a higher chance of the patella displacing laterally and subluxing or dislocating [50, 51].

The movement of the patella in relation to the femoral trochlea may be likened to sliding down a slide as shown in the next figure.

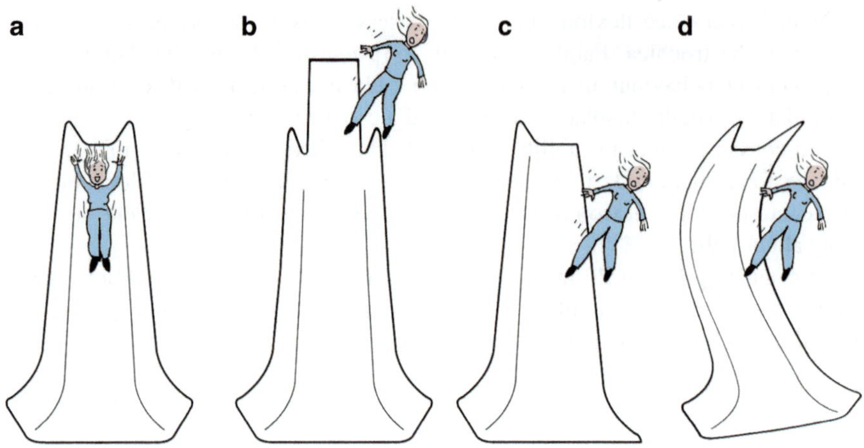

The movement of the patella in relation to the femoral trochlea is analogous to sliding down a slide. **(a)** If you are starting with the feet in the slide, and the slide has deep side walls then one is likely to have a smooth slide. **(b)** However, if one has to slide on a flat surface before entering the slide(equivalent to patella alta) there is the possibility of falling over and missing the slide. **(c)** Similarly, if the slide walls are deficient and the slide is flat (equivalent to trochlear dysplasia) or **(d)** if the slide is twisted on one site (equivalent to internal femoral rotation) the slider may roll out of the slide rather than making it down smoothly.

Functional [8–16]

- Weakness of hip abductors and external rotators—leading to femoral adduction and internal rotation of the femur under the patella
- Foot pronation due to muscle/ligamentous imbalance—leading to tibial and femoral internal rotation and knee valgus
- Dynamic knee valgus
- Soft tissue factors—muscle imbalance, lateral ligamentous tightness, medial ligamentous laxity/dysfunction

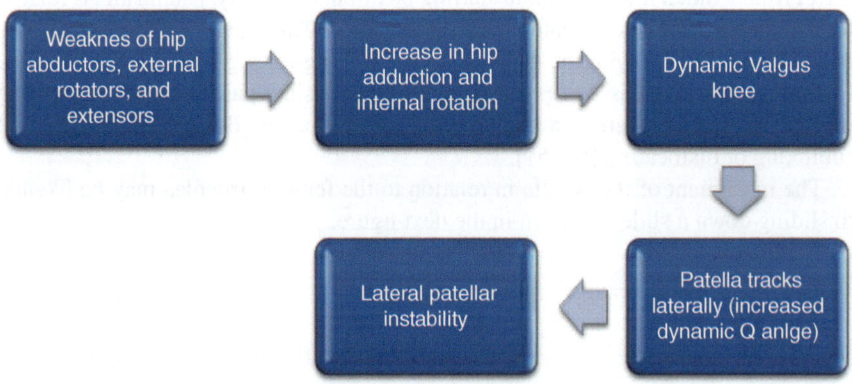

Hip weakness may lead to lateral patellofemoral joint instability

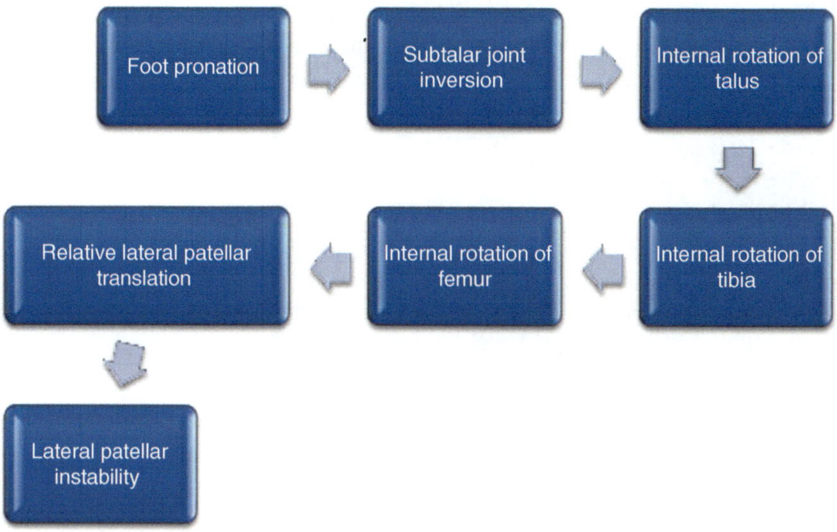

Foot pronation may lead to lateral patellofemoral joint instability

4.11 Biomechanics of Patellofemoral Degeneration

Any condition which leads to increased pressures on the PF joint is likely to be associated with PF degeneration and arthritis [30, 53–56].

Hence, the above described biomechanical conditions that have been shown to cause:

- Increased PF contact pressures in the absence of PF instability
- PF instability leading to altered PF pressures

have also been related to a higher rate of PF degeneration.

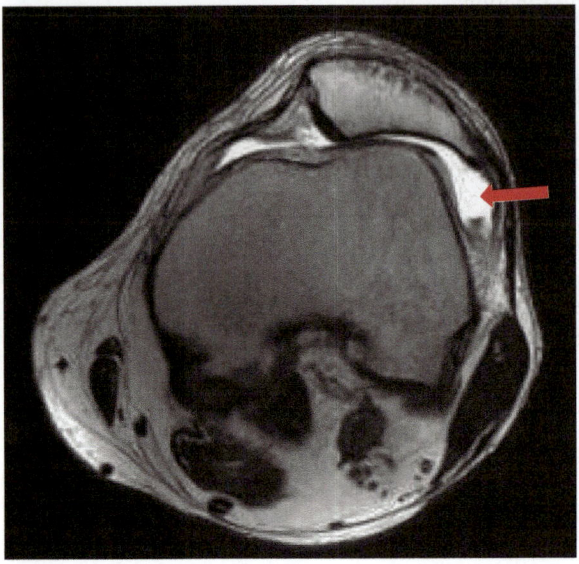

Effusion associated with patellofemoral degeneration and lateral patellar subluxation

4.11.1 *Osteoarthritis Associated with Posterior Cruciate Ligament/Posterolateral Corner Deficiency* [54–56]

Chronic posterior cruciate ligament (PCL) and posterolateral corner (PLC) deficiency has been related to increased risk of knee osteoarthritis (OA), mainly of the PF compartment and medial compartment:

- Cadaveric studies have shown that sectioning the PCL/PLC increases the contact pressures in the medial and PF compartments
- The lateral facet of the PF joint is particularly affected
- In PCL/PLC deficiency the tibia translates posteriorly and externally rotates in relation to the femur. Posterior translation of the tibia drags the patella backwards, increasing the patella compression against the trochlea and raising PF contact pressures. External rotation of the tibia in relation to the femur leads to lateralization of the tibial tubercle which drags the patella laterally, thus increasing lateral patellar loading.

References

1. Loudon JK. Biomechanics and pathomechanics of the patellofemoral joint. Int J Sports Phys Ther. 2016;11(6):820–30.
2. Schindler OS, Scott WN. Basic kinematics and biomechanics of the patello-femoral joint. Part 1: the native patella. Acta Orthop Belg. 2011;77(4):421–31.
3. Iranpour F, Merican AM, Teo SH, Cobb JP, Amis AA. Knee biomechanics—patellofmeroal articulation—Femoral articular geometry and patellofemoral stability. Knee. 2017;24(3):555–63.
4. Hadidi O, Ellanti P, Lincoln M, Hogan N. The J-sign in patellar maltracking. BMJ Case Rep. 2018, 2018. pii: bcr-2017-222887; https://doi.org/10.1136/bcr-2017-222887.
5. Sheehan FT, Derasari A, Fine KM, Brindle TJ, Alter KE. Q-angle and J-sign: indicative of maltracking subgroups in patellofemoral pain. Clin Orthop Relat Res. 2010;468(1):266–75.
6. Lin F, Makhsous M, Chang AH, Hendrix RW, Zhang LQ. In vivo and noninvasive six degrees of freedom patellar tracking during voluntary knee. Clin Biomech (Bristol, Avon). 2003;18(5):401–9.
7. Trepczynski A, Kutzner I, Kornaropoulos E, Taylor WR, Duda GN, Bergmann G, Heller MO. Patellofemoral joint contact forces during activities with high knee flexion. J Orthop Res. 2012;30(3):408–15.
8. Costigan PA, Deluzio KJ, Wyss UP. Knee and hip kinetics during normal stair climbing. Gait Posture. 2002;16(1):31–7.
9. Ericson MO, Nisell R. Patellofemoral joint forces during ergometric cycling. Phys Ther. 1987;67(9):1365–9.
10. Meira EP, Brumitt J. Influence of the hip on patients with patellofemoral pain syndrome: a systematic review. Sports Health. 2011;3(5):455–65.
11. Willson JD, Kernozek TW, Arndt RL, Reznichek DA, Scott SJ. Gluteal muscle activation during running in females with and without patellofemoral pain syndrome. Clin Biomech (Bristol, Avon). 2011;26(7):735–40.
12. Kaya D, Citaker S, Kerimoglu U, Atay OA, Nyland J, Callaghan M, Yakut Y, Yüksel I, Doral MN. Women with patellofemoral pain syndrome have quadriceps femoris volume and strength deficiency. Knee Surg Sports Traumatol Arthrosc. 2011;19(2):242–7.
13. Earl JE, Hoch AZ. A proximal strengthening program improves pain, function, and biomechanics in women with patellofemoral pain syndrome. Am J Sports Med. 2011;39(1):154–63.
14. Gross MT, Foxworth JL. The role of foot orthoses as an intervention for patellofemoral pain. J Orthop Sports Phys Ther. 2003;33(11):661–70.
15. Tiberio D. The effect of excessive subtalar joint pronation on patellofemoral joint mechanics: a theoretical model. J Orthop Sports Phys Ther. 1987;9:160–9.
16. Barton CJ, Menz HB, Crossley KM. The immediate effects of foot orthoses on functional performance in individuals with patellofemoral pain syndrome. Br J Sports Med. 2011;45(3):193–7.
17. Barton CJ, Munteanu SE, Menz HB, Crossley KM. The efficacy of foot orthoses in the treatment of individuals with patellofemoral pain syndrome: a systematic review. Sports Med. 2010;40(5):377–95.
18. Barton CJ, Menz HB, Levinger P, Webster KE, Crossley KM. Greater peak rearfoot eversion predicts foot orthoses efficacy in individuals with patellofemoral pain syndrome. Br J Sports Med. 2011;45(9):697–701.
19. Souza RB, Draper CE, Fredericson M, Powers CM. Femur rotation and patellofemoral joint kinematics: a weight-bearing magnetic resonance imaging analysis. J Orthop Sports Phys Ther. 2010;40(5):277–85.
20. Ward SR, Powers CM. The influence of patella alta on patellofemoral joint stress during normal and fast walking. Clin Biomech (Bristol, Avon). 2004;19(10):1040–7.
21. Luyckx T, Didden K, Vandenneucker H, Labey L, Innocenti B, Bellemans J. Is there a biomechanical explanation for anterior knee pain in patients with patella alta?: influence of patellar

height on patellofemoral contact force, contact area and contact pressure. J Bone Joint Surg Br. 2009;91(3):344–50.
22. Singerman R, Davy DT, Goldberg VM. Effects of patella alta and patella infera on patellofemoral contact forces. J Biomech. 1994;27(8):1059–65.
23. Stefanik JJ, Zhu Y, Zumwalt AC, Gross KD, Clancy M, Lynch JA, Frey Law LA, Lewis CE, Roemer FW, Powers CM, Guermazi A, Felson DT. Association between patella alta and the prevalence and worsening of structural features of patellofemoral joint osteoarthritis: the multicenter osteoarthritis study. Arthritis Care Res (Hoboken). 2010;62(9):1258–65.
24. Maeo S, Yamamoto M, Kanehisa H, Nosaka K. Prevention of downhill walking-induced muscle damage by non-damaging downhill walking. PLoS One. 2017;12(3):e0173909. https://doi.org/10.1371/journal.pone.0173909.
25. Maeo S, Ochi Y, Yamamoto M, Kanehisa H, Nosaka K. Effect of a prior bout of preconditioning exercise on muscle damage from downhill walking. Appl Physiol Nutr Metab. 2015;40(3):274–9.
26. Eston RG, Lemmey AB, McHugh P, Byrne C, Walsh SE. Effect of stride length on symptoms of exercise-induced muscle damage during a repeated bout of downhill running. Scand J Med Sci Sports. 2000;10(4):199–204.
27. Amis AA. Current concepts on anatomy and biomechanics of patellar stability. Sports Med Arthrosc Rev. 2007;15(2):48–56.
28. Zaffagnini S, Grassi A, Zocco G, Rosa MA, Signorelli C, Muccioli GMM. The patellofemoral joint: from dysplasia to dislocation. EFORT Open Rev. 2017;2(5):204–14.
29. Keshmiri A, Schöttle P, Peter C. Trochlear dysplasia relates to medial femoral condyle hypoplasia: an MRI-based study. Arch Orthop Trauma Surg. 2020;140(2):155–60.
30. Van Haver A, De Roo K, De Beule M, Labey L, De Baets P, Dejour D, Claessens T, Verdonk P. The effect of trochlear dysplasia on patellofemoral biomechanics: a cadaveric study with simulated trochlear deformities. Am J Sports Med. 2015;43(6):1354–61.
31. Lin F, Makhsous M, Chang AH, Hendrix RW, Zhang LQ. In vivo and noninvasive six degrees of freedom patellar tracking during voluntary knee movement. Clin Biomech (Bristol, Avon). 2003;18(5):401–9.
32. Nisell R, Ericson M. Patellar forces during isokinetic knee extension. Clin Biomech (Bristol, Avon). 1992;7(2):104–8.
33. Lee TQ, Morris G, Csintalan RP. The influence of tibial and femoral rotation on patellofemoral contact area and pressure. J Orthop Sports Phys Ther. 2003;33(11):686–93.
34. Panagiotopoulos E, Strzelczyk P, Herrmann M, Scuderi G. Cadaveric study on static medial patellar stabilizers: the dynamizing role of the vastus medialis obliquus on medial patellofemoral ligament. Knee Surg Sports Traumatol Arthrosc. 2006;14(1):7–12.
35. Kaleka CC, Aihara LJ, Rodrigues A, de Medeiros SF, de Oliveira VM, de Paula Leite Cury R. Cadaveric study of the secondary medial patellar restraints: patellotibial and patellomeniscal ligaments. Knee Surg Sports Traumatol Arthrosc. 2017;25(1):144–51.
36. Stephen JM, Lumpaopong P, Dodds AL, Williams A, Amis AA. The effect of tibial tuberosity medialization and lateralization on patellofemoral joint kinematics, contact mechanics, and stability. Am J Sports Med. 2015;43(1):186–94.
37. Dejour H, Walch G, Nove-Josserand L, Guier C. Factors of patellar instability: an anatomic radiographic study. Knee Surg Sports Traumatol Arthrosc. 1994;2(1):19–26.
38. Bollier M, Fulkerson JP. The role of trochlear dysplasia in patellofemoral instability. J Am Acad Orthop Surg. 2011;19(1):8–16.
39. Wibeeg G. Roentgenographs and Anatomic Studies on the Femoropatellar Joint: With Special Reference to Chondromalacia Patellae. Acta Orthop Scand. 1941;12(1–4):319–410.
40. Saragaglia D, Mader R, Blaysat M, Mercier N. Medial facet patelloplasty in patellar instability associated with patellofemoral dysplasia: a report of 26 cases. Orthop Traumatol Surg Res. 2012;98(2):167–72.
41. Manske RC, Davies GJ. Examination of the patellofemoral joint. Int J Sports Phys Ther. 2016;11(6):831–53.

42. Caton JH, Dejour D. Tibial tubercle osteotomy in patello-femoral instability and in patellar height abnormality. Int Orthop. 2010;34(2):305–9.
43. Teitge R. Osteotomy in the Treatment of Patellofemoral Instability. Tech Knee Surg. 2006;5:2–18.
44. Galland O, Walch G, Dejour H, Carret JP. An anatomical and radiological study of the femoropatellar articulation. Surg Radiol Anat. 1990;12(2):119–25.
45. Colvin AC, West RV. Patellar instability. J Bone Joint Surg Am. 2008;90(12):2751–62.
46. Merchant AC, Mercer RL, Jacobsen RH, Cool CR. Roentgenographic analysis of patellofemoral congruence. J Bone Joint Surg Am. 1974;56(7):1391–6.
47. Caton J, Deschamp G, Chambat P, Lerat JL, Dejour H. Les rotules basses (Patellae inferae)—a propos de 128 observations. Rev Chir Orthop. 1982;68:317–25.
48. Caton J. Méthode de mesure de la hauteur de la rotule. Acta Orthop Belg. 1989;55:385–6.
49. Huntington LS, Webster KE, Devitt BM, Scanlon JP, Feller JA. Factors associated with an increased risk of recurrence after a first-time patellar dislocation: a systematic review and meta-analysis. Am J Sports Med. 2019;11:363546519888467. https://doi.org/10.1177/0363546519888467.
50. Watson NA, Duchman KR, Grosland NM, Bollier MJ. Finite element analysis of patella alta: a patellofemoral instability model. Iowa Orthop J. 2017;37:101–8.
51. Ward SR, Terk MR, Powers CM. Patella alta: association with patellofemoral alignment and changes in contact area during weight-bearing. J Bone Joint Surg Am. 2007;89(8):1749–55.
52. Dewan V, Webb MSL, Prakash D, Malik A, Gella S, Kipps C. When does the patella dislocate? A systematic review of biomechanical & kinematic studies. J Orthop. 2019;20:70–7.
53. Farahmand F, Tahmasbi MN, Amis AA. Lateral force-displacement behaviour of the human patella and its variation with knee flexion—a biomechanical study in vitro. J Biomech. 1998;31(12):1147–52.
54. MacDonald P, Miniaci A, Fowler P, Marks P, Finlay B. A biomechanical analysis of joint contact forces in the posterior cruciate deficient knee. Knee Surg Sports Traumatol Arthrosc. 1996;3(4):252–5.
55. Logan M, Williams A, Lavelle J, Gedroyc W, Freeman M. The effect of posterior cruciate ligament deficiency on knee kinematics. Am J Sports Med. 2004;32(8):1915–22.
56. Gill TJ, DeFrate LE, Wang C, Carey CT, Zayontz S, Zarins B. Li G The effect of posterior cruciate ligament reconstruction on patellofemoral contact pressures in the knee joint under simulated muscle loads. Am J Sports Med. 2004;32(1):109–15.

42. Caton JH, Dejour D. Tibial tubercle osteotomy in patello-femoral instability and in patellar height abnormality. Int Orthop. 2010;34(2):305–9.
43. Teitge R. Osteotomy in the Treatment of Patellofemoral Instability. Tech Knee Surg. 2006;5 [illegible]
44. Galland O, Walch G, Dejour H, Carret JP. An anatomical and radiological study of the femoropatellar articulation. Surg Radiol Anat. 1990;12(2):119–25.
45. Colvin AC, West RV. Patellar instability. J Bone Joint Surg Am. 2008;90(12):2751–62.
46. Marchant M, Mercer RL, Jacobson RH, Cook CR. [illegible]
47. Caton J, Deschamps G, Chambat P, Lerat JL, Dejour H. Les rotules basses. Patella infera. A propos de 128 observations. Rev Chir Orthop. 1982;68(5):317–25.
48. [illegible]
49. [illegible]
[illegible]

Chapter 5
Clinical History for Knee Conditions

When making a clinical diagnosis the initial step is taking a thorough history of the patient's complaints and symptoms. This may be achieved by using open questions (so that patients are given the opportunity to express the difficulties they face in their own words and in their own priorities) but also more direct questions, which aim to elicit specific facts that the patient may not otherwise volunteer.

Clinical history taking for knee conditions takes the formal structure involving questions about the presenting complaint, events that may have led to the onset of the complaint, and its effects upon the patient in terms of pain, limitation of function or other disturbance.

The clinician then questions about the treatments which may have already been tried and what the patient's response has been to those. Furthermore, information is obtained about the overall health of the patient, any other musculoskeletal problems, previous and current medications, and any relevant family history. The patient's personal circumstances, including recreational and occupational activities, are also elicited.

This chapter describes some of the enquiries [1–18] that may be made in obtaining a clinical history for the troublesome knee.

5.1 Presenting Complaint

Information is gathered for each of the patient's complaints as described next.

C. Panayiotou Charalambous, *The Knee Made Easy*,
https://doi.org/10.1007/978-3-030-54506-2_5

5.1.1 Nature of Complaint

- Pain
  - Location
  - Type
    - Dull
    - Sharp
    - Burning
  - Severity
    - On a scale of 0 to 10 (0—no pain, 10-severe pain)
    - Effect on sleep—difficulty going to sleep/awakening
- Locking
  - What does patient mean by locking
    - Catching
    - Giving way
    - Abnormal motion
    - Abnormal noise
    - Jamming
    - Knee getting stuck
  - Onset
    - Slowly
    - Sudden
    - After prolonged sitting/after knee kept in flexion, at rest, any time, upon turning/twisting
  - What position is knee left at
    - Flexion/extension
    - Inability to further flex or extend or both
  - How does it unlock
    - Gradually
    - Suddenly, with a snap
  - Associated with
    - Pain
    - Knee swelling
    - Clicking, snapping or other noise
- Giving way
  - "Sudden loss of control", "buckles", "wobbly", "shifts"
  - Fallen down/short of falling down
  - Onset
    - Whilst standing still, walking straight, turning, twisting, descending stairs, pivoting, squatting
- Stiffness
  - Global versus a specific movement direction
- Weakness
  - Global vs. specific movement direction

  - Global vs. specific leg position
  - Affecting high vs. low demand activities
  - Severity
    - Absence of power vs. less power than expected vs. early fatigue
  - Endurance vs. repetition
- Clicking/Clucking
  - Type of noise
  - Heard versus felt
    - By patient or others
  - Location/source
- Paraesthesia
  - Nature
    - Altered sensation
    - Pins and needles
    - Reduced sensation
    - Tingling
    - Numbness
    - "Dead" leg
  - Location
  - Severity
  - Painful versus painless
  - Constant versus intermittent
- Swelling
  - Description
    - Prominence
    - Deformity
    - Asymmetry between sides
    - Something out of place, something sticking out
    - Shape, size, colour, temperature
  - Noticed by patient or others
- Isolated symptom or in combination

5.1.2 Onset of Complaint

- Speed of onset
  - Sudden
  - Gradual

Possible precipitating event:

- Nil obvious
- Chronic repetitive strain
- Chronic repetitive loading
- Change in type of activities or activity level prior to onset of symptoms

- Onset due to sudden loading
- If symptoms started post-injury
  - What was patient doing?—Sports—football, rugby, skiing (wearing cleats?)
  - How did injury happen?
  - Non-contact injury—such as changing direction, stopping suddenly, landing from a jump
  - Contact injury—direct impact
  - What exactly happened to the leg?
    - Twisting
    - Forced in a particular direction (hyperextension, valgus, varus, hyperflexion, tibia pushed backwards/forwards)
    - Axial loading (such as on the car pedal)
    - Foot on floor at the time of impact or off floor
- Associated sound—snap/tear/pop/clicking/clunk
- Associated swelling
  - Straight away –this is suggestive of intra-articular bleeding–secondary to
    - Ligamentous tear
    - Intra-articular fracture
    - Peripheral meniscal tear
  - After a short interval/overnight—suggestive of inflammatory cause –such as secondary to meniscal tear
- Ability to mobilise in the immediate time post injury
  - Able to stand up after injury and continue previous activity—suggestive of not a major injury
  - Able to weightbear but had to stop activity
  - Unable to weightbear

5.1.3 *Progress of Complaint*

- Duration
  - Length
  - Continuous/intermittent

Change in size or shape (such as of a swelling or lump):

- Getting bigger/smaller/up and down—intermittently changing size
- Speed of change—fast/slow
- Size does not alter with joint position vs. changing with joint motion/position

5.1.4 *Exacerbating and Relieving Factors*

- Leg position
- Rest vs. exertion, staying still vs. leg motion

- At rest or on activity
- Weight bearing vs. non-weight bearing
- Walking vs. running
- Walking on a flat surface vs. ascending stairs vs. descending stairs
- Walking on even vs. uneven surface
- Specific activities
  - Kneeling
  - Turning
  - Jumping
- Timing—night vs. day, morning vs. rest of day

5.1.5 Impact of Presenting Complaint

Understanding the effect of the presenting complaint on the patient and the limitations it confers is essential to help consider the level of intervention necessary, and any potential benefits of any such intervention. These include:

- Functional limitations
  - Activities of daily living
  - Occupational limitations
  - Recreational limitations
- What does it stop you from doing that you want to do?
- Effect on personal/social life
- Effect on psychological well being

5.1.6 Up to Date Management of Presenting Complaint

An enquiry is made about previous management of the complaint. This may be gathered from the patient and their close ones, or, where relevant, from previous medical or surgical records:

- What has been tried?
  - How?
  - By whom?
  - How many times?
- What has been tried and helped symptoms?
- What has been tried but failed to improve symptoms?

5.2 Previous Musculoskeletal History

In this part of clinical history, information is obtained about any other musculoskeletal problems:

- Symptomatic knee/leg
- Opposite knee/leg
- Other joints
- Inflammatory or other arthropathy
- Previous injuries—fractures or otherwise

5.3 Activities History

- Participating sports
- Regular activity
  - Intensity
  - Frequency
  - Duration
- Recent change in pattern of activities
- Pre-warming patterns
- Change in foot wear, worn footwear

5.4 Previous Medical History

The previous medical history of the patient is examined to identify disorders that may be associated with the development of knee symptoms, to determine the patient's overall health and their ability to undergo surgery or other interventions:

- Diabetes mellitus
  - Link to perioperative complications such as infection
  - Risk of hyperglycaemia following steroid injection therapy
- Cardiovascular and respiratory fitness if considering surgery
- Malignancy—possibility of metastatic cause of symptoms, fitness for surgery
- Infection in other parts of the body
- Osteonecrosis in other parts of the body
- Conditions associated with steroid use—osteonecrosis
- Deep venous thrombosis/pulmonary embolism—increased risk post-surgery
- Mouth ulcers (in Reiter's syndrome, reactive arthritis)
- Skin rash—scaly (e.g. psoriasis), erythema migrans (Lyme disease), butterfly rash (lupus), vasculitic rash (rheumatoid arthritis)

- Eye symptoms—conjunctivitis, uveitis (e.g. in rheumatoid arthritis, Reiter's syndrome, reactive arthritis)
- Urological symptoms (in reactive arthritis, Reiter's syndrome)

5.5 Previous Surgical History

Enquiries are made about any previous surgical history both with regards to the knee and leg in question, the rest of the musculoskeletal system and non-musculoskeletal problems, to help determine:

- Condition of the knee that may confer difficulties if surgery were to be carried out- such as previous knee surgery and thus associated scarring
- Fitness for surgery
- Potential surgery/anaesthetic complications the patient may be predisposed to
  - Any previous surgery
  - What type of anaesthesia
  - Timing of previous surgery
  - Development of post-surgical complications

5.6 Medication History

Information about current and previous medications, details of any allergies, as well as alcohol and tobacco use:

- History of steroid use—link with osteonecrosis
- Medications that may influence anaesthetic risk or injection therapy
- Other drugs if relevant—anabolic steroids, stimulants, antibiotics (fluoroquinolones)
- Allergies
  - Agent
  - Reaction
  - Alternatives—tried and safe?
  - May be associated with predisposition to joint stiffness
  - Allergy to metallic material (if contemplating implant use)
    - Reaction to cheap jewellery, other metal
    - What reaction –localised itching, redness, blisters, extensive body reaction
- Alcohol use
  - Link with osteonecrosis
  - May influence compliance with treatment
- Smoking

5.7 Family Musculoskeletal History

Certain musculoskeletal conditions may exhibit familial association and these are sought:

- Family history of knee conditions which may affect the patient's knowledge, preconceptions or expectations
- Familial association of osteonecrosis, inflammatory arthropathy
- Familial association of conditions associated with arthropathy such as gout, inflammatory bowel disease

Learning Pearls

- A systematic history taking may ensure that all important information is gathered and important facts are not overlooked
- Maintain lateral thinking, even when the diagnosis seems very obvious
- Even an accurate history may not give the definite answer and complimentary radiological or other investigations are usually needed. Swain MS et al [19] carried out a systematic review to identify diagnostic studies comparing the accuracy of clinical examination items for anterior cruciate ligament (ACL) injury to the level achieved by arthroscopic evaluation, or magnetic resonance imaging. They examined the diagnostic accuracy 9 items gathered from the clinical history (including popping sound at the time of injury, giving way, effusion, pain, ability to continue activity). They concluded that none of these provided useful diagnostic information in a clinical setting. Their conclusion was that despite being widely used and accepted in clinical practice, the results of individual history items or physical tests do not meaningfully change the probability of ACL injury.

References

1. Calmbach WL, Hutchens M. Evaluation of patients presenting with knee pain: Part I. History, physical examination, radiographs, and laboratory tests. Am Fam Physician. 2003;68(5):907–12.
2. Katz JN, Smith SR, Yang HY, Martin SD, Wright J, Donnell-Fink LA, Losina E. Value of history, physical examination, and radiographic findings in the diagnosis of symptomatic meniscal tear among middle-aged subjects with knee pain. Arthritis Care Res (Hoboken). 2017;69(4):484–90.
3. Kim JG, Han SW, Lee DH. Diagnosis and treatment of discoid meniscus. Knee Surg Relat Res. 2016;28(4):255–62.
4. Yan R, Wang H, Yang Z, Ji ZH, Guo YM. Predicted probability of meniscus tears: comparing history and physical examination with MRI. Swiss Med Wkly. 2011;141:w13314. https://doi.org/10.4414/smw.2011.13314.
5. Bunt CW, Jonas CE, Chang JG. Knee pain in adults and adolescents: the initial evaluation. Am Fam Physician. 2018;98(9):576–85.

6. Wagemakers HP, Luijsterburg PA, Boks SS, Heintjes EM, Berger MY, Verhaar JA, Koes BW, Bierma-Zeinstra SM. Diagnostic accuracy of history taking and physical examination for assessing anterior cruciate ligament lesions of the knee in primary care. Arch Phys Med Rehabil. 2010;91(9):1452–9.
7. Kastelein M, Luijsterburg PA, Wagemakers HP, Bansraj SC, Berger MY, Koes BW, Bierma-Zeinstra SM. Diagnostic value of history taking and physical examination to assess effusion of the knee in traumatic knee patients in general practice. Arch Phys Med Rehabil. 2009;90(1):82–6.
8. Wagemakers HP, Heintjes EM, Boks SS, Berger MY, Verhaar JA, Koes BW, Bierma-Zeinstra SM. Diagnostic value of history-taking and physical examination for assessing meniscal tears of the knee in general practice. Clin J Sport Med. 2008;18(1):24–30.
9. Näslund J, Näslund UB, Odenbring S, Lundeberg T. Comparison of symptoms and clinical findings in subgroups of individuals with patellofemoral pain. Physiother Theory Pract. 2006;22(3):105–18.
10. Fulkerson JP. Office evaluation of patients with anterior knee pain. Am J Knee Surg. 1997;10(3):181–3.
11. Merchant AC, Fulkerson JP, Leadbetter W. The diagnosis and initial treatment of patellofemoral disorders. Am J Orthop (Belle Mead NJ). 2017;46(2):68–75.
12. Smith BW, Green GA. Acute knee injuries: part I. History and physical examination. Am Fam Physician. 1995;51(3):615–21.
13. Ayre C, Hardy M, Scally A, Radcliffe G, Venkatesh R, Smith J, Guy S. The use of history to identify anterior cruciate ligament injuries in the acute trauma setting: the 'LIMP index'. Emerg Med J. 2017;34(5):302–7.
14. Burnett R, Allum RL. Relevance of history of injury to the diagnosis of meniscal tears. Ann R Coll Surg Engl. 1993;75(4):229–30.
15. Baum J. Joint pain. It isn't always arthritis. Postgrad Med. 1989;85(1):311–3. 316, 321
16. Wallis JA, Taylor NF, Bunzli S, Shields N. Experience of living with knee osteoarthritis: a systematic review of qualitative studies. BMJ Open. 2019;9(9):e030060. https://doi.org/10.1136/bmjopen-2019-030060.
17. Meding JB, Klay M, Healy A, Ritter MA, Keating EM, Berend ME. The prescreening history and physical in elective total joint arthroplasty. J Arthroplast. 2007;22(6 Suppl 2):21–3.
18. Peat G, Wood L, Wilkie R, Thomas E, KNE-SCI Study Group. How reliable is structured clinical history-taking in older adults with knee problems? Inter- and intraobserver variability of the KNE-SCI. J Clin Epidemiol. 2003;56(11):1030–7.
19. Swain MS, Henschke N, Kamper SJ, Downie AS, Koes BW, Maher CG. Accuracy of clinical tests in the diagnosis of anterior cruciate ligament injury: a systematic review. Chiropr Man Therap. 2014;22:25. https://doi.org/10.1186/s12998-014-0025-8.

Chapter 6
Clinical Examination of the Knee

Clinical examination aims to elicit signs that can supplement the clinical symptoms gathered from the clinical history, and prove or disprove the working diagnosis.

Examination of any joint in Orthopaedics may follow a Look/Feel/Move/Special tests sequence [1–3] and this order is also applied to examination of the knee. The examiner inspects the patient and their knees, palpates the knee and then determines the active and passive range of knee motion. Individual muscle strength is subsequently examined along with special tests that are guided towards specific underlying conditions. The lumbosacral spine, hip, ankle, and foot joints are also examined as indicated.

This chapter presents a structured knee clinical examination with special emphasis on some of the many special tests described for knee assessment. A structured clinical approach may ensure that any significant findings are not overlooked. A selection of special tests may be utilised according to the working diagnosis.

Clinical examination of the knee follows a structured *look*, *feel*, *move*, and *special tests* approach and this is described next.

6.1 Look

The patient's lower trunk and lower limbs are exposed. The patient is inspected overall:

- Comfortable at rest or in discomfort?
- The patient is asked to stand and take a few steps to assess the overall dynamic posture, balance and mobility of lower and upper limbs
- Ability to walk with or without a walking aid is noted

The patient is asked to stand so that the examiner can move around the patient to inspect the spine, pelvis, and lower limbs (hips, knees, ankles, and feet).

C. Panayiotou Charalambous, *The Knee Made Easy*,
https://doi.org/10.1007/978-3-030-54506-2_6

Look at the:

- Front
- Side
- Back

Look for:

- Surgical or traumatic scars
- Lumps or bumps
- Abnormal or asymmetrical posture (flexion hip or knee, hyperextension knee, planovalgus/high arched feet)
- Abnormal or asymmetrical alignment—spine, pelvis, and lower limbs (hips, knees, ankles, feet)—coronal, sagittal, axial planes:
  - Static and dynamic
  - On loading (standing or walking, standing on tip-toes to assess if any foot deformity such as planovalgus is correctable)
  - On unloading
- Muscle wasting
- Skin—colour, rash or other cutaneous lesions
- Look at the patient's footwear—uneven wear?

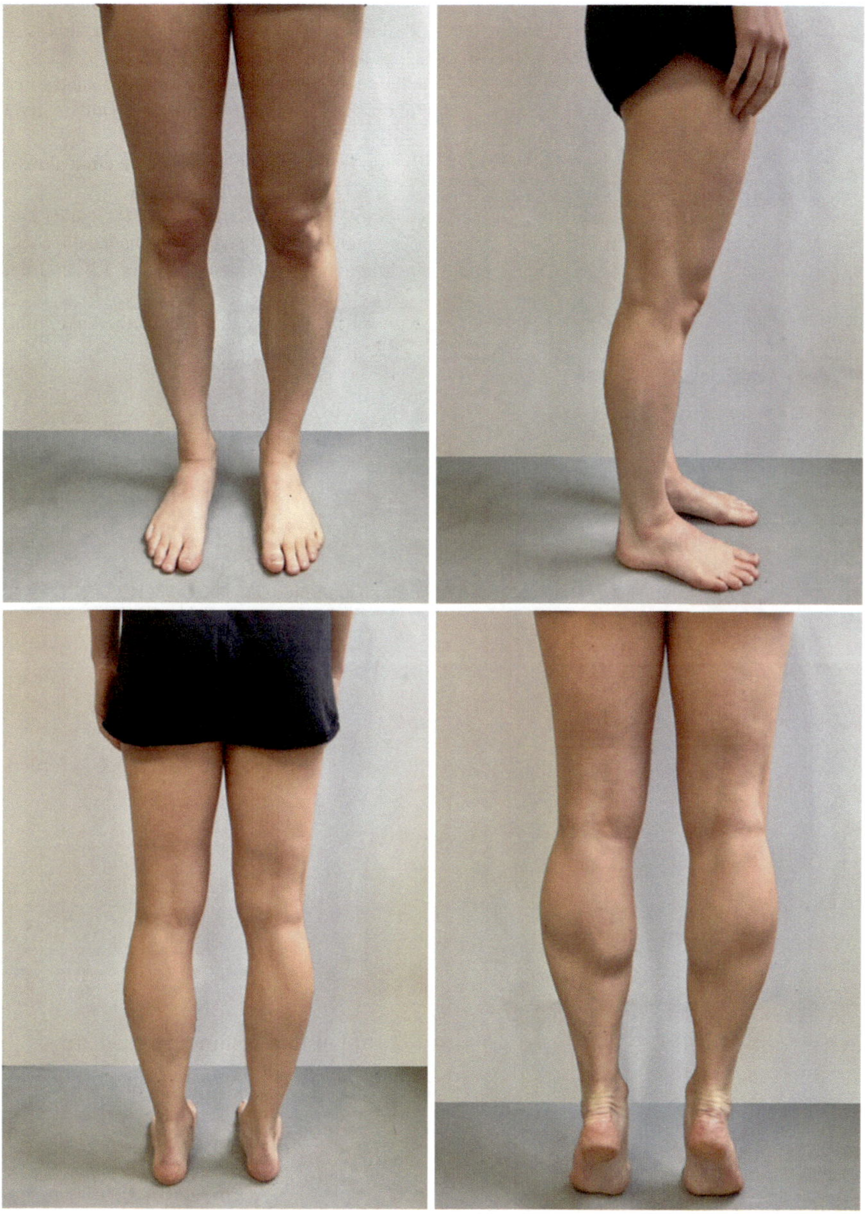

Look from the front, side and back

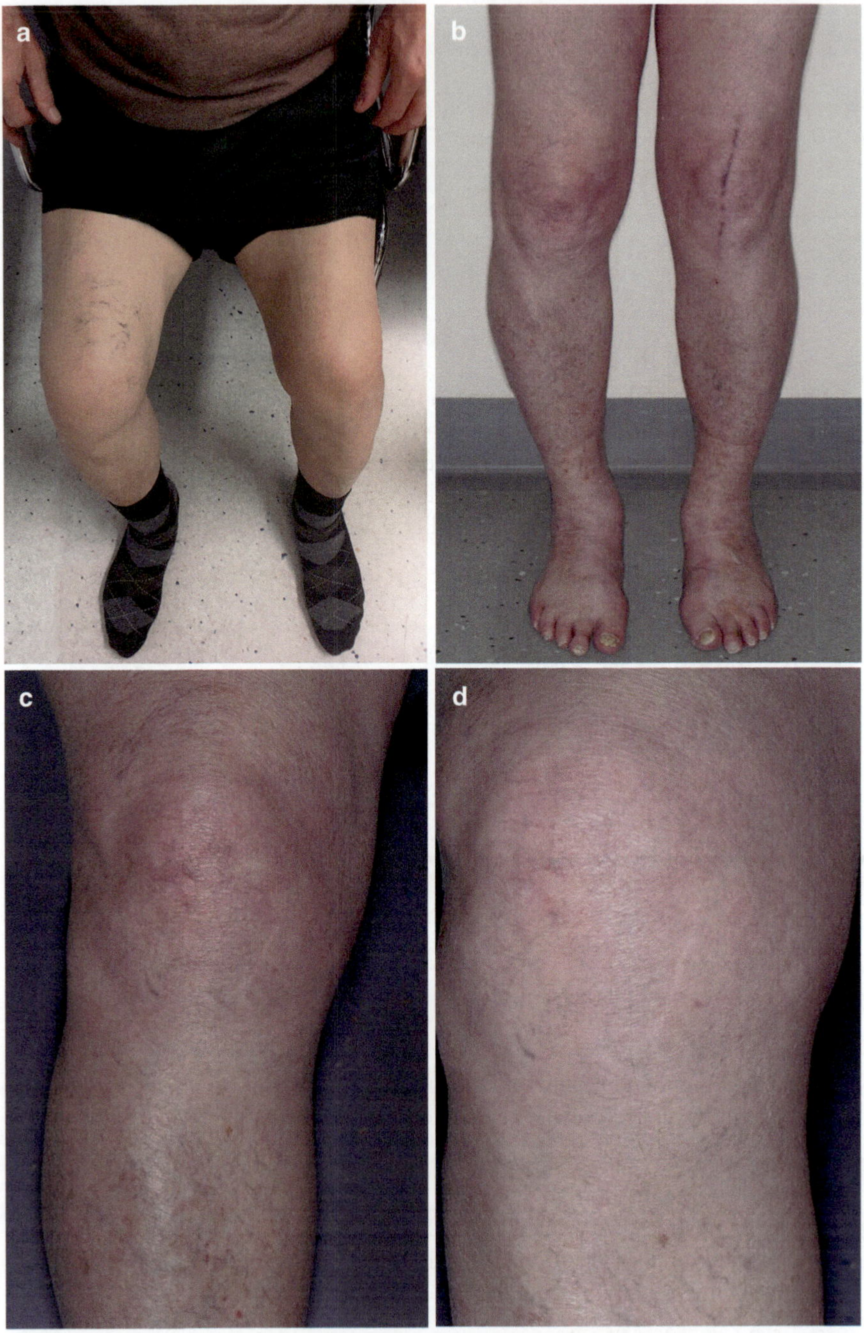

(**a**) Left knee quadriceps wasting. (**b**) Anterior knee surgical scar used in total knee replacement arthroplasty. (**c, d**) Antero-medial scar used in open medial meniscectomy

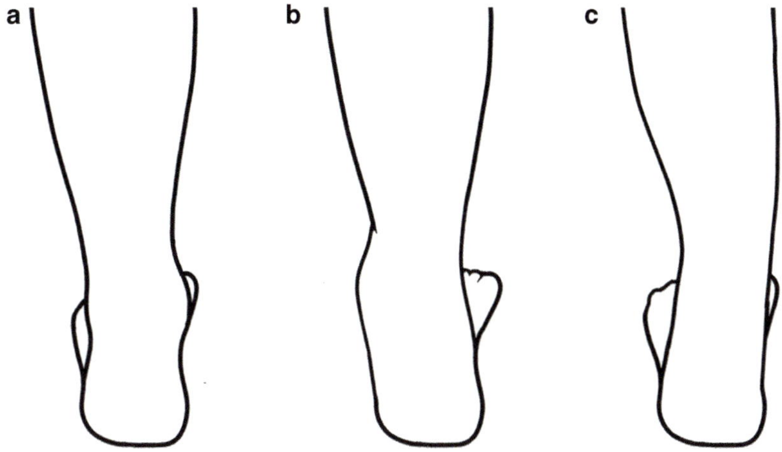

The alignment of the feet is assessed from the back (**a**) Neutral (**b**) Foot supination (**c**) Foot pronation

Special attention is paid to the alignment of the knee when:

1. Standing still, weightbearing, with the knee placed as straight as possible
2. Supine, non-weightbearing

- Coronal alignment—varus/valgus (unilateral vs. bilateral)
- Sagittal alignment—flexion posture, hyperextension posture
- Axial alignment—patellae pointing towards each other, away from each other

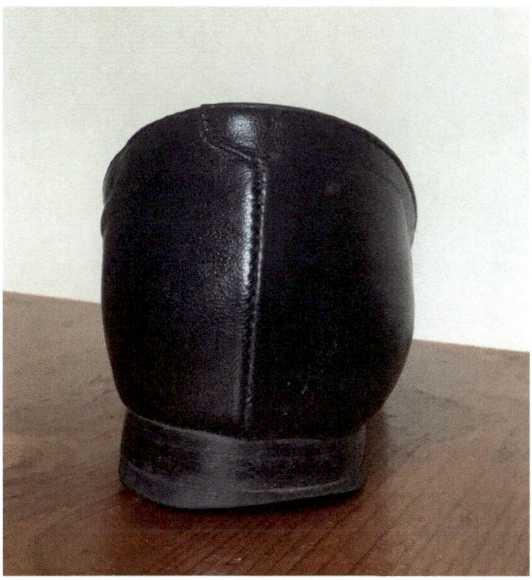

Examination of the footwear reveals uneven wear of the shoe's heel

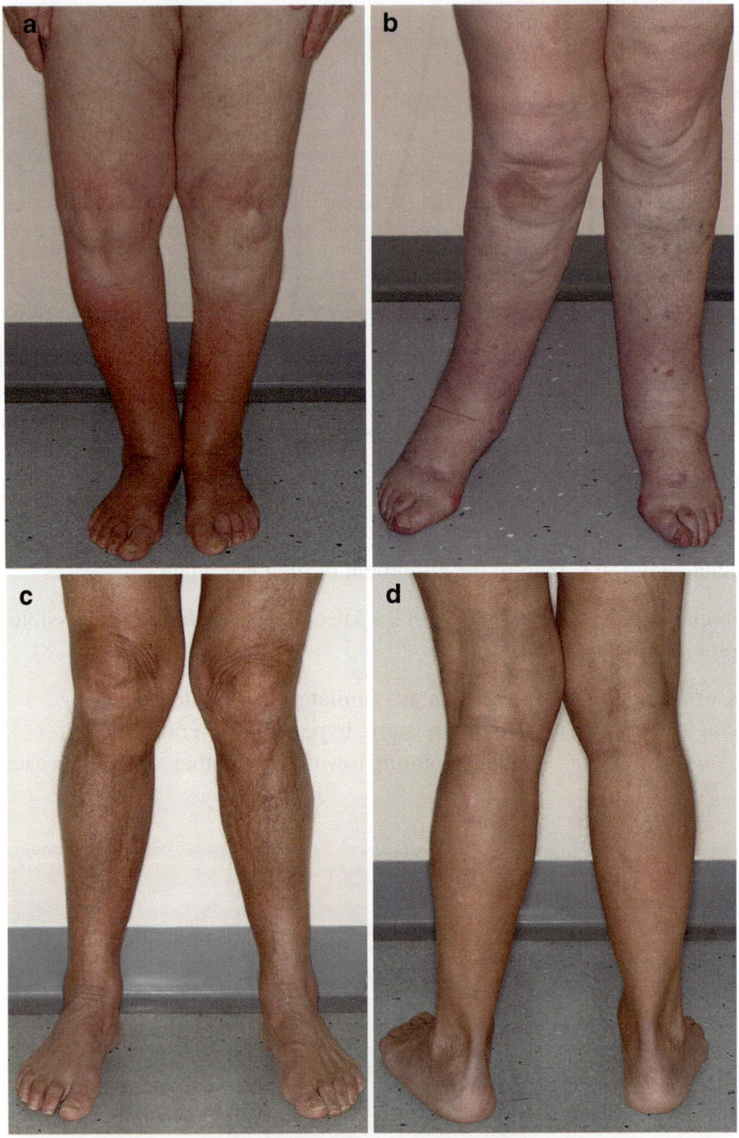

(**a**) Knee varus (**b–d**) Knee valgus

If any malalignment is noted with the patient standing, this is further examined with the patient supine, to help determine if:

- It is fully or partially correctable
- It can be worsened by application of a stress force

The ability to correct coronal malalignment is assessed in both knee extension and flexion; this may guide as to which structures are contributing to the malalignment (and hence may need addressing during surgery).

- Inability to correct a valgus deformity in both knee flexion and knee extension suggests a tight lateral collateral ligament, popliteus tendon or posterolateral capsule
- Inability to correct a valgus deformity in knee extension but not in flexion suggests a tight iliotibial band

Malalignment may be due to:

- Soft tissues
- Bony
- Combined

At the knee, coronal deformity may be due to:

- Intra-articular cause
  - Articular surface morphology
  - Articular cartilage loss
  - Meniscal loss
- Extra-articular (femoral or tibial) cause
  - Metaphyseal
  - Diaphyseal
- Ligamentous dysfunction
- Combination of the above

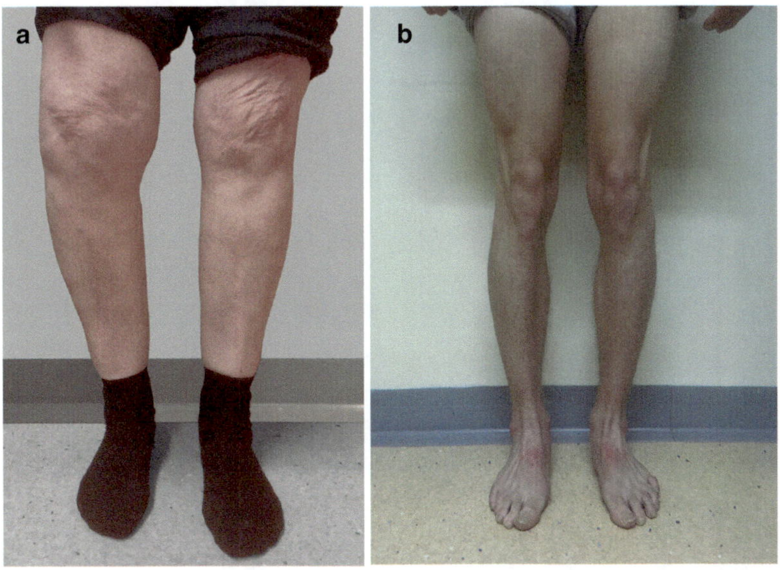

(**a**) Knee varus due to intra-articulae degeneration. (**b**) Left knee varus to metaphyseal deformity

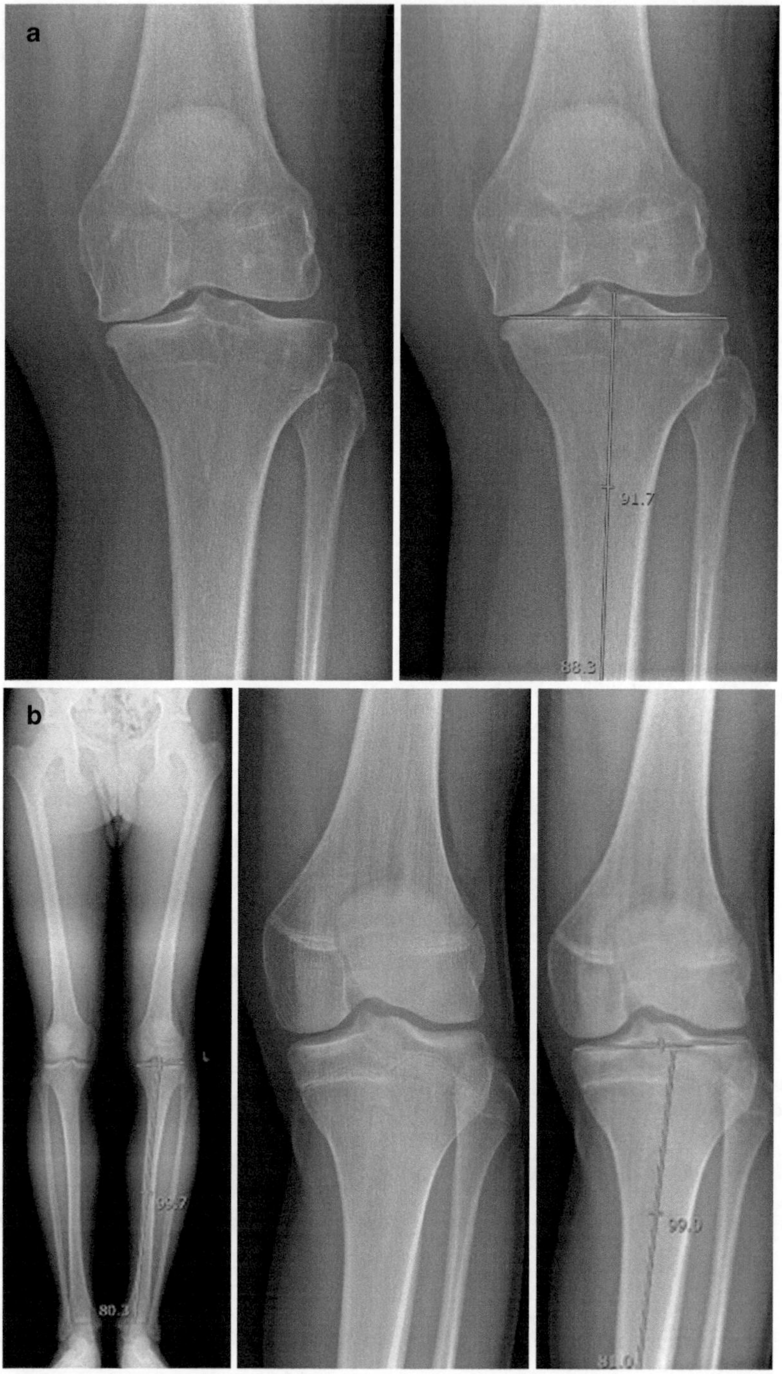

(**a**) Knee varus due to loss of medial compartment joint space and no proximal tibial deformity. (**b**) Proximal tibial vara, due to metaphyseal deformity and preservation of joint space

6.2 Feel

Palpate potential sources of pain:

- Lumbosacral spine along with paraspinal muscles
- Hips—greater trochanter, groin
- Knee
  - Tibial tuberosity
  - Patellar tendon (with the knee straight)
  - Lower and upper pole of the patella
  - Medial and lateral tibiofemoral joint line
  - Pes anserinus area
  - Medial and lateral retinaculae, medial plica
  - Proximal tibiofibular joint
  - Posterior aspect of the patella—patellar facets
  - Femoral and tibial condyles
  - Tendons around the knee
    - Medial and lateral hamstrings
    - Gastrognemius heads
    - Distal quadriceps
  - Lower leg—calf, shin

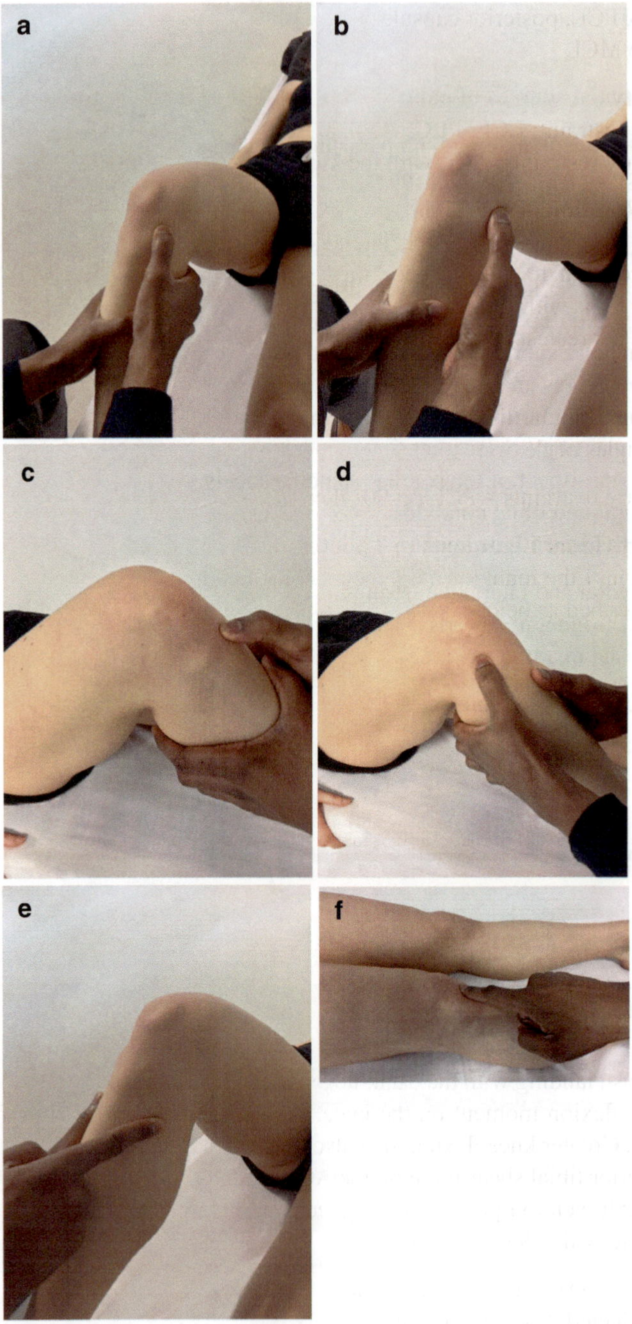

Palpation looking for localised tenderness: (**a**) Antero-medial joint line tenderness. (**b**) Postero-medial joint line tenderness. (**c**) Antero-lateral joint line tenderness. (**d**) Postero-lateral joint line tenderness. (**e**) Pes anserinus tenderness. (**f**) Patellar tendon origin tenderness

Check for effusion [4–6].

- *Patellar tap test* (for moderate effusion)—the patient lies supine with the knee straight and relaxed. With one hand the examiner compresses the suprapatellar pouch, translating any intra-articular fluid distally (and hence lifting the patella off the femur). With the opposite thumb the examiner presses briskly the patella towards the femur and then lets go whilst feeling for the patella tapping on the femur and then bouncing off. It has been shown that 14–45 cc of fluid are needed to allow a positive test. The patellar tap may disappear with higher volumes [7].
- *Fluid fluctuation test* (for a small effusion)—the patient lies supine with the knee straight and relaxed. With one hand the examiner compresses the suprapatellar pouch, translating any intra-articular fluid distally. With the opposite hand the examiner strokes upwards the medial pat of the knee from just below the joint line to the suprapatellar pouch (thus milking any fluid laterally). With the back of the same hand, the examiner then strokes downwards the lateral side of the knee looking for a fluid wave (shift) medially. This may be repeated fluctuating the fluid from one side to the other.

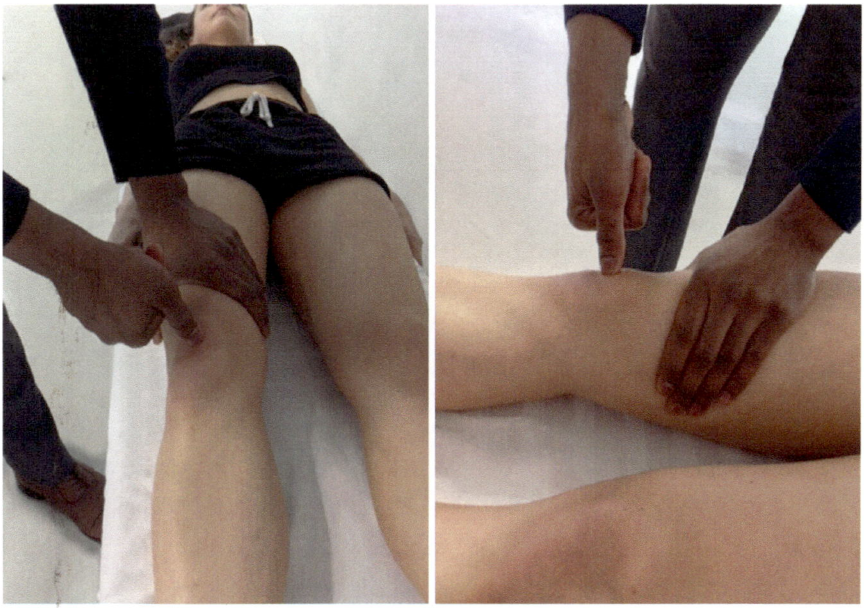

Patellar tap test

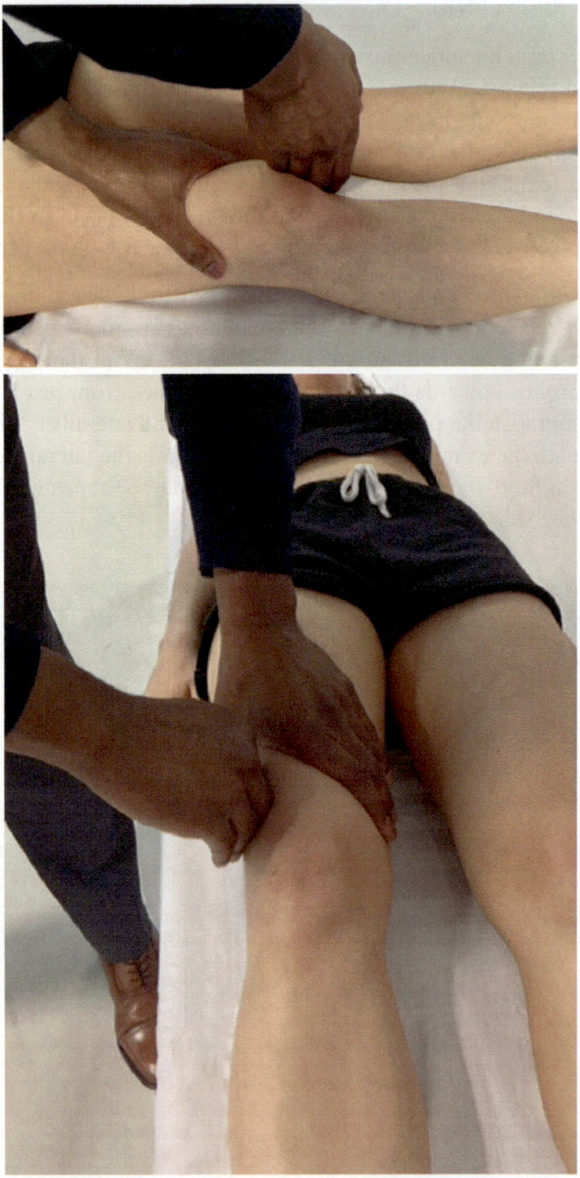

Fluid fluctuation test

Muscle bulk—muscle bulk of the thigh may be quantified by measuring the thigh circumference 10 cm proximal to the patella.

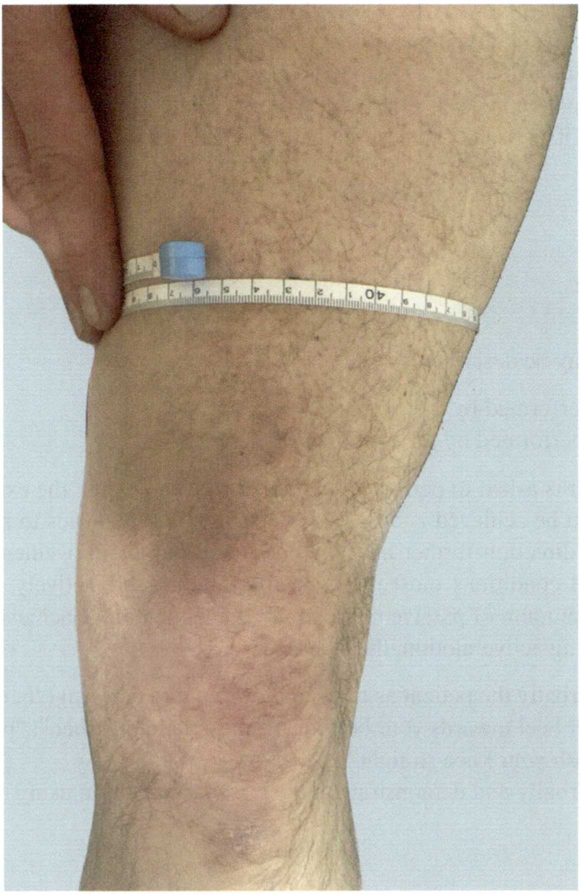

Tape measurement of thigh muscle bulk

Palpate for neurovascular status

- Sensation
- Distal pulses
  - Posterior Tibial artery
  - Dorsalis pedis
- Capillary refill

Quadriceps (Q) Angle
This is measured with the knee in 30° flexion, so the patella is centred in the trochlea. It is the angle between a line drawn from the anterior superior iliac spine to the centre of the patella and a line drawn from the centre of the tibial tubercle to the

centre of the patella. It may be assessed with the patient standing or supine. It may also be performed with the quadriceps relaxed or tense.

However, the value of the Q angle is questionable as it is not reliably reproducible, and has not been consistently shown to correlate to clinical symptoms [8–10]. Furthermore, it is a static measurement, whereas patellar tracking is a dynamic process.

6.3 Move

Movement may be described as:

- Active—performed by the patient
- Passive—performed by the examiner

The patient is asked to perform a particular movement and the extent (range) to which this can be achieved is observed. The examiner then tries to push the leg in the specified direction further and any additional passive movement is observed. Under normal conditions most motion will be achievable actively, but in certain disorders the amount of passive motion may exceed the range achieved actively.

In examining active motion, the examiner may:

- Instruct verbally the patient as to what movement to perform ("bend your knee", "bring your heel towards your bottom", "straighten your knee", "push your knee back", "push your knee straight")
- Instruct verbally and demonstrate to the patient the motion using own legs

6.3.1 Overall Gait

The patient is asked to walk and is observed from the front, back and side. Abnormal motions in the trunk, pelvis or lower limbs are determined. The following gait parameters are evaluated.

Coronal Plane

Varus thrust—this refers to an increase in varus alignment of the knee that occurs upon weightbearing (stance phase of gait), as compared to the non-weightbearing state. It indicates dynamic instability in the frontal plane. In the presence of varus thrust there is visible bowing out of the knee laterally upon weightbearing, with return to a less varus position during the swing phase (non-weightbearing). This may be better appreciated by observing the patient from behind during walking.

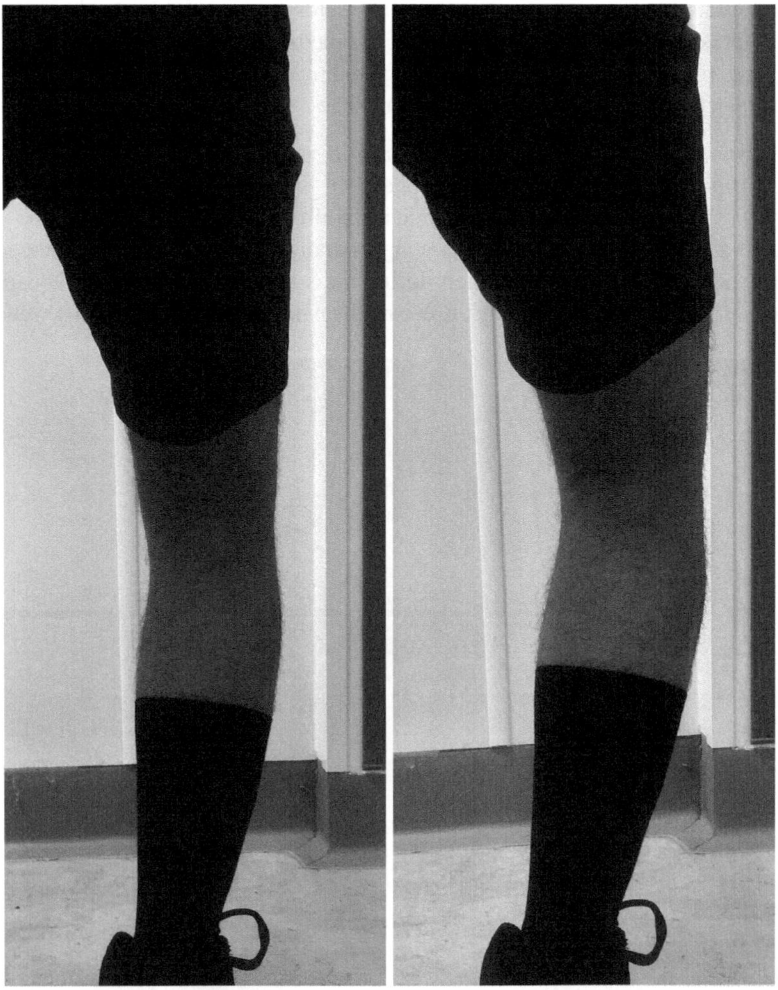

Varus thrust – upon weightbearing the knee goes into more varus (and appears to project more laterally when viewed from the back)

Varus thrust leads to an acute increase in the load of the medial compartment with each weightbearing step. Gait analysis has shown that the knee adduction moment is greater in the presence of varus thrust [11] suggesting higher loading of the medial compartment. Such thrust may increase the shear and compressive forces on the medial compartment, increasing the risk of medial compartment OA progression.

Varus thrust causes include:

- Idiopathic
- Neuromuscular deficiency such as quadriceps weakness
- Extra-articular tibiofemoral varus

- Bony/articular causes—articular cartilage loss/meniscal loss with increased compression (and hence narrowing) of the medial compartment
- Elongation/disruption of the lateral ligamentous restraints to varus, with resultant opening up of the lateral side of the knee

Valgus thrust—this refers to an increase in valgus alignment of the knee that occurs upon weightbearing (stance phase of gait), as compared to the non-weightbearing state. It indicates dynamic instability in the frontal plane. In the presence of valgus thrust there is visible bowing medially of the knee upon weightbearing, with return to a less valgus position during the swing phase (non-weightbearing). This may be better appreciated by observing the patient from behind during walking.

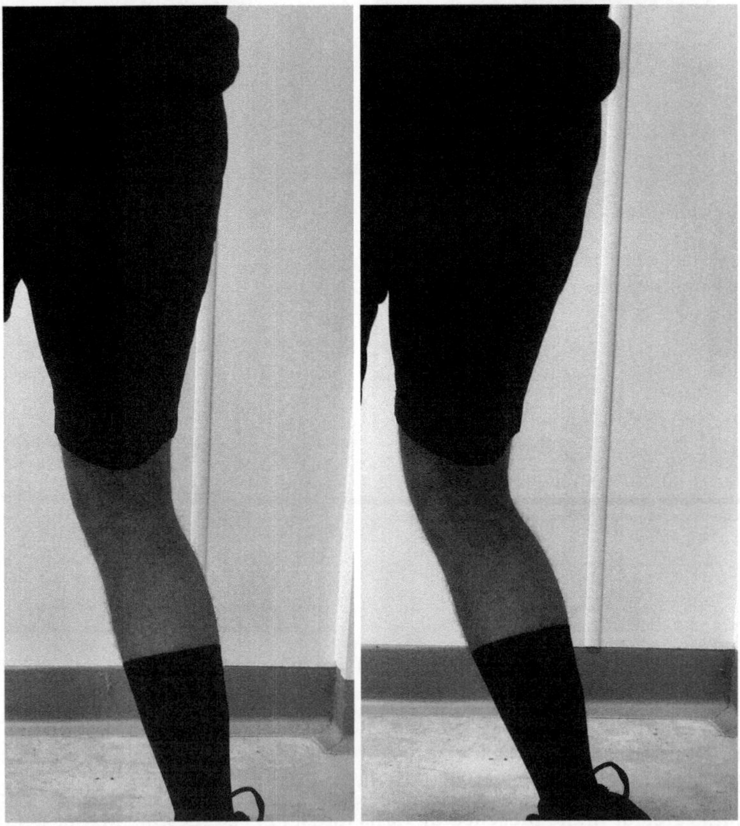

Valgus thrust – looking at left knee from the back upon weightbearing the knee goes into more valgus (and appears to project more medially)

Valgus thrust is much less common than varus thrust.

Valgus thrust may be:

- Idiopathic
- Due to deficiency of the medial collateral ligament (MCL)
- Neuromuscular deficiency such as quadriceps weakness
- Extra-articular valgus
- Intra-articular causes—articular cartilage loss/meniscal loss with increased compression (and hence narrowing) of the lateral compartment on weightbearing

Chang et al [12] looked at the frequency of varus and valgus thrust and factors associated with thrust presence in persons with or at higher risk of developing knee osteoarthritis.

Varus thrust was seen in 32% of those without radiographic evidence of OA and in 37% of those with radiographic evidence of OA. Valgus thrust was seen in 7% and 9% respectively.

In those with no radiographic OA the following factors were associated with the presence of varus thrust:

- Caucasians > African-Americans
- Older age
- Higher BMI
- Varus malalignment
- Male gender
- Reduced knee extensor strength

In those with OA the following factors were associated with the presence of varus thrust:

- Varus malalignment, severe OA, male gender

Valgus thrust was seen more commonly in African–Americans compared to Caucasians and in valgus malalignment.

Sagittal plane

- Hip, Knee, ankle and foot
  - Flexion/extension

Axial plane

- Foot static alignment—in-toeing, out-toeing
- Foot progression angle—in-toeing, out-toeing
- Patellae static/dynamic alignment-pointing inwards/outwards

Some gaits to note are:

- Antalgic gait—this may be seen in the presence of lower limb pain. The patient avoids weightbearing on the painful leg, hence the stance time is shortened and the swing time is increased.
- Foot drop gait—the patient bends the knee and hip much more during the swing phase (almost as if climbing stairs) to help clear the foot off the floor. A slap may be heard when the foot makes contact with the ground as ankle dorsiflexion at heel contact is not possible, and contact with the ground is uncontrolled.
- Trendelenburg gait—the pelvis drops on the non-weight bearing side or the patient leans the trunk towards the affected side.
- Knee recurvatum gait—the knee goes into hyperextension upon weightbearing

6.3.2 Knee Movements Assessed

- Flexion
  - Patient is supine and is asked to bend the knee and bring the foot towards the buttock (active flexion). The examiner then grasps the tibia and tries to flex the knee further to see if any further (passive) motion is possible. The amount of flexion is described in relation to the angle between the lower leg and thigh (tibia in relation to femur) or in terms of the distance between the heel and buttock.
- Extension
  - Patient is supine and is asked to straighten the knee pressing it down onto the couch (active extension). The examiner then stabilises the femur with one hand and grasps the tibia and tries to extend the knee further to see if any further (passive) motion is possible. The amount of extension is described in relation to the angle between the lower leg and thigh (tibia in relation to femur). This is negative if short of full extension, positive if hyperextension. During active knee extension, the examiner may place the hand under the knee to determine if there is any gap between the knee and couch, as an indication of loss of extension.

- Straight leg raising (with foot in dorsiflexion, as it improves the efficiency of the knee extensors)—"pull your foot towards your face, and now try and lift your leg up"

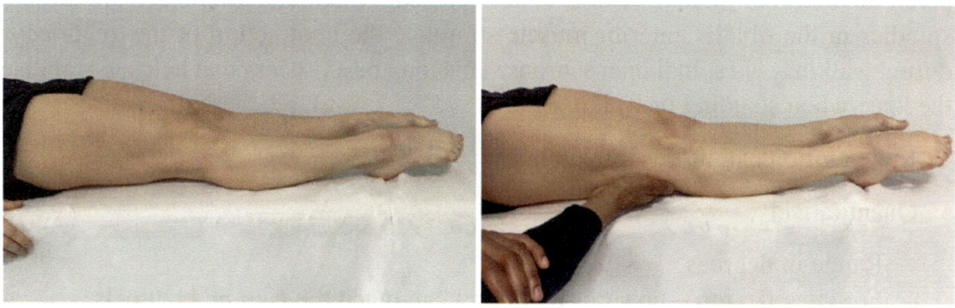

Assessment of knee extension

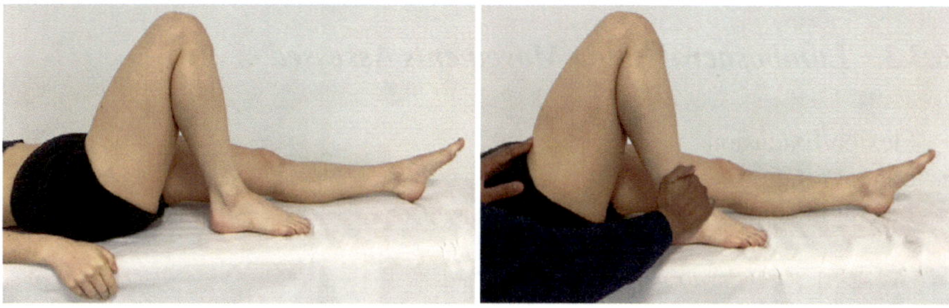

Assessment of active and passive knee flexion

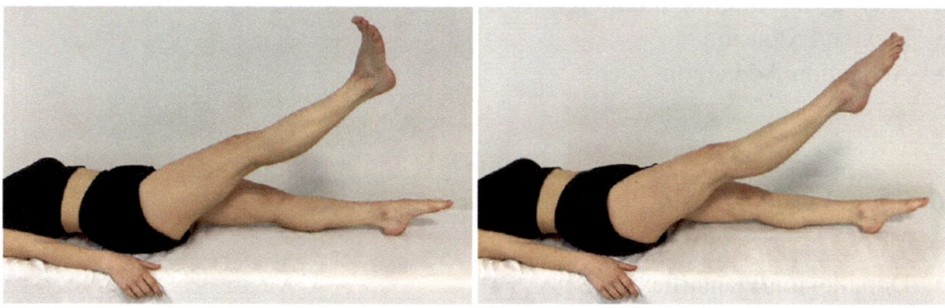

Active straight leg raising with dorsiflexion and plantarflexion of the foot

It has been shown that ankle dorsiflexion facilitates knee extension [13, 14]. Maximum electromyographic activity of the quadriceps during ankle dorsiflexion is greater than with the ankle in neutral position. Ankle dorsiflexion has been shown to enhance quadriceps activity during isokinetic or isometric strengthening as compared to neutral or plantar flexion. It has been suggested that afferents from muscle spindles in the tibialis anterior muscle stimulate the contraction of the quadriceps during walking, via spinal interneurons. This may be a process that helps to stabilise the knee when standing or walking.

Knee motion can be described:

- Quantitatively:
  - Range in degrees
  - For knee flexion—how close the heel can reach the patient's buttock
- Qualitatively—smooth, interrupted

6.3.3 Lumbosacral Spine Movements Assessed

- Flexion/Extension
- Lateral rotation
- Lateral flexion

6.3.4 Hip Movements Assessed

- Internal and external rotation
- Flexion/Extension
- Abduction/Adduction

6.3.5 Ankle Movements Assessed

- Dorsiflexion/Plantarflexion
- Ability to stand on tip toes/ability to stand on heels

Testing for internal and external rotation of the hip (looking for limitation of motion and pain upon movement) is a good screening test for hip movements and in most cases that will suffice.

6.4 Special Tests in Knee Examination

Special tests are clinical examination manoeuvres that aim to assess the presence of specific disorders or the specific source of an individual's symptoms. Such tests may examine:

- Muscle strength
- Muscle stiffness
- Pain provocation
- Apprehension provocation
- Instability provocation
- Other symptom provocation

In an ideal situation, special tests aim to isolate and specifically test one structure or group of structures at a time such as:

- One muscle at a time in assessing muscle strength
- One pain source structure at a time in assessing pain provocation
- One process at a time in assessing apprehension
- One group of structures in assessing instability

An ideal special test is one which has high:

- Sensitivity—the ability of a test to correctly identify diseased states
- Specificity—the ability of a test to correctly identify non-diseased states

However, the qualities of commonly used special tests in Orthopaedic examinations and specifically in examination of the knee have been questioned. Such tests are often not highly sensitive or specific [15–18]. This may be due to:

- Close anatomical relationship of various structures which make it difficult to isolate and test a single structure.
- Multiple structures having common innervation, hence causing similar pain upon provocation.
- Multiple structures may have similar functions and, hence, compensate for the loss of one of those—such as one ligament compensating for the loss of another ligament.
- A test may point towards the area of origin of symptoms, but not identify the pathology in that area—such as tibiofemoral joint pain being the final result of multiple pathological conditions in the joint.
- The mechanism of why some tests are positive in certain disorders may not be fully understood.

- The extent of symptoms such as pain upon provocation tests may not be all or none but vary widely, with no cut off point as to when a test is considered positive. Hence, there is often a subjective component in quantifying what is substantial pain, what is exacerbated pain, or what is pain out of proportion.
- Some tests may be unreliable or very difficult to perform in the presence of concomitant pathology, as that pathology may:
- Prevent the individual from placing the knee in the position required to carry out the test (such as flexing the acutely injured knee to 90° to assess the cruciate ligaments with the drawer test)
- Cause symptoms similar to the ones that the special test aims to elicit (such as testing for a meniscal tear in the presence of extensive tibiofemoral arthritis)

A systematic review into special knee tests has shown that many tests for meniscal pathology, laxity and instability are inaccurate, have substantial variation between clinicians and may thus not be useful in clinical practise [3].

These limitations of special tests must be taken into account in clinical examination. Special tests should thus be used with caution, and considered as an additional piece to the diagnostic jigsaw rather than a process that gives an absolute answer.

A plethora of special tests have been described for knee disorders but a description of all of these is beyond the scope of this book. In addition, the use of a multitude of knee tests is often practically impossible in routine clinical practise. Hence, clinicians often choose and utilise certain tests in their routine examination. Special tests used by the author in clinical examination of the knee are presented here.

6.5 Assessing Muscle Strength in Knee Examination

Assessing muscle strength is challenging as:

- It is essential to distinguish between true and apparent weakness (weakness due to pain or stiffness)
- Several muscles may contribute to a motion, and loss of one may be compensated by others

In grading muscle strength the following are considered:

Medical Research Council grading system whereby muscle strength is graded 0–5 [19]:

- Grade 0—No muscle contraction.
- Grade 1—Flicker or trace of muscle contractions.
- Grade 2—Contraction enabling movement with gravity eliminated.
- Grade 3—Contraction enabling movement against gravity.
- Grade 4—Active movement against gravity and resistance.
- Grade 5—Normal motor function.

Alternatively, a more simplified grading system may be utilised, whereby three grades of muscle strength are described as:

- Strong
- Weak but can maintain preposition
- Severely week—cannot maintain preposition

In assessing muscle strength the following approach may be utilised:

- Ask the patient to perform the motion actively. This will guide as to whether there is severe weakness or only some weakness
- Then place the leg passively to the position you would expect the patient to achieve and ask them to keep it there. In the case of straight leg raising be ready to catch the patient's leg, to stop it from dropping suddenly and causing discomfort, if the patient cannot maintain straight leg raising.
- If the patient can maintain the position then proceed to further examine strength and quantify it or compare it to the opposite healthy knee where applicable. This is achieved by asking the patient to keep the leg in the position whilst you apply an opposing force.

6.5.1 Testing Muscle Strength—Individual Muscles

6.5.1.1 Quadriceps

Active Extension Lag

The patient sits at the side of the bed with the knee flexed and is asked to straighten the knee actively. An attempt is then made to further straighten the knee by the examiner passively. The difference between the two is the active extension lag. Some degree of active extension lag is physiological and normal (2–4°, the higher limit reached with more prolonged active knee extension) [20].

Quadriceps Resistance Strength Test

The patient sits at the side of the bed with the knee flexed and is asked to extend the knee and maintain that position resisting a downward force on the tibia applied by the examiner. It is preferable for the examiner to apply the force close to the knee, to minimise the moment arm effect (moment exerted at the joint is equal to the applied force multiplied by the distance at which this force is exerted from the joint).

For either test, the patient may be able to demonstrate that in order to extend their bad knee, they have to assist it with the opposite good one, which is suggestive of substantial weakness of knee extension.

6.5.1.2 Hamstrings

Flexion Strength

Whilst sitting or lying flat, the patient is asked to flex the knee and maintain that position resisting a straightening force on the tibia applied by the examiner. It is preferable for the examiner to apply the force close to the knee.

- The test may be repeated with the patient lying prone (to assess the ability to flex against gravity)
- By prepositioning the lower leg it may be possible to test the medial and lateral hamstrings selectively (higher hamstring activity with ipsilateral rotation—medial hamstrings with medial tibial rotation, lateral hamstrings with lateral tibial rotation) [21, 22]. Mohamed et al. [21] looked at tibial rotation at 70° of knee flexion and found statistically greater torque production and electromyography activation of the medial and lateral hamstrings during ipsilateral rotation (for the semimembranosus and semitendinosus prepositioning of the tibia in internal rotation, and biceps femoris prepositioning of the tibia in external rotation). Beyer et al. [22] showed that the greatest force production in the lateral hamstrings occurs at 30° knee flexion and decreases with higher flexion (whilst activation of the medial hamstrings was not affected by knee flexion).

6.6 Pain Provoking Tests

In these tests the examiner performs a manoeuvre and asks the patient to report as to whether new pain is experienced or ongoing pain is worsened. The patient' face is observed for any sign to suggest apprehension or pain.

6.6.1 *Patellofemoral Compression Test* [2, 23]

Passive—the patient lies supine. The examiner presses downwards on the anterior surface of the patella (pressing the patella onto the trochlea) with both thumbs or palm of one hand, whilst passively flexing and extending the knee. Pain and grinding may suggest patellofemoral dysfunction (including degeneration, chondral lesions).

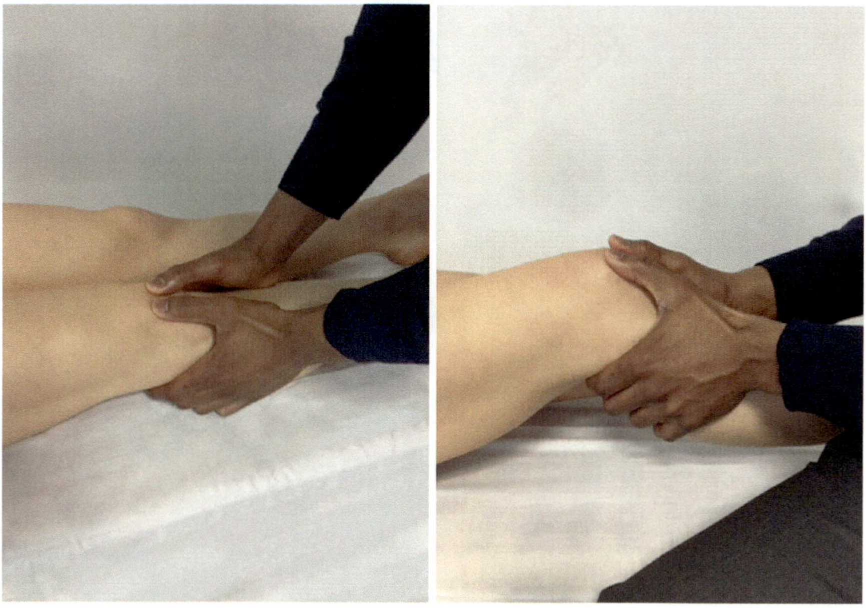

Passive patellofemoral compression test

Active—above is repeated but with patient actively flexing and extending the knee.

Alternatively, instead of flexing the knee, the patella is held with the thumb and index finger by the examiner. With the patient's leg relaxed and straight the patella is pressed against the medial and lateral femoral condyles. By moving the patella in an upward and downward direction most of its articular surface may be assessed. Pain or an unpleasant sensation are sought.

6.6.2 Meniscal Tear Pain Provoking Tests

McMurray's Test [24]

Medial meniscal tear—The patient lies flat, relaxed. The examiner grasps the patient's foot on the affected side. The knee and hip are fully flexed until the heel approaches the buttock. Whilst holding the leg in external rotation the knee is passively extended. The examiner palpates the medial joint line. Pain and clicking on the medial tibiofemoral joint suggests a possible tear of the posterior horn of the medial meniscus.

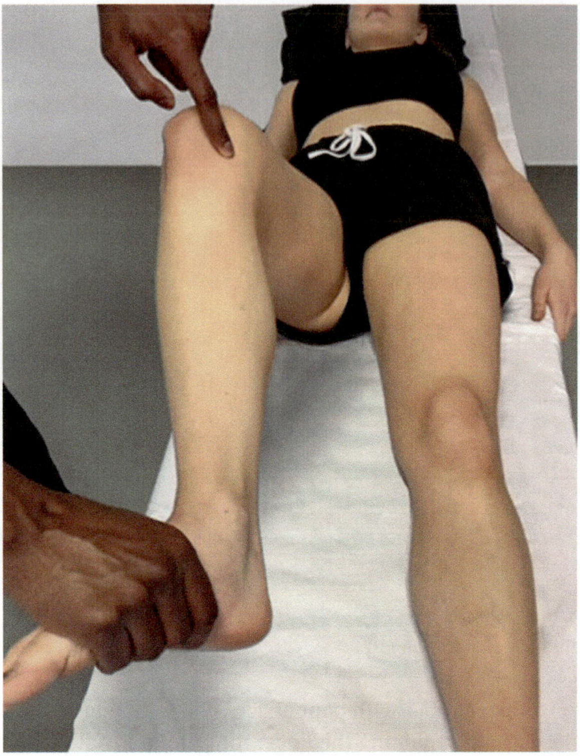

McMurray's test for medial meniscal tear

Lateral meniscal tear—The patient lies flat, relaxed. The examiner grasps the patient's foot on the affected side. The knee and hip are fully flexed until the heel approaches the buttock. Whilst holding the leg in internal rotation the knee is passively extended. The examiner palpates the lateral joint line. Pain and clicking on the lateral tibiofemoral joint suggests a possible tear of the lateral meniscus.

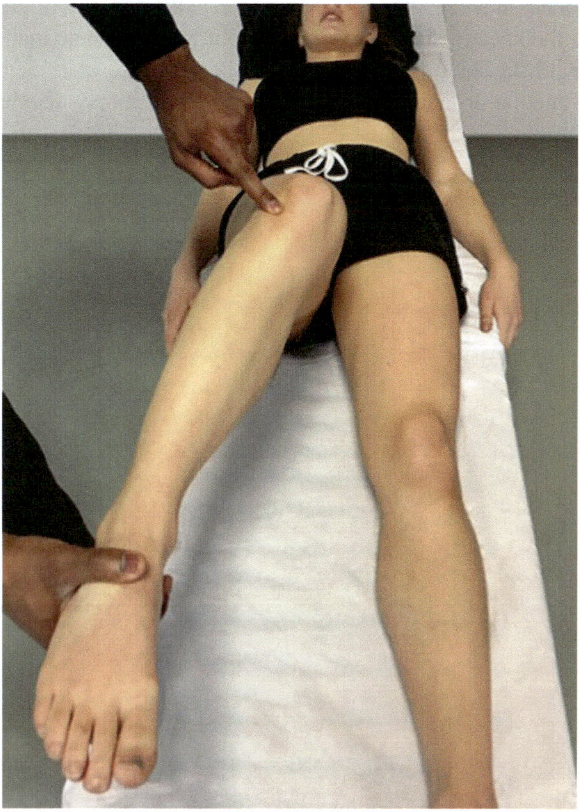

McMurray's test for lateral meniscal tear

In the initial description, a painful palpable click was essential for a positive test. However, it is recognised that a click may not be present, and instead localised pain, reproducing the patient's symptoms may suffice for a positive test. A non-painful click may be seen even with an intact meniscus.

In this test, the principle is that with leg rotation the torn meniscal fragment becomes entrapped between the femoral and tibial condyles causing pain or clicking. External rotation tests the medial meniscus, whilst internal rotation tests the lateral meniscus. However, it has been shown that paradoxical findings may occur, with external rotation identifying a lateral meniscal tear and vice versa.

McMurray's test has been shown to have a high specificity especially with regards to the lateral meniscus but low sensitivity and low inter-rater reliability.

Thesally Test [25]

This test aims to load the meniscus and reproduce the patient's symptoms in the presence of a meniscal tear. The examiner supports the patient by holding his/her outstretched hands, whilst the patient stands with one foot flat on the floor. The patient then rotates his/her knee and body, internally and externally, three times, whilst keeping the knee in slight flexion (of about 5°). The same manoeuvre is then repeated but with the knee flexed at 20°. In the presence of a meniscal tear, the patient reports medial or lateral joint-line discomfort and may also have a sense of locking/catching.

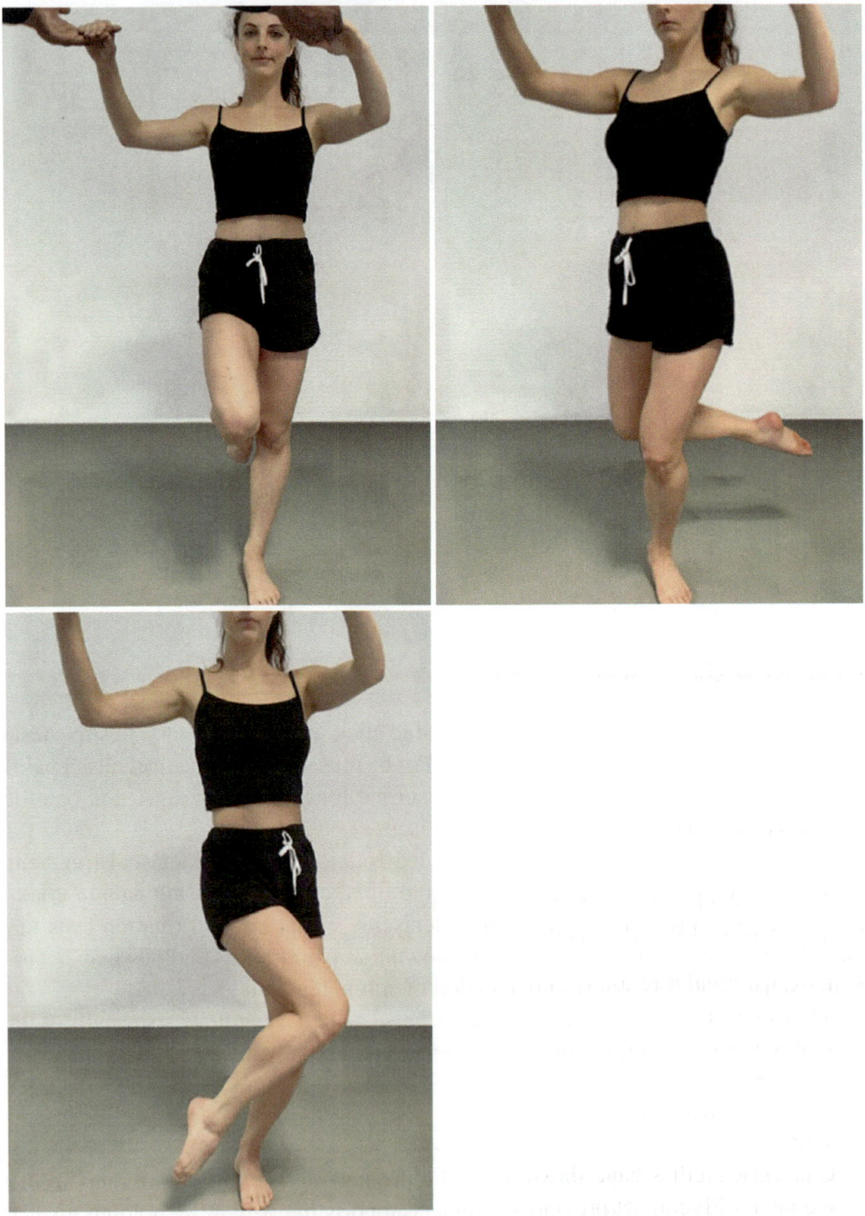

Thesally test

6.6.3 *Hoffa's Test [26]*

The patient lies supine with the hip and knee flexed about 45°. The examiner presses with both thumbs on either side of the patellar tendon, just below the inferior pole of the patella, whilst the patient extends the knee actively. The test is positive if it causes pain at the level of the patellar tendon, due to impingement of the infrapatellar fat pad between the femur, tibia and patella.

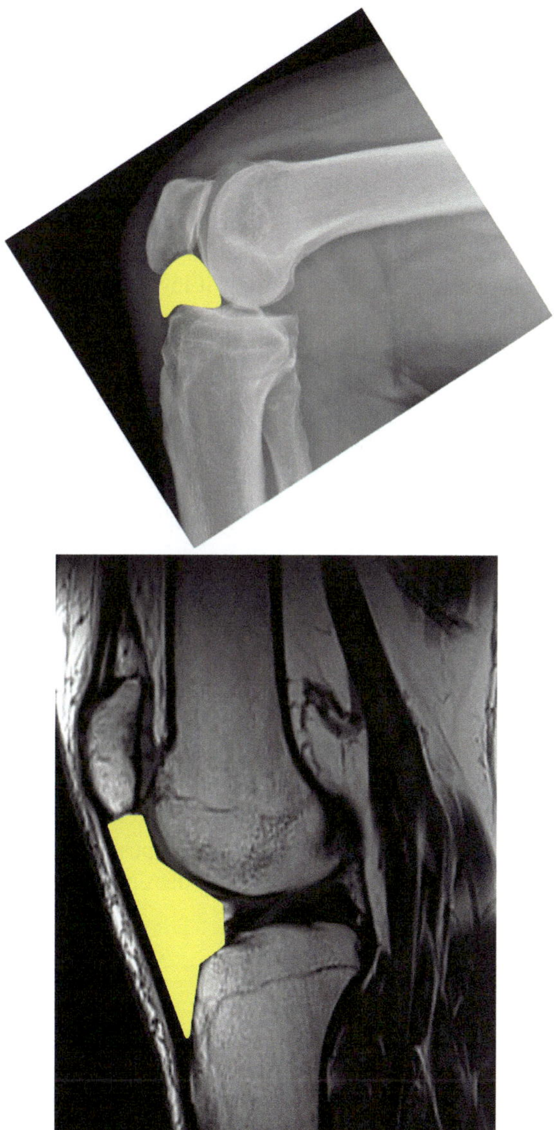

Change in the position of the fat pad with knee flexion and extension. In flexion the fat pad is accommodated by the femoral notch. In contrast, in extension the fat pat is squeezed between the patellar tendon and distal femoral condyle

6.6.4 Medial Patellar Plica (MPP) Test [27]

The patient is supine with the knee extended. The examiner's thumb presses the inferomedial part of the patellofemoral joint, compressing the medial plica between the medial femoral condyle and the patella. While maintaining the pressure by the thumb, the knee is flexed to 90°. The knee is positive when it causes pain with the knee in extension, but minimal or no pain with the knee in 90° flexion.

6.7 Laxity Assessment

Hyperlaxity refers to the presence of excessive joint laxity (excessive joint translation or motion). This may be described with regards to the tibiofemoral joint of the knee as excessive translation of the tibia in relation to the femur, or in the patellofemoral joint as excessive translation of the patella in relation to the trochlea. It may also be described as generalised hyperlaxity if it involves multiple joints. The following tests may be used in the assessment of laxity.

6.7.1 Assessment of Tibiofemoral Knee Laxity

6.7.1.1 Anterior Knee Laxity

Lachman Test [28]

The patient is lying supine. The knee is flexed to about 30°. The examiner is sat by the patient, places one hand behind the posteromedial part of the tibia (just below the knee) and the other on the patient's anterior thigh (just above the knee), and pulls the tibia anteriorly noting:

- The extend of anterior translation of the tibia in relation to the femur
- The presence of a firm end point to this translation

Excessive anterior translation compared to the opposite site, or a soft or absent end point to the translation, is suggestive of ACL disruption.

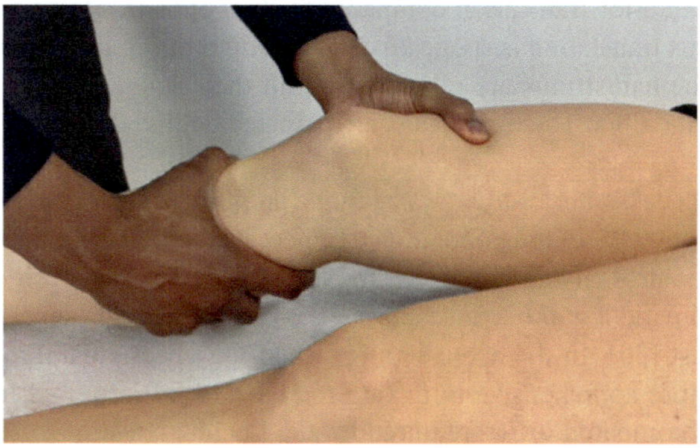

Lachman test for anterior knee laxity

Anterior Drawer Test [29]

The patient is lying supine. The knee is flexed to 90°. The examiner is sat on the patient's foot, places the hands behind the tibia (just below the knee), and pulls the tibia forwards noting:

- The extend of anterior translation of the tibia in relation to the femur
- The presence of a firm end point to this translation

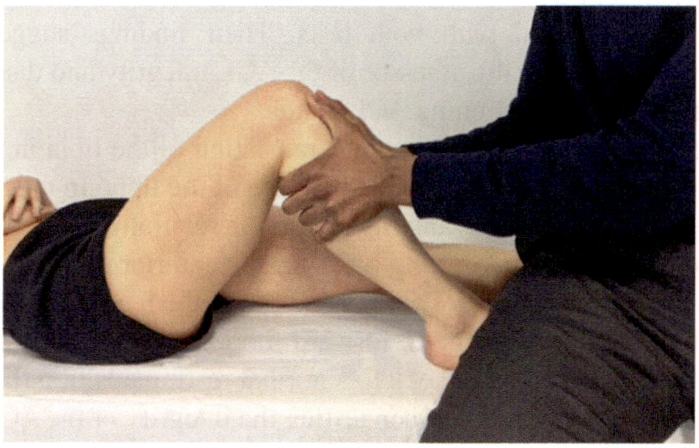

Anterior drawer test for anterior knee laxity

Excessive anterior translation compared to the opposite site or a soft or absent end point to this translation is suggestive of ACL disruption. It is important that during this test the hamstrings are relaxed, to limit their active opposition to anterior translation of the tibia. The hamstrings are palpated behind the knee to confirm they are relaxed.

In normal knees, anterior tibial translation varies very little between left and right knees (<2 mm in 95% of the population). Hence, it is important to use the contralateral knee as control (if uninjured). In the acute setting it has been shown that (if examining the patient without anaesthesia) the Lachman test is superior to the anterior drawer test [30]. In the acute setting, when the knee is painful, the patient is likely to be more apprehensive in flexing the knee to 90° required for the anterior drawer test as compared to 30° required for the Lachman test.

It has been suggested that the:

- Anteromedial (AM) band of the ACL is the primary restraint to anterior tibial translation at 90° of flexion, hence tested by the anterior drawer test.
- Posterolateral (PL) band is the primary restraint at 20° of flexion, hence tested by the Lachman test.

However, Rosenberg TD and Rasmussen GL [31] assessed the tension of the ACL arthroscopically in young adult patients with intact knee ligaments and menisci. They assessed tension in the AM, central, and PL parts of the ACL before and during an anterior drawer test (90° knee flexion) and a Lachman test (15° knee flexion). Baseline tension was greater at 15° of flexion than at 90°. A Lachman test produced maximal tension in most of the ligament, whilst the anterior drawer did not produce maximum tension in any part of the ligament. Tension in the AM and central parts predominated with both tests. Their findings suggested that the Lachman test is a more specific assessor of the ACL integrity and disputed the concept of two reciprocally functioning ACL bands.

When assessing the amount of anterior translation of the tibia in relation to the femur, it is vital to determine the starting position of the tibia. In neutral position of the intact knee, the tibia shows an anterior step-off in relation to the femur (5–10 mm) which must be considered the starting point for the anterior drawer test. If the tibia starts in a posteriorly displaced position in relation to the femur (as seen in posterior cruciate ligament (PCL) deficiency), forward motion of the tibia by the examiner may simply signify its relocation back to a normal resting position (but mistaken as excessive anterior laxity). Hence, when testing the integrity of the ACL, it is important to relocate the tibia to a normal resting position (anterior to the femur) and then determine any further anterior laxity from that point forwards. Otherwise, the relocation motion back to a normal resting position may be mistaken for anterior knee laxity.

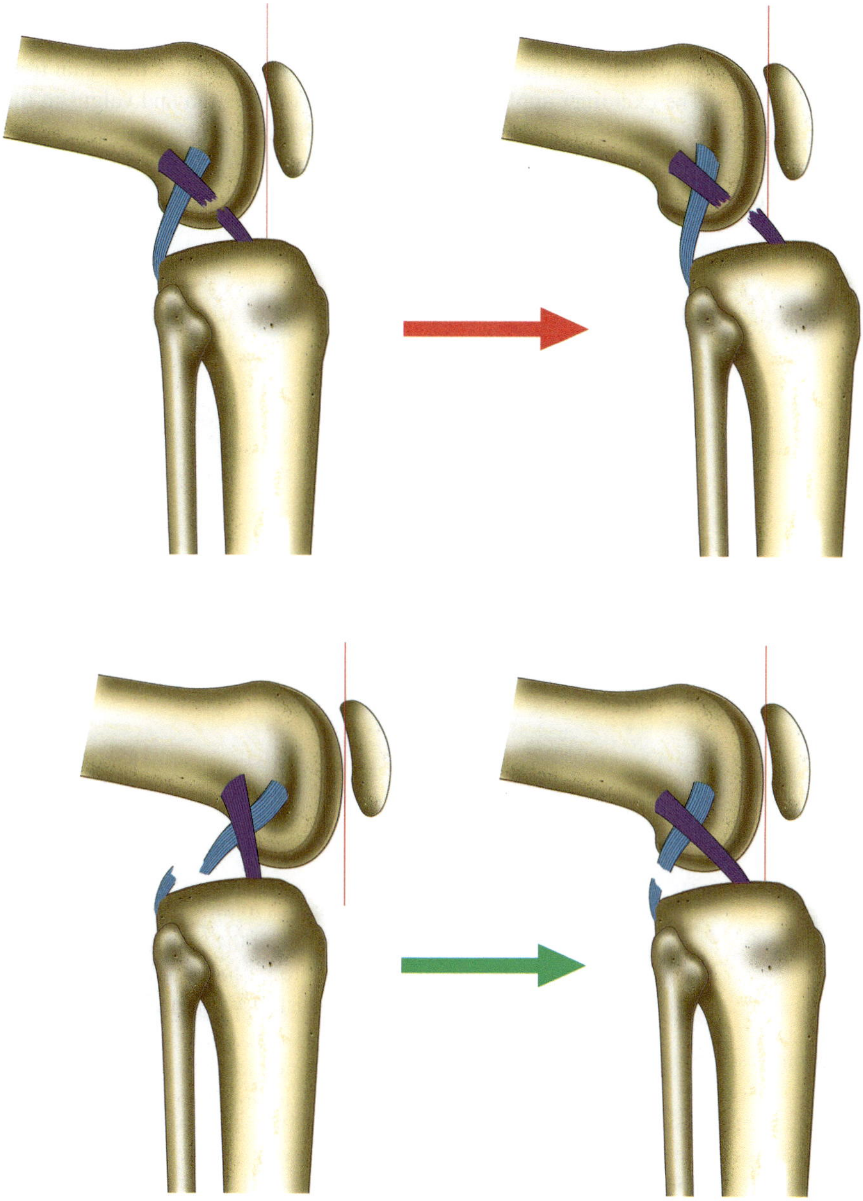

When performing the anterior drawer test, any posterior sag must be corrected prior to applying an anterior force to test the ACL. Anterior translation of a posteriorly sagged tibia, may be misinterpreted as an ACL disruption

Pivot Shift Test [32]

The patient is supine. The examiner holds the leg straight and places the distal tibia under the arm. The examiner applies internal rotation of the tibia and valgus to the knee, and then flexes the knee. The test is positive if, as the knee flexes from full extension to about 20–30°, the tibia translates backwards in relation to the femur (with a smooth glide or a sudden clunk).

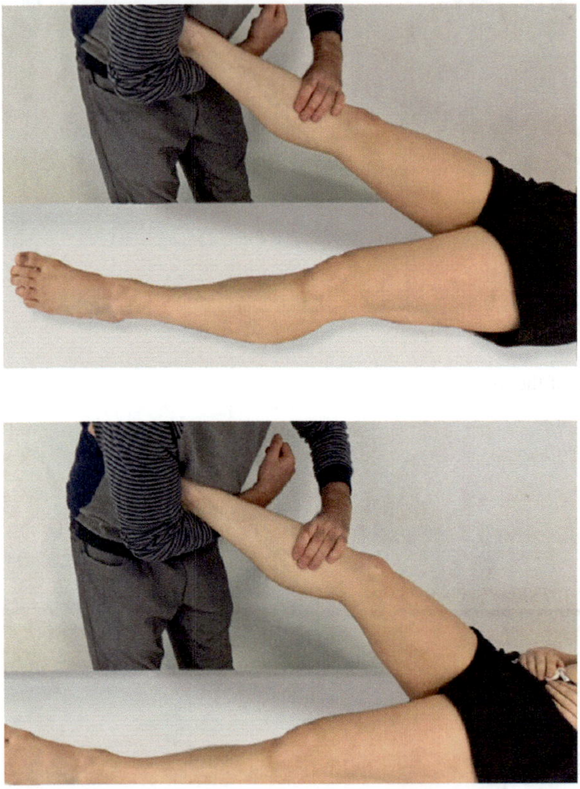

Pivot shift test maneuvre

During the pivot shift, with the knee just short of full extension and the tibia held by the examiner and internally rotated, the effect of gravity on the femur results in anterior subluxation of the tibia in relation to the femur (if there is ACL deficiency). As the knee flexes beyond 20° the iliotibial band pulls the tibia posteriorly reducing its anterior subluxation. Hence, the pivot shift depends on the integrity of the iliotibial tract. If the iliotibial band is insufficient it will not cause reduction and will allow continued tibial subluxation throughout flexion. In complete extension, tightening of the posterior capsule causes reduction, hence in full extension there is no pivot shift. The knee is most unstable at 10–20° flexion.

In the presence of OA, the rotation and subluxation required for the pivot shift to be effective can be limited, and hence may influence the reliability of the test. It is also of note that displaced meniscal tears may falsely give a negative anterior translation test or pivot shift test, as they limit tibiofemoral motion [33].

Markolf et al. [34] studied the relationship between the pivot shift and Lachman tests in a cadaver study. The magnitude of the pivot shift test and anterior laxity of the ACL did not show a linear correlation. They concluded that:

- The magnitude of laxity of an injured knee, when considered alone, may not accurately predict the magnitude of the pivot shift.
- However, the difference in anterior laxity between the injured knee and the normal knee (the injured-normal difference) may be a good clinical predictor of the injured-normal difference in the pivot shift.
- An insufficiently tensioned ACL graft may substantially reduce anterior laxity, whilst leaving the pivot shift assessment unchanged.

A metanalysis [35] has compared the accuracy of the three commonly utilised tests for anterior knee laxity and showed the following:

Sensitivity overall without anaesthesia
- Lachman 85%
- Anterior drawer 55% (for chronic)
- Pivot shift 24%

Specificity overall without anaesthesia
- Lachman 94%
- Anterior drawer 92% (for chronic)
- Pivot shift 98%

Sensitivity overall with anaesthesia
- Lachman 97%
- Anterior drawer 77% (for chronic)
- Pivot shift 74%

Specificity overall with anaesthesia
- Lachman 93%
- Anterior drawer 87% (for chronic)
- Pivot shift 99%

6.7.1.2 Posterior Knee Laxity

Posterior Tibial Sag Sign [36, 37]

The patient lies supine with the hip flexed to 45° and the knee flexed to 90°. In this position, the tibia sags backwards on the femur, in the presence of PCL dysfunction. Normally, the medial tibial plateau extends about 5–10 mm anteriorly beyond the femoral condyle with the knee flexed to 90°. If this step-off is lost it is considered a positive sag test. The presence or loss of this step may be determined by visual inspection and palpation.

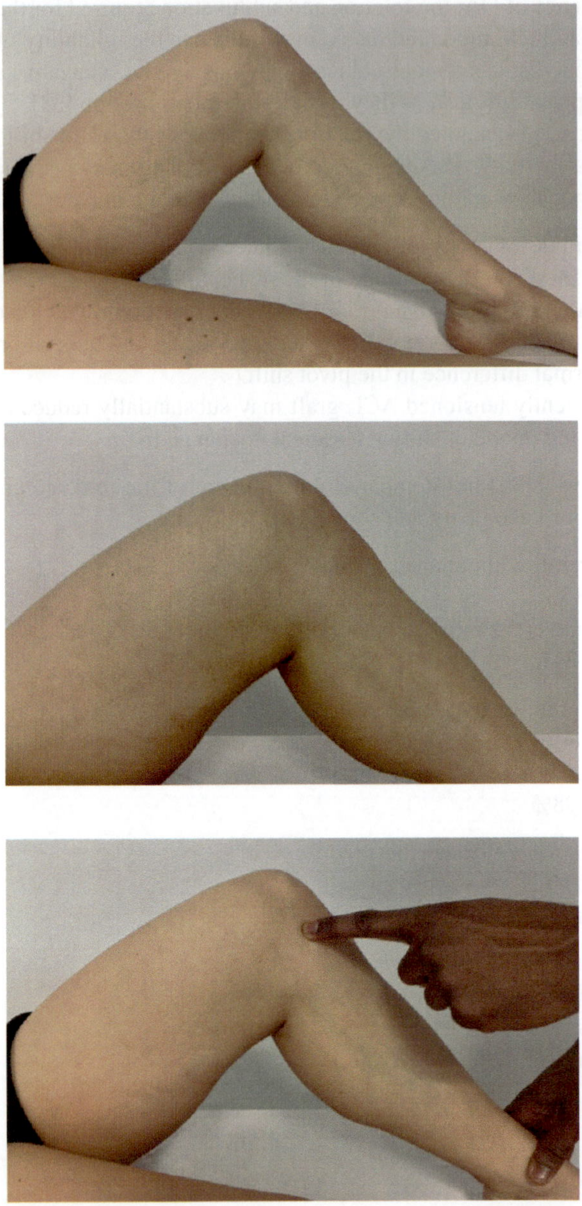

Looking and palpating for a posterior sag of the tibia in relation to the femur

Posterior Drawer Test [38, 39]

The subject lies supine with the flexed to 45°, knee flexed to 90°, and foot in neutral position. The examiner sits on the patient's foot, and grasps the anterior proximal part of the tibia (just below the knee) with the thumbs placed on the joint line. The examiner then pushes the tibia backwards noting:

- The extend of posterior translation of the tibia in relation to the femur (the medial tibial plateau step-off may be observed or palpated to help further determine posterior tibial translation)
- The presence of a firm end point to this translation

Excessive posterior tibial translation compared to the opposite site, or a soft/absent end point is indicative of posterior knee laxity and is suggestive of PCL disruption.

When assessing the amount of posterior translation of the tibia in relation to the femur, it is vital to determine the starting position of the tibia. If the tibia starts in a more posteriorly displaced position in relation to the femur as compared to the normal resting position (as seen in PCL deficiency), a posteriorly directed force on the tibia by the examiner may not produce much further translation. This may be mistaken as absent or not excessive posterior laxity. Hence, it is important to relocate the tibia to a normal resting position (anterior to the femur) and then determine any posterior laxity from that point backwards.

The posterior drawer test may be graded:

- Grade 1—0–5 mm posterior translation but with the tibia remaining anterior to the femur
- Grade 2—5–10 mm posterior tibial translation but with the tibia aligned with the femur
- Grade 3— >10 mm posterior tibial translation, with the tibia displacing posterior to the femur

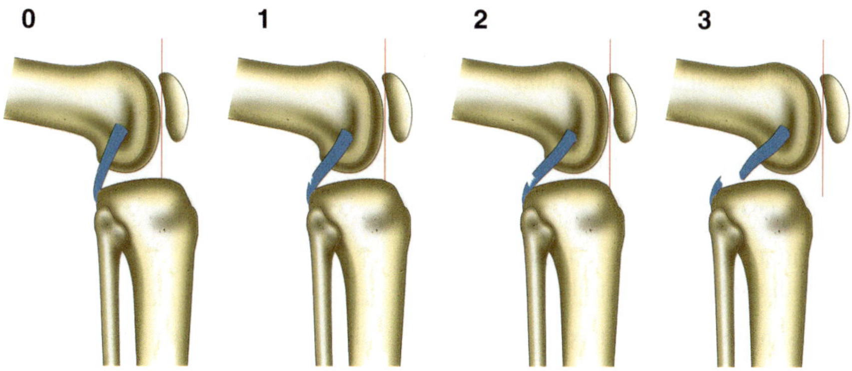

PCL intact (**0**) and disrupted (grade **1**–**3**)

Quadriceps active test [40]—patient lies supine with the knee in 90° of flexion. The patient is asked to contract the quadriceps, which pulls the tibia forwards reducing or abolishing the posterior tibial sag.

Reverse Pivot Shift Test [41, 42]

The patient is supine. The examiner holds the leg with the knee flexed at 90° and places the distal tibia under the arm. The examiner applies external rotation of the tibia and valgus at the knee, and then extends the knee. The test is positive if with knee extension the tibia moves forwards with a smooth glide or a sudden clunk (that may be felt or seen).

With the knee in flexion the tibia is subluxed posteriorly in relation to the femur (if there is PCL deficiency). As the knee extends the tibia moves forwards and reduces in relation to the femur. Repeat flexion of the knee causes again the tibia to sublux backwards.

It has been shown in cadavers [42] that combined sectioning of the PCL and posterolateral corner (PLC) ligaments produces an increase in the reverse pivot shift test whilst isolated division of either has no effect. On the basis of this it is suggested that a reverse pivot shift test may be suggestive of a combined PCL and PLC disruption.

6.7.1.3 Valgus/Varus Laxity

Valgus Laxity

Valgus Test [43, 44]

The patient is supine. The knee is straight. The examiner places one hand over the outer (lateral) part of the distal femur (just above the knee), to stabilise the femur. With the other hand placed on the inner part of the distal tibia, the tibia is pushed in a valgus (lateral direction) noting:

- The extend of lateral translation/angulation of the tibia in relation to the femur
- The presence of a firm end point to this translation/angulation

The test is repeated:

- With the knee in 30° of flexion
- With the knee in 0° (full extension)

Testing in 30° and 0° flexion may guide as to the extent of ligamentous disruption:

- Increased laxity in 30° flexion is suggestive of MCL disruption
- Increased laxity in 0° flexion is suggestive of combined MCL and posteromedial capsule (posterior-oblique ligament) and/or ACL disruption

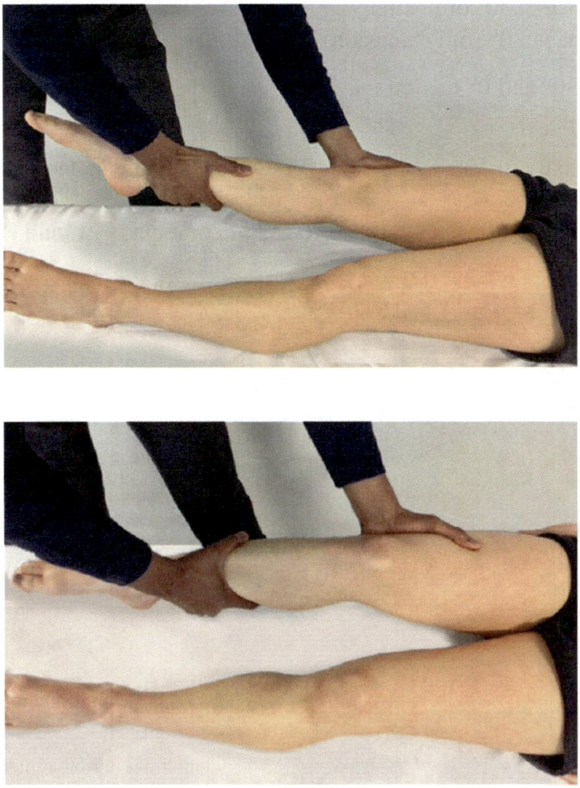

Valgus laxity testing

Valgus Thrust

As described above.

Varus Laxity [45]

Varus Test

The patient lies supine, relaxing the muscles of the knee. The knee is straight. The examiner grasps with one hand the inner (medial) part of the distal femur (just above the knee) to stabilise the femur. With the other hand placed on the outer part of the distal tibia, the tibia is pushed in a varus (inwards direction-adduction) noting:

- The extend of medial translation/angulation of the tibia in relation to the femur
- The presence of a firm end point to this translation/angulation

The test is repeated:

- With the knee in 30° of flexion
- With the knee in 0° (full extension)

Testing in 30° and 0° flexion may guide as to the extent of ligamentous disruption [46, 47]:

- Increased laxity in 30° flexion is suggestive of lateral collateral ligament (PLC) disruption
- Increased laxity in 0° flexion is suggestive of combined PLC and PCL disruption

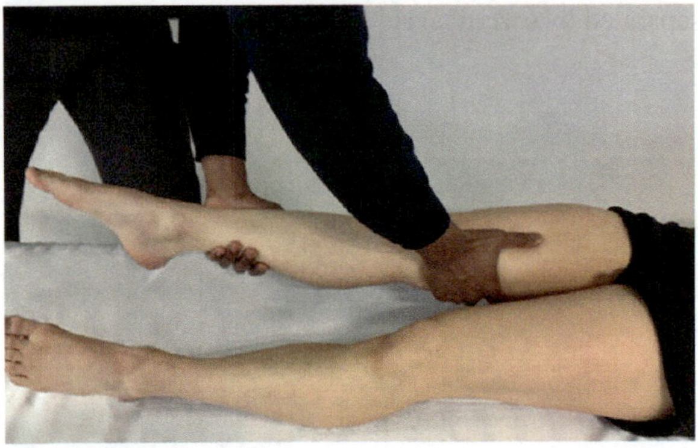

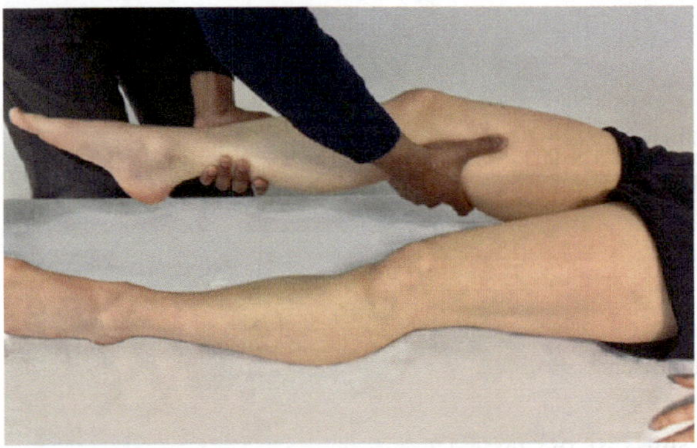

Varus laxity testing

Varus Thrust

As described above.

When testing for valgus/varus laxity—by flexing the knee 30° the posterior capsule and tendons are relaxed allowing the MCL and LCL respectively to be tested in isolation.

Valgus/varus laxity may be graded according to the American Medical Association grading system [48]:

- Grade 1: 0–5 mm opening, hard end point (stretched ligament)
- Grade 2: 5–10 mm opening, hard end point (partial ligament tear)
- Grade 3: >10 mm opening, soft end point (complete ligament tear)

6.7.1.4 Rotatory Laxity [49–51]

Dial test- the patient is lying prone, with the knees closely apposed. With the knees flexed 30° the examiner holds both feet and externally rotates the tibiae. Excessive external rotation or an asymmetry of 10° more in the affected knee is considered important (smaller asymmetries may be physiological and be seen in the absence of any ligamentous disruption). The test is repeated with the knees flexed 90°.

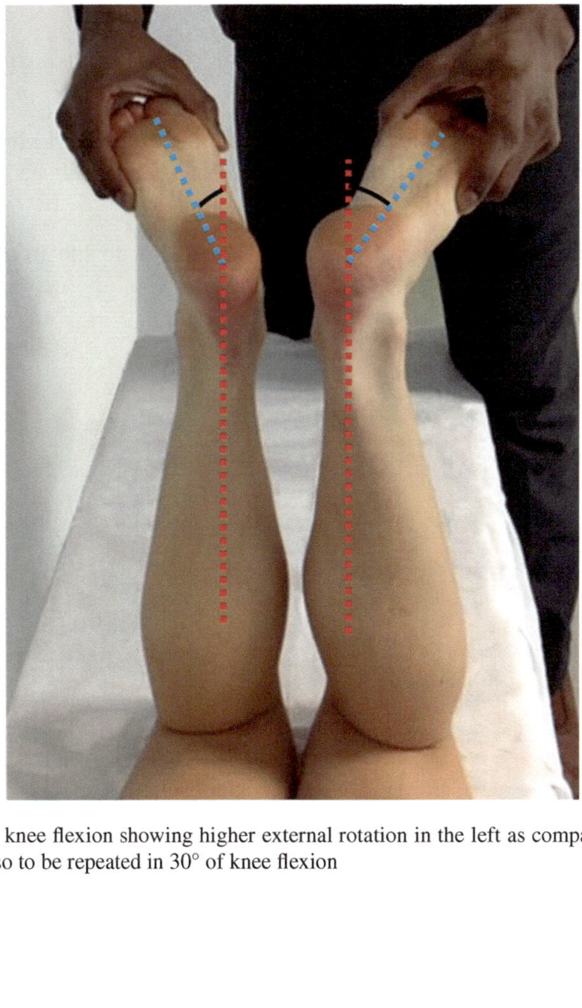

Dial test in 90° knee flexion showing higher external rotation in the left as compared to the right knee. Test is also to be repeated in 30° of knee flexion

External rotation increase observed in:

- 30° of knee flexion is suggestive of PLC disruption
- 90° of knee flexion is suggestive of combined PLC and PCL disruption.

Increased external rotation may be seen in other conditions including [52–54]:

- MCL disruption
- ACL disruption

In ACL disruption with an intact PLC, an increase in external rotation of up to 7° in both 30° and 90° of knee flexion has been reported, leading to suggestions that a side to side difference of >15° should be considered indicative of PLC disruption [53, 54]. Similarly, MCL disruption may lead to dial test changes similar to those seen in PLC disruptions at both 30° and 90°.

6.7.2 Assessment of Patellofemoral Laxity [55]

Lateral/Medial Patellar Laxity

The patient lies supine with the knee straight and the extensor mechanism relaxed. The examiner grasps the patella between thumb and index finger. The patella is sequentially translated laterally and medially, noting:

- The extend of translation of the patella in relation to the trochlea (may be described in terms of the patellar width equivalent)
- The presence of a firm end point to this translation

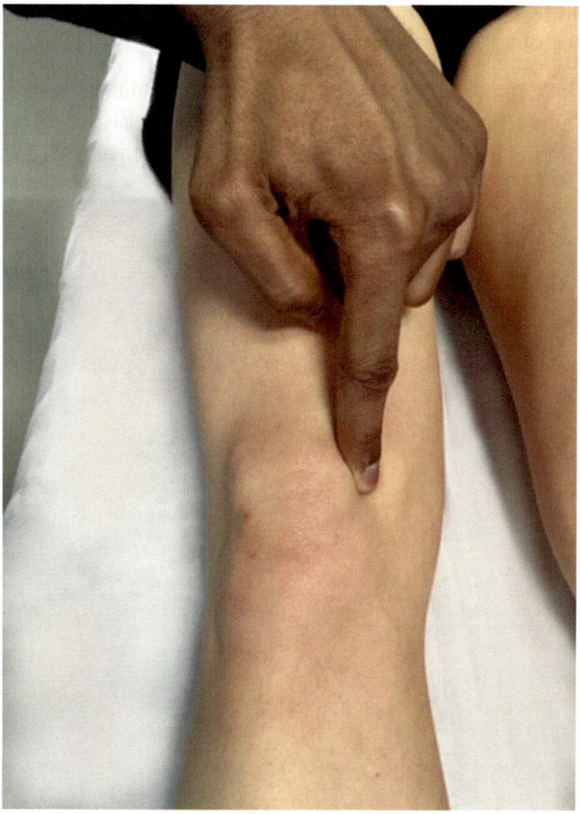

Assessment of medial patellar laxity

The test may be repeated:

- With the knee in full extension
- With the knee in 30° flexion
- With the knee in 60° flexion

With the knee extended:

- A lateral translation of more than ¾ of patellar width is suggestive of medial retinaculum laxity
- A medial translation of less than ¼ of patellar width is suggestive of lateral retinaculum tightness

Patellar Eversion Laxity

Medial Patellar Eversion Test

The patient lies supine, with the knee straight and the extensor mechanism relaxed. The examiner pushes the patella medially with both thumbs and with the index fingers everts the medial part of the patella in relation to the trochlea noting:

- The extend of eversion of the medial part of the patella away from the trochlea
- The presence of a firm end point to this eversion

If the patella cannot be everted beyond the horizontal then it is suggestive of medial retinaculum tightness. If it can be everted excessively as compared to the opposite site, it may indicate medial patellofemoral ligament (MPFL) disruption.

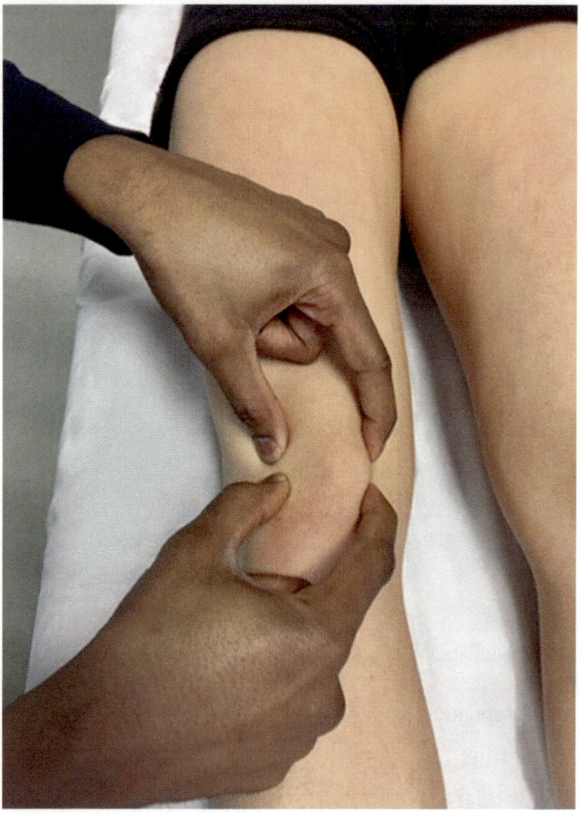

Medial patellar eversion test

Lateral Patellar Eversion Test

The patient is supine, with the knee straight and the extensor mechanism relaxed. The examiner with both index fingers pushes the patella laterally and with the thumbs everts the outer part of the patella in relation to the trochlea noting:

- The extend of eversion of the lateral part of the patella away from the trochlea
- The presence of a firm end point to this eversion

If the patella cannot be everted beyond the horizontal then it is suggestive of lateral retinaculum tightness.

J Sign [56, 57]

The patient sits at the end of the bed with the knee in 90° flexion. The patient actively extends the knee slowly, whilst the examiner observes the motion of the patella. Upon extension from knee flexion, as the patella comes out of the trochlear groove, it translates proximally and then laterally. This path is inverse J shaped. This is suggestive of excessive lateral patellar shift in extension which could be due to:

- Laxity of medial retinaculum
- Lateral retinaculum tightness
- Vastus medialis weakness

It is of note that surgeons have been shown to visually correctly identify patellar maltracking in less than 70% of time [58].

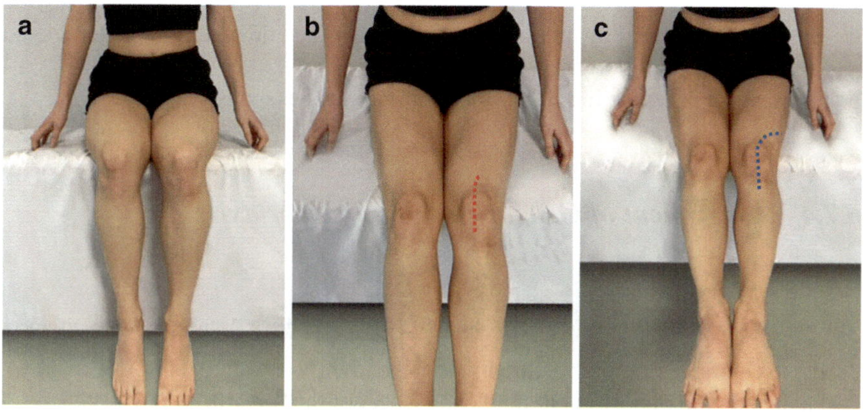

Looking for J sign upon knee extension. With the knee in flexion the patella is usually centred (**a**) and with knee extension it moves proximally and slightly laterally (red line, **b**). In lateral patellar instability, excessive lateral patellar motion may be seen with knee extension (blue line, **c**)

Patellar gravity subluxation test to access medial patella subluxation [59]—the patient lies in the lateral decubitus position with the affected leg up. The leg is then abducted passively by the examiner with the quadriceps relaxed and the knee extended. This allows the patella to sublux medially out of the trochlear groove under the effect of gravity. A sulcus may be seen at the anterolateral part of the knee.

- The patella may then be relocated into the trochlear groove by the examiner applying a laterally directed pressure on the medial border of the patella.
- The patient is also asked to actively pull the patella into the trochlear groove by contracting the quadriceps; if this cannot be achieved it is suggestive that the lateral part of quadriceps (vastus lateralis) is detached from the patella or that the lateral retinaculum is lax or deficient.

It is of note that medial patellar subluxation may also be observed in patients with hypermobile joints, in the absence of previous surgery or injury. However, in those cases, as the quadriceps and lateral retinaculum are intact, voluntary contraction of the quadriceps may pull the patella back into the trochlear groove.

6.7.3 Assessment of Proximal Tibiofibular Joint Laxity [60]

The patient flexes the knee to hyperflexion (to relax the biceps femoris), whilst the proximal tibiofibular joint is observed for a visible displacement of the fibular head (anterior translation being the most common).

The above is repeated whilst the examiner applies an anterior force to the proximal fibula, again looking for a translation of the fibular head.

- Internal rotation may also be applied along with knee flexion, if the latter fails to elicit obvious fibular translation.
- In assessing posterior instability the examiner applies a posterior force.

6.7.4 Assessment of Generalised Joint Hyperlaxity

Beighton Score [61, 62]
The subject is examined for the presence of the following:

1. Passive dorsiflexion of the little finger beyond 90°
2. Passive thumb opposition to the flexor aspect of the forearm
3. Active elbow hyperextension beyond 10°—patient is asked to straighten elbows as much as possible
4. Active knee hyperextension beyond 10°- patient is asked to straighten knees as much as possible
5. Forward flexion of the trunk—patient is asked to lean forwards and touch the palms of the hands flat on the floor whilst keeping the knees straight

The presence of each of the first four components scores one point for the left and one for the right side, and the presence of the fifth component scores one point, thus giving a maximum potential score of nine. A score greater than 6 in adults is suggestive of hyperlaxity.

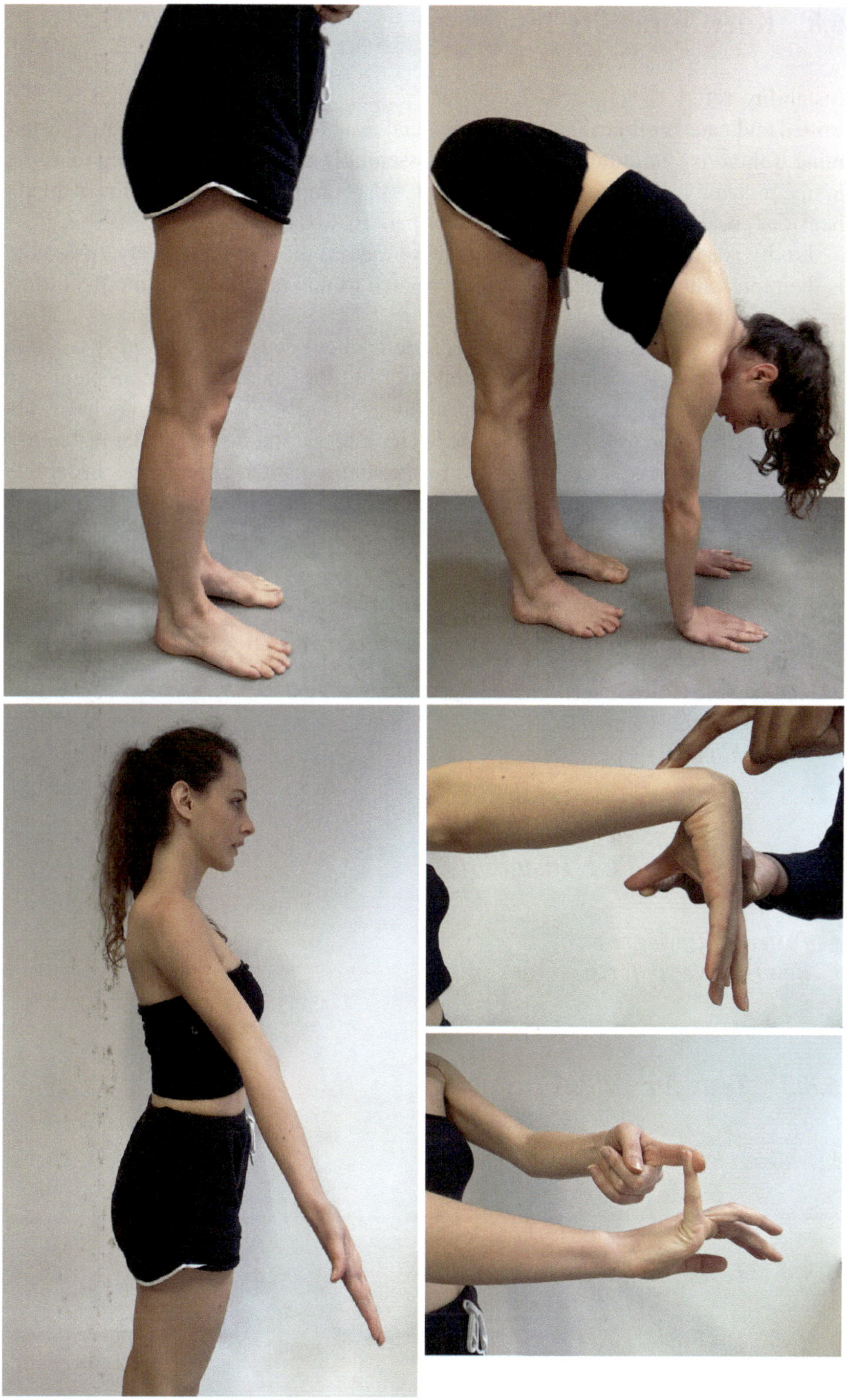

Assessment of Beighton score

6.8 Knee Instability Tests

Instability refers to joint translation that regardless of its degree cannot be controlled and causes clinical symptoms. Special tests for knee instability aim to determine if there is symptomatic instability. Essentially the tests that are used to assess laxity, indicate instability if excessive laxity is accompanied by symptoms of apprehension, protective muscle contraction or pain [63, 64].

Laxity is a clinical sign (objective measurement) measured passively. Instability is the represented of clinical symptoms related to that laxity (sensation of shifting, buckling, giving way, pain).

Ligamentous deficiency (such as ACL deficiency) does not necessarily result in instability. Patients may have substantial anterior tibiofemoral laxity consistent with ACL deficiency, but experience no instability. Similarly, the patient may have substantial laxity of the patellar retinaculae but have no symptoms of patellar instability.

If during the tests described above for laxity the patient experiences instability symptoms, then instability is said to accompany any identified increase in laxity.

6.8.1 *Tests for ACL Instability*

- *Lachman test*
- *Anterior drawer test*
- *Pivot shift test*

6.8.2 *Tests for PCL Instability*

- *Posterior drawer test*
- *Reverse pivot shift test*

6.8.3 *Tests for Valgus Instability*

- *Valgus test*

6.8.4 *Tests for Varus Instability*

- *Varus test*

6.8.5 Tests for Posterolateral Corner Instability

- *Dial test*

6.8.6 Tests for Patellofemoral Instability

Lateral patellar apprehension test [65]—the patient lies supine with the knee extended. The examiner moves the patient's leg by the side of the bed (so the knee can be flexed). The examiner then applies a lateral directed force on the patella with one hand, whilst flexing the knee with the opposite hand. Experience of apprehension by the patient that the patella may dislocate is suggestive of lateral patellar instability (the patient may tell the examiner to stop, seize the examiner's hands to stop the push on the patella, complain of pain).

Relocation test for medial patellar instability [66]—the patient lies supine with the knee extended. The examiner stands on the same side as the symptomatic knee. The examiner applies a medial directed force on the patella with one hand (to sublux the patella medially). The examiner then flexes the knee with the opposite hand and lets the patella go. The test is positive if as the knee flexes the patient experiences pain, apprehension or reproduction of their symptoms (as the knee flexes the extensor mechanism tensions and pulls the patella laterally into the trochlea; the patella relocates by jumping over the medial trochlear facet). The patella is seen moving laterally but essentially this is repositioning from an over-medialized position.

6.8.7 Tests for Proximal Tibiofibular Joint Instability

Patient reports instability symptoms when flexing the knee or when a force is applied by the examiner to the proximal fibula.

6.9 Lumbosacral Spine Tests

Femoral Nerve Stretch Test [67]
The patient lies prone. The examiner flexes the patient's knee and extends the patient's hip. A positive test occurs when this causes substantial pain in the anterior part of the thigh and groin, and is suggestive of femoral nerve dysfunction.

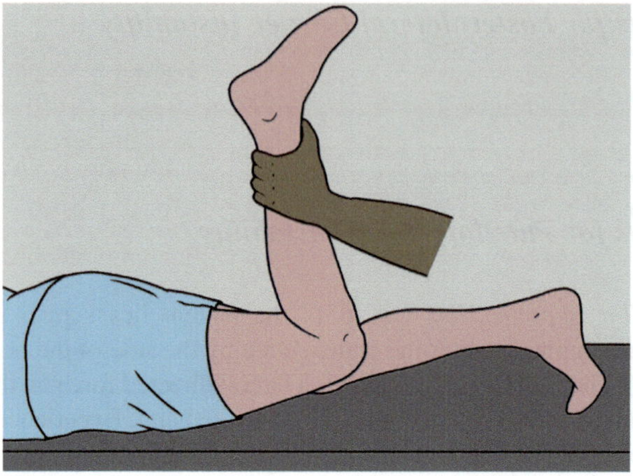

Femoral nerve stretch test

Straight-Leg Raise Test—Sciatic Stretch Test [68]

The patient lies supine. The examiner raises the patient's leg by flexing the hip with the knee in extension. The test is considered positive if it reproduces pain in the lower leg in the distribution of the sciatic nerve roots (L5/S1) and is suggestive of irritation or compression of those nerve roots. The pain may be aggravated by dorsiflexion of the foot.

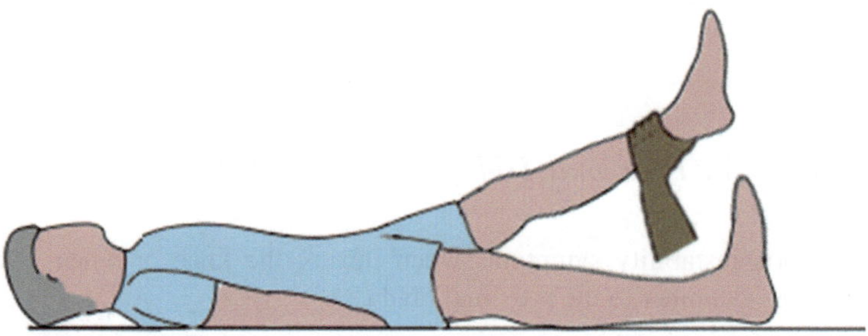

Straight leg test

6.10 Core Balance Tests [69–71]

Several tests may be used to screen for core weakness or unbalance. These include:

Single Leg Stance

The patient is asked to stand on one leg at a time. Inability to achieve or maintain this position in a balanced way is suggestive of core weakness or unbalance. Use of the patient's arms to balance and maintain the stance, flexion or twisting of the weightbearing leg may also indicate core weakness.

Single Leg Squat

The patient is asked to stand on one leg and do a quarter to half squat. Inability to achieve or maintain this position in a balanced way is suggestive of core weakness or unbalance. Use of the patient's arms to balance and maintain the stance, flexion or twisting of the weightbearing leg may also indicate core weakness.

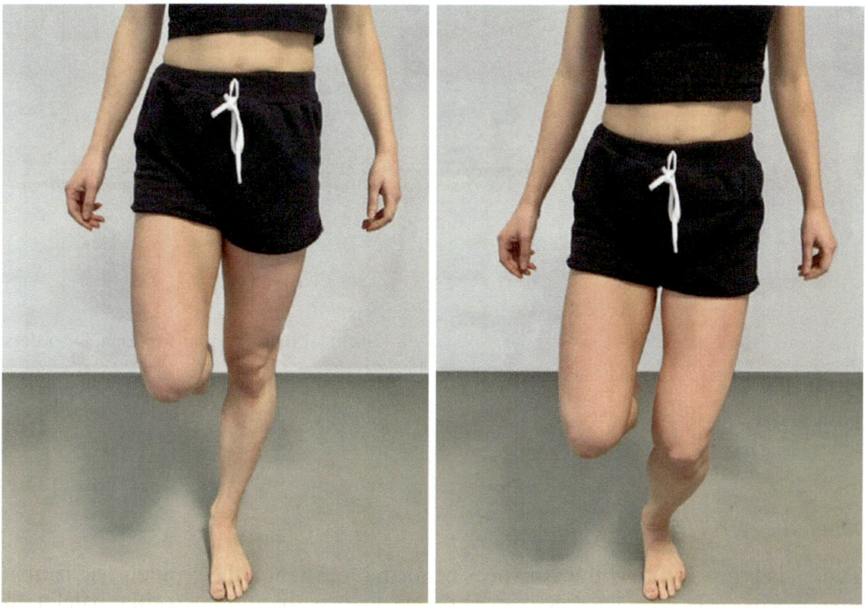

Single leg squat

Basic Bridge

The patient lies supine with both knees bent and feet flat on the ground. The hips are lifted off the floor creating a straight line from the knees to the shoulders. The position is held for about 10 s, and then slowly lowered back down. The patient is observed for any weakness in lifting off or maintaining the position (pelvis not staying level, wobbling, hamstrings cramping). This action relies on the core (spinal muscles, abdominal muscles, hip abductors and external rotators) as well as hamstrings.

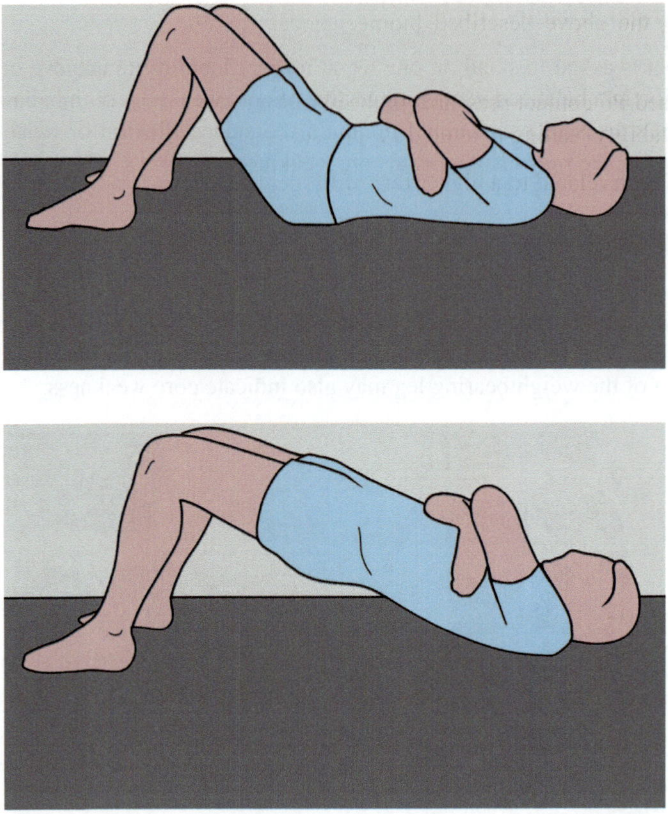

Basic bridge

Single Leg Bridge

Patient is lying supine with both knees bent, and feet flat on the ground. The patient places their arms across the chest and lifts off the torso until it is parallel to the floor (creating a straight line from the knees to the shoulders). One leg is then extended and raised while keeping the pelvis level. The position is held for 10 s, and then the patient returns to the starting position with the knees bent. The patient is observed for any weakness in lifting off or maintaining the position in both the horizontal and vertical planes (pelvis not staying level, wobbling, hamstrings cramping).

6.11 Knee Muscle/Tendon Flexibility Tests

Rectus femoris flexibility—Ely's Test [72]: Patient lies prone with the knees extended. The examiner passively flexes the patient's knee. The test is positive (suggestive of rectus femoris tightness) if the hip on the same side passively rises off the table as the examiner flexes the knee.

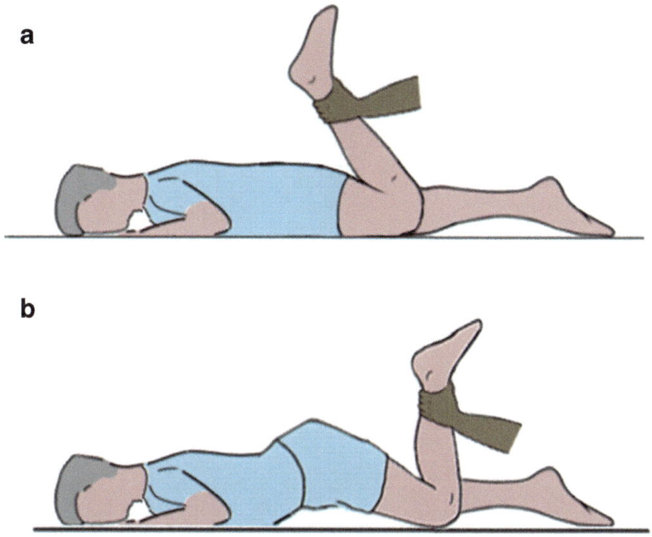

Assessment of rectus femoris flexibility. (**a**) Normal rectus femoris. (**b**) Tight rectus femoris with resultant hip flexion

Hamstring Flexibility [73, 74]

1. *Passive knee extension test*: Patient is lying supine with the ipsilateral hip flexed to 90°. The examiner extends the ipsilateral knee until reaching the maximal tolerable stretch of the hamstring muscles and at this point measures the knee flexion angle (angle short of extension), which is normally about 40° in men and 30° in women.

2. *Active knee extension test* [73–75]: Patient is lying supine. The ipsilateral hip is flexed to 90° by the examiner. The patient is instructed to straighten the knee until reaching the maximal tolerable stretch of the hamstrings (until a stretch sensation is felt), whilst the examiner holds the ipsilateral hip in 90° of flexion. The examiner measures the knee flexion angle (angle short of extension) which is normally about 40° in both sexes.

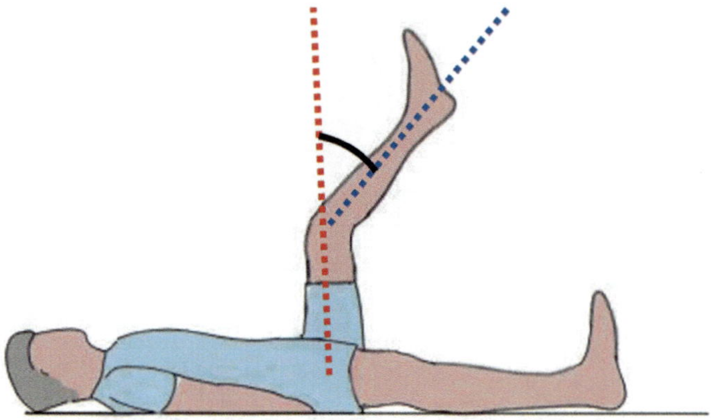

Active knee extension test. The angle short of full knee extension is measured

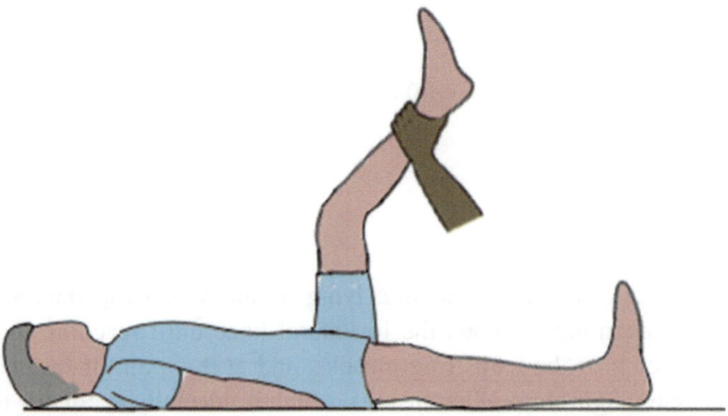

Passive knee extension test

Iliotibial band (ITB) flexibility test

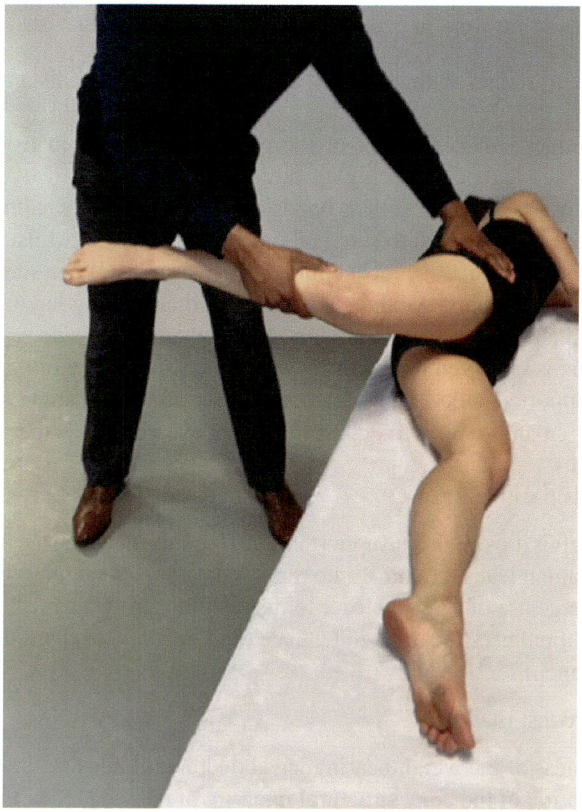

Assesment of Iliotibial band flexibility

Patient is lying on the side with the affected up. The bottom knee and hip are slightly flexed. The examiner stabilizes the pelvis or greater trochanter with one hand, and holds the patient's examined leg with the other hand, flexing the knee to 90°. The examiner extends and abducts the hip. The leg is then lowered towards the floor until resistance is felt. The leg should be able to adduct with the thigh dropping down slightly below horizontal. In the presence of ITB tightness, the leg remains in an abducted position or the patient experiences lateral knee pain.

6.12 Hip Abductors' Strength

Trendelenburg's Test [76]

- The patient stands with the feet apart (similar to the distance between the shoulders).
- The examiner stands in front of the patient, with arms in front of the waist, elbows flexed and palms facing upwards.
- The patient is asked to rest their hands onto the examiner's palms.
- The patient is then asked to stand on one leg (testing leg) whilst flexing the contralateral knee about 30° (but keeping the hip straight). When standing on one leg the patient relies on the abductor muscles of the standing leg to keep the pelvis horizontal and stop it from dropping on the unsupported side.
- The pelvis is observed to determine whether it stays level or whether it dips on the unsupported side. The pressure exerted by the patient's hands on the examiner's hands is felt, to determine if it is even or unequal as the patient tries to balance)
- The test is positive if:
  - The pelvis dips on the unsupported side (the side on which leg is off the ground)
  - The patient leans the trunk onto the standing side (to achieve balance by shifting the centre of gravity closer to the weightbearing leg)
  - The patient uses the arms to balance (and thus presses hard onto the examiner's hands)
- A positive test is seen in:
  - Weakness of the weightbearing leg abductors (gluteus medius)
  - Disruption of the bony structural integrity of the weightbearing hip joint (dislocation/subluxation, femoral head collapse)

Forward Step-Down Test [77]

The patient stands on a 20 cm box with arms folded across the chest and squats down on one leg 5–10 times consecutively until the heel touches the floor, maintaining balance. The patient is observed for any deviation of the trunk, pelvis, hip or knee which is suggestive of weakness of the hip abductors.

Single Hop Test [78]

In this test, the aim is to jump as far as possible on a single leg, without losing balance, and landing firmly. The distance is measured from the start line to the heel of the landing leg. The goal is to have a less than 10% difference in hop distance between both limbs.

6.13 Rotational Profile [79]

Several parameters may be assessed in evaluating the rotational profile of the lower limbs.

This aims at assessing the rotational profile of the femur, tibia, and the presence of metatarsus adductus/abductus at the foot.

- Version refers to rotation which is within normal range (95% of the population)
- Torsion refers to rotation which is >2 standard deviations lower or higher than the population mean

Femoral version describes the rotation of the proximal part of the femur in relation to the distal femur (a line passing through the posterior part of the distal femoral condyles). This rotation may be influenced by the:

- Inclination (version) of the femoral neck in relation to the shaft of the femur
  - Anteversion = anterior inclination
  - Retroversion = posterior inclination
- Version of the proximal part of the femoral shaft in relation to the posterior distal femoral condyles

Tibial version describes the rotation of the proximal part of the tibia in relation to a line intersecting the distal fibula and distal tibia (at the level of the ankle joint).

Changes in version may be influenced by rotation of any segments between these two levels (metaphyseal or diaphyseal).

The following evaluations may be used in assessing the rotational profile. The presence of clinical findings which are suggestive of altered rotational profile, may lead to specialised radiological investigations (Computed Tomography or Magnetic Resonance Imaging (MRI)) to quantify the rotational profile and determine the level of any rotational changes.

Look—on inspection from the front:

1. The patient is asked to stand with the feet pointing forwards and the ability to achieve that is noted.
2. The positioning of the patellae is noted (patellae should be pointing forwards):
   - Squinting patella—patella points inwards, towards the other patella—this may be unilateral or bilateral. It is indicative of internal rotation of the femur in relation to the tibia—it may be due to:
     - Primary internal femoral torsion (excessive femoral anteversion/femoral shaft deformity) or
     - Compensatory, secondary to primary external tibial torsion

- Out-pointing patella—patella points outwards, away from the midline—this may be unilateral or bilateral. It may be due to:
  - External femoral torsion (excessive femoral retroversion/femoral shaft deformity, hip soft tissue contractures)
  - External tibial torsion

3. The patient is asked to walk forwards and the foot progression angle (FPA) is noted. This is the angle between the direction of progression (walking) and the long axis of the foot (line between tip of heel and second toe).
   - In-toeing—foot points inwards
   - Out-toeing—foot points outwards
     A negative FPA indicates in-toeing and a positive FPA indicates out-toeing.
   - Internal rotation of the hip, internal femoral torsion, and internal tibial torsion are associated with greater in-toeing.

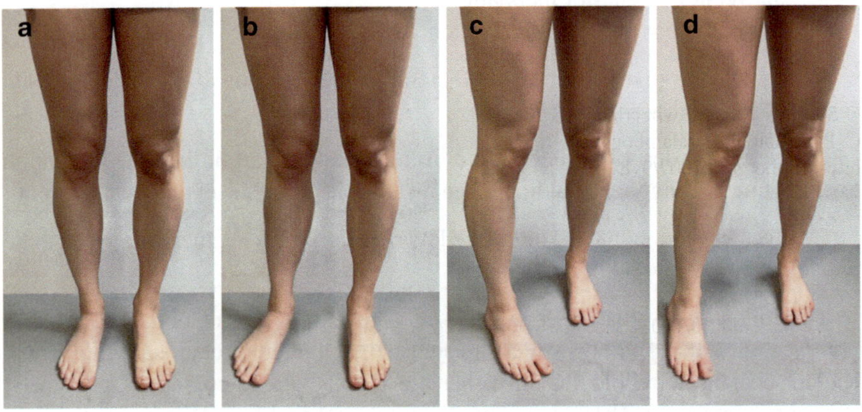

(**a**) Normal alignment with patella and foot pointing forwards. (**b**) External tibial torsion with patella pointing forwards and foot outwards. (**c**) Internal femoral torsion with patella and foot pointing inwards. (**d**) Internal femoral tossion with patella pointing inwards and external tibial torsion with foot pointing forwards (Miserable malalignment) (edited photos)

   - External rotation of the hip, external femoral torsion, and external tibial torsion are associated with greater out-toeing during gait.

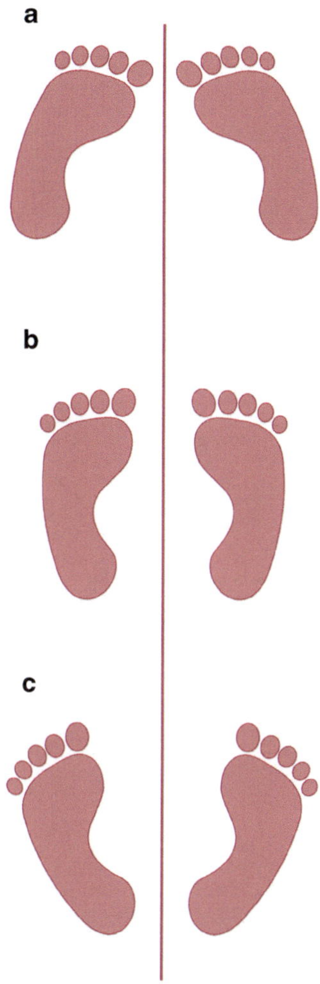

Foot progression angle. (**a**) In-toeing. (**b**) Neutral. (**c**) Out-toeing

With the patient prone, femoral version, tibial version and foot alignment are assessed as below:

Femoral Version

Hip rotation—internal/external rotation is assessed. The patient lies prone, the knee is flexed to 90° and the lower leg (tibia) is rotated maximally outwards (away from the midline). The angle between the longitudinal axis of the tibia and a vertical reference line is a measure of hip internal rotation. When the tibia is rotated inwards (towards the midline, crossing the legs) this angle is a measure of hip external rotation.

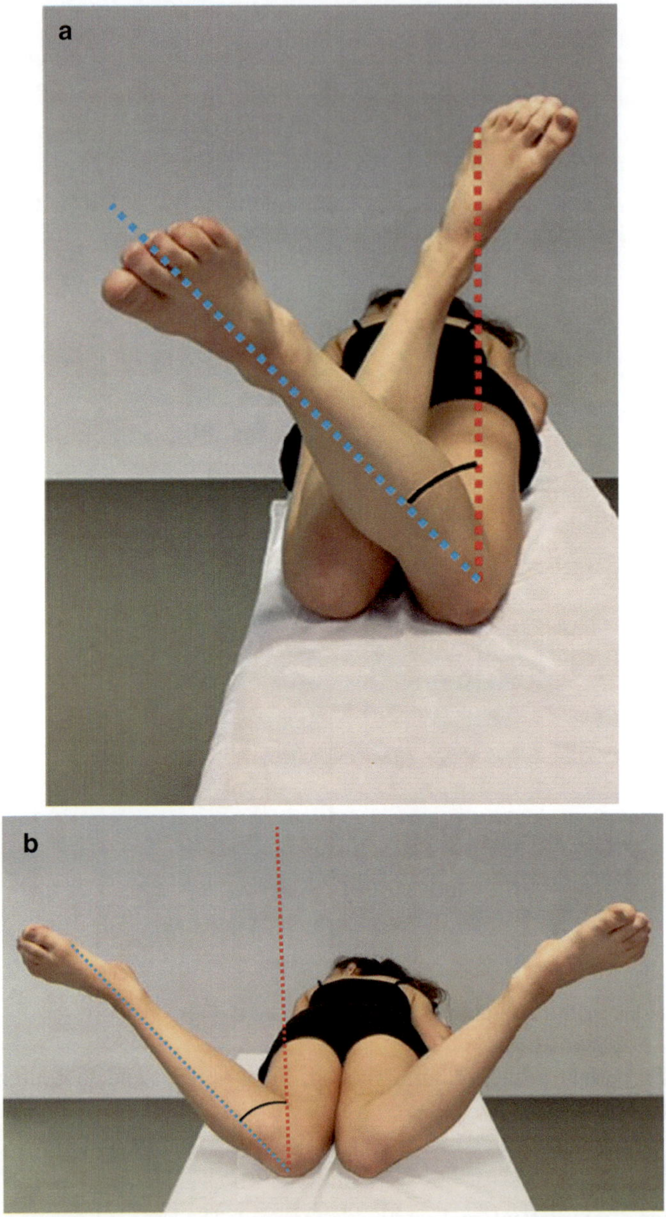

Assessment of external (**a**) and internal (**b**) hip rotation in the prone position

When looking at a prone patient it is often difficult to picture which direction of tibial rotation assesses internal and which assesses external rotation of the hip. As a memory aid consider that rotation of the tibia signifies a rotation of the hip in an opposite direction to what one might expect by looking at the tibia:

- Outer rotation of the tibia (away from midline) signifies internal rotation of the femur
- Inner rotation of the tibia (towards midline) signifies external rotation of the femur

Alternatively, consider that the femoral neck is horizontal with the femoral head at its tip and try to work out which way the femoral head will move by rotating the tibia as above:

- Anterior motion of the femoral head occurs in inner rotation of the tibia—equivalent to external rotation of the hip
- Posterior motion of the femoral head occurs in outer rotation of the tibia—equivalent to internal rotation of the hip

Passive hip rotation is used as a proxy measurement of femoral version and can help estimate the direction and the estimated amount of femoral version. Total hip motion (IR + ER) should be similar on each side (about 90° in adults). However, use of hip rotation values to provide the exact amount of femoral version is not a very accurate method.

Internal rotation of the hip in the prone position has been shown to correlate with anteversion of the femoral neck and acetabulum. Hence, although hip rotation may be also assessed in the supine position (with hip and knee at 0° or with the hip and knee flexed 90°) or in a sitting position (with hip and knee flexed 90°) the prone position is preferred. It is of note that different hip positions may give different values of hip rotation, as the tightness of soft tissues may vary between positions, and impingement between the femoral neck and acetabulum may also differ between positions.

Femoral neck version angle—the patient lies prone, the knee is flexed to 90°. The examiner rotates the lower leg (tibia) inwards and outwards whilst palpating the tip of the greater trochanter. At the point the palpable greater trochanter is most prominent, the neck of the femur is considered to be horizontal (parallel to the floor), and the angle between the longitudinal axis of the tibia and a vertical reference line is considered a measure of the femoral neck version angle (internal rotation = anteversion angle, external rotation = retroversion angle).

Tibial version—the patient lies prone, the knee is flexed to 90° and the ankle is positioned in neutral dorsiflexion. Consider:

- A line passing along the long axis of the thigh
- A line passing along the long axis of the foot

The angle between the two lines is the thigh-foot angle, which is a measure of tibial version (internal tibial version if foot pointing inwards, external tibial version if foot pointing outwards). Normal value in adults is about 10° of external rotation.

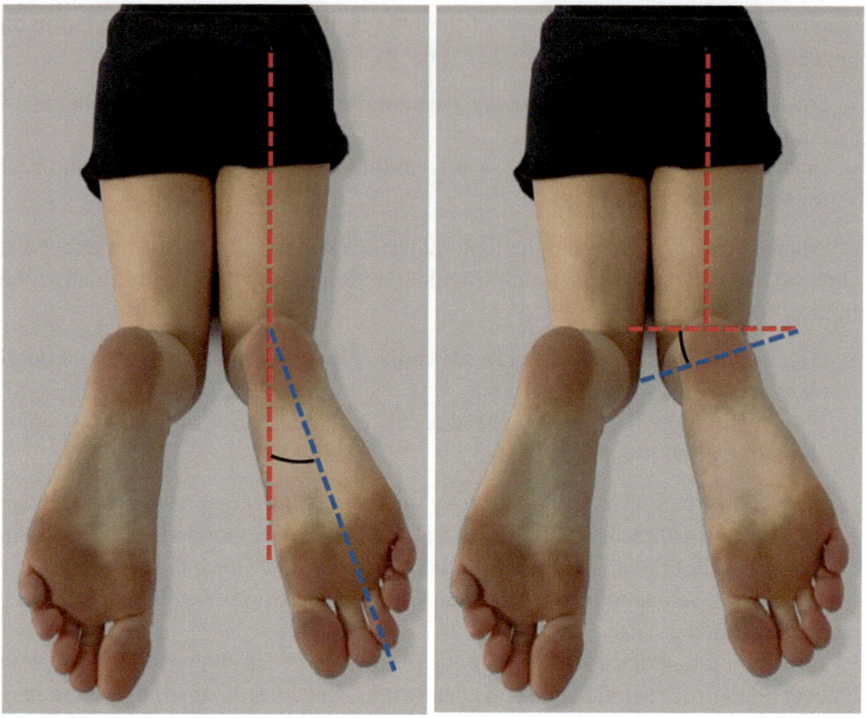

Assessment of tibial version

An alternative angle to be measured (if it is felt difficult to determine the long axis of the foot) is the angle between:

- A line perpendicular to a line passing along the length of the thigh (equivalent to the transcondylar axis)
- A line intersecting the distal tibia and fibula at the level of the ankle joint (trans-malleolar axis)

Metatarsus Adductus

This is a common foot deformity in children that causes the forefoot to turn inwards. The outer border of the foot is convex instead of straight. The hind foot is well aligned. A line bisecting the heel passes through the second web space if the foot in well aligned. In metatarsus adductus this line moves laterally at the forefoot. Metatarsus adductus is one of the causes of in-toeing.

Learning Pearls

- Each special test is usually carried out first on the normal knee so that the patient gets used to what is required, and also to allow comparison between the two knees.
- Even an accurate history may not give the definite answer and complimentary radiological or other investigations are usually needed. Swain et al. [80] carried out a systematic review to identify diagnostic studies comparing the accuracy of clinical examination items for ACL injury (to the level achieved by arthroscopic evaluation, or MRI imaging). They examined the diagnostic accuracy of several clinical examination tests (anterior drawer test, Lachman's test and pivot shift test). They concluded that none of these provided useful diagnostic information in a clinical setting. Their conclusion was that despite being widely used and accepted in clinical practice, the results of individual history items or physical tests do not meaningfully change the probability of ACL injury.
- The pattern of injury of a specific structure may influence the clinical findings-paradoxical findings have been observed when using the McMurray's test and these may be related to the meniscal type present [81].
- Tests which have been classically described as assessing particular ligamentous structures, are increasingly recognised to be influenced by injuries of other ligamentous restraints.
- The dial test has been extensively used to assess the PLC and PCL. However, more recently, it has been shown that the dial test may also be influenced by ACL [82, 83] and MCL [54] tears. Forsythe B et al. [53] showed that ACL tear accounts for nearly 7° tibial external rotation when performing the dial test, and recommended that a positive dial test should be treated with caution as to its associated underlying pathology. Griffith CJ et al. [54] showed in a cadaveric study that significant increases occur in external rotation at 30° of knee flexion, following division of the superficial part of the MCL, indicating that a positive dial test may be seen not only with PLC but also medial knee injuries.
- Slichter et al. [82] evaluated the inter- and intra-related agreement on performing the dial test in patients with ACL tears, to assess for a concomitant PLC injury. The inter-rater agreement was 70% whereas the intra-rater agreement was statistically not significant.

References

1. Solomon L, Apley A. Physical examination in orthopaedics: Taylor & Francis; 1997.
2. Reider B. The knee. In: Reider B, editor. The orthopaedic physical examination. Philadelphia, PA: WB Saunders Company; 1999.
3. Bronstein RD, Schaffer JC. Physical examination of the knee: meniscus, cartilage, and patellofemoral conditions. J Am Acad Orthop Surg. 2017;25(5):365–74.
4. Sturgill LP, Snyder-Mackler L, Manal TJ, Axe MJ. Interrater reliability of a clinical scale to assess knee joint effusion. J Orthop Sports Phys Ther. 2009;39(12):845–9.

5. Hauzeur JP, Mathy L, De Maertelaer V. Comparison between clinical evaluation and ultrasonography in detecting hydrarthrosis of the knee. J Rheumatol. 1999;26:2681–3.
6. Mann G, Finsterbush A, Frankl U, Yarom J, Matan Y. A method of diagnosing small amounts of fluid in the knee. J Bone Joint Surg Br. 1991;73(2):346–7.
7. Jung-Ro Yoon MD, Taik-Seon Kim MD, Han S-B. Quantitative analysis of the patellar tap test for knee joint effusion. Knee Surg Relat Res. 2006;18(1):102–6.
8. Silva Dde O, Briani RV, Pazzinatto MF, Gonçalves AV, Ferrari D, Aragão FA, de Azevedo FM. Q-angle static or dynamic measurements, which is the best choice for patellofemoral pain? Clin Biomech (Bristol, Avon). 2015;30(10):1083–7.
9. Greene CC, Edwards TB, Wade MR, Carson EW. Reliability of the quadriceps angle measurement. Am J Knee Surg. 2001;14(2):97–103.
10. France L, Nester C. Effect of errors in the identification of anatomical landmarks on the accuracy of Q angle values. Clin Biomech (Bristol, Avon). 2001;16(8):710–3.
11. Mahmoudian A, van Dieen JH, Bruijn SM, Baert IA, Faber GS, Luyten FP, Verschueren SM. Varus thrust in women with early medial knee osteoarthritis and its relation with the external knee adduction moment. Clin Biomech (Bristol, Avon). 2016;39:109–14.
12. Chang A, Hochberg M, Song J, Dunlop D, Chmiel JS, Nevitt M, Hayes K, Eaton C, Bathon J, Jackson R, Kwoh CK, Sharma L. Frequency of varus and valgus thrust and factors associated with thrust presence in persons with or at higher risk of developing knee osteoarthritis. Arthritis Rheum. 2010;62(5):1403–11.
13. Kim DH, Lee JH, Yu SM, An CM. The effects of ankle position on torque and muscle activity of the knee extensor during maximal isometric contraction. J Sport Rehabil. 2019;11:1–6.
14. Mikaili S, Khademi-Kalantari K, Rezasoltani A, Arzani P, Baghban AA. Quadriceps force production during straight leg raising at different hip positions with and without concomitant ankle dorsiflexion. J Bodyw Mov Ther. 2018;22(4):904–8.
15. Décary S, Ouellet P, Vendittoli PA, Desmeules F. Reliability of physical examination tests for the diagnosis of knee disorders: evidence from a systematic review. Man Ther. 2016;26:172–82.
16. Lange T, Freiberg A, Dröge P, Lützner J, Schmitt J, Kopkow C. The reliability of physical examination tests for the diagnosis of anterior cruciate ligament rupture—A systematic review. Man Ther. 2015;20(3):402–11.
17. Leblanc MC, Kowalczuk M, Andruszkiewicz N, Simunovic N, Farrokhyar F, Turnbull TL, Debski RE, Ayeni OR. Diagnostic accuracy of physical examination for anterior knee instability: a systematic review. Knee Surg Sports Traumatol Arthrosc. 2015;23(10):2805–13.
18. Nijs J, Van Geel C, Van der Auwera C, Van de Velde B. Diagnostic value of five clinical tests in patellofemoral pain syndrome. Man Ther. 2006;11(1):69–77.
19. Medical Research Council. Aids to the investigation of the peripheral nervous system. Memorandum No. 45. Her Majesty's Stationary Office. London. 1981. https://www.mrc.ac.uk/documents/pdf/aids-to-the-examination-of-the-peripheral-nervous-system-mrc-memorandum-no-45-superseding-war-memorandum-no-7/
20. Stillman BC. Physiological quadriceps lag: its nature and clinical significance. Aust J Physiother. 2004;50(4):237–41.
21. Mohamed O, Perry J, Hislop H. Synergy of medial and lateral hamstrings at three positions of tibial rotation during maximum isometric knee flexion. Knee. 2003;10(3):277–81.
22. Beyer EB, Lunden JB, Russell Giveans M. Medial and lateral hamstrings response and force production at varying degrees of knee flexion and tibial rotation in healthy individuals. Int J Sports Phys Ther. 2019;14(3):376–83.
23. Nijs J, Van Geel C, Van der Auwera C, Van de Velde B. Diagnostic value of five clinical tests in patellofemoral pain syndrome. Man Ther. 2006;11(1):69–77. Epub 2005 Jun 13
24. McMurray TP. Internal derangements of the knee joint. Ann R Coll Surg Engl. 1948;3(4):210–9.
25. Karachalios T, Hantes M, Zibis AH, Zachos V, Karantanas AH, Malizos KN. Diagnostic accuracy of a new clinical test (the Thessaly test) for early detection of meniscal tears. J Bone Joint Surg Am. 2005;87(5):955–62.
26. Hoffa A. The influence of the adipose tissue with regard to the pathology of the knee joint. JAMA. 1904;XLIII(12):795–6.

27. Kim SJ, Jeong JH, Cheon YM, Ryn SW. MPP Tejf in the diognosis of medial patettor plica syndnome. Arthroslopy. 2004;20(10):1101–3.
28. Frank C. Accurate interpretation of the Lachman test. Clin Orthop Relat Res. 1986;213:163–6.
29. Marshall JL, Wang JB, Furman W, Girgis FG, Warren R. The anterior drawer sign: what is it? J Sports Med. 1975;3(4):152–8.
30. Mitsou A, Vallianatos P. Clinical diagnosis of ruptures of the anterior cruciate ligament: a comparison between the Lachman test and the anterior drawer sign. Injury. 1988;19(6):427–8.
31. Rosenberg TD, Rasmussen GL. The function of the anterior cruciate ligament during anterior drawer and Lachman's testing. An in vivo analysis in normal knees. Am J Sports Med. 1984;12(4):318–22.
32. Galway HR, MacIntosh DL. The lateral pivot shift: a symptom and sign of anterior cruciate ligament insufficiency. Clin Orthop. 1980;(147):45–50.
33. Kong KC, Hamlet MR, Peckham T, Mowbray MA. Displaced bucket handle tears of the medial meniscus masking anterior cruciate deficiency. Arch Orthop Trauma Surg. 1994;114(1):51–2.
34. Markolf KL, Jackson SR, McAllister DR. Relationship between the pivot shift and Lachman tests: a cadaver study. J Bone Joint Surg Am. 2010;92(11):2067–75.
35. Benjaminse A, Gokeler A, van der Schans CP. Clinical diagnosis of an anterior cruciate ligament rupture: a meta-analysis. J Orthop Sports Phys Ther. 2006;36(5):267–88.
36. Mayo Robson AW. Ruptured crucial ligaments and their repair by operation. Ann Surg. 1903;37:716–8.
37. Magee DJ. Orthopedic physical assessment. 3rd ed. Philadelphia, PA: WB Saunders; 1997. p. 506–98.
38. McMaster WC. Isolated posterior cruciate ligament injury: literature review and case reports. J Trauma. 1975;15(11):1025–9.
39. Moore HA, Larson RL. Posterior cruciate ligament injuries. Results of early surgical repair. Am J Sports Med. 1980;8(2):68–78.
40. Daniel DM, Stone ML, Barnett P, Sachs R. Use of the quadriceps active test to diagnose posterior cruciate-ligament disruption and measure posterior laxity of the knee. J Bone Joint Surg Am. 1988;70(3):386–91.
41. Larson RL. Physical examination in the diagnosis of rotatory instability. Clin Orthop Relat Res. 1983;172:38–44.
42. Petrigliano FA, Lane CG, Suero EM, Allen AA, Pearle AD. Posterior cruciate ligament and posterolateral corner deficiency results in a reverse pivot shift. Clin Orthop Relat Res. 2012;470(3):815–23.
43. Fetto JF, Marshall JL. Medial collateral ligament injuries of the knee: a rationale for treatment. Clin Orthop Relat Res. 1978;132:206–18.
44. Encinas-Ullán CA, Rodríguez-Merchán E. Isolated medial collateral ligament tears: an update on management. EFORT Open Rev. 2018;3:398–407. 5241.3.170035
45. Lunden JB, Bzdusek PJ, Monson JK, Malcomson KW, Robert F. Laprade current concepts in the recognition and treatment of posterolateral corner injuries of the knee. J Orthop Sports Phys Ther. 2010;40:8. 502-516
46. Gollehon DL, Torzilli PA, Warren RF. The role of the posterolateral and cruciate ligaments in the stability of the human knee. A biomechanical study. J Bone Joint Surg Am. 1987;69: 233–42.
47. Grood ES, Stowers SF, Noyes FR. Limits of movement in the human knee. Effect of sectioning the posterior cruciate ligament and posterolateral structures. J Bone Joint Surg Am. 1988;70:88–97.
48. American Medical Association, Committee on the medical aspect of sports. Subcommittee on classification of sports injuries. Standard nomenclature of athletic inuries. Chicago II, 1966:157.
49. Loomer RL. A test for knee posterolateral rotatory instability. Clin Orthop Relat Res. 1991;264:235–8.
50. Veltri DM, Warren RF. Isolated and combined posterior cruciate ligament injuries. J Am Acad Orthop Surg. 1993;1(2):67–75.

51. LaPrade RF, Wentorf F. Diagnosis and treatment of posterolateral knee injuries. Clin Orthop Relat Res. 2002;402:110–21.
52. Pritsch T, Blumberg N, Haim A, Dekel S, Arbel R. The importance of the valgus stress test in the diagnosis of posterolateral instability of the knee. Injury. 2006;37(10):1011–4.
53. Forsythe B, Saltzman BM, Cvetanovich GL, Collins MJ, Arns TA, Verma NN, Cole BJ, Bach BR Jr. Dial test: unrecognized predictor of anterior cruciate ligament deficiency. Arthroscopy. 2017;33(7):1375–81.
54. Griffith CJ, LaPrade RF, Johansen S, Armitage B, Wijdicks C, Engebretsen L. Medial knee injury: part 1, static function of the individual components of the main medial knee structures. Am J Sports Med. 2009;37(9):1762–70.
55. Merchant AC, Fulkerson JP, Leadbetter W. The diagnosis and initial treatment of patellofemoral disorders. Am J Orthop (Belle Mead NJ). 2017;46(2):68–75.
56. Sheehan FT, Derasari A, Fine KM, Brindle TJ, Alter KE. Q-angle and J-sign: indicative of maltracking subgroups in patellofemoral pain. Clin Orthop Relat Res. 2010;468(1):266–75.
57. Hadidi O, Ellanti P, Lincoln M, Hogan N. The J-sign in patellar maltracking. BMJ Case Rep. 2018;2018. pii: bcr-2017-222887 https://doi.org/10.1136/bcr-2017-222887.
58. Best MJ, Tanaka MJ, Demehri S, Cosgarea AJ. Accuracy and reliability of the visual assessment of patellar tracking. Am J Sports Med. 2020;48(2):370–5.
59. Nonweiler DE, DeLee JC. The diagnosis and treatment of medial subluxation of the patella after lateral retinacular release. Am J Sports Med. 1994;22(5):680–6.
60. Owen R. Recurrent dislocation of the superior tibio-fibular joint. A diagnostic pitfall in knee joint derangement. J Bone Joint Surg Br. 1968;50(2):342–5.
61. Beighton P, Horan F. Orthopaedic aspects of the Ehlers-Danlos syndrome. J Bone Joint Surg. 1969;51B:444.
62. Beighton P, Solomon L, Soskolne CL. Articular mobility in an African population. Ann Rheum Dis. 1973;32(5):413–8.
63. Maffulli N. Laxity versus instability. Orthopedics. 1998;21(8):837. 842
64. Schmitt LC, Fitzgerald GK, Reisman AS, Rudolph KS. Instability, laxity, and physical function in patients with medial knee osteoarthritis. Phys Ther. 2008;88(12):1506–16.
65. Fairbank HA. Internal derangement of the knee in children and adolescents. Proc R Soc Med. 1936;30:427–32.
66. Fulkerson JP. A clinical test for medial patella tracking. Tech Orthop. 1997;12:144.
67. Ohryi A. Dr Jacob Mackiewicz (1887-1966) and his sign. J Med Biogr. 2007;15(2):102–3.
68. Camino Willhuber GO, Piuzzi NS. Straight leg raise test. [Updated 2019 Nov 15]. In: StatPearls [Internet]. Treasure Island, FL: StatPearls Publishing; 2020. https://www.ncbi.nlm.nih.gov/books/NBK539717/.
69. Butowicz CM, Ebaugh DD, Noehren B, Silfies SP. Validation of two clinical measures of core stability. Int J Sports Phys Ther. 2016;11(1):15–23.
70. Gianola S, Castellini G, Stucovitz E, Nardo A, Banfi G. Single leg squat performance in physically and non-physically active individuals: a cross-sectional study. BMC Musculoskelet Disord. 2017;18(1):299. Published 2017 Jul 14. https://doi.org/10.1186/s12891-017-1660-8.
71. Weir A, Darby J, Inklaar H, Koes B, Bakker E, Tol JL. Core stability: inter- and intraobserver reliability of 6 clinical tests. Clin J Sport Med. 2010;20(1):34–8.
72. Peeler J, Anderson JE. Reliability of the Ely's test for assessing rectus femoris muscle flexibility and joint range of motion. J Orthop Res. 2008;26(6):793–9.
73. Reurink G, Goudswaard GJ, Oomen HG, Moen MH, Tol JL, Verhaar JA, Weir A. Reliability of the active and passive knee extension test in acute hamstring injuries. Am J Sports Med. 2013;41(8):1757–61.
74. Davis DS, Quinn RO, Whiteman CT, Williams JD, Young CR. Concurrent validity of four clinical tests used to measure hamstring flexibility. J Strength Cond Res. 2008;22(2):583–8.
75. Kuilart KE, Woollam M, Barling E, Lucas N. The active knee extension test and slump test in subjects with perceived hamstring tightness. Int J Osteopathic Med. 2005;8(3):89–97.

76. Hardcastle P, Nade S. The significance of the Trendelenburg test. J Bone Joint Surg Br. 1985;67(5):741–6.
77. Park KM, Cynn HS, Choung SD. Musculoskeletal predictors of movement quality for the forward step-down test in asymptomatic women. J Orthop Sports Phys Ther. 2013;43(7):504–10.
78. Sekiya I, Muneta T, Ogiuchi T, Yagishita K, Yamamoto H. Significance of the single-legged hop test to the anterior cruciate ligament-reconstructed knee in relation to muscle strength and anterior laxity. Am J Sports Med. 1998;26(3):384–8.
79. Balcarek P, Radebold T, Schulz X, Vogel D. Geometry of torsional malalignment syndrome: trochlear dysplasia but not torsion predicts lateral patellar instability. Orthop J Sports Med. 2019;7(3):2325967119829790. https://doi.org/10.1177/2325967119829790.
80. Swain MS, Henschke N, Kamper SJ, Downie AS, Koes BW, Maher CG. Accuracy of clinical tests in the diagnosis of anterior cruciate ligament injury: a systematic review. Chiropr Man Therap. 2014;22:25.
81. Kim SJ, Min BH, Han DY. Paradoxical phenomena of the McMurray test. An arthroscopic investigation. Am J Sports Med. 1996;24(1):83–7.
82. Slichter ME, Wolterbeek N, Auw Yang KG, Zijl JAC, Piscaer TM. Rater agreement reliability of the dial test in the ACL-deficient knee. J Exp Orthop. 2018;5(1):18. https://doi.org/10.1186/s40634-018-0131-y.
83. Rossi MJ. Editorial commentary: a positive "Half Dial Test" is seen in anterior cruciate ligament injury, so get out your goniometer. Arthroscopy. 2017;33(7):1382–3.

Chapter 7
Investigations for Knee Disorders

Once a clinical impression is made as to the likely source of the patient's symptoms, the aim is to investigate this further, to evaluate the working and alternative diagnoses. Radiological and neurophysiological examinations are utilised for the symptomatic knee.

The chapter describes the potential radiological and neurophysiological tests available in the diagnosis of knee conditions, helping to guide the reader as to what information they may provide and hence when they could be used. The role of diagnostic local anaesthetic injections and gait analysis is also discussed.

7.1 Radiological Investigations

Several radiological investigations are available to the knee clinician. Their choice is influenced by the question to be answered, working diagnosis, structures to assess (bony or soft tissue) as well as radiological resources and radiological expertise availability. Some of the radiological investigations that may be utilised in assessing the knee and the scenarios where they would be preferable are presented next. However, discussion between knee clinicians and local radiologists may help guide as to the best radiological modality available to answer a specific question.

7.1.1 Plain Radiographs

Preferable for the assessment of bony, calcium containing and other radio-opaque structures, hence they are utilised in the imaging of:

- Arthritis
- Fractures

C. Panayiotou Charalambous, *The Knee Made Easy*,
https://doi.org/10.1007/978-3-030-54506-2_7

- Abnormal joint displacement (knee instability)
- Soft tissue calcification

Plain radiographs may be described as:

- Non-weightbearing vs weightbearing/loading views
- Stress views

Several knee views have been described [1–6] but five commonly used are:

1. Anteroposterior (AP) weightbearing view with the knee straight (in extension)

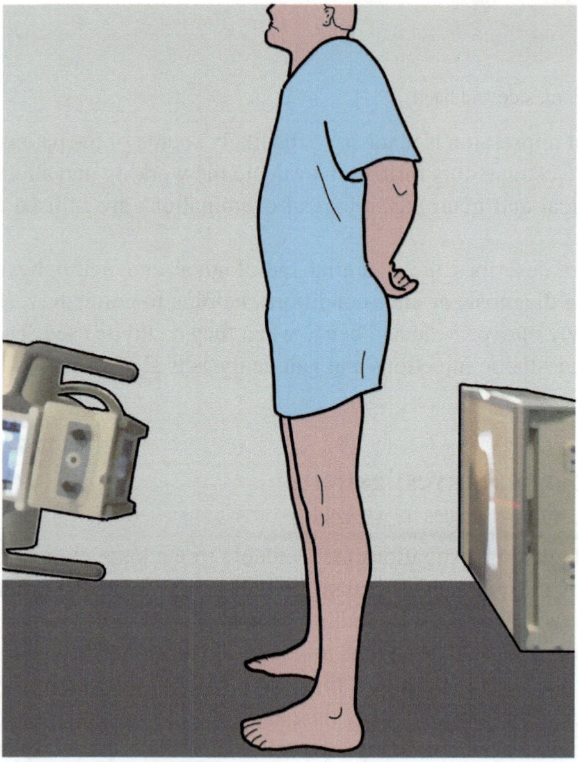

Obtaining an anteroposterior weightbearing knee radiograph

- Equivalent to looking at the knee from the front
- May be obtained with the patient
  - Standing—weightbearing
  - Lying flat, supine

The radiation beam is angled 10° caudal from the front in relation to the knee, with the cassette held behind the knee.

A weightbearing view is preferable when evaluating the tibiofemoral joint for cartilage loss, as it allows full compression of the articular surfaces.

- Assesses the tibiofemoral joint and proximal tibiofibular joint and adjacent bony structures
- Localises calcification and other radio-opaque structures in a superior-inferior and medial-lateral direction

2. Lateral view

- Equivalent to looking at the knee from the side
- May be obtained with the patient:
  - Supine, the knee flexed and the lower leg externally rotated
  - Supine, knee straight
  - Standing

A lateral view with the patient supine and knee straight (horizontal view) allows assessment for lipohaemarthrosis—fat released into the joint from the bone marrow, as a result of an intra-articular fracture, rises on top of the blood and gives a radiolucent (black) line in the suprapatellar pouch

- Assesses the tibiofemoral, patellofemoral (PF) and proximal tibiofibular joints
- Assesses the distal femur, proximal tibia, fibula, patella and fabella
- Assesses the relation of the patella to the femur and tibia in a superior to inferior direction (patellar height)
- Localises calcification and other radio-opaque structures in an anterior-posterior and superior-inferior direction

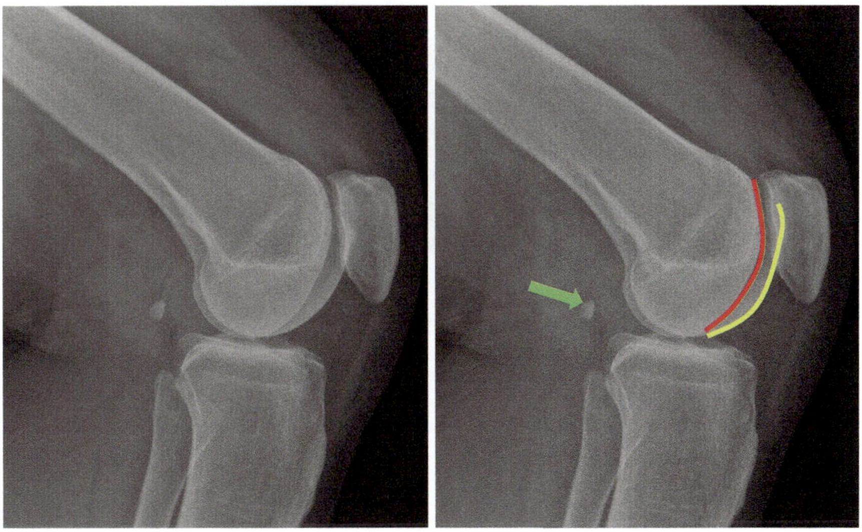

Lateral view of the knee—the medial femoral condyle (yellow) projects more distally than the lateral femoral condyle (red). The fabella (green arrow) may be seen in the back of the knee

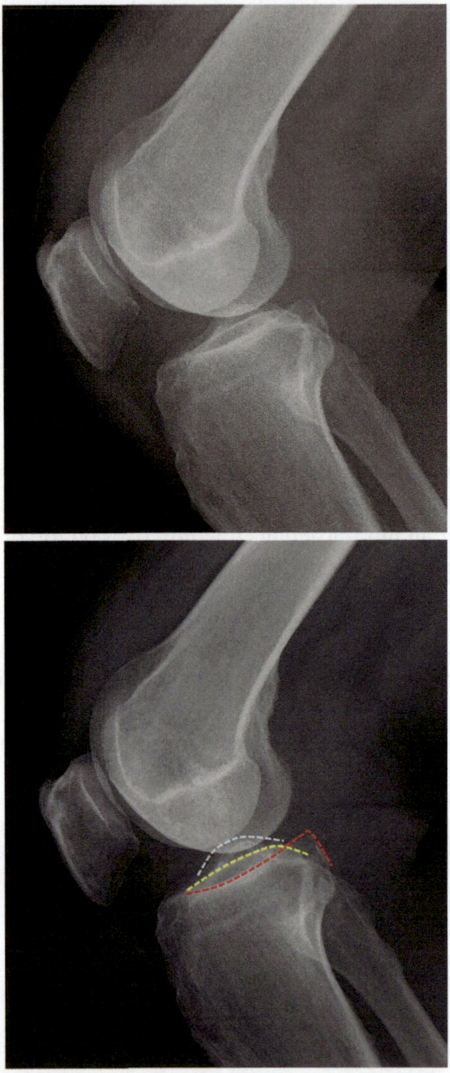

Lateral view of the knee—the medial tibial plateau (red) is concave, whereas the lateral tibial plateau (yellow) is convex. The lateral distal tibial spine (blue) projects higher than either of the tibial condyles

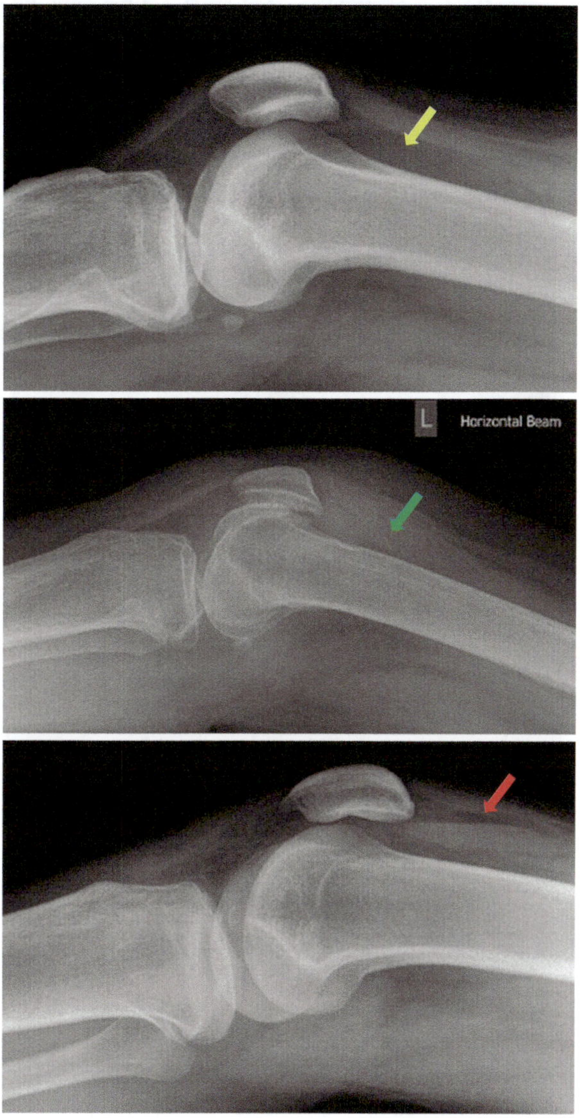

Suprapatellar pouch showing no effusion (yellow arrow), effusion with no obvious lipohaemarthrosis (green arrow), effusion with lipohaemarthrosis (red arrow) (plain radiograph-horizontal beam)

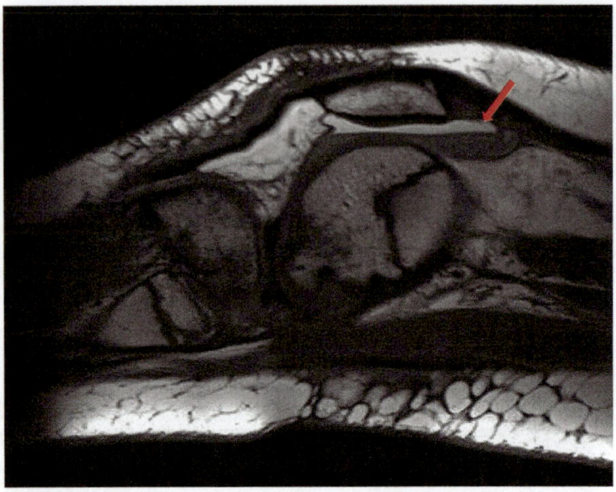

MRI examination of a lipohaemarthrosis allows recognition of what appears as a radiolucent line in the suprapatellar pouch (red arrow). The floating fat has the same appearance as the infrapatellar fat pat and subcutaneous fat.

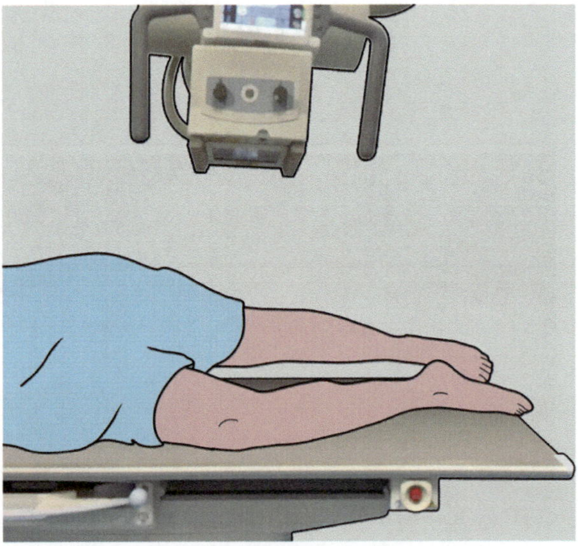

Obtaining a lateral non-weightbearing knee radiograph

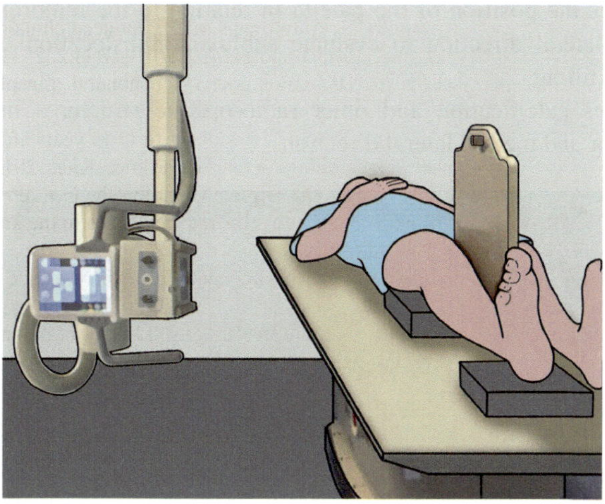

Obtaining a horizontal beam lateral non-weightbearing knee radiograph

3. Skyline view
   - May be obtained with the patient:
     - Supine, the knee flexed about 40°
     - Cassette held vertical on the distal thigh, by the patient
     - The radiation beam is directed cranially through the patellofemoral joint straight on or angled about 20° from the horizontal

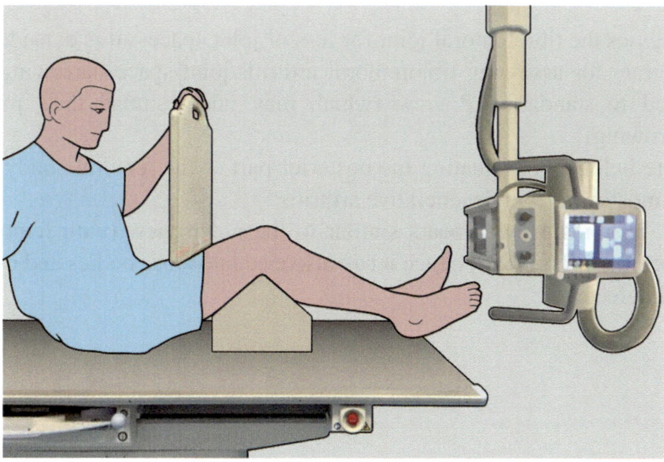

One of the ways of obtaining a skyline view radiograph of the patellofemoral joint

   - Equivalent to looking at the femoral trochlea and patella end on, to evaluate trochlear dysplasia, patellar dysplasia, PF arthritis

- Assesses the position of the patella in relation to the femoral trochlea in a medial-lateral direction to evaluate subluxation/dislocation of the patella, patellar tilting
- Localises calcification and other radio-opaque structures in an anterior-posterior and medial-lateral direction

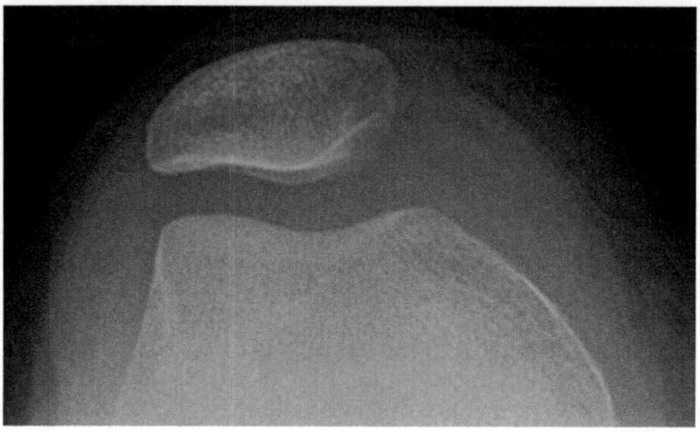

Skyline view

4. Posteroanterior (PA) weightbearing view with the knee in flexion

   - Equivalent to looking at the knee from the back
   - Obtained with the patient

     – Standing, knee flexed 45°, weightbearing
     – Radiation beam angled from the back, 10° caudal in relation to the knee
     – Cassette held vertical in front of knee

   - Assesses the tibiofemoral joint for loss of joint space—it is considered more accurate for assessing tibiofemoral arthritis/joint space narrowing as compared to standard AP view (which may underestimate/miss joint space narrowing)
   - More helpful in evaluating the posterior part of the femoral condyles which are mostly worn in degenerative arthritis
   - The resulting view appears similar to the notch view (with femoral notch appearing prominent), hence it can also evaluate loose bodies and osteochondral defects

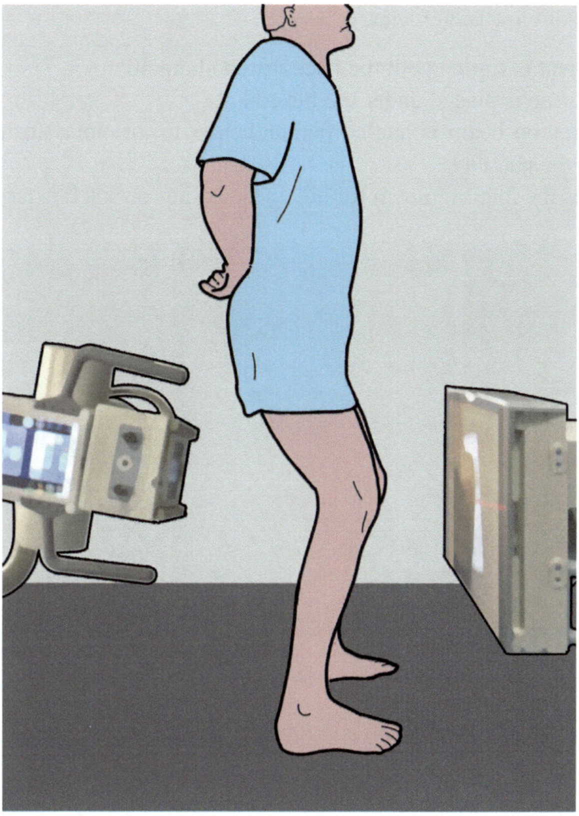

Obtaining a posterior-anterior weightbearing knee radiograph with the knee in 45° flexion

Rosenberg et al. [3] compared PA weightbearing radiographs taken with the knee in 45° of flexion with conventional AP radiographs in 55 patients who had surgical treatment for a lesion causing knee pain. Narrowing of the cartilage space of 2 mm or more was defined as indicative of major degeneration. Comparison of the intraoperative findings (degeneration) with the joint space narrowing observed in preoperative radiographs showed that the PA weightbearing view with the knee in 45° flexion was:

- More accurate
- More specific
- More sensitive

than the conventional AP weightbearing view with the knee in extension. They demonstrated that more than 80% of the cases showed joint narrowing with the PA flexion view but only 30% with the AP view.

5. Intercondylar view (notch view)

   - The patient is supine with the knee flexed about 40°
   - The cassette is placed under the flexed knee
   - The radiation beam is angled perpendicular to the tibia, at the level of the apex of the patella
   - Assesses the femoral notch for any loose bodies or notch osteophytes

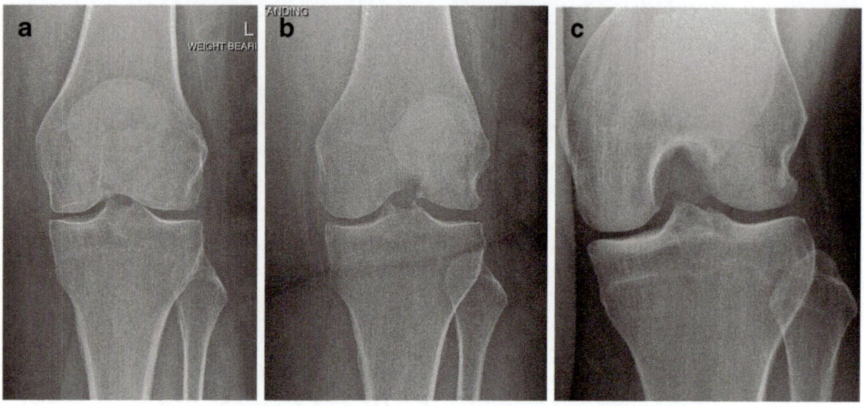

(**a**) AP weight bearing view. (**b**) Rosenberg view. (**c**) Notch view

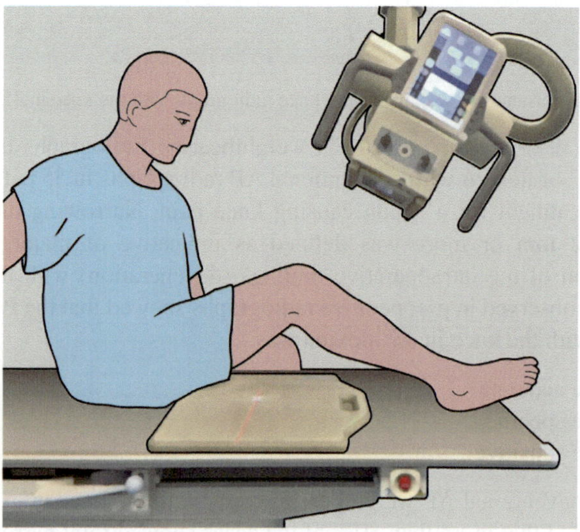

One of the ways of obtaining a notch view radiograph

7.1.2 Plain Radiographs Stress Views [7–14]

These involve the application of a force to the knee and comparing radiographs obtained before and post application of such a force to determine changes in alignment or relative position of the:

- Tibia and femur at the tibiofemoral joint
- Patella and femur at the PF joint

They may be used to assess:

Collateral ligament disruption

- AP radiograph, with the knee in extension and 30° flexion, to determine the coronal relation between tibia and femur whilst applying a:
  - Valgus force to the tibia—to assess the medial collateral ligament (MCL)
  - Varus force to the tibia to assess the lateral collateral ligament (LCL)

Posterior cruciate ligament (PCL) disruption

- Lateral radiograph to determine the sagittal relationship between tibia and femur (looking for posterior translation of the tibia in relation to the femur):
  - Kneeling stress view—the patient kneels on the knee with the knee flexed 90°
  - Gravity sag view—the knee is flexed 90°

7.1.3 Ultrasound [15–17]

Uses ultrasound waves to assess soft tissues around the knee. It is used to:

- Assess the superficial soft tissue envelope—skin, subcutaneous fat, tendons, muscles
- Evaluate the presence and nature of knee joint effusion
- Distinguish between solid and cystic soft-tissue swellings. Ultrasound may also determine if such swellings are vascularised which may indicate an active inflammatory lesion, infective changes, or neoplasia
- Guide the insertion of needles into or round the knee for introducing injectates or for fluid aspiration—such as in injecting the patellar tendon sheath to avoid injection into the patellar tendon

During ultrasound examination the leg may be actively or passively flexed and extended to help stretch the knee tendons (such as quadriceps or patellar tendon) and hence evaluate their continuity. The leg may also be moved to assess any abnormal displacement of the tendons—such as tendon snapping [4].

Ultrasound is relatively quick and simple to perform but its accuracy is operator dependent.

7.1.4 Plain Magnetic Resonance Imaging [18–20]

In plain magnetic resonance imaging (MRI), the patient is placed in a scanner which applies a magnetic field to help create a picture of the structures of the body. Coils may also be placed around the knee to allow an additional local application of a magnetic field and hence higher image quality.

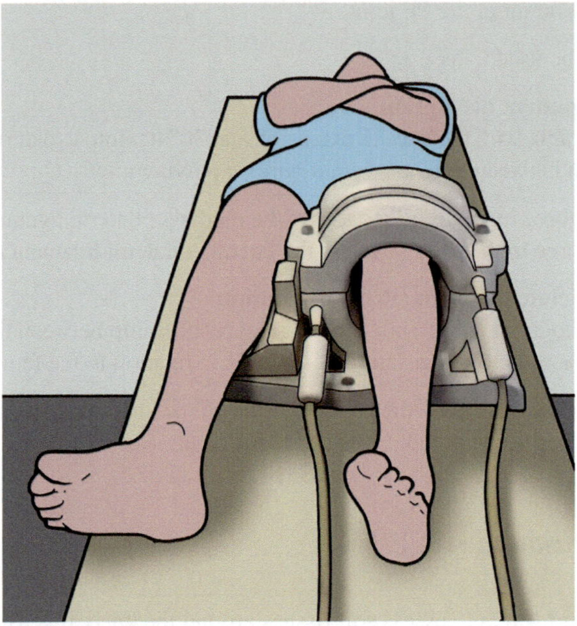

Local magnetic coil applied to the knee when obtaining an MRI

Images are formed using shades of white, grey and black, which can be altered to give multiple versions (sequences) to help assess the presented structures. Some commonly utilised MRI sequences are:

- T1 weighted—Fluid looks black, muscle grey, fat white
  - Evaluates anatomy—structure
- T2 weighted—Fluid looks white, muscle grey, fat white
  - Evaluates pathology—inflammation, infection show increased fluid levels

- STIR sequence—Fat looks dark, fluid looks bright
  - Evaluates edema in soft tissue and bones

  Images can be obtained in multiple planes, with three commonly used:

- Coronal—Equivalent to looking at the knee from the front
- Sagittal—Equivalent to looking at the knee from the side
- Axial—Equivalent to looking at the knee from the top down

  MRI is preferable for the detailed and accurate assessment of:

- Superficial soft tissues of the knee—skin, subcutaneous tissue, tendons (continuity, inflammation, degeneration), muscles (atrophy)
- Deep soft tissues of the knee—menisci, ligaments
- Bone consistency (marrow)—bone oedema, osteonecrosis, infection, inflammation, neoplasia, occult fracture
- Articular cartilage—early degenerative or other chondral changes not evident on plain radiographs
- Morphology of bone and articular cartilage—trochlear dysplasia in PF instability
- Relation of bones—patellar tilting, subluxation, tibial tubercle-trochlear groove (TT-TG) distance in evaluating the position of the tibial tuberosity in the assessment of PF instability
- Assessment of lower leg axial and rotational alignment

7.1.5 Contrast Enhanced MRI [21–23]

This is MRI performed following the intravenous administration of a contrast (dye) fluid, such as gadolinium. Contrast may accumulate in pathological areas which have leaky blood vessels making them appear bright.

Preferable for evaluating the presence of:

- Infection
- Inflammation
- Neoplasia

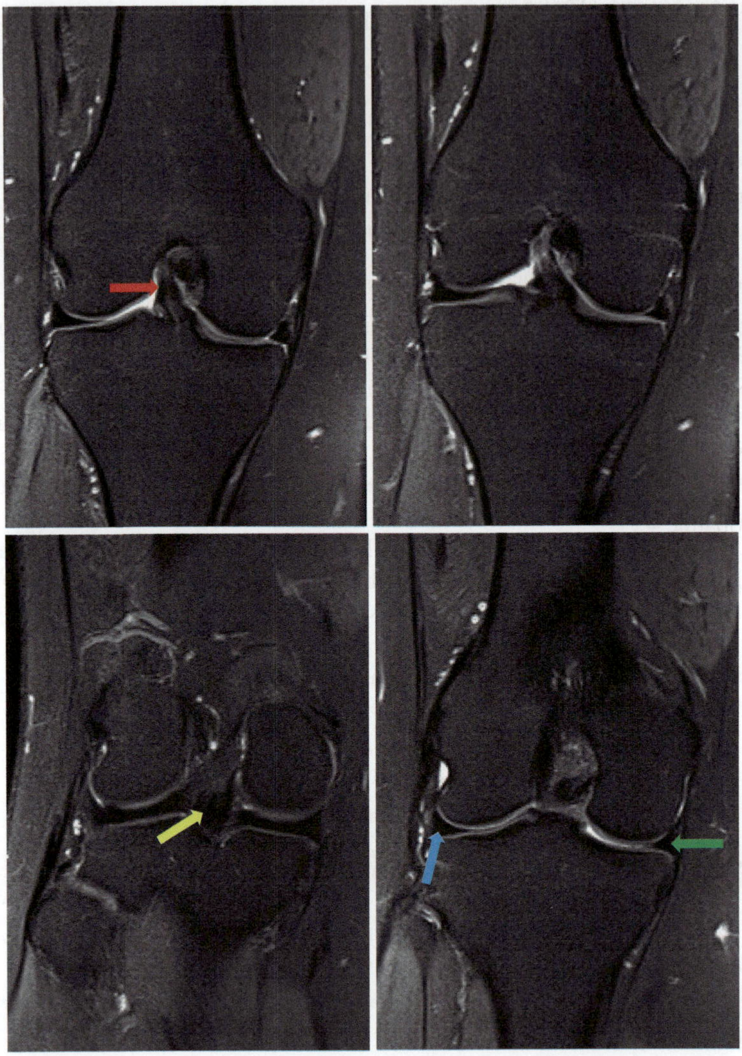

ACL (red arrow), PCL (yellow arrow), medial (green arrow) and lateral (blue arrow) meniscus

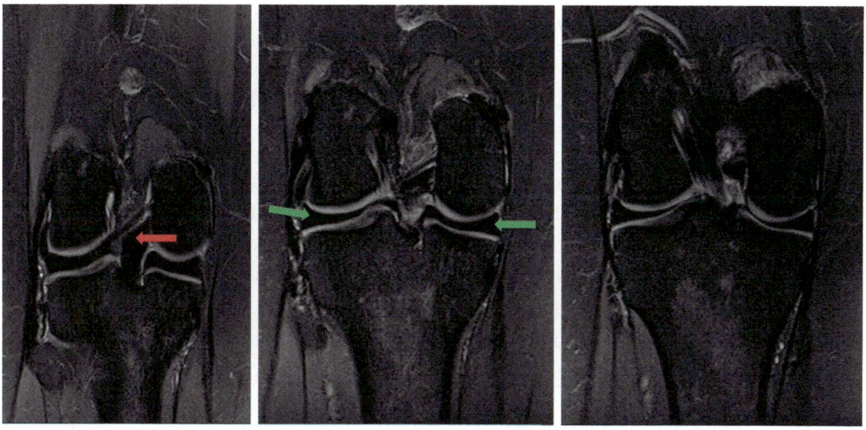

Posterior cruciate ligament (green) and posterior horns of menisci (red arrows)

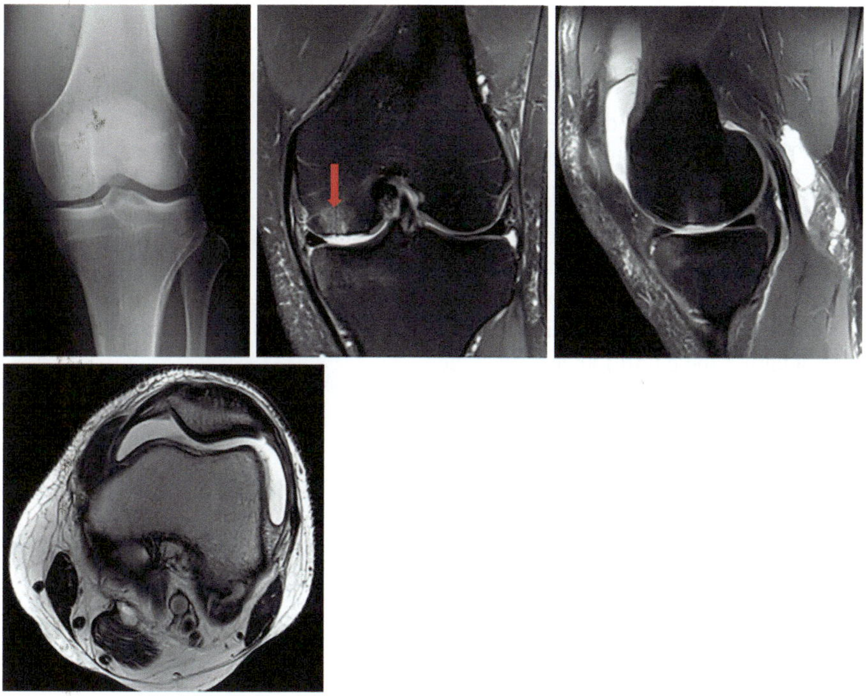

Medial articular cartilage loss, with medial femoral condyle oedema (red arrow), joint effusion and popliteal bursa on MRI, despite normal looking plain radiographs

7.1.6 MRI Arthrography [24–26]

MRI performed following the injection of a contrast (dye) fluid into the tibiofemoral joint [5, 6].

- Use of contrast may increase the accuracy of assessing knee lesions such as meniscal tears. The injected contrast inflates the joint and may separate the torn ends of a meniscus, demonstrating a gap between the two, and hence confirming the tear. This may be of value in the presence of previous meniscal surgery.
- An effusion, in the acute stage following an injury, may have the same effects as intra-articular contrast in aiding visualisation of intra-articular structures.

7.1.7 Computed Tomography

Computed tomography (CT) assesses mainly the morphology and structure of bone, although soft tissue evaluation (with or without contrast) is also possible.

- Preferable in the evaluation of bone morphology in planning surgery:
  - Tibial or femoral defects in joint arthroplasty
  - Tunnel position—in cruciate ligament revision surgery
  - Trochlear dysplasia—in PF instability
- Assessment of fractures (confirm presence, determine morphology)
- Evaluation of bone union in fractures
- Assessment of lower leg axial and rotational alignment—as in planning osteotomy surgery, or in assessing the position of knee replacement components in evaluating the painful knee replacement

7.1.8 CT Arthrography [24, 25]

CT performed following the injection of a contrast (dye) fluid into the knee joint.

- Use of contrast may increase the accuracy of assessing knee lesions such as chondral lesions
- Contrast may fill any cartilage surface defects making them easier to delineate

7.1.9 Bone Scan [27, 28]

- Knee bone scan—assesses the perfusion of the knee, to determine if there is any increased perfusion (hot spot) consistent with an increased osteoblastic activity (that occurs in bone regeneration, inflammation or infection). Increased activity may be seen in altered force loading or loosening of knee replacement components
- Whole body bone scan—assesses the whole skeleton for hot spots
  - May help determine if a lesion seen in the knee, is isolated to the knee or is associated with similar lesions in other parts of the skeleton. It may thus help determine:
    - If a neoplastic lesion is isolated to the knee (hence likely to be a primary lesion) or associated with other skeletal lesions (hence likely to be a metastatic lesion)
    - If knee infection is isolated or associated with other foci of infection in the skeleton, suggestive of a source (such as endocarditis or spinal discitis) shedding infective emboli
    - If there is a widespread metabolic bone lesion involving the knee and other parts of the skeleton

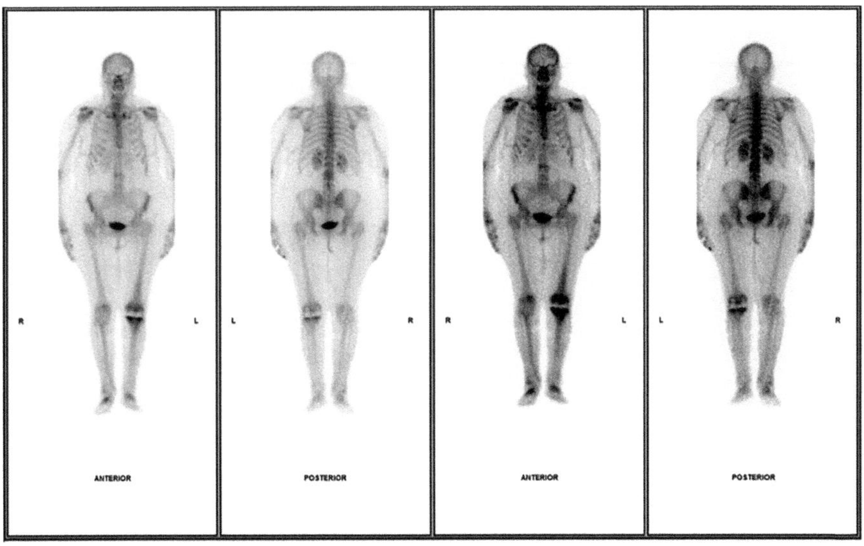

Whole body bone scan

7.1.10 Radio-Labelled White Cell Bone Scan

White blood cells are obtained from the individual and are labelled with radio-active dye. These labelled white cells are then injected into the bloodstream and their distribution around the knee under evaluation is assessed. Abnormal accumulation of labelled white cells suggests underlying infection or inflammation. Radio-labelled white cell bone scan may thus help:

- Distinguish between inflammation and infection (higher white cell accumulation seen in the latter)
- Distinguish between aseptic (not infective) and infective loosening of knee arthroplasty implants (higher white cell accumulation seen in the latter)

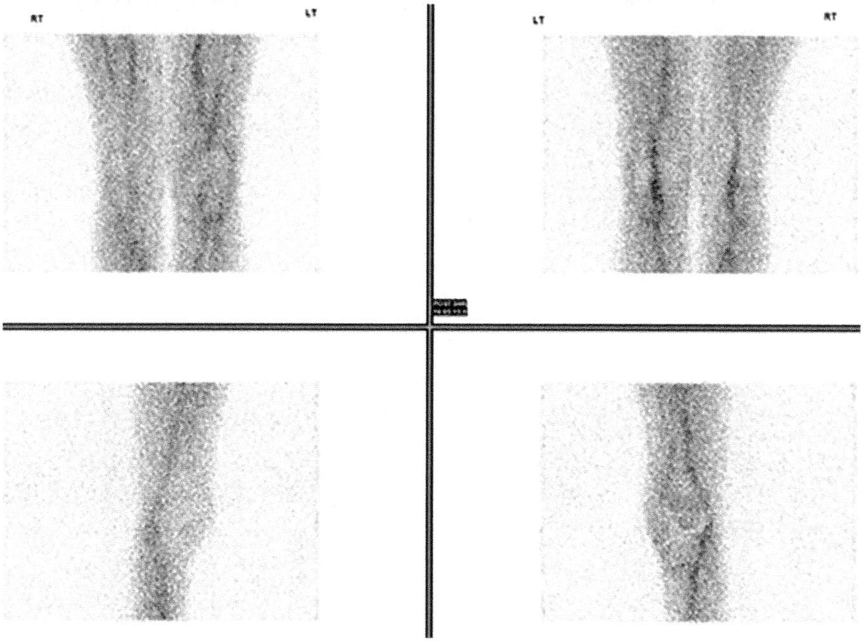

White cell bone scan

7.1.11 Single-Photon Emission Computed Tomography SPECT (+/– arthrography) [29–32]

A SPECT scan involves the combination of a 3D bone scan and a CT scan of the knee.

The images from both scans are then fused together to give a combined image [7, 8].

Conventional bone scans may show an area of increased activity in the knee but are difficult to localise the area of the knee that the increased activity involves. SPECT allows a more accurate localisation, and may thus help determine the source of pain where clinical symptoms are not specific.

This may be amongst others to identify:

- Compartment overloading
- Non-healing chondral or osteochondral lesions
- Arthroplasty implant loosening/infection

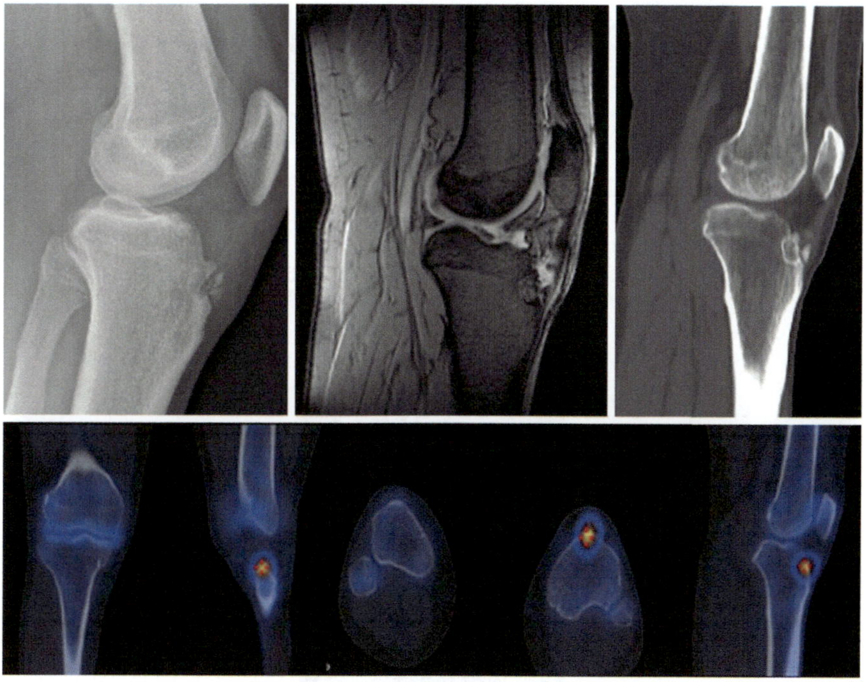

Tibial tubercle apophysitis (MRI, CT), with hot spot on SPECT scan

7.2 Assessment of Lower Limb/Knee Alignment [33–37]

- Plain radiographs—whole leg (long leg) weightbearing films (AP)—coronal, sagittal alignment
- CT scan lower limbs—coronal, sagittal, rotational alignment (knee, long leg)
- MRI lower limbs—coronal, sagittal, rotational alignment (knee, long leg)

The advantage of plain radiographs in assessing alignment in the coronal plane is that they can be obtained weightbearing as opposed to CT and MRI which are usually non-weightbearing (although weightbearing scanners are now available, but still of limited use).

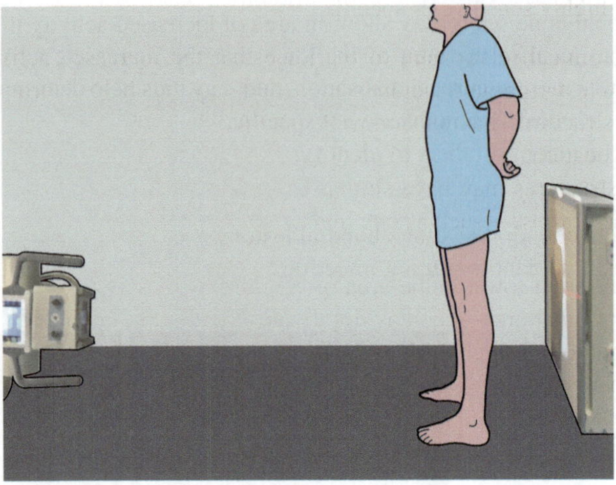

Obtaining a long leg plain radiograph with patient standing about 3m from the radiation beam

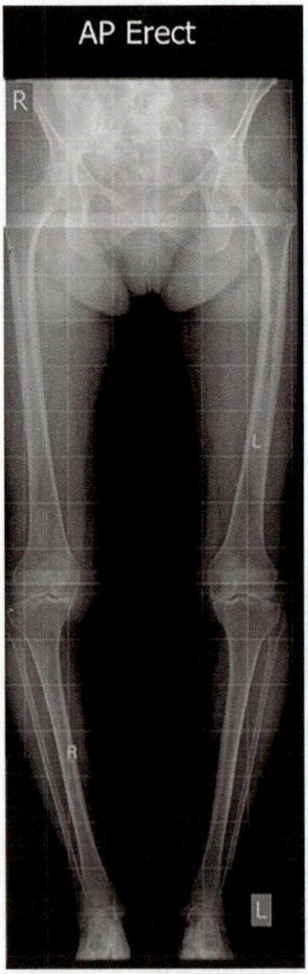

Long leg plain radiograph

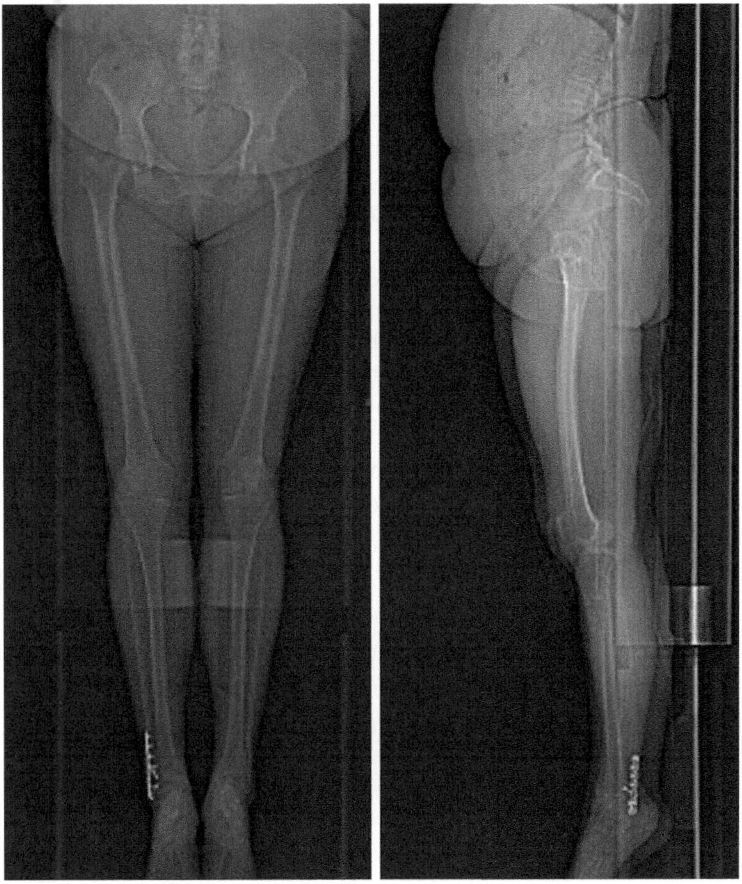

Long leg CT tomogram to assess leg length and alignment

7.2.1 *Lower Limb Alignment*

Certain radiological parameters are used to describe lower limb alignment and these are described below:

7.2.1.1 Coronal Alignment

Radiographs of the whole leg, from hip to ankle, taken when standing are used. Assessments may also be made on non-standing CT or MRI.

The following is assessed on full leg weightbearing radiograph:

- Weightbearing axis—a line connecting the centre of the femoral head to the centre of the distal tibial plafond. This normally passes through, or very near to the centre of the knee. This makes an angle of 3°with the vertical axis (a vertical line passing down from the symphysis pubis)

- Mechanical axis of the femur—line connecting the centre of the femoral head to the centre of the distal femur (centre of knee)
- Mechanical axis of the tibia—line connecting the centre of the tibial plateau (knee) to the centre of the distal tibial plafond
- Anatomical axis of the femur—line connecting the centre of the femoral shaft in the subtrochanteric area and the centre of the femoral trochlea
- Femoral anatomical-mechanical angle—the angle between the mechanical and anatomical axes of the femur (about 6° valgus)
- Anatomical axis of the tibia—line connecting the centre of the tibial plateau to the centre of the tibial plafond. This coincides with the mechanical axis
- Distal femoral articular axis—line connecting the most distal points of the medial and lateral femoral condyles
- Proximal tibial articular axis—line connecting the most proximal points of the medial and lateral tibial plateau condyles
- Angle between femoral mechanical axis—distal femoral articular axis—the angle between the femoral mechanical axis and the distal femoral articular axis (about 3° in valgus)
- Angle between femoral anatomical axis—distal femoral articular axis—the angle between the femoral anatomical axis and the distal femoral articular axis (about 9° in valgus)
- Angle between proximal tibial articular axis and tibial mechanical (or anatomical) axis (about 2–3° varus)
- Mechanical tibiofemoral angle—the angle between the femoral mechanical axis and the tibial mechanical axis—these usually coincide
- Anatomical tibiofemoral angle—the angle between the anatomical axis of the femur and the anatomical axis of the tibia (about 6° valgus, lower in men)

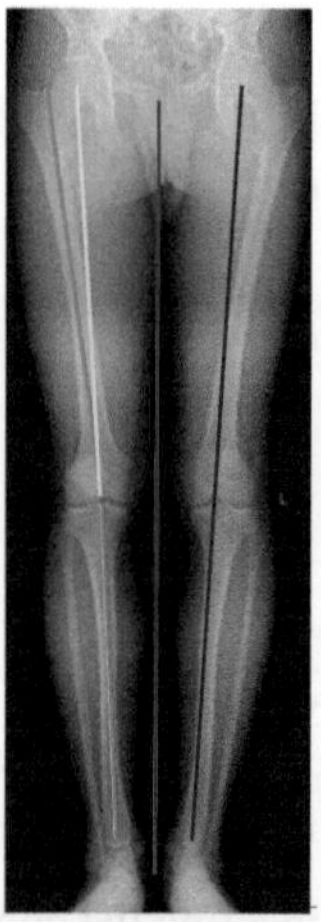

Long leg films—normal alignment (anatomical axis femur—green, mechanical axis femur—yellow, anatomical axis and mechanical axis tibia—orange, vertical line—red). Weightbearing axis—purple coincides with mechanical axis of femur and tibia in well aligned lower limb

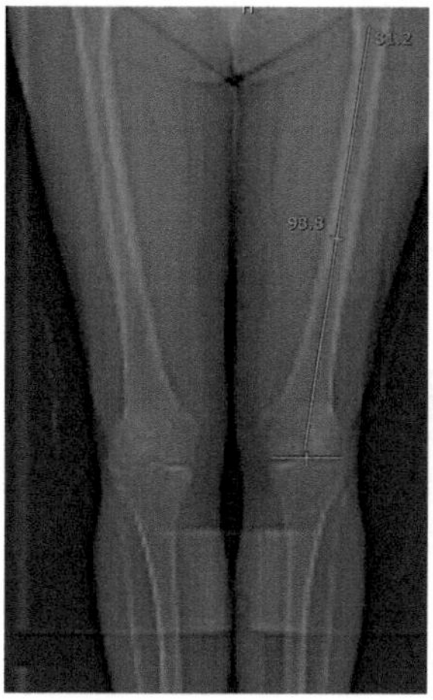

Long leg CT tomogram assessing the angle between the femoral anatomical axis and distal femoral articular line axis

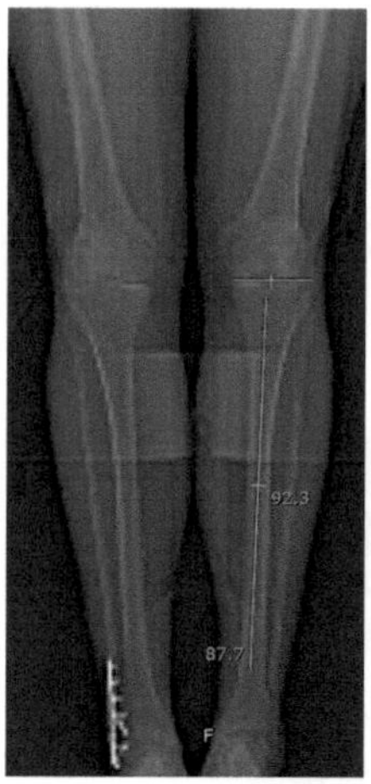

Long leg CT tomogram assessing the angle between the tibial anatomical axis and proximal tibial articular line axis

7.2.1.2 Sagittal Alignment

1. Caton-Deschamps ratio—assessed on lateral plain radiographs. It measures the distance between the inferior edge of the patellar articular surface and the anterosuperior angle of the tibia, on a sagittal plain radiograph (AT) divided by the length of the patellar articular surface (AP). AT/AP is normally equal to 1.

   - A ratio equal or superior to 1.2 is defined as patella alta
   - A ratio less than or equal to 0.6 is defined as patella infera (patella baja)

The Caton-Deschamps ratio relies on readily identifiable and reproducible anatomical landmarks and is not affected by:

- The quality of X-rays
- Knee size
- Radiological enlargement
- Position of the tibial tubercle
- Knee flexion (within 10° and 80° of knee flexion)

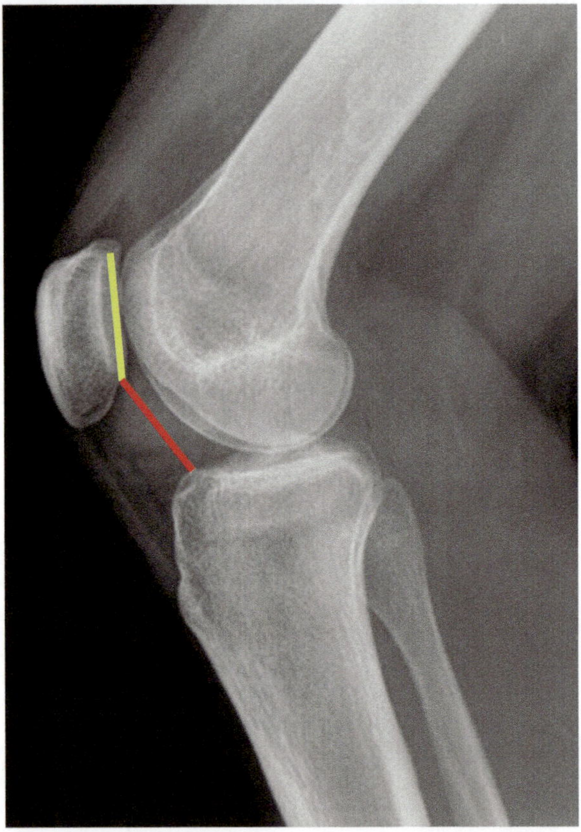

Caton-Deschamps index: The distance from the inferior border of the patellar articular surface to the superior/anterior border of the tibial plateau (length of the red line) is divided over the length of the patellar articular surface (yellow line)

2. Patellar articular overlap—on sagittal MRI the patellar articular length is measured. The length of the patellar cartilage that overlaps the trochlear cartilage is also measured. This overlap cartilage may be expressed as absolute value (with <6 mm considered indicative of patella alta) or as a percentage of the total patellar articular cartilage.

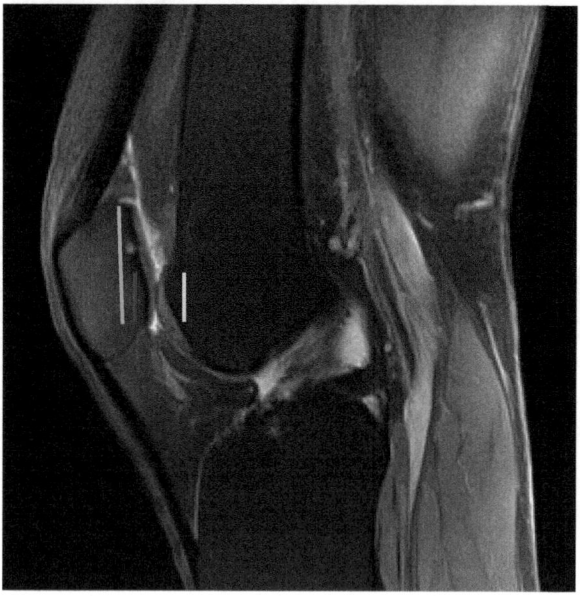

Patellar overlap index measurements—a measure of the patellar cartilage length (red) overlapping with the trochlear cartilage (yellow) in extension. This may be expressed as the proportion of the total patellar articular cartilage length (green)

7.2.1.3 Rotational Alignment

- Femoral anteversion angle is between the:
  - Axis of the femoral neck (mid-point between the anterior and posterior femoral neck cortices to the centre of the femoral head)
  - Line connecting the posterior condyles of the distal femur
  - Reported ranges in adults about 15°± 7°
- Tibial torsion angle is the angle between a:
  - Line connecting the posterior condyles of the proximal tibia
  - Line passing through the transmalleolar axis
  - Reported ranges in adults about 25°± 7°

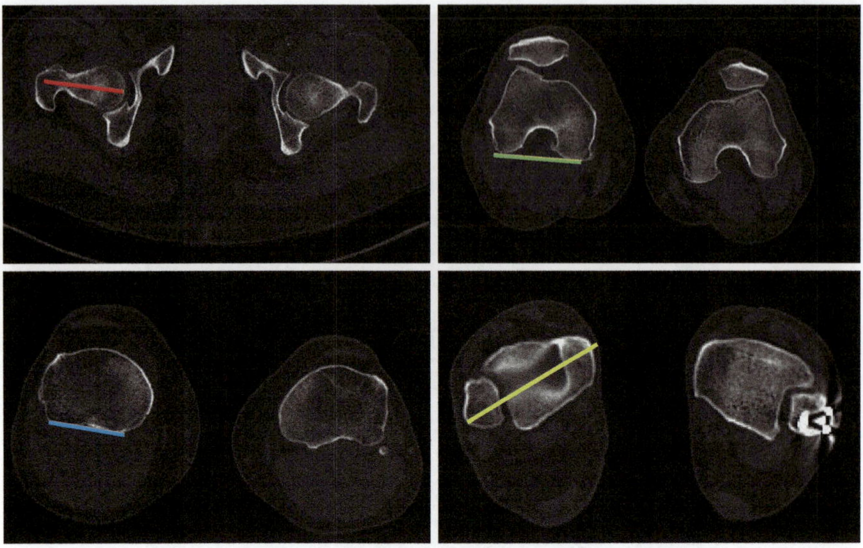

CT assessment of rotational profile. The lines passing through the middle of the femoral neck (red line), along the posterior femoral condyles (green line), posterior condyles of the widest part of the proximal tibia (blue line) and transmalleolar axis (yellow line) are determined and the angle between them is measured

7.2.1.4 Bone Morphology

1. TT-TG distance—assesses the position (lateralisation) of the tibial tubercle in relation to the trochlear groove. It may be determined on axial MRI or CT images. The deepest point of the trochlear groove is identified on the first cranio-caudal image that shows a complete cartilaginous trochlea (for MRI examinations). A line (trochlear line) is drawn through this, perpendicular to the posterior condylar line. A second line is drawn parallel to the trochlear line through the most anterior part of the tibial tubercle. The distance between the two lines is measured (TT-TG distance). Reported values in non-symptomatic knees are: 15.5 ± 1.5 mm on CT, 12.5 ± 2 mm on MRI.

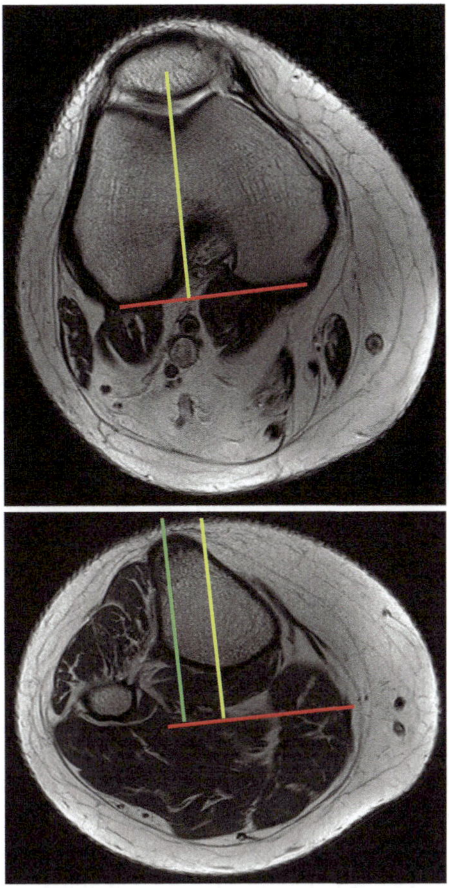

TT-TG assessment—this is the distance from a line passing through the deepest part of the trochlear sulcus (yellow line) and perpendicular to the posterior condylar line (red line) to a line passing through the most prominent part of the tibial tubercle (green line) and perpendicular to the posterior condylar line.

2. Trochlear sulcus angle—this is the angle between a line drawn from the centre of the deepest part of the trochlea along the medial trochlear facet and a similar line drawn along the lateral trochlear facet. It may be assessed on plain radiographs (skyline view), axial CT (bony sulcus angle) or axial MRI (cartilaginous sulcus angle) scans. Reported values for non-symptomatic knees are:

- Cartilaginous sulcus angle 142° (95% CI: 140°–144°)
- Bony sulcus angle 134° (95% CI:131°–136°)

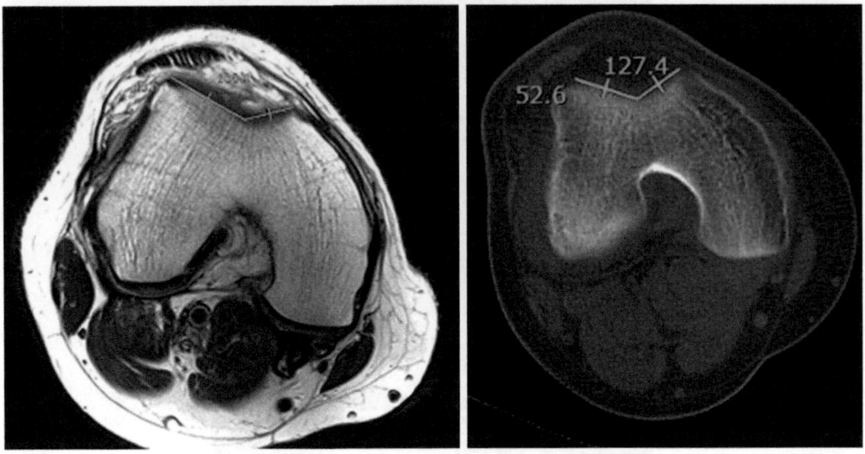

Chondral and bony sulcus angles in a case of trochlear dysplasia with symptomatic patellar instability

7.3 MRI Subchondral Oedema [38, 39]

"Subchondral oedema" is a term used to describe the presence of high signal on T1 and T2 images in the bone of the knee and is a frequent finding on MRI examinations of the knee [9–11].

Such a finding may be due to multiple causes including:

- Post-traumatic
- Degenerative arthritis
- Inflammatory arthritis
- Osteomyelitis
- Osteonecrosis
- Neoplasia
- Haematological conditions
- Metabolic conditions
- Mechanical-overloading

In some of these conditions the appearances may be characteristic such as:

- In secondary osteonecrosis the lesions are wedge shaped subchondral lesions
- In spontaneous osteonecrosis of the knee (SPONK) the lesion often appears as localised oval area in the subchondral bone with flattening of the convexity of the condyle

However, in many of these underlying causes the appearance of changes on MRI are often macroscopically similar. Furthermore, this radiological finding may not necessarily represent bone "oedema" but a spectrum of histological appearances varying from increased local fluid levels to cell necrosis and regeneration.

Hence, to help distinguish the nature and clinical significance of such MRI oedema, its presence must be correlated with the clinical history and clinical findings as well as the presence of associated MRI findings such as intra-articular lesions (meniscus, ligamentous, articular cartilage dysfunction).

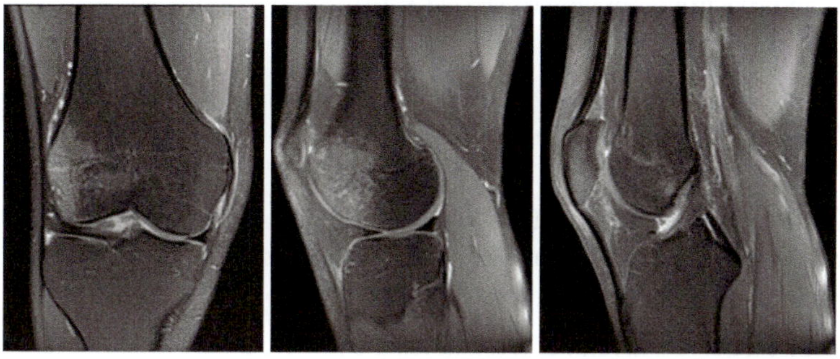

Post patellar dislocation, oedema in lateral femoral condyle and patella

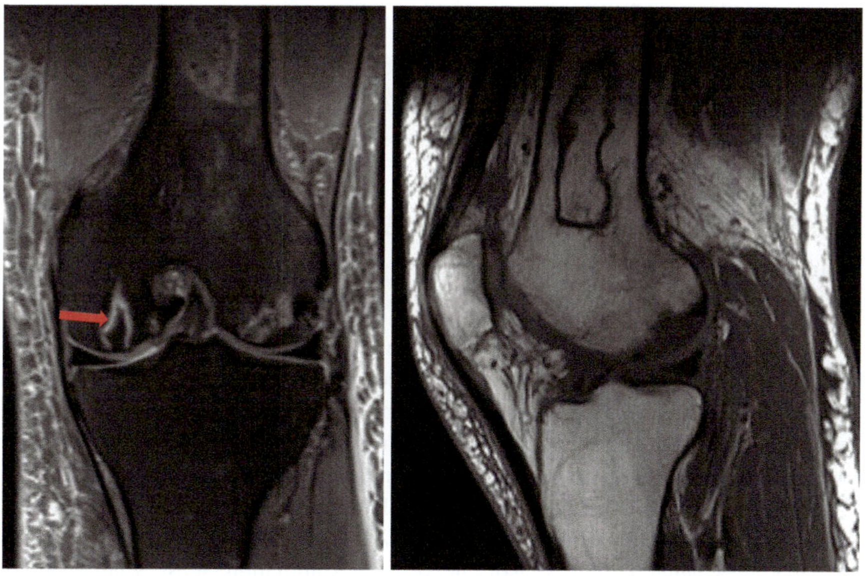

Avascular necrosis of the distal femur—geographic appearence (red arrow) (MRI)

7.4 Neurophysiological Investigations for Knee Conditions [40, 41]

Neurophysiological investigations of the knee and lower limb may be used in conjunction with clinical findings, to diagnose dysfunction of nerves and muscles which may account for knee symptoms. They consist of nerve conduction (NC) studies and Electromyography (EMG) [12–14].

7.4.1 Nerve Conduction Studies

This is the examination of conduction along motor and sensory nerves.

Nerve conduction studies may help identify the presence of nerve dysfunction and determine its likely cause. These may determine:

- Whether a nerve's myelin or axon fibres are involved
- Whether one or more nerves are involved
- The site of nerve dysfunction (nerve root, plexus, peripheral nerve)
- The pattern of nerve dysfunction
  - Long vs. short fibre nerves
  - Large vs. small fibre nerves
  - Focal, multi-focal, random nerve involvement

A nerve conduction study involves:

1. Stimulating and recording over 2 separate points of a peripheral sensory nerve
2. Stimulating a peripheral motor nerve and recording over a muscle

In this way:

1. The time taken for electrical impulses to travel along two points on the nerve (latency) can be determined, and hence the speed of electrical transmission (conduction velocity) can be calculated. Slow conduction may be seen in demyelinating neurological disorders or may be secondary to prolonged transmission at the neuromuscular junction. Focal, well localised reduction in conduction velocity may indicate external compression of the nerve
2. The size of electrical activity in the muscle upon nerve stimulation is recorded (compound muscle action potential—CMAP). Similarly, the size of the electrical activity generated in a sensory nerve by its stimulation (sensory nerve action potential—SNAP) is measured. A reduction in the magnitude of such electrical

activities (lower than expected) may suggest that there is loss of axon fibres rather than simply loss of myelin. Severe compression of a nerve for prolonged time may lead to axon loss

7.4.2 EMG

EMG is the detection of electrical activity from muscles. This is determined by inserting percutaneously fine needle electrodes into muscles. EMG has two main roles:

1. Differentiate between a primary muscle disorder versus a neurogenic disorder as the cause of muscle weakness or atrophy
2. Determine whether there is involvement of a nerve's myelin sheath or axon fibres; axonal loss signifies a more severe dysfunction
3. When dealing with a neurogenic disorder, sampling of several muscles, determining the extent and pattern of the muscle involvement, and taking into account their anatomical innervation, EMG may help localise the lesion and distinguish between:

    a. Spinal root involvement
    b. Plexus lesion
    c. Peripheral nerve lesion

EMG recordings mainly aim to assess:

1. The presence of spontaneous muscle electrical activity—that is activity generated in the absence of any voluntary effort to contract the muscle. The morphology of such spontaneous electrical activity may guide as to the presence and type of neurogenic or myopathy disorders:

    a. Denervated muscle (due to axonal loss) may show spontaneous discharges of electrical activity—fibrillations and fasciculations
    b. Myotonic discharges—seen in certain myotonias

2. Muscle unit electrical activity
3. Electrical recruitment of muscle fibres upon attempted voluntary contraction

7.5 Diagnostic Knee Injections

Local anaesthetic injections may help guide a clinician as to the origin of a patient's pain [42–44]. A local anaesthetic is injected into the area of the knee (intra-articular, or specific extra-articular location) that is considered to be the origin of a patient's pain and time is allowed for the local anaesthetic to start working (usually a few minutes depending on how fast acting the local anaesthetic is). The patient may be asked to move the knee or walk and see whether the injection has helped the pain.

Reduction in pain suggests that the pain is likely coming from the area that has been injected. If no reduction in pain is reported, then one needs to consider that the pain may not be coming from the injected area.

In cases where the pain is thought to be referred from the hip or lumbosacral spine, a diagnostic local anaesthetic injection may be administered to the hip or lumbosacral spine and any improvement in knee pain noted.

Reduction in pain by a local anaesthetic injection may also allow one to distinguish between true and apparent (pain mediated) weakness, or between true and apparent (pain mediated) stiffness. Apparent weakness and apparent stiffness may improve following a reduction in pain (for the duration that the local anaesthetic remains active), whereas true weakness or true stiffness are not helped by pain reduction.

Local anaesthetic injections may be combined with a steroid injection to try and improve long term pain. Hence, injections can have a diagnostic but also a therapeutic effect.

Local anaesthetic injections may help temporarily relax muscles to determine if that improves a patient's symptoms which may then be attributed to muscular overactivity (such as injecting the hamstring muscles to help distinguish between true and apparent stiffness (loss of extension) [18].

7.6 Gait Analysis

This is a method used to analyse several gait patterns which may help guide to the force distribution at the knee, help determine the underlying diagnosis, and guide treatment. This analysis is usually performed in a gait laboratory [45–47].

Gait analysis data are captured non-invasively using:

- Cameras—to capture motion
- Force plates—to measure the forces exerted on the ground
- EMG measurements—to assess muscle activity

The patient moves (walks/runs) whilst motion is captured on a camera and the force exerted on the ground is measured.

External sensors (reflective markers) are attached to the patient's skin (e.g. using adhesive tape) at certain anatomical positions which correspond to the patient's pelvis and limbs. In this way the 3D position of the patient's bones are represented in space, and an anatomical model of the patient is constructed. The angles of joint motion can thus be determined from the orientation of the lower limb components in space. By taking into account the forces exerted by the foot on the ground, the moments (equal to force multiplied by distance) related to joint motion can then be determined. EMG activity may also be measured simultaneously to help relate the activity of specific muscles to other gait parameters.

Although not widely used in the routine management of knee conditions, gait analysis may be utilised in complex cases. In the future, gait analysis may have a more widespread use in working out gait specific deficits in individual cases to help determine who will benefit from specific interventions (such as unloading bracing), the outcomes of which are not consistently predictable.

Learning Pearls

- Different radiological modalities may be considered complimentary rather than mutually exclusive, as each may be better at assessing specific components of the musculoskeletal system. Hence, multiple radiological investigations may be utilised in the diagnostic work up
- "Less" is on occasion "more"—a plain radiograph may be more informative than MRI in evaluating advanced arthritis of the knee joint.
- Although various "normal values" and "normal ranges" have been described for several radiological indices, these should be interpreted with caution and over-reliance on these should be avoided as they may be affected by:
  - Position of the limb (flexion/extension, rotation)
  - Weightbearing vs. non-weightbearing state
  - Static or dynamic limb state
  - Position of the knee components in relation to each other in physiological and pathological conditions
  - Angulation of radiology source and position of cassette in relation to the knee (for plain radiographs)
  - Subchondral bone morphology may differ from the morphology of its overlying articular cartilage (hence plain radiographs/CT evaluations may give different values compared to MRI evaluations of the same parameters)
  - Intra- and inter-rater variation in measurement of indices
- Muscle denervation changes may not be apparent for 2–3 weeks post-nerve injury. Hence, neurophysiological studies are better obtained after 3 weeks post injury or other nerve insult

References

1. Keogh P, Masterson E, Murphy B, McCoy CT, Gibney RG, Kelly E. The role of radiography and computed tomography in the diagnosis of acute dislocation of the proximal tibiofibular joint. Br J Radiol. 1993;66(782):108–11.
2. Jones AC, Ledingham J, McAlindon T, Regan M, Hart D, MacMillan PJ, Doherty M. Radiographic assessment of patellofemoral osteoarthritis. Ann Rheum Dis. 1993;52(9):655–8.
3. Rosenberg TD, Paulos LE, Parker RD, Coward DB, Scott SM. The forty-five-degree posteroanterior flexion weight-bearing radiograph of the knee. J Bone Joint Surg Am. 1988;70(10):1479–83.
4. Brattstrom H. Roentgen examination of the distal femur end and the femoro-patellar joint by so called axial picture. Acta Orthop Scand. 1964;68(Suppl):53–78.
5. Merchant AC. Patellofemoral imaging. Clin Orthop Relat Res. 2001;389:15–21.
6. Buckland-Wright C. Which radiographic techniques should we use for research and clinical practice? Best Pract Res Clin Rheumatol. 2006;20(1):39–55.
7. James EW, Williams BT, LaPrade RF. Stress radiography for the diagnosis of knee ligament injuries: a systematic review. Clin Orthop Relat Res. 2014;472(9):2644–57.
8. Laprade RF, Wijdicks CA. The management of injuries to the medial side of the knee. J Orthop Sports Phys Ther. 2012;42(3):221–33.
9. Kappel A, Mortensen JF, Nielsen PT, Odgaard A, Laursen M. Reliability of stress radiography in the assessment of coronal laxity following total knee arthroplasty. Knee. 2020;27(1):221–28.
10. Laprade RF, Bernhardson AS, Griffith CJ, Macalena JA, Wijdicks CA. Correlation of valgus stress radiographs with medial knee ligament injuries: an in vitro biomechanical study. Am J Sports Med. 2010;38(2):330–8. https://doi.org/10.1177/0363546509349347.
11. LaPrade RF, Heikes C, Bakker AJ, Jakobsen RB. The reproducibility and repeatability of varus stress radiographs in the assessment of isolated fibular collateral ligament and grade-III posterolateral knee injuries. An in vitro biomechanical study. J Bone Joint Surg Am. 2008;90(10):2069–76.
12. Garofalo R, Fanelli GC, Cikes A, N'Dele D, Kombot C, Mariani PP, Mouhsine E. Stress radiography and posterior pathological laxity of knee: comparison between two different techniques. Knee. 2009;16(4):251–5.
13. Shino K, Mitsuoka T, Horibe S, Hamada M, Nakata K, Nakamura N. The gravity sag view: a simple radiographic technique to show posterior laxity of the knee. Arthroscopy. 2000;16(6):670–2.
14. Osti L, Papalia R, Rinaldi P, Denaro V, Bartlett J, Maffulli N. The kneeling view: evaluation of the forces involved and side-to-side difference. Knee. 2009;16(6):463–5.
15. Friedman L, Finlay K, Jurriaans E. Ultrasound of the knee. Skelet Radiol. 2001;30(7):361–77.
16. Hung CY, Chang KV, Lam S. Dynamic sonography for snapping knee syndrome caused by the gracilis tendon. J Ultrasound Med. 2018;37(3):803–4.
17. Guillin R, Marchand AJ, Roux A, Niederberger E, Duvauferrier R. Imaging of snapping phenomena. Br J Radiol. 2012;85(1018):1343–53.
18. Nacey NC, Geeslin MG, Miller GW, Pierce JL. Magnetic resonance imaging of the knee: an overview and update of conventional and state of the art imaging. J Magn Reson Imaging. 2017;45(5):1257–75.
19. Sanders TG, Miller MD. A systematic approach to magnetic resonance imaging interpretation of sports medicine injuries of the knee. Am J Sports Med. 2005;33(1):131–48.
20. Kijowski R, Roemer F, Englund M, Tiderius CJ, Swärd P, Frobell RB. Imaging following acute knee trauma. Osteoarthr Cartil. 2014;22(10):1429–43.
21. Shakoor D, Demehri S, Roemer FW, Loeuille D, Felson DT, Guermazi A. Are contrast-enhanced and non-contrast MRI findings reflecting synovial inflammation in knee osteoarthritis: a meta-analysis of observational studies. Osteoarthr Cartil. 2020;28(2):126–36.
22. Geith T, Niethammer T, Milz S, Dietrich O, Reiser M, Baur-Melnyk A. Transient bone marrow edema syndrome versus osteonecrosis: perfusion patterns at dynamic contrast-

enhanced MR imaging with high temporal resolution can allow differentiation. Radiology. 2017;283(2):478–85.
23. Lee JH, Dyke JP, Ballon D, Ciombor DM, Tung G, Aaron RK. Assessment of bone perfusion with contrast-enhanced magnetic resonance imaging. Orthop Clin North Am. 2009;40(2):249–57.
24. Kalke RJ, Di Primio GA, Schweitzer ME. MR and CT arthrography of the knee. Semin Musculoskelet Radiol. 2012;16(1):57–68. https://doi.org/10.1055/s-0032-1304301.
25. Baker JC, Friedman MV, Rubin DA. Imaging the postoperative knee meniscus: an evidence-based review. AJR Am J Roentgenol. 2018;211(3):519–27.
26. Smith TO, Drew BT, Toms AP, Donell ST, Hing CB. Accuracy of magnetic resonance imaging, magnetic resonance arthrography and computed tomography for the detection of chondral lesions of the knee. Knee Surg Sports Traumatol Arthrosc. 2012;20(12):2367–79.
27. Love C, Palestro CJ. Nuclear medicine imaging of bone infections. Clin Radiol. 2016;71(7):632–46.
28. Gemmel F, Van den Wyngaert H, Love C, Welling MM, Gemmel P, Palestro CJ. Prosthetic joint infections: radionuclide state-of-the-art imaging. Eur J Nucl Med Mol Imaging. 2012;39(5):892–909.
29. Hirschmann A, Hirschmann MT. Chronic knee pain: clinical value of MRI versus SPECT/CT. Semin Musculoskelet Radiol. 2016;20(1):3–11.
30. Murer AM, Hirschmann MT, Amsler F, Rasch H, Huegli RW. Bone SPECT/CT has excellent sensitivity and specificity for diagnosis of loosening and patellofemoral problems after total knee arthroplasty. Knee Surg Sports Traumatol Arthrosc. 2019; https://doi.org/10.1007/s00167-019-05609-w.
31. Barnsley L, Barnsley L. Detection of aseptic loosening in total knee replacements: a systematic review and meta-analysis. Skelet Radiol. 2019;48(10):1565–72.
32. Lu SJ, Ul Hassan F, Vijayanathan S, Gnanasegaran G. Radionuclide bone SPECT/CT in the evaluation of knee pain: comparing two-phase bone scintigraphy, SPECT and SPECT/CT. Br J Radiol. 2018;91(1090):20180168. https://doi.org/10.1259/bjr.20180168.
33. Winter A, Ferguson K, Syme B, McMillan J, Holt G. Pre-operative analysis of lower limb coronal alignment—a comparison of supine MRI versus standing full-length alignment radiographs. Knee. 2014;21(6):1084–7.
34. Abu-Rajab RB, Deakin AH, Kandasami M, McGlynn J, Picard F, Kinninmonth AW. Hip-Knee-Ankle radiographs are more appropriate for assessment of post-operative mechanical alignment of total knee arthroplasties than standard AP knee radiographs. J Arthroplast. 2015;30(4):695–700.
35. Guggenberger R, Pfirrmann CW, Koch PP, Buck FM. Assessment of lower limb length and alignment by biplanar linear radiography: comparison with supine CT and upright full-length radiography. AJR Am J Roentgenol. 2014;202(2):W161–7.
36. Parikh S, Noyes FR. Patellofemoral disorders: role of computed tomography and magnetic resonance imaging in defining abnormal rotational lower limb alignment. Sports Health. 2011;3(2):158–69.
37. Gromov K, Korchi M, Thomsen MG, Husted H, Troelsen A. What is the optimal alignment of the tibial and femoral components in knee arthroplasty? Acta Orthop. 2014;85(5):480–7.
38. Steinbach LS, Suh KJ. Bone marrow edema pattern around the knee on magnetic resonance imaging excluding acute traumatic lesions. Semin Musculoskelet Radiol. 2011;15(3):208–20.
39. Fowkes LA, Toms AP. Bone marrow oedema of the knee. Knee. 2010;17(1):1–6.
40. Mohassel P, Chaudhry V. Neurophysiology simplified for imagers. Semin Musculoskelet Radiol. 2015;19(2):112–20.
41. Mills KR. The basics of electromyography. J Neurol Neurosurg Psychiatry. 2005;76(Suppl 2):ii32–5.
42. Flierl MA, Sobh AH, Culp BM, Baker EA, Sporer SM. Evaluation of the painful total knee arthroplasty. J Am Acad Orthop Surg. 2019;27(20):743–51.
43. Al-Hadithy N, Rozati H, Sewell MD, Dodds AL, Brooks P, Chatoo M. Causes of a painful total knee arthroplasty. Are patients still receiving total knee arthroplasty for extrinsic pathologies? Int Orthop. 2012;36(6):1185–9.

44. Lesher JM, Dreyfuss P, Hager N, Kaplan M, Furman M. Hip joint pain referral patterns: a descriptive study. Pain Med. 2008;9(1):22–5.
45. Minns RJ. The role of gait analysis in the management of the knee. Knee. 2005;12(3):157–62.
46. Oppelt K, Hogan A, Stief F, Grützner PA, Trinler U. Movement analysis in orthopedics and trauma surgery—measurement systems and clinical applications. Z Orthop Unfall. 2019; https://doi.org/10.1055/a-0873-1557.
47. Hart HF, Culvenor AG, Collins NJ, Ackland DC, Cowan SM, Machotka Z, Crossley KM. Knee kinematics and joint moments during gait following anterior cruciate ligament reconstruction: a systematic review and meta-analysis. Br J Sports Med. 2016;50(10):597–612.

Chapter 8
Challenges in Managing Knee Disorders

There is no such uncertainty as a sure thing—Robert Burns [1]

Once a diagnosis is made, taking into account clinical findings and relevant investigations, the next step is to plan and initiate appropriate treatment. The aim of treatment is to reduce troublesome symptoms and improve function. The clinician has multiple options in how to manage knee conditions and it is a vital skill to decide which to employ.

This chapter discusses some of the challenges faced in deciding when and how to intervene when faced with knee complaints. The need to consider the underlying natural history of some conditions, and the need to distinguish between incidental asymptomatic findings and findings that are likely to be the source of a patient's symptoms are also discussed.

This chapter also presents some of the management options in treating knee conditions with special reference to the intervention ladder.

In managing knee conditions there are several considerations to be made, which are described next.

8.1 Natural History of Knee Disorders

Many knee disorders have a natural history of improvement which must be taken into account in planning management. Hence, when discussing treatment with a patient one ought to explain that the aim of intervening is to improve current symptoms and speed up recovery rather than necessarily influence the final outcome:

- It is recognised that many cases of pain due to meniscal tears improve with time. Noble and Erat [2] showed that in 50 of 250 patients scheduled for meniscectomy the clinical symptoms subsided and operation was deferred. Intervention

C. Panayiotou Charalambous, *The Knee Made Easy*,
https://doi.org/10.1007/978-3-030-54506-2_8

may thus aim to improve current troublesome pain that interferes with activities of daily living rather than altering the final long term outcome. Similarly, this natural history suggests that a trial of non-surgical management may be adopted.

In contrast, some conditions may have a natural history of deterioration, and worsen with time. Hence, in such circumstances the clinician may discuss the need to intervene to halt or slow a natural history of further deterioration, rather than simply to help with current symptoms:

- Knee osteoarthritis may worsen with time [3, 4] leading to ligamentous contractures and clinical deformities as well as worsening of symptoms. Hence, there may be an argument for intervening early and replacing the joint prior to such changes occurring, which may make surgery more challenging. However, the results of knee arthroplasty are often unpredictable and may deteriorate with time [5–7].
- Following tear of the anterior cruciate ligament (ACL) in young active individuals there is a high risk of developing further meniscal tears and chondral damage due to ongoing knee instability [8, 9]. Such further meniscal or chondral damage could have a deleterious effect on the knee structure and function, and predispose to osteoarthritis. Hence, there may be an argument for intervening early with ACL surgery, to stabilise the knee, to prevent further deterioration. However, long term studies have failed to show a protective role of ACL reconstruction on the development of osteoarthritis [10, 11].

8.2 Incidental Clinical Findings in the Evaluation of the Knee

Certain findings on clinical examination of the knee may not directly contribute to a patient's symptoms. Hence, it is important to correlate such clinical examination findings to clinical symptoms before deciding whether they need addressing. The mere presence of such clinical findings does not necessarily mean they need medical attention. In contrast, intervening in an area that is not symptomatic may itself cause new trouble.

8.3 Incidental Investigation Findings in the Evaluation of the Knee

Certain knee radiological or arthroscopic findings may be incidental rather than truly account for a patient's symptoms [12–14]. Hence, it is important to correlate such radiological or arthroscopic findings to clinical findings before deciding whether they need addressing. The mere presence of such findings does not necessarily mean they need medical attention. In contrast, intervening in an area that is not the source of the patient's symptoms may itself cause trouble. It is recognised that:

- Degenerate medial meniscal tears are commonly encountered in the general asymptomatic population and their incidence increases with age. Their presence on MRI should thus be correlated with clinical symptoms and signs in considering medical intervention.
- Englund et al. [12] evaluated the prevalence of a meniscal tear or of meniscal destruction using magnetic resonance imaging (MRI), and reported that this ranged from 19% (95% confidence interval (CI) 15–24%) among women of 50–59 years of age to 56% (95% CI, 46–66%) among men 70–90 years of age. 61% of those with a meniscal tear on MRI had not had any pain, aching, or stiffness during the previous month.

8.4 Not all Pathological Knee Findings Need Addressing

A symptomatic knee may exhibit multiple pathological findings. There is a need to understand which of these contribute to clinical symptoms and which are less relevant. Addressing the major contributors may help one's symptoms whereas dealing with other findings may confer no additional benefit:

- Degenerative meniscal tears are associated with knee osteoarthritis and the patient's symptoms are more likely to be due to the arthritis rather than the meniscal tear per se.
- In the study by Englund et al. [12] it was shown that:
  - The prevalence of meniscal damage was significantly higher among those with radiographic evidence of tibiofemoral osteoarthritis than among those without arthritis (82% vs. 25%). The rate of meniscal tears was higher in the presence of more advanced arthritis (95% of cases with radiographic evidence of severe osteoarthritis had meniscal damage).
  - In cases with osteoarthritis, the presence of clinical symptoms was not influenced by the presence of a meniscal tear:
    - Meniscal tear was present in 63% of those with knee pain, aching, or stiffness vs. in 60% of those with no symptoms

Hence, in the presence of severe arthritis addressing the arthritis rather than other associated findings may be the main component of intervention.

8.5 Clinical Symptoms Originating from Multiple Knee Sources

Symptoms may originate from multiple sources and failure to address all of those may lead to persistent trouble. Such recognition may also help manage patient expectations as part of shared decision making:

- Meniscal tears may be associated with tibiofemoral chondral damage or tibiofemoral arthritis [15, 16]. Hence, arthroscopic excision of meniscal tears may not relieve the patient's symptoms. Instead, if the arthritis is severe it may be essential to address the arthritis with joint replacement arthroplasty rather than addressing the meniscal tear.

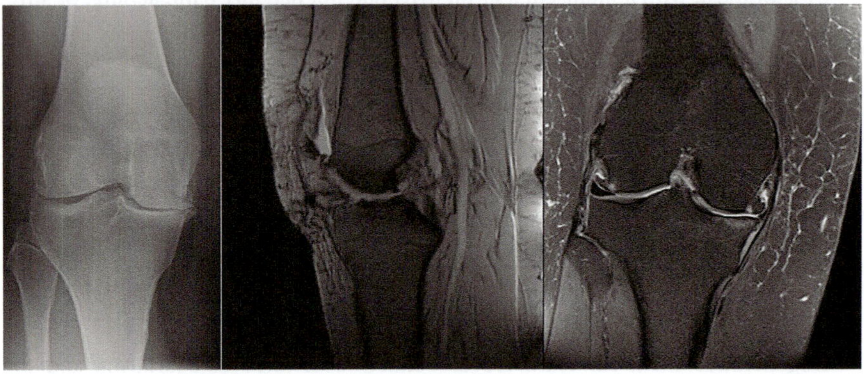

Osteoarthritis of the tibiofemoral joint, associated with ACL tear and medial meniscal tear (plain radiograph and MRI)

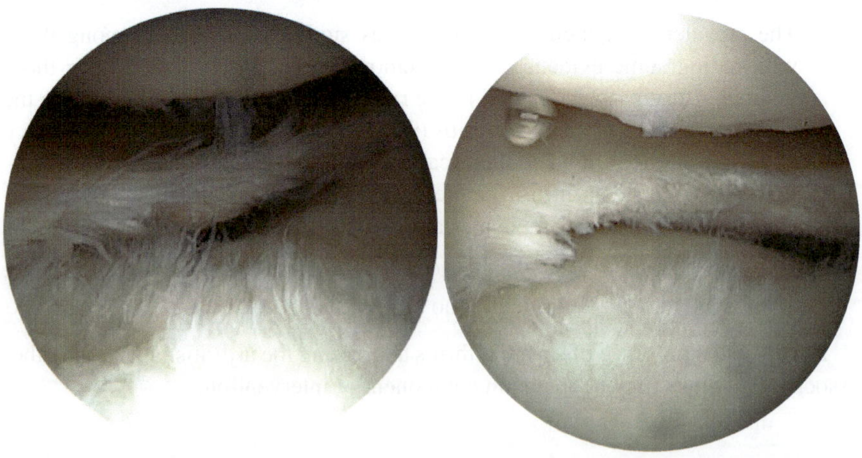

Degenerate meniscal tear associated with articular cartilage degeneration. Following partial meniscectomy the articular degeneration continues to exist which may account for continuing pain (and hence inability of partial meniscectomy to improve symptoms)

- Anterolateral knee pain in patella alta may originate from the patellofemoral (PF) articular surface (excessive compression/chondral damage), patellar tendon (tendinopathy), or fat pad (inflammation due to impingement). Hence, identification of the main source of pain may be difficult. Similarly, addressing only some of the potential sources of pain may not improve clinical symptoms.

8.6 Systemic/Distant Disorders Causing Knee Clinical Symptoms

In dealing with knee symptoms it is essential to enquire about systemic or other multi-focal conditions that could involve the knee area. Non-knee conditions may also be mistaken for knee conditions due to referred or similarly presenting symptoms. Hence, broad thinking should be utilised in history taking and clinical examination to help guide appropriate investigations:

- Pain in the knee may be referred pain from nearby or distant structures—ipsilateral hip, lumbosacral spine [17].
- A double or triple "crush" syndrome may exist, with part of the pain originating from the knee and part of the pain having some other cause. Differentiation and relative quantification of these may be difficult. Pain originating from the knee may co-exist with pain originating from the hip or lumbosacral spine. Hence, in such situations knee intervention would be expected to improve only part of one's symptoms.
- Constant night knee pain may be referred from the hip or may be due to a more sinister cause such as a neoplastic lesion, rather than be attributed to knee arthritis seen on plain radiographs.
- Knee arthropathy may not be degenerative but inflammatory, involving multiple joints
- A rapid knee joint destruction may not be due to degenerative changes, but due to osteomyelitis and septic arthritis, as part of multi-focal septic arthritis

8.7 Consider Clinical Symptoms Rather than Pathology in Knee Evaluation

The clinical symptoms and signs may not be those expected, given the main underlying pathology or precipitating event. Hence, it is important to obtain a thorough clinical history to clarify the presenting symptoms and carry out a systematic clinical examination to detect relevant signs:

- Following ACL tear, patients often continue with recurrent knee instability. However, on occasions a patient may develop substantial knee stiffness due to a soft tissue inflammatory reaction to the trauma and arthrofibrosis associated with

the initial injury. In the latter case, surgical release of the arthrofibrosis rather than reconstruction of the torn ACL may be the preferred initial surgical intervention.
- Koornat et al. [17] evaluated the relationship between clinical features and structural abnormalities on MRI of patients with knee osteoarthritis. Of the parameters examined only the presence of an effusion or a PF osteophyte were associated with pain. Other findings including cartilage abnormalities, subchondral cysts, bone marrow oedema, meniscal tears, or baker cysts were not related to pain. Yusuf et al. [18] in a systematic review reported that only MRI bone marrow lesions and effusion/synovitis were related to pain in knee osteoarthritis.

8.8 Uncertainty as to How Some Clinical Knee Symptoms Are Mediated

In some situations we may not fully understand how clinical symptoms are mediated and why similar pathologies may cause a wide spectrum of symptom severity amongst patients.

There is evidence that the perception of pain and hence the response to any interventions applied may be influenced by [19–21]:

- Central processing
- Psychological disorders
- Ongoing compensation disputes

This must be taken into account in proposing treatments or in evaluating treatment outcomes.

8.9 Uncertainty as to How Knee Interventions Work

In some situations we may not fully understand how our interventions work, and hence why the effects of the same intervention may vary amongst patients:

- In carrying out arthroscopic excision of a meniscal tear potential ways by which the pain may be relieved include:
  - Removal of the unstable torn meniscal piece per se
  - Excision of surrounding degenerate meniscal tissue
  - Partial synovectomy to remove pain receptors, pain transmission nerve endings and mediators
  - Washout of the knee joint reducing the load of inflammatory mediators

- Debridement of associated chondral flaps
- Central pain processing
- Placebo effect [22, 23]

Appreciating such limitations is essential to:

- Plan the relative components of any applied intervention
- Counsel patients with regards to any proposed management

8.10 Lack of Evidence Supporting Knee Interventions

When it comes to treatment of a particular condition we may have limited high quality evidence as to the effectiveness of the available interventions, and the superiority of one intervention over another. Similarly, although an intervention may positively influence some parameters, it may not be able to alter the natural history of the disorder with regards to others. ACL reconstruction as compared to non-surgical treatment for ACL tears, has been shown to be associated with fewer subsequent meniscal injuries, less need for further surgery, and better activity levels, but has not been shown to be associated with a lower rate of development of radiographically evident osteoarthritis [24].

Hence:

- It may be preferable to try the least invasive and least risky interventions first
- It is essential to communicate such uncertainty to patients

8.11 Inability to Accurately Predict those Who Will Benefit from an Intervention

Although studies may identify factors associated with better outcomes following an intervention, as well as groups of patients that may benefit the most, it is often difficult at an individual level to accurately predict the response to an intervention.

Skou et al. [25] showed that in patients with knee osteoarthritis the ability of non-surgical treatment to improve pain was not related to the degree of radiographic severity of the arthritis, and concluded such patients may be treated non-surgically even if they have severe radiographic arthritis.

Hence:

- The least invasive interventions may be tried first

8.12 Intervention Management Ladder for Knee Disorders

In dealing with knee conditions one may consider the intervention management ladder [26] whereby simple non-invasive interventions are tried prior to proceeding with more complex invasive interventions such as arthroscopic or open knee surgery.

This management ladder needs to be discussed with the patient and it is on occasions preferable that one step in the ladder is tried before the next step is ascended. However, some patients may prefer going straight on to the more invasive interventions, to avoid time loss and associated functional loss that may occur if the less invasive procedures do not work. Some patients may also have strong views against some interventions or not being able to tolerate some interventions (such as injection therapy in needle phobia) and this should also be taken into account in discussing treatment.

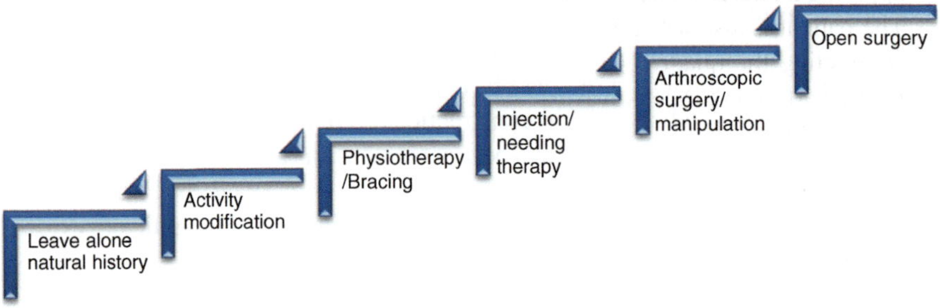

Intervention management ladder for knee conditions

Learning Pearls

- There is uncertainty in much of what we do
- One solution does not fit all
- Shared decision making may manage expectations and improve patient experience

References

1. https://www.goodreads.com/quotes/tag/certainty, accessed on 5/5/20.
2. Noble J, Erat K. In defence of the meniscus. A prospective study of 200 meniscectomy patients. J Bone Joint Surg Br. 1980;62-B(1):7–11.
3. Dieppe PA, Cushnaghan J, Shepstone L. The Bristol 'OA500' study: progression of osteoarthritis (OA) over 3 years and the relationship between clinical and radiographic changes at the knee joint. Osteoarthr Cartil. 1997;5(2):87–97.
4. Felson DT, Zhang Y, Hannan MT, Naimark A, Weissman BN, Aliabadi P, Levy D. The incidence and natural history of knee osteoarthritis in the elderly. The Framingham Osteoarthritis Study. Arthritis Rheum. 1995;38(10):1500–5.
5. Baker PN, Rushton S, Jameson SS, Reed M, Gregg P, Deehan DJ. Patient satisfaction with total knee replacement cannot be predicted from pre-operative variables alone: a cohort study from the National Joint Registry for England and Wales. Bone Joint J. 2013;95-B(10):1359–65.

6. Baker PN, van der Meulen JH, Lewsey J, Gregg PJ, National Joint Registry for England and Wales. The role of pain and function in determining patient satisfaction after total knee replacement. Data from the National Joint Registry for England and Wales. J Bone Joint Surg Br. 2007;89(7):893–900.
7. Williams DP, Blakey CM, Hadfield SG, Murray DW, Price AJ, Field RE. Long-term trends in the Oxford knee score following total knee replacement. Bone Joint J. 2013;95-B(1):45–51.
8. Brambilla L, Pulici L, Carimati G, Quaglia A, Prospero E, Bait C, Morenghi E, Portinaro N, Denti M, Volpi P. Prevalence of associated lesions in anterior cruciate ligament reconstruction: correlation with surgical timing and with patient age, sex, and body mass index. Am J Sports Med. 2015;43(12):2966–73.
9. Mok YR, Wong KL, Panjwani T, Chan CX, Toh SJ, Krishna L. Anterior cruciate ligament reconstruction performed within 12 months of the index injury is associated with a lower rate of medial meniscus tears. Knee Surg Sports Traumatol Arthrosc. 2019;27(1):117–23.
10. Lohmander LS, Englund PM, Dahl LL, Roos EM. The long-term consequence of anterior cruciate ligament and meniscus injuries: osteoarthritis. Am J Sports Med. 2007;35(10):1756–69.
11. Leyland KM, Hart DJ, Javaid MK, Judge A, Kiran A, Soni A, Goulston LM, Cooper C, Spector TD, Arden NK. The natural history of radiographic knee osteoarthritis: a fourteen-year population-based cohort study. Arthritis Rheum. 2012;64(7):2243–51.
12. Englund M, Guermazi A, Gale D, Hunter DJ, Aliabadi P, Clancy M, Felson DT. Incidental meniscal findings on knee MRI in middle-aged and elderly persons. N Engl J Med. 2008;359(11):1108–15.
13. Tornbjerg SM, Nissen N, Englund M, Jørgensen U, Schjerning J, Lohmander LS, Thorlund JB. Structural pathology is not related to patient-reported pain and function in patients undergoing meniscal surgery. Br J Sports Med. 2017;51(6):525–30.
14. Guermazi A, Niu J, Hayashi D, Roemer FW, Englund M, Neogi T, Aliabadi P, McLennan CE, Felson DT. Prevalence of abnormalities in knees detected by MRI in adults without knee osteoarthritis: population based observational study (Framingham Osteoarthritis Study). BMJ. 2012;345:e5339. https://doi.org/10.1136/bmj.e5339.
15. Englund M, Guermazi A, Lohmander LS. The meniscus in knee osteoarthritis. Rheum Dis Clin N Am. 2009;35(3):579–90.
16. Englund M, Guermazi A, Lohmander SL. The role of the meniscus in knee osteoarthritis: a cause or consequence? Radiol Clin N Am. 2009;47(4):703–12.
17. Kornaat PR, Bloem JL, Ceulemans RY, Riyazi N, Rosendaal FR, Nelissen RG, Carter WO, Hellio Le Graverand MP, Kloppenburg M. Osteoarthritis of the knee: association between clinical features and MR imaging findings. Radiology. 2006;239(3):811–7.
18. Yusuf E, Kortekaas MC, Watt I, Huizinga TW, Kloppenburg M. Do knee abnormalities visualised on MRI explain knee pain in knee osteoarthritis? A systematic review. Ann Rheum Dis. 2011;70(1):60–7.
19. Akin-Akinyosoye K, Sarmanova A, Fernandes GS, Frowd N, Swaithes L, Stocks J, Valdes A, McWilliams DF, Zhang W, Doherty M, Ferguson E, Walsh DA. Baseline self-report 'central mechanisms' trait predicts persistent knee pain in the Knee Pain in the Community (KPIC) cohort. Osteoarthr Cartil. 2020;28(2):173–81.
20. Iijima H, Aoyama T, Fukutani N, Isho T, Yamamoto Y, Hiraoka M, Miyanobu K, Jinnouchi M, Kaneda E, Kuroki H, Matsuda S. Psychological health is associated with knee pain and physical function in patients with knee osteoarthritis: an exploratory cross-sectional study. BMC Psychol. 2018;6(1):19. https://doi.org/10.1186/s40359-018-0234-3.
21. Gowd AK, Lalehzarian SP, Liu JN, Agarwalla A, Christian DR, Forsythe B, Cole BJ, Verma NN. Factors associated with clinically significant patient-reported outcomes after primary arthroscopic partial meniscectomy. Arthroscopy. 2019;35(5):1567–1575.e3. https://doi.org/10.1016/j.arthro.2018.12.014.
22. Sihvonen R, Paavola M, Malmivaara A, Itälä A, Joukainen A, Nurmi H, Kalske J, Järvinen TL. Finnish Degenerative Meniscal Lesion Study (FIDELITY) Group. Arthroscopic partial meniscectomy versus sham surgery for a degenerative meniscal tear. N Engl J Med. 2013;369(26):2515–24.

23. Moseley JB, O'Malley K, Petersen NJ, Menke TJ, Brody BA, Kuykendall DH, Hollingsworth JC, Ashton CM, Wray NP. A controlled trial of arthroscopic surgery for osteoarthritis of the knee. N Engl J Med. 2002;347(2):81–8.
24. Chalmers PN, Mall NA, Moric M, Sherman SL, Paletta GP, Cole BJ, Bach BR Jr. Does ACL reconstruction alter natural history?: a systematic literature review of long-term outcomes. J Bone Joint Surg Am. 2014;96(4):292–300.
25. Skou ST, Derosche CA, Andersen MM, Rathleff MS, Simonsen O. Nonoperative treatment improves pain irrespective of radiographic severity. A cohort study of 1,414 patients with knee osteoarthritis. Acta Orthop. 2015;86(5):599–604.
26. Charalambous CP. Professionalism in surgery, in career skills for surgeons: Springer; 2017. p. 5–46.

Chapter 9
Surgical Interventions for Knee Disorders

Surgery lies at the top of the intervention management ladder [1] in dealing with knee disorders. This chapter discusses how surgical interventions aim to reduce troublesome symptoms and improve knee function, to help guide the clinician patient communication. It also describes the principles of arthroscopic surgery and the various open approaches that may be utilised in knee surgery. Some of the common knee surgical procedures are presented, along with a description as to what they entail.

9.1 Principles of Surgical Interventions

Surgical interventions may be considered based on what they aim to achieve. This may be to:

- *Restore* the normal structure of the knee as close as possible such as by:
  - Repairing a torn meniscal tear
  - Reconstructing the anterior cruciate ligament (ACL) to stabilise an unstable tibiofemoral joint
- *Replace* a joint to help pain and improve function
  - Replace the tibiofemoral joint in osteoarthritis or inflammatory arthropathy
- *Salvage* an unfavourable situation—accept that it is not possible to restore the normal structure of the knee but use alternative means to improve one's symptoms
  - Partial meniscectomy in torn meniscal tear
  - Fusion arthroplasty of the tibiofemoral joint in severe degeneration where other modalities have failed or not deemed appropriate

C. Panayiotou Charalambous, *The Knee Made Easy*,
https://doi.org/10.1007/978-3-030-54506-2_9

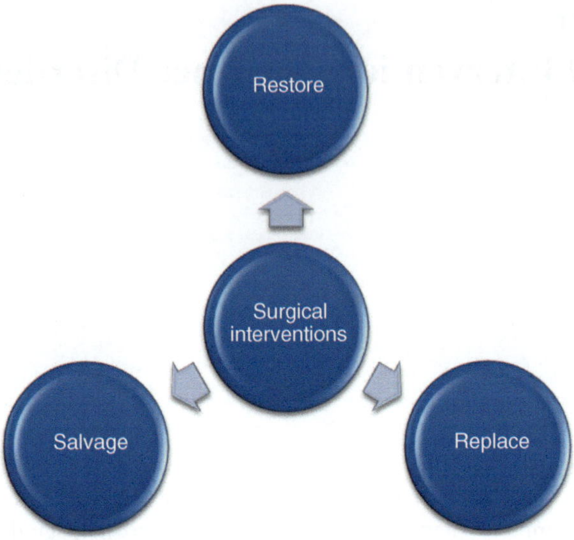

Aims of surgical interventions

Knee surgical procedures may be broadly divided into:

- Soft tissue procedures
- Cartilage/Bone procedures
- Combined

Knee procedures may also be described:

According to the number of times a procedure has been performed as:

- Primary procedure

This refers to the first time of performing a procedure in the knee under consideration.

- Revision procedure

This refers to the second or higher time of performing a procedure in the knee under consideration. This may be performed in cases where the preceding procedure has failed or is not functioning adequately, and the patient is having ongoing symptoms related to that.

Revision surgery may be performed as:

- One stage—previously inserted implants/devices are removed and new implants/devices are inserted on the same setting
- Two stage—previously inserted implants/devices are removed and an interval is allowed (few weeks to months), before the new implants/devices are inserted. This interval may be necessary to allow for infection to be treated, or soft tissues to settle.

According to their effect on the articulation as:

- Joint preserving—Osteotomy, cartilage regeneration techniques
- Joint sacrificing—Replacement arthroplasty

9.2 Arthroscopic and Open Knee Surgery

Certain surgical procedures are commonly used in dealing with knee conditions and these are described next.

9.2.1 Arthroscopic Knee Surgery

Arthroscopic surgery (keyhole surgery) utilises portals (small incisions) [2–5] through which:

- A camera is passed to allow visualisation of the tibiofemoral and patellofemoral (PF) joints
- Instruments are passed to carry out a surgical procedure (power shaver for shaving and removing bone, vapour device for dividing or coagulating soft tissue, repair instruments for suturing tears)

  During arthroscopic surgery the knee is inflated with fluid (normal saline) to:

- Improve visualisation
- Minimise bleeding (by increasing the intra-articular pressure)

9.2.1.1 Surgical Portals in Arthroscopic Knee Surgery

Several portals are available for arthroscopic knee surgery, including:

<u>Anterolateral Portal</u>

Provides access to the:

- Tibiofemoral and PF joints

Location
- Anterior part of the knee, just lateral to the patellar tendon, just proximal to the tibiofemoral joint level (anterolateral soft spot)

<u>Anteromedial Portal</u>

Provides access to the tibiofemoral and PF joints

Location
- About 1 cm medial to the medial edge of the patellar tendon, just above the superior surface of the medial meniscus (portal made under direct visualisation using a needle to confirm planned position prior to incision)

Superomedial Portal

Provides access to the:

- PF joint

Location

- Medial part of knee, about 3 cm proximal to the superior pole of the patella, in line with the medial patellar border
- Percutaneous needle can help guide the exact position under direct arthroscopic visualisation

Posteromedial Portal

Provides access to the posterior horn of the medial meniscus and posterior cruciate ligament (PCL).

Location

- About 1 cm proximal to the tibiofemoral joint line, posterior to the medial collateral ligament (MCL)

Posterolateral Portal

Provides access to the posterior horn of the lateral meniscus and PCL.

Location

- About 1 cm proximal to the tibiofemoral joint line, between the lateral collateral ligament (LCL) and the biceps tendon

9.2.2 *Open Knee Surgery*

Open surgery refers to the use of longer incisions to allow access to the knee joint, whereby surgery is performed under direct visualisation. Several approaches are available for open knee surgery [6, 7], including:

- *Anterior—medial parapatellar approach*

  Access:

  - Knee joint

  Incision:

  - From the superior pole of the patella to the tibial tuberosity

  Superficial dissection:

  - Fascia of the thigh

- Prepatellar and infrapatellar bursa, patellar tendon sheath
- The quadriceps tendon is incised longitudinally proximally, the medial patellar retinaculum distally

Deep dissection:

The patella is retracted laterally or is everted
If more extensive access is required—this may be achieved by:

- Quadriceps snip
- Patellar tendon insertion osteotomy

- *Anterior—lateral-parapatellar approach*

  Access:

  - Knee joint

  Incision:

  - From the superior pole of the patella to the tibial tuberosity

  Superficial dissection:

  - Thigh fascia
  - Prepatellar and infrapatellar bursa, patellar tendon sheath
  - The quadriceps tendon is incised longitudinally proximally, the lateral patellar retinaculum distally

  Deep dissection:

  - Retract the patella medially or evert the patella

- *Lateral approach to the knee*

  Access:

  - To the lateral ligaments of the knee for stabilisation surgery

  Incision:

  - In line with the lateral part of the distal femur curving towards and distal to the Gerdy's tubercle of the tibia

  Dissection:

Three windows may be utilised:

- Window 1—Fascia—Incision between the iliotibial band anteriorly and biceps femoris posteriorly, which are retracted to expose the LCL and popliteofibular ligament.
- Window 2—Incision along the anterior border of the iliotibial band gives access at the level of the lateral epicondyle (allowing approach to the origin of the LCL and insertion of the popliteus tendon).
- Window 3—Incision along the posterior border of the biceps femoris (with retraction and protection of the common peroneal nerve) gives access to the insertion of the LCL and popliteofibular ligament to the head of the fibula

- *Medial approach to the knee*

  Access:

  - To the MCLs of the knee

  Incision:

  - From proximal to the adductor tubercle to the anteromedial part of the tibia

  Dissection:

  - Superficially, identify and protect the saphenous nerve and long saphenous vein
  - Fascia—Incision along the anterior border of sartorius (identified best close to its tibial insertion or proximal to the joint line)
  - Retract sartorius, gracilis and semitendinosus posteriorly, to expose the superficial part of the MCL, capsule and posterior oblique ligament

- Various *posterior approaches* to the knee for approaching the posterior structures have also been described but their use are limited in orthopaedic practise, hence a detailed description is beyond the scope of this chapter.

9.3 Patient Positioning for Knee Surgery

- This aims to facilitate access to the necessary area

  Patient positioning includes:

- Patient supine—leg straight
- Patient supine—knee flexed
- Patient prone—for access to the posterior part of the knee

9.4 Minimising Bleeding in Knee Surgery

This aims to:

- Minimise any haematological or cardiovascular adverse effects on the patient
- Improve the arthroscopic or open surgical view to facilitate surgery

  Certain approaches may be adopted to help minimise intraoperative bleeding [8–14]:

- Thigh tourniquet
- Joint/space inflation with pressurised fluid in arthroscopic surgery
- Chemical agents
  - Intravenous/intra-articular tranexamic acid
  - Local (extra-articular and intra-articular) adrenaline

- Surgical techniques—minimise fluid turbulence, apply direct pressure
- Anaesthesia induced
  - Hypotension

9.5 Types of Knee Surgical Procedures

Several surgical procedures are available in dealing with knee conditions and the following describes what these involve. Most of these (with the exception of realignment osteotomies, arthroplasty procedures, and medial or lateral ligament repair/reconstruction) may be performed with either arthroscopic or open surgery.

9.5.1 Soft Tissue Procedures

Some of the soft tissue procedures to consider include the following:

Tendon/ligament repair—if a tendon or ligament is torn through its substance it may be stitched together by passing sutures through the torn ends. However, in many knee conditions tendon or ligament tears are avulsions from their bony insertions rather than mid-substance tears. Such avulsions may be reattached back to bone by using:

- Suture anchors—these are screw like implants (made of metal or non-metallic material) that have sutures attached to them. The anchor is inserted into the bone and the suture is used to stitch the tendon onto the bone. These may be:
  - Knotted –require the sutures to be tied
  - Knotless—do not require the tying of knots
- Bone tunnels—tunnels are drilled trough the bone through which sutures are passed which then reattach the tendon or ligament back to bone.

Tendon transfer—this refers to detaching a tendon from its normal insertion, moving it and reattaching it somewhere else.

Tenotomy—the division of a tendon which is then left free (not reattached).

Tenodesis—the reattachment of a tendon at a site different to its normal insertion point.

Ligament Reconstruction Surgery:

This may be achieved using an:

- Autograft
  - Hamstring tendons (gracilis and semitendinosus)

- Patellar tendon (the central part of the patellar tendon is harvested along with a bony block from its patellar origin and tibial insertion)
- Quadriceps tendon (the central superficial part of the quadriceps tendon is harvested along with a bony block from its patellar insertion)

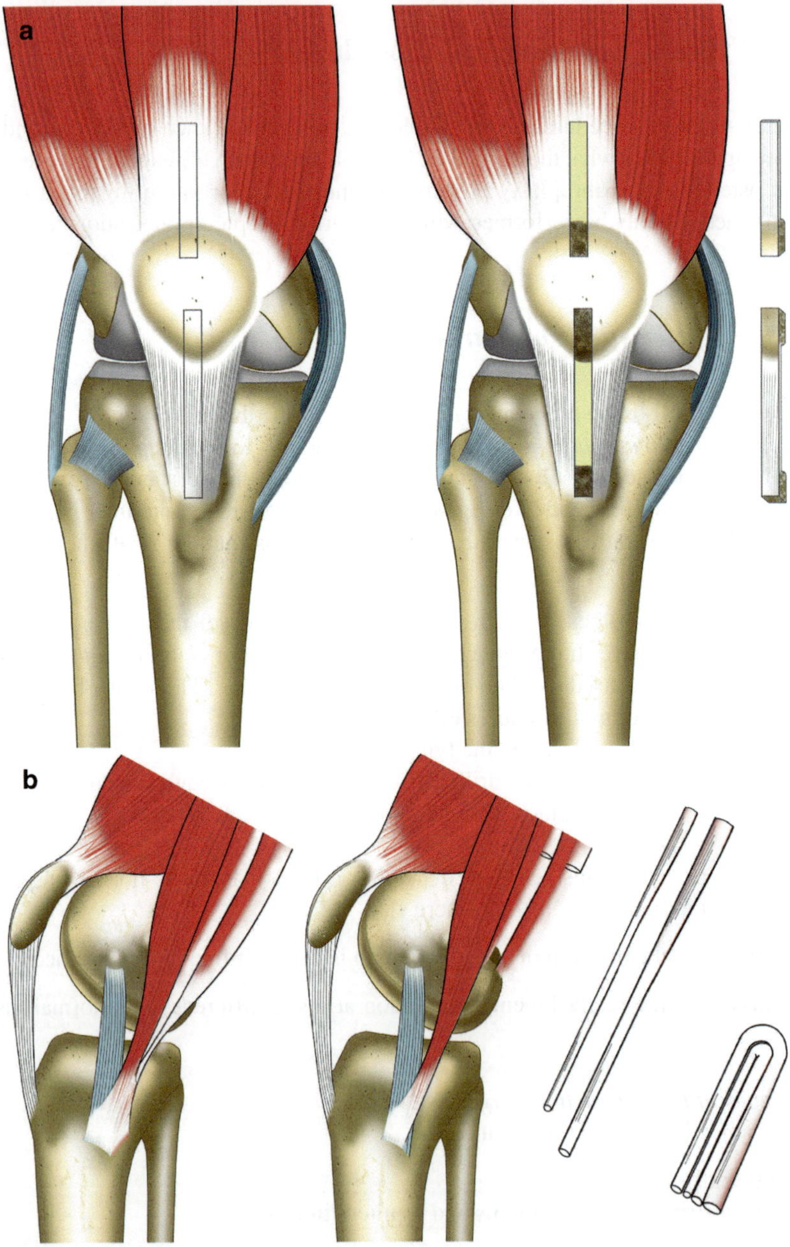

Autografts used in knee ligament reconstruction—(**a**) Bone-patellar-bone, Quadriceps tendon, (**b**) Hamstring tendons

- Allograft
- Synthetic ligament

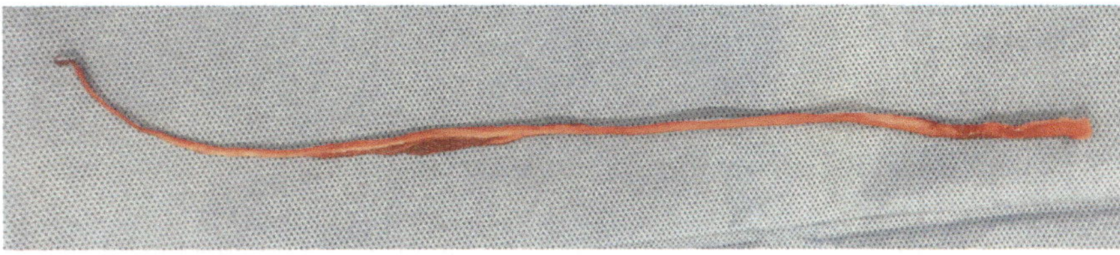

Harvested gracilis used in ligament reconstruction

The graft is secured into bone tunnels or onto the bone surface of the femur and tibia. The graft acts as a scaffold for laying down new collagen and thus turning it into a new ligament.

Multiple types of fixation of the graft onto the bone may be utilised including:

- Interference screws
- Suspensory devices
- Bone anchors

In cruciate ligament reconstruction surgery both single and double bundle techniques have been described. Double bundle techniques tend to be technically more demanding and have not consistently shown to confer any clinical advantage when compared to single bundle reconstructions [15].

- Single bundle ACL reconstruction:
  - Reconstruction of the anteromedial bundle of the ACL
- Double bundle ACL reconstruction:
  - Reconstruction of the anteromedial and posterolateral bundles of the ACL using separate grafts

Internal bracing—this refers to the use of a tissue repair technique whereby a ligament or tendon is repaired, and it is also bridged using a synthetic suture tape fixed in line with the repair (close to the origin and insertion sites of the repaired ligament or tendon). This bridge aims to protect the repair until healing occurs [16, 17].

9.5.2 *Cartilage/Bone Procedures*

Some of the cartilage/bone procedures to consider include the following.

9.5.2.1 Partial Meniscectomy

This is a procedure whereby part of the meniscus (such as a torn or troublesome part) is excised.

9.5.2.2 Meniscal Repair

This is a procedure whereby a tear within the meniscus, or a detachment of the peripheral margin of the meniscus from the capsule, is repaired. Various arthroscopic techniques have been described [18–22] which may be divided into:

- *Outside-in*—sutures are inserted through the meniscus using needles inserted from outside the knee (under arthroscopic visualisation and assistance) which are then retrieved and tied outside the knee capsule
- *Inside out*—sutures are inserted arthroscopically with needles from the inside of the knee, through the meniscus and pulled outside the knee capsule and tied
- *All inside*—sutures are inserted arthroscopically through the meniscus and tied arthroscopically within the knee joint

9.5.2.3 Articular Cartilage Restoration Procedures

Articular cartilage restoration is utilised in full thickness chondral defects. The aim is to replace the lost cartilage with hyaline cartilage or fibrocartilage.

Bone Marrow Stimulation Techniques

Bone marrow stimulation techniques involve the release of mesenchymal cells from the bone marrow which can then differentiate and lay down new cartilage in the area of the chondral defect.

This technique involves an initial debridement of the base of the chondral defect. The subchondral bone at the base of the defect is then penetrated with a sharp instrument (microfractured) which leads to bleeding and fibrin clot formation in the chondral defect. Pluripotent mesenchymal cells from the underlying bone marrow migrate into this defect, and differentiate into fibrocartilage cells and chondrocytes. This leads to the formation of fibrocartilaginous tissue that covers the defect to provide a smoother and more congruent surface, with the aim of improving symptoms. However, the repair tissue consists mainly of type 1 collagen (unlike hyaline cartilage which is type 2). This has inferior biomechanical properties to hyaline cartilage with lower compressive strength, elasticity, and resistance to wear. The area microfractured is usually protected by limiting weightbearing for 6–8 weeks whilst allowing joint motion.

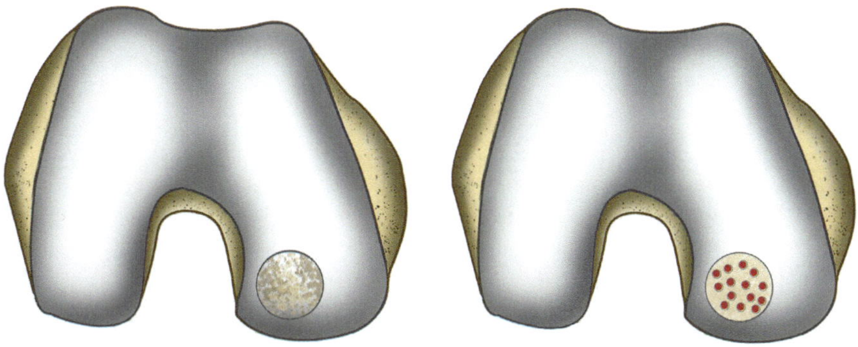

Microfacture for cartilage defects

Microfracture techniques may confer better outcomes in smaller lesions. It has been shown that:

- Lesions larger than about 4 cm^2
- Degenerative lesions
- Lesions in older patients

do not do well with microfracture [23, 24].

Autologous Matrix-Induced Chondrogenesis (AMIC)—this is a technique whereby microfracture of the subchondral bone at the base of a chondral defect, is followed by the fixation (with glue or sutures) of an artificial sponge like material (chondrogel) to the chondral crater. This aims to capture the cells migrating from the bone marrow and prevent their leakage away from the defect [25, 26].

Cartilage Implantation Techniques

Autologous osteochondral grafts—this is a technique whereby osteochondral grafts are harvested as pegs (cylinders) from the non-weightbearing part of the knee with the chondral defect (such as from the margins of the intercondylar notch). The base of the chondral defect is debrided. Cylindrical tunnels are then created in the base of the defect into which the osteochondral graft pegs are inserted under press fit, filling and covering the defect. The resultant defect surface is thus covered with a mixture of hyaline cartilage (surface of pegs) and fibrocartilage (between pegs).

This technique tends to be used for small defects due to limited availability of autologous osteochondral graft that can be harvested. It tends to be used for lesions less than 3–4 cm^2. For larger chondral defects, allograft tissue (which can be obtained in greater amounts) may be used [27–29].

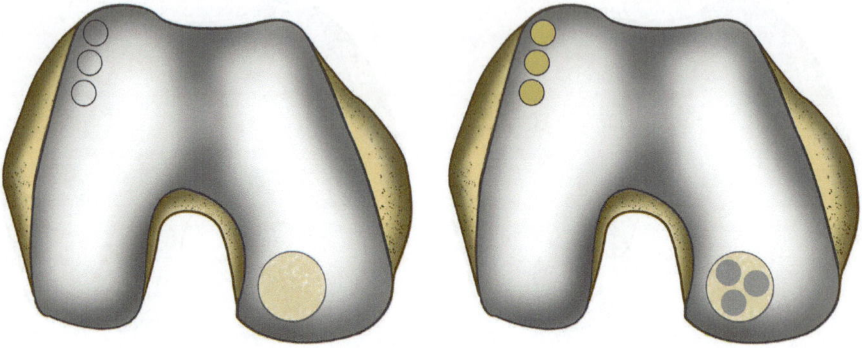

Autologous osteochondral grafting for chondral defect

Osteochondral Allografts

These are obtained from human cadaver knees. There are two main types [30]:

- Shell type grafts—include less than 10 mm of subchondral bone
- Deep type graphs—include more than 10 mm of subchondral bone

Allografts can also be described according to the type of their preservation technique [31]:

- Fresh allografts—stored at about 4° and implanted within a week of harvesting
- Cryo-preserved allografts—preserved in a chemical agent to help maintain chondrocytes
- Fresh frozen allografts—frozen to about −80° soon after harvesting

Fresh allografts contain active chondrocytes but are prone to immunogenic reactions and can only be used shortly after harvesting. Preserved grafts (cryo- or fresh frozen) may confer less immunogenic reactions but also have decreased chondrocyte numbers. In addition, preservation may impair the biomechanical properties (such as strength) of the graft's extracellular matrix.

In this technique the cartilage defect is debrided and sized, and a corresponding osteochondral allograft is prepared from the donor. The graft is then impacted into the defect, using press fit or other means of fixation. The aim is for the graft's subchondral bone to heal onto the bed of the defect (equivalent to bone to bone fracture healing).

Autologous Cartilage Implantation (ACI)

This is a technique whereby cartilage cells are obtained from the knee with the defect, multiplied in the laboratory, and then introduced in the defect, with the aim of making new cartilage to fill and cover the defect. The cells are held in the area of the defect usually by covering the defect with a natural or artificial membrane.

This technique may be used for defects between 2 and 10 cm^2 which do not have substantial subchondral bone loss (less than 6–8 mm).

The technique involves multiple steps including:

- The base of the defect is debrided with removal of the calcified layer
- Penetration of the subchondral bone is avoided to prevent bone marrow cells migrating and laying down fibrocartilage
- Cartilage is obtained from the same knee (non-weightbearing area)
- Chondrocytes are obtained from the harvested cartilage and multiplied (grown) in the laboratory. Once sufficient number of cells has been obtained, they are injected into the defect (usually at 4–6 weeks following the initial harvest)
- A natural (such as a periosteal flap harvested from the proximal medial tibia) or synthetic membrane is sutured to the surrounding cartilage to produce a water tight compartment, and the chondrocytes are injected underneath it [31, 32].

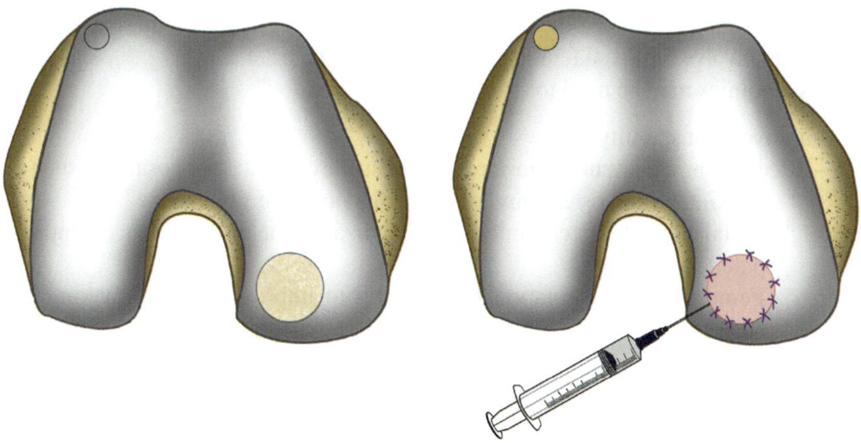

Autologous matrix implantation for chondral defect

Matrix guided autologous chondrocyte implantation (MACI)—This technique aims to improve the way in which cartilage cells are delivered to the defect. The defect is prepared and the cartilage cells are harvested and grown as in ACI. In this technique however, the cartilage cells are incorporated into a sponge like artificial scaffold (collagen membrane, agarose-alginate matrix) which is then secured to the defect (with glue or sutures). Hence, local leakage of the cells may be minimised [33–35].

Fixation of Detached Osteochondral Fragments

In cases where an osteochondral fragement has partially or completely detached (due to trauma or spontaneously), such a fragment may be relocated and fixed to its base with screws, pins, or pegs (metallic or non-metallic). The aim in such cases is to encourage the detached fragment to heal [36, 37].

Articular debridement—this is a procedure, usually performed arthroscopically, whereby the joint is debrided (cleansed out). Such debridement may involve:

- Removal of unstable articular cartilage flaps
- Smoothening of articular cartilage fibrillations
- Excision of unstable tendinous flaps
- Excision of inflamed/hyperplastic synovium

9.5.3 Bone Procedures

9.5.3.1 Osteotomy

This refers to surgical division of a bone. It is part of a realignment procedure whereby the bone is divided, its alignment or orientation is altered, and the bone is then fixed in the new position. The bone then heals in this new position. Osteotomies around the knee may involve the distal femur, proximal tibia or the patella.

Osteotomies may be used to:

- Improve joint stability by:
  - Redirecting a joint surface towards a more stable orientation or position—such as:
    - Proximal tibial osteotomy to reduce the posterior tibial slope
    - Tibial tubercle osteotomy and medialization or distalization to improve patellar stability
    - Femoral external rotational osteotomy to improve patellar tracking and stability
- Unload/reduce the load on a diseased area by shifting the transmitted forces to a healthy area, and hence improve pain [38–44]

Osteotomy may be used to realign bones in the coronal, sagittal or axial planes. An opening or closing wedge osteotomy may be utilised for the coronal or sagittal planes, whereas a rotational osteotomy may be utilised to address the axial plane. Osteotomy techniques include:

Closing wedge osteotomy—a wedge of bone is removed and the gap is closed by moving the distal bone surface closer to the proximal bone surface to close the gap. In this way the alignment of the part of the bone distal to the osteotomy is altered in relation to the part of the bone proximal to the osteotomy.

Opening wedge osteotomy—the bone is divided and the two bony surfaces are separated leaving an empty wedge between the two (this empty space may be filled with bone graft). The gap is maintained in an open position by using internal (plate and screws) or external fixation. In this way the alignment of the part of the bone distal to the osteotomy is altered in relation to the part of the bone proximal to the osteotomy.

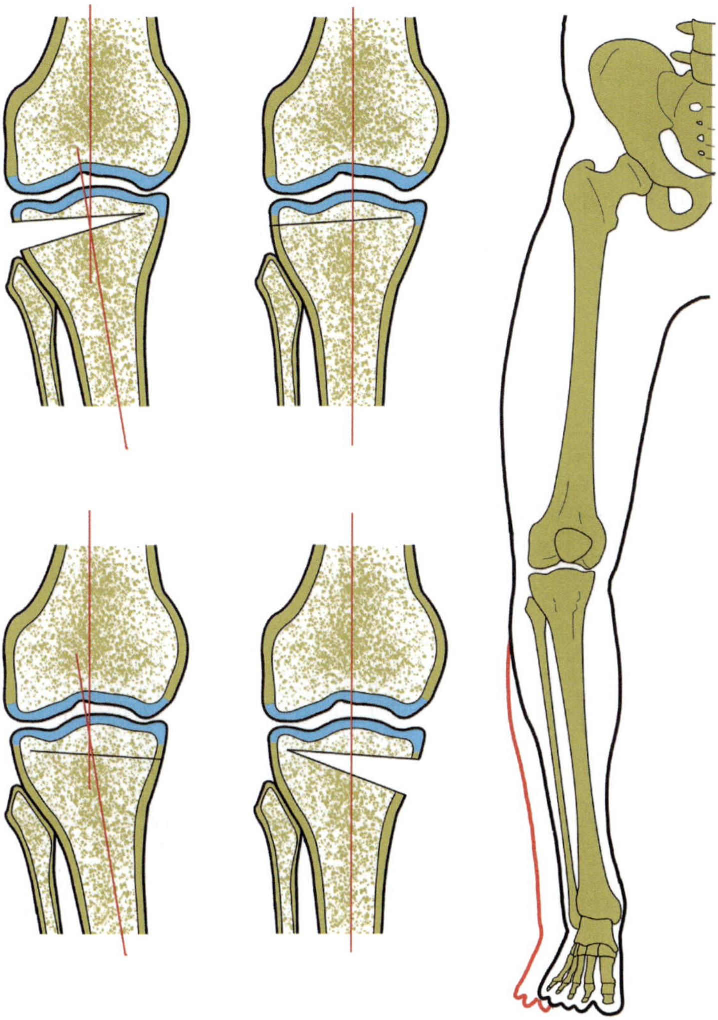

Closing and opening wedge osteotomies of the tibia

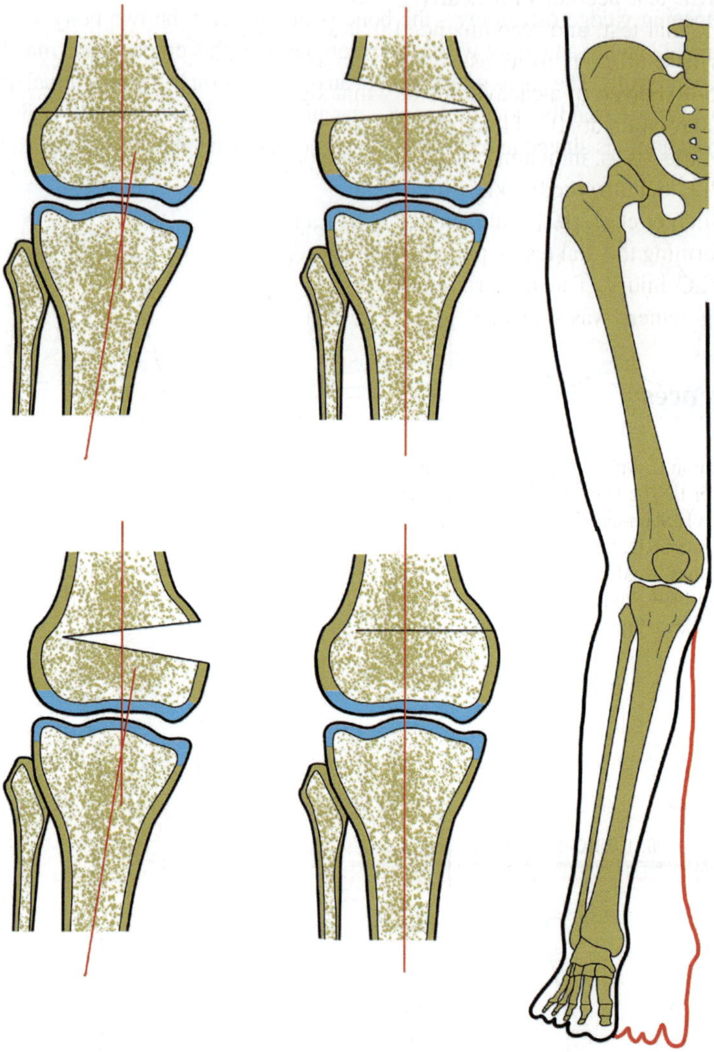

Opening and closing wedge osteotomies of the femur

Progressive callus distraction osteotomy—this is a procedure whereby an opening wedge osteotomy is made, but separation of the divided bony surfaces is done gradually. An external fixator is applied to stabilise the osteotomy site and the patient can commence early weightbearing. Gradual distraction is applied using the external fixator to open up the osteotomy site and thus correct the deformity.

Level of Osteotomy

When considering osteotomy surgery for the correction of a clinical deformity it is necessary to consider the level/cause of deformity. This is because an osteotomy of the bone involved, and at the level of the deformity, is preferable.

A varus deformity is often treated with a proximal tibial osteotomy (high tibial osteotomy). It is of note that a metaphyseal varus deformity is different from acquired tibial varus (due to cartilage wear or meniscal tear). A high tibial osteotomy corrects the actual deformity in the former, but is only compensatory in acquired varus.

Valgus deformity at the knee is often due to distal femoral condyle deficiency rather than tibial wear or deformity. In such cases, a distal femoral osteotomy is preferable as it may help to correct an underlying joint line obliquity (as a result of the femoral condyle deficiency). Maintaining neutral joint line is necessary to avoid increasing the shear stresses on the joint. In contrast, in such situation, a tibial osteotomy may not correct but instead exacerbate such joint line obliquity.

It is of note that an osteotomy may not only influence the osteotomised bone, but also adjacent soft tissue and bony structures. In relation to this, a high tibial osteotomy may influence patellar height [41, 42]. It has been shown that:

- Patella infera may increase after opening wedge HTO
- Patella alta may increase after closing wedge HTO
- Hence in the presence of:
  - Patella infera—closing wedge OT is recommended
  - Patella alta—opening wedge OT is recommended

Patellar osteotomy—this is a procedure whereby the patella is osteotomised [45, 46]. It is used in patellar dysplasia where there is a flat or concave patella, to help recreate two patellar facets. Possible techniques include:

- Anterior sagittal closing wedge osteotomy
- Lateral closing wedge osteotomy

9.5.3.2 Knee Joint Arthroplasty

This refers to altering the joint in one of several ways. It may be described according to:

1. Its effects upon the knee joint
   - Excision arthroplasty—part of the joint is excised—this may stop two arthritic areas rubbing against each other and causing pain, such as in proximal tibiofibular joint excision
   - Fusion arthroplasty—the articular surfaces of a joint are excised and the articulating bones are fixed together to encourage bone union between the two. This aims to stop two arthritic areas rubbing against each other and causing pain. Improvement in pain occurs at the expense of joint motion. Tibiofemoral

fusion may be performed but this has very limited indications as it confirms substantial loss of function to the patient. It tends to be reserved for cases of knee infection that cannot be controlled by other means, or in cases of severe bone loss.

Siller TN and Hadjipavlou A [47] reviewed 41 patients in whom knee fusion was performed mainly for degenerative arthritis and knee infection. They showed that:

- Only 15% of patients were without post-surgical complications
- Persistent knee and back pain were the most common complications
- Many patients were unable to return to work or participate in social activities
- The optimal position for fusion was 15–20° of flexion to allow a smoother gait and make it easier to drive a car. Siller TN and Hadjipavlou A [47] reviewed 41 patients in whom knee fusion was performed mainly for degenerative arthritis and knee infection. They showed that:
- Only 15% of patients were without post-surgical complications
- Persistent knee and back pain were the most common complications
- Many patients were unable to return to work or to participate in social activities
- The optimal position for fusion was 15–20° of flexion to allow a smoother gait and make it easier to drive a car

- Distraction arthroplasty—an external fixator is applied across the joint and it is adjusted so that it slowly distracts the tibiofemoral joint (pulling the tibia away from the femur). This is done over a period of 6–8 weeks, after which the external fixator is removed and the patient is allowed to mobilise freely. This aims to improve pain in arthritis by:
  - Temporarily unloading the articular cartilage which may encourage its repair
  - Stretching of the periarticular soft tissues (ligaments and tendons)
- Replacement arthroplasty—one or both articular surfaces of a joint are replaced
  - Hemiarthroplasty—only one of the two articulating surfaces are replaced—such as the femoral trochlea in PF arthritis
  - Partial knee replacement—one or two of the knee's three compartments (medial, lateral, PF) are replaced (unicompartmental, bicompartmental)
  - Total knee replacement (TKR)—all articular surfaces are replaced

Knee replacement arthroplasty usually consists of metallic femoral and tibial components, with a polyethylene insert in between. Ceramic femoral components are also utilised. Furthermore, tibial components made entirely of polyethylene may be used.

Of the various arthroplasty options, TKR is the one most commonly used in the management of arthritis. Several types of TKR are described [48–58] depending on the characteristics of the prosthesis utilised, and the technique employed. Such descriptions may be:

- According to the timing of the arthroplasty procedure:
  - Primary arthroplasty
    - This refers to the first time arthroplasty of a particular joint
  - Revision arthroplasty
    - This refers to the second or higher time arthroplasty of a particular joint. In revision replacement arthroplasty this may involve:
      - Exchange of one or more of the implants inserted at the time of the preceding arthroplasty
      - Additional insertion of implants (such as patellar resurfacing following isolated tibiofemoral joint replacement arthroplasty)
- According to the parts of the knee replaced
  - Tibiofemoral joint
  - Tibiofemoral replacement and patellar resurfacing (with a patellar button-prosthesis)

It is of note that in many cases of TKR the patella is not replaced (hence the term “total” is a misnomer). This need to be explained to the patient prior to surgery (as part of shared decision making). There is no strong evidence that patellar resurfacing improves outcomes following TKR and may instead increase the risk of operative complications. Patellar resurfacing may be indicated in the presence of extensive PF degeneration, or in inflammatory arthritis. In the presence of isolated PF arthritis, TKR without patellar resurfacing is an acceptable option.

- According to the management of the posterior cruciate ligament (PCL) in TKR
  - Cruciate retaining—PCL retained
  - Cruciate sacrificing—PCL excised and the components of the prosthesis are shaped to compensate for this (compensate for the reduction in stability)
- According to the presence of a prosthesis stem:
  - Stemless—the femur, tibia and patella are reshaped to accommodate a cap which is used to cover the joint surface. The component has no stem inserting into the bone. The component may be stabilised by cemented or cementless (press fit) methods.
  - Stemmed prosthesis—the replacement component has a stem that inserts into the femur or tibia and is stabilised by cemented or cementless methods (press fit) methods.
- According to the resistance to translation of one articulating surface in relation to the other, provided by the morphology (shape) of the articulating surfaces of the prosthesis:
  - Unconstrained—the articular surfaces of the tibial and femoral components show minimal conformity, allowing a large amount of motion, but at the expense of stability
  - Constrained—the articular surfaces of the tibial and femoral components are conforming to improve stability (but this may limit motion, and increase stresses at the prosthesis bone interface)
- According to the presence of a connection between the femoral and tibial components:

  - Unlinked—the tibial and femoral components are not linked
  - Linked—the tibial and femoral components are linked by a hinge to improve knee stability
- According to the mobility of the tibial polyethylene bearing:
  - All poly tibia—the whole of the tibial component is made of polyethylene
  - Fixed bearing—the bearing is fixed in relation to the tibial metallic component
  - Mobile bearing—the bearing is mobile in relation to the tibial and femoral components—to increase conformity between the tibial and femoral components across the range of motion, to reduce wear. Reduction in wear may also be achieved by distributing the stresses between two mobile articulations:
  - Femur and superior surface of insert
  - Inferior surface of insert and tibial tray
- According to the mode of implantation of the prosthesis in relation to the surrounding articular cartilage or bone:
  - Inlay—the prosthesis is inserted into a carved pocket on the articular surface (such as the trochlear component in PF arthroplasty, being inserted in a bed created in the trochlear cartilage and subchondral bone, so it lays flush with the surrounding trochlear cartilage)
  - Onlay—a bony cut is made, and the component is placed on top of that bony cut

Inlay designs are more anatomical (in that they aim to reproduce the native anatomy), hence they may have the theoretical advantage of altering to a lesser extent the tension of the surrounding soft tissues and extensor mechanism. They may thus be associated with a smaller risk for overstuffing the replaced joint.

- According to the use of computer guidance or robotic assistance for performing the surgery
  - Computer assisted surgery
  - Robotic surgery

These aim to improve the accuracy at which bone cuts are made and at which components are implanted.

- According to the use of off-the shelf or patient specific implants
  - Gender specific designs have been described (to allow for differences in the morphology of the distal femur between sexes—narrower distal femoral diameter in relation to anteroposterior size seen in females as compared to males)
  - Custom made designs—using preoperative scans to assess joint morphology, and manufacture components specific to that morphology, rather than use one of already premade, off the shelf components.

Learning Pearls

- Replacement arthroplasty surgery needs to be treated with caution, especially in young active patients in whom the risk of revision is much higher. However, this needs to be balanced against uncontrolled pain hindering quality of life. It is of note that it is the level of activity rather than patient's age per se that may be related to prosthesis longevity. In patients with inflammatory arthritis, with lots of joint destruction, knee arthroplasty may be performed at a younger age as such patients may have limited mobility and function due to multiple joint involvement.
- Revision replacement arthroplasty surgery is much more complex than primary surgery because of extensive soft tissue scarring (as a result of the previous surgery), but also because it may be associated with bone loss which in some cases may make further joint replacement impossible. This is equivalent to having a crown over a bad tooth. Every time the crown loosens and falls off, there is often less tooth to deal with, and eventually there may not be enough tooth left to allow crowning.
- Knee osteotomy procedures may act as the definitive treatment or as a treatment aimed at delaying surgery in those in whom a joint arthroplasty would be associated with a much higher risk of early revision (younger, high demand patients).
- Similarly, unicompartmental knee arthroplasty procedures may act as the definitive treatment or as a treatment aimed at delaying surgery in those in whom a joint arthroplasty would be associated with a much higher risk of early revision (younger, high demand patients).

References

1. Charalambous CP. Professionalism in surgery, in career skills for surgeons: Springer; 2017. p. 5–46.
2. Thompson SR. Diagnostic knee arthroscopy and partial meniscectomy. JBJS Essent Surg Tech. 2016;6(1):e7. https://doi.org/10.2106/JBJS.ST.N.00095.
3. Ward BD, Lubowitz JH. Basic knee arthroscopy part 1: patient positioning. Arthrosc Tech. 2013;2(4):e497–9. https://doi.org/10.1016/j.eats.2013.07.010. eCollection 2013 Nov
4. Ward BD, Lubowitz JH. Basic knee arthroscopy part 2: surface anatomy and portal placement. Arthrosc Tech. 2013;2(4):e501–2. https://doi.org/10.1016/j.eats.2013.07.013.
5. Ward BD, Lubowitz JH. Basic knee arthroscopy part 3: diagnostic arthroscopy. Arthrosc Tech. 2013;2(4):e503–5.
6. Hoppenfeld S, Deboer P, Buckley R. Surgical exposures in orthopedics: the anatomic approach. 4th edition. Lippincott Williams and Wilkins, 2009.
7. The multiple ligament injured knee: a practical guide to management. Gregory C. Fanelli Ed. Springer 2004.
8. Papalia R, Zampogna B, Franceschi F, Torre G, Maffulli N, Denaro V. Tourniquet in knee surgery. Br Med Bull. 2014;11(1):63–76.
9. Arthur JR, Spangehl MJ. Tourniquet use in total knee arthroplasty. J Knee Surg. 2019;32(8):719–29.

10. Fillingham YA, Ramkumar DB, Jevsevar DS, Yates AJ, Shores P, Mullen K, Bini SA, Clarke HD, Schemitsch E, Johnson RL, Memtsoudis SG, Sayeed SA, Sah AP, Della Valle CJ. The efficacy of tranexamic acid in total knee arthroplasty: a network meta-analysis. J Arthroplast. 2018;33(10):3090–8.
11. Felli L, Revello S, Burastero G, Gatto P, Carletti A, Formica M, Alessio-Mazzola M. Single intravenous administration of tranexamic acid in anterior cruciate ligament reconstruction to reduce postoperative hemarthrosis and increase functional outcomes in the early phase of postoperative rehabilitation: a randomized controlled trial. Arthroscopy. 2019;35(1):149–57.
12. Bhutta MA, Ajwani SH, Shepard GJ, Ryan WG. Reduced blood loss and transfusion rates: additional benefits of local infiltration anaesthesia in knee arthroplasty patients. J Arthroplast. 2015;30(11):2034–7.
13. Anderson LA, Engel GM, Bruckner JD, Stoddard GJ, Peters CL. Reduced blood loss after total knee arthroplasty with local injection of bupivacaine and epinephrine. J Knee Surg. 2009;22(2):130–6.
14. Karaoglu S, Dogru K, Kabak S, Inan M, Halici M. Effects of epinephrine in local anesthetic mixtures on hemodynamics and view quality during knee arthroscopy. Knee Surg Sports Traumatol Arthrosc. 2002;10(4):226–8.
15. Dong Z, Niu Y, Qi J, Song Y, Wang F. Long term results after double and single bundle ACL reconstruction: is there any difference? A meta—analysis of randomized controlled trials. Acta Orthop Traumatol Turc. 2019;53(2):92–9.
16. Jonkergouw A, van der List JP, DiFelice GS. Arthroscopic primary repair of proximal anterior cruciate ligament tears: outcomes of the first 56 consecutive patients and the role of additional internal bracing. Knee Surg Sports Traumatol Arthrosc. 2019;27(1):21–8.
17. van der List JP, DiFelice GS. Primary repair of the medial collateral ligament with internal bracing. Arthrosc Tech. 2017;6(4):e933–7.
18. Malinowski K, Góralczyk A, Hermanowicz K, LaPrade RF. Tips and pearls for all-inside medial meniscus repair. Arthrosc Tech. 2019;8(2):e131–9.
19. Nelson CG, Bonner KF. Inside-out meniscus repair. Arthrosc Tech. 2013;2(4):e453–60.
20. Menge TJ, Dean CS, Chahla J, Mitchell JJ, LaPrade RF. Anterior horn meniscal repair using an outside-in suture technique. Arthrosc Tech. 2016;5(5):e1111–6.
21. Henning CE. Arthroscopic repair of meniscal tears. Orthopaedics. 1983;6:1130–2.
22. Warren RF. Arthroscopic meniscus repair. Arthroscopy. 1985;1(3):170–2.
23. Weber AE, Locker PH, Mayer EN, Cvetanovich GL, Tilton AK, Erickson BJ, Yanke AB, Cole BJ. Clinical outcomes after microfracture of the knee: midterm follow-up. Orthop J Sports Med. 2018;6(2):2325967117753572. https://doi.org/10.1177/2325967117753572.
24. Gobbi A, Karnatzikos G, Kumar A. Long-term results after microfracture treatment for full-thickness knee chondral lesions in athletes. Knee Surg Sports Traumatol Arthrosc. 2014;22(9):1986–96.
25. Benthien JP, Behrens P. Autologous Matrix-Induced Chondrogenesis (AMIC): combining microfracturing and a collagen I/III matrix for articular cartilage resurfacing. Cartilage. 2010;1(1):65–8.
26. Gao L, Orth P, Cucchiarini M, Madry H. Autologous matrix-induced chondrogenesis: a systematic review of the clinical evidence. Am J Sports Med. 2019;47(1):222–31.
27. Karataglis D, Green MA, Learmonth DJ. Autologous osteochondral transplantation for the treatment of chondral defects of the knee. Knee. 2006;13(1):32–5.
28. Solheim E, Hegna J, Øyen J, Harlem T, Strand T. Results at 10 to 14 years after osteochondral autografting (mosaicplasty) in articular cartilage defects in the knee. Knee. 2013;20(4):287–90.
29. Familiari F, Cinque ME, Chahla J, Godin JA, Olesen ML, Moatshe G, LaPrade RF. Clinical outcomes and failure rates of osteochondral allograft transplantation in the knee: a systematic review. Am J Sports Med. 2018;46(14):3541–9.
30. Seo SS, Kim CW, Jung DW. Management of focal chondral lesion in the knee joint. Knee Surg Relat Res. 2011;23(4):185–96.
31. Richardson JB, Caterson B, Evans EH, Ashton BA, Roberts S. Repair of human articular cartilage after implantation of autologous chondrocytes. J Bone Joint Surg Br. 1999;81(6):1064–8.

32. Biant LC, Bentley G, Vijayan S, Skinner JA, Carrington RW. Long-term results of autologous chondrocyte implantation in the knee for chronic chondral and osteochondral defects. Am J Sports Med. 2014;42(9):2178–83.
33. Nawaz SZ, Bentley G, Briggs TW, Carrington RW, Skinner JA, Gallagher KR, Dhinsa BS. Autologous chondrocyte implantation in the knee: mid-term to long-term results. J Bone Joint Surg Am. 2014;96(10):824–30.
34. Bartlett W, Skinner JA, Gooding CR, Carrington RW, Flanagan AM, Briggs TW, Bentley G. Autologous chondrocyte implantation versus matrix-induced autologous chondrocyte implantation for osteochondral defects of the knee: a prospective, randomised study. J Bone Joint Surg Br. 2005;87(5):640–5.
35. Ebert JR, Schneider A, Fallon M, Wood DJ, Janes GC. A comparison of 2-year outcomes in patients undergoing tibiofemoral or patellofemoral matrix-induced autologous chondrocyte implantation. Am J Sports Med. 2017;45(14):3243–53.
36. Schlechter JA, Nguyen SV, Fletcher KL. Utility of bioabsorbable fixation of osteochondral lesions in the adolescent knee: outcomes analysis with minimum 2-year follow-up. Orthop J Sports Med. 2019;7(10):2325967119876896. https://doi.org/10.1177/2325967119876896.
37. Grimm NL, Ewing CK, Ganley TJ. The knee: internal fixation techniques for osteochondritis dissecans. Clin Sports Med. 2014;33(2):313–9.
38. Amis AA. Biomechanics of high tibial osteotomy. Knee Surg Sports Traumatol Arthrosc. 2013;21(1):197–205. https://doi.org/10.1007/s00167-012-2122-3.
39. Herman B, Litchfield R. Getgood a role of osteotomy in posterolateral instability of the knee. J Knee Surg. 2015;28(6):441–9. https://doi.org/10.1055/s-0035-1558856.
40. Schuster P, Geßlein M, Schlumberger M, Mayer P, Richter J. The influence of tibial slope on the graft in combined high tibial osteotomy and anterior cruciate ligament reconstruction. Knee. 2018;25(4):682–91.
41. Bin SI, Kim HJ, Ahn HS, Rim DS, Lee DH. Changes in patellar height after opening wedge and closing wedge high tibial osteotomy: a meta-analysis. Arthroscopy. 2016;32(11):2393–400.
42. El-Azab H, Glabgly P, Paul J, Imhoff AB, Hinterwimmer S. Patellar height and posterior tibial slope after open- and closed-wedge high tibial osteotomy: a radiological study on 100 patients. Am J Sports Med. 2010;38(2):323–9.
43. Dejour D, Le Coultre B. Osteotomies in patello-femoral instabilities. Sports Med Arthrosc Rev. 2018;26(1):8–15.
44. Imhoff FB, Cotic M, Liska F, Dyrna FGE, Beitzel K, Imhoff AB, Herbst E. Derotational osteotomy at the distal femur is effective to treat patients with patellar instability. Knee Surg Sports Traumatol Arthrosc. 2019;27(2):652–8.
45. Choufani C, Barbier O, Versier G. Patellar lateral closing-wedge osteotomy in habitual patellar dislocation with severe dysplasia. Orthop Traumatol Surg Res. 2015;101(7):879–82.
46. Jiang C, Liu Z, Wang Y, Bian Y, Feng B, Weng X. Posterior cruciate ligament retention versus posterior stabilization for total knee arthroplasty: a meta-analysis. PLoS One. 2016;11(1):e0147865. https://doi.org/10.1371/journal.pone.0147865.
47. Siller TN, Hadjipavlou A. Knee arthrodesis: long-term results. Can J Surg. 1976;19(3):217–9.
48. Barlow BT, Oi KK, Lee YY, Joseph AD, Alexiades MM. Incidence, indications, outcomes, and survivorship of stems in primary total knee arthroplasty. Knee Surg Sports Traumatol Arthrosc. 2017;25(11):3611–9.
49. Pećina M, Ivković A, Hudetz D, Smoljanović T, Janković S. Sagittal osteotomy of the patella after Morscher. Int Orthop. 2010;34(2):297–303.
50. Gehrke T, Kendoff D, Haasper C. The role of hinges in primary total knee replacement. Bone Joint J. 2014;96-b(11 Suppl. A):93–5.
51. Sabatini L, Risitano S, Rissolio L, Bonani A, Atzori F, Massè A. Condylar constrained system in primary total knee replacement: our experience and literature review. Ann Transl Med. 2017;5(6):135.
52. Verra WC, van den Boom LG, Jacobs W, Clement DJ, Wymenga AA, Nelissen RG. Retention versus sacrifice of the posterior cruciate ligament in total knee arthroplasty for treating osteoar-

thritis. Cochrane Database Syst Rev. 2013;(10):CD004803. https://doi.org/10.1002/14651858.CD004803.pub3.

53. Hofstede SN, Nouta KA, Jacobs W, van Hooff ML, Wymenga AB, Pijls BG, Nelissen RG, Marang-van de Mheen PJ. Mobile bearing vs fixed bearing prostheses for posterior cruciate retaining total knee arthroplasty for postoperative functional status in patients with osteoarthritis and rheumatoid arthritis. Cochrane Database Syst Rev. 2015;(2):CD003130. https://doi.org/10.1002/14651858.CD003130.pub3.
54. Feucht MJ, Cotic M, Beitzel K, Baldini JF, Meidinger G, Schöttle PB, Imhoff AB. A matched-pair comparison of inlay and onlay trochlear designs for patellofemoral arthroplasty: no differences in clinical outcome but less progression of osteoarthritis with inlay designs. Knee Surg Sports Traumatol Arthrosc. 2017;25(9):2784–91.
55. Picard F, Deakin AH, Riches PE, Deep K, Baines J. Computer assisted orthopaedic surgery: past, present and future. Med Eng Phys. 2019;72:55–65.
56. Xie X, Zhong Y, Lin L, Li Q. No clinical benefit of gender-specific total knee arthroplasty: a systematic review and meta-analysis of 6 randomized controlled trials. Acta Orthop. 2015;86(2):274–5.
57. Meheux CJ, Park KJ, Clyburn TA. A retrospective study comparing a patient-specific design total knee arthroplasty with an off-the-shelf design: unexpected catastrophic failure seen in the early patient-specific design. J Am Acad Orthop Surg Glob Res Rev. 2019;3(11):pii: e10.5435. https://doi.org/10.5435/JAAOSGlobal-D-19-00143. eCollection 2019 Nov
58. Reimann P, Brucker M, Arbab D, Lüring C. Patient satisfaction—A comparison between patient-specific implants and conventional total knee arthroplasty. J Orthop. 2019;16(3):273–7.

Chapter 10
External Devices for Disorders of the Knee

External devices may be applied to the lower limb to increase proprioception, improve stability, modify load distribution, control range of motion, or apply a stretching force. They aim to improve knee biomechanics, pain and function. Several types of external devices may be utilised, applied either at the knee or the foot. Such devices may be pre-fabricated (off the shelf, chosen from a commercially available range) or specifically made for an individual (custom made).

10.1 Knee External Devices

External devices applied to the knee may be utilised to:

- Control range of motion
- Control the position of one bone in relation to another to improve joint stability:
  - Patella in relation to the femur
  - Tibia in relation to the femur
- Improve neuromuscular control by:
  - Enhancing proprioception
  - Providing a feeling of joint support, giving confidence to the patient
- Modify weight distribution:
  - Unload diseased compartments by redirecting forces to healthy compartments
- Stretch soft tissues to improve range of motion in stiffness

C. Panayiotou Charalambous, *The Knee Made Easy*,
https://doi.org/10.1007/978-3-030-54506-2_10

External devices applied to the knee may be described according to:

Material composition
- Taping, simple sleeves made of cloth
- Soft material
- Rigid material

Presence of rigid vertical posts
- None
- Unilateral
- Bilateral

Presence of hinge
- None
- Non-adjustable hinge
- Adjustable hinge

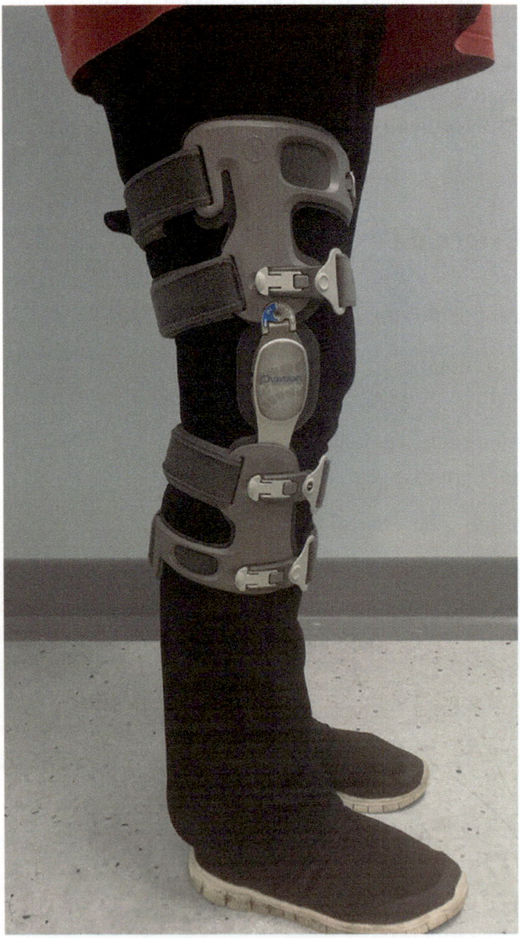

Knee brace with adjustable hinge

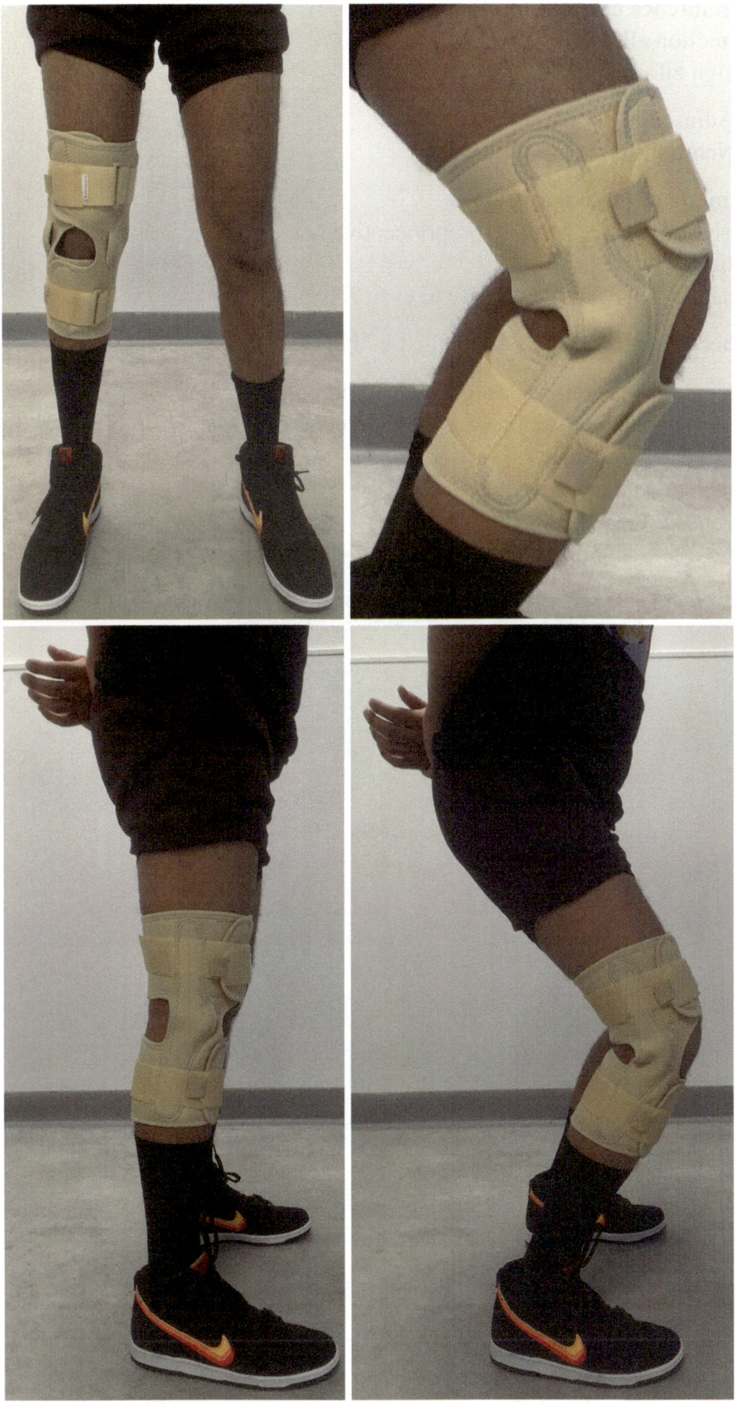

Knee brace with non-adjustable hinge

Their influence on joint motion

- No motion allowed
- Motion allowed
  - Adjustable
  - Non-adjustable

Their mode of force application

- Passive—no force applied, proprioceptive braces
- Static
- Dynamic—use muscle activity to exert forces

A mechanical force may be applied in the:

- Coronal plane—varus or valgus unloading braces
- Sagittal plane—posterior cruciate ligament (PCL)/anterior cruciate ligament (ACL) dynamic braces
- Axial plane—patellar instability braces

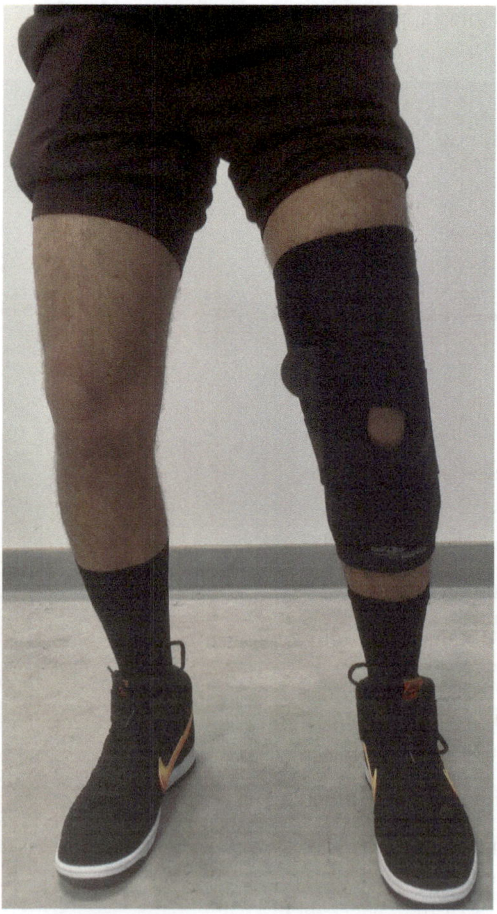

Patellar brace applying medial patella force

A force may be exerted to:

- Limit motion
- Alter the relationship of one bone in relation to another to:
  - Limit forces on a ligament to protect its integrity (such as ACL brace limiting forces on an ACL graft following ACL reconstruction)
  - Unload an articular compartment—such as unloading the medial tibiofemoral compartment in medial knee arthritis
- Stretch soft tissues and restore motion
  - Posterior force on the tibia in relation to the femur to improve flexion
  - Anterior force on the tibia in relation to the femur to improve extension
  - Medial force on the patella to stretch the lateral patellar retinaculum

Braces aim to provide forces using a 3 or 4 point fixation system across the knee [1–4]. A force may be applied using various constructions including:

- In coronal plane—forces may be applied using a combination of one or more vertical posts located on the side of the knee, and straps which pass around the tibia and femur and provide a counterproductive force. A varus or valgus force may be thus applied to the tibia in relation to the femur to offload the medial or lateral compartments respectively.
- In sagittal plane—rigid shells, straps and pressure pads are placed on the front and back of the tibia and femur in such a way as to apply a force on the tibia in relation to the femur (often across the range of motion). This may help limit posterior sagging of the tibia in PCL deficiency or limit anterior tibial translation in ACL deficiency.

It is of note that:

- It is more difficult for braces to control limbs with larger soft tissue volume
- The amount of strap tension that may be applied is limited by patient comfort and blood circulation.

Some types of knee braces are described in greater detail next.

10.1.1 Medial Compartment Unloading Braces

Medial compartment unloading braces (valgus braces) aim to unload the medial compartment of the knee to help reduce knee pain and improve function [5–12].

Knee braces used in medial compartment osteoarthritis (OA) may exert their effect by:

- Direct application of an external force to create a valgus angulation of the tibia on the femur, to cause a reduction in the adduction moment applied to the knee

- Altering gait parameters
- Altering muscle activation

Application of an external force is achieved by a combination of hinges and straps. Such a brace often consists of a hinge applied at the medial aspect of the knee, which is secured to the thigh and lower leg with a series of straps that produce a three point contact bending system. This brace arrangement produces a medially directed force to the lateral aspect of the knee joint (where the apex of the deformity is) and laterally directed forces to the femur and tibia proximal and distal to the knee. In this way a valgus moment is produced around the knee.

A change in gait parameters, or alterations in muscle activation as a result of brace wear may also influence medial compartment loading. In knee osteoarthritis, loss of cartilage and loss of meniscal tissue with resultant loss of joint space may lead to joint laxity. This may cause co-contraction of antagonist muscles around the knee (vastus lateralis and lateral hamstrings, vastus medialis and medial hamstrings), in an attempt to improve knee stability. However, such muscle contraction may also increase contact pressures, potentially aggravating degeneration and worsening knee pain. Unloading knee braces have been shown to reduce such co-contractions.

However, biomechanical studies have suggested that these may be less important than the application of a valgus force. Brandon et al. [13] evaluated two braces used in knee arthritis to apply a valgus moment. They showed that bracing reduced medial loads by about 10% bodyweight (BW) and increased lateral loads by 0.03–0.2 BW. Changes in gait kinematics and knee activation were subtle. They concluded that knee braces reduced medial tibiofemoral loads primarily by applying a direct, and substantial, valgus moment to the knee.

Clinical results have shown that medial compartment unloading braces are effective in decreasing pain, improving function, improving range of knee motion, speed of walking and step length.

Varus unloading braces have the opposite effect, and are used in unloading the lateral compartment.

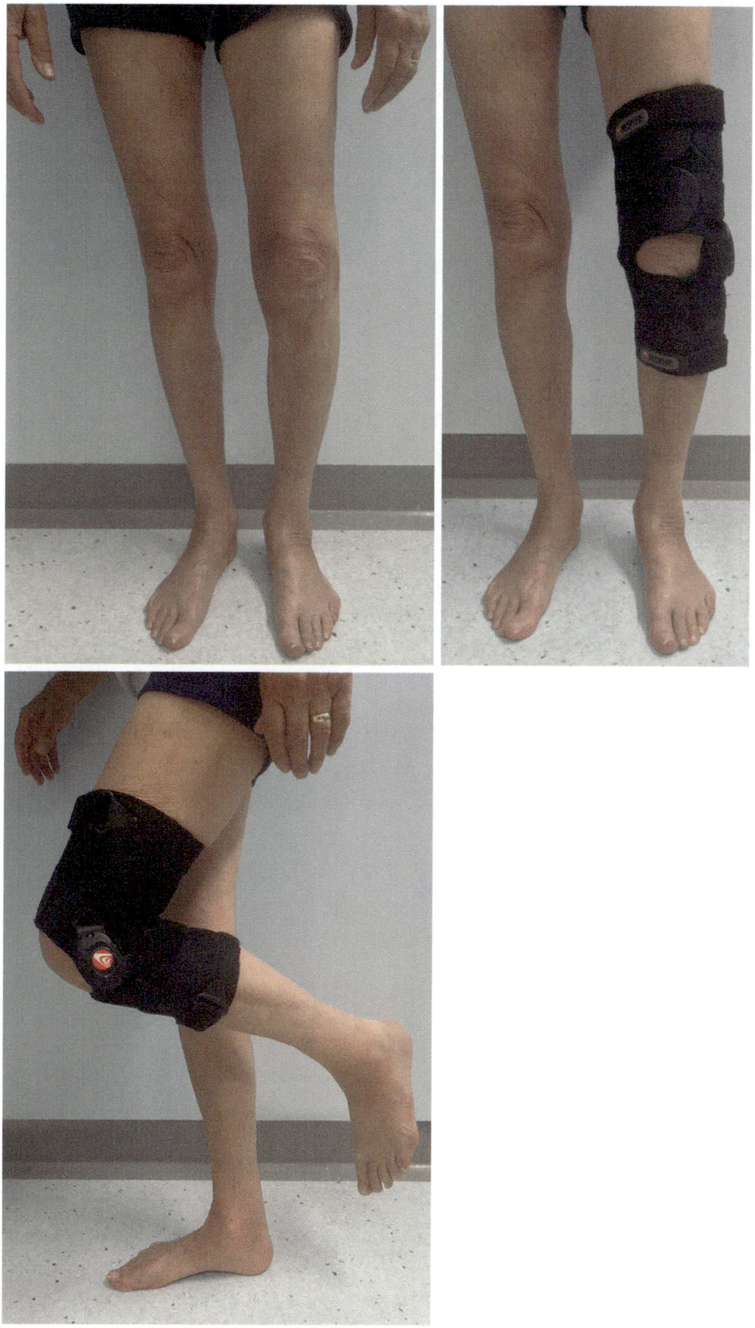

Medial compartment unloading knee brace

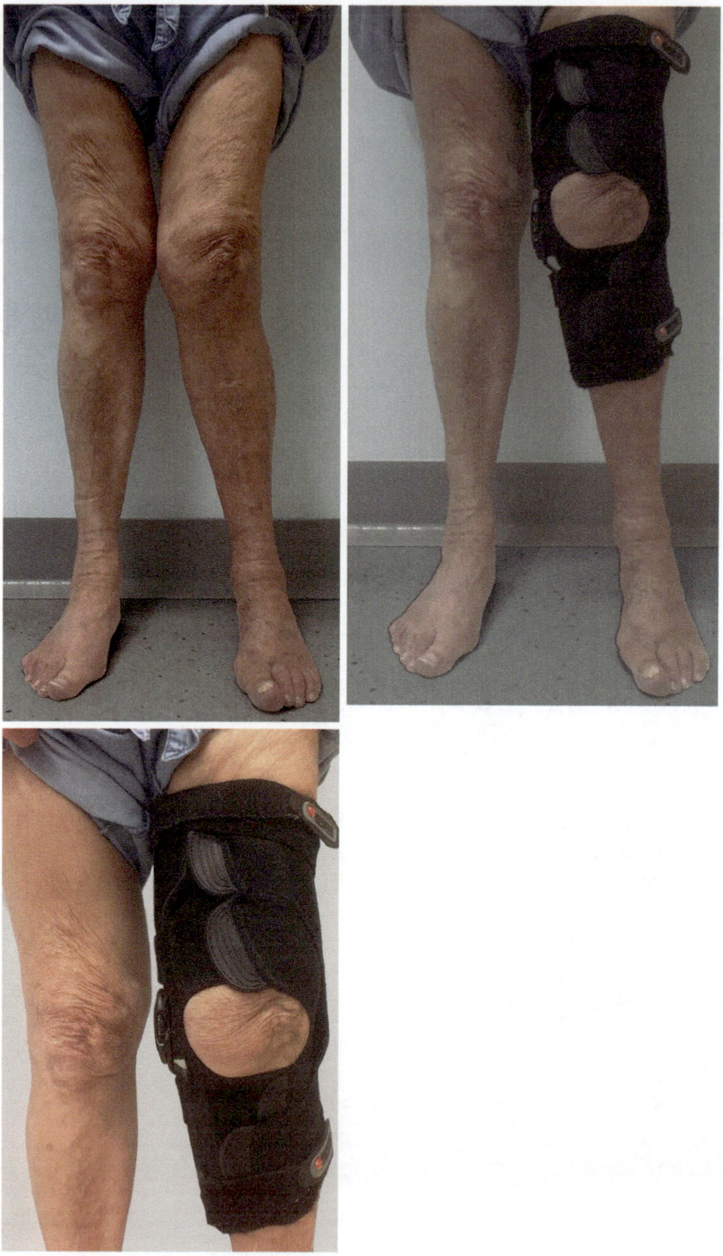

Lateral compartment unloading knee brace

10.1.2 Functional ACL Braces

In ACL deficiency, anterior translation of the tibia in relation to the femur may cause symptomatic instability. Similarly, in the early period following surgical ACL reconstruction, a tendency of the tibia to translate anteriorly in relation to the femur (due to the normal effect of weightbearing or activation of quadriceps) may increase the forces on the ACL graft. This may predispose to graft stretching out, or the graft translating in relation to its fixation site (slipping), leading to graft dysfunction.

ACL functional braces [14, 15] aim to:

- Improve stability in the ACL deficient knee to improve symptoms
- Improve stability in the ACL deficient knee to minimise further intra-articular damage (meniscal, chondral) whilst awaiting delayed reconstruction surgery
- Protect an ACL graft following reconstruction surgery by reducing the forces and strain on the graft

ACL braces aim to limit the anterior translation of the tibia on the femur through a combination of straps, sleeves and bars, connected to posts and hinges usually applied on either side of the knee. These apply a posterior force on the tibia and anterior directed counter force on the femur.

Different types of ACL braces are described:

- Static force brace—applies a constant posterior force to the anterior tibia in relation to the femur
- Dynamic force brace—applies a posterior force on the tibia in relation to the femur which varies with knee flexion (higher force in extension- where the ACL is known to experience higher anterior forces under physiological conditions)

10.1.3 PCL Braces

Flexion of the knee increases the tension on the PCL up to about 90°. When the PCL is disrupted the tibia sags backwards in relation to the femur (posterior sag) as a result of the effect of gravity and the action of the hamstrings. If this posterior sag is allowed, the PCL may heal in a lengthened (stretched out) position and hence, although healed it may be dysfunctional.

PCL braces [16, 17] aim to apply an anterior force to the tibia, to reduce posterior sag and limit tension on the PCL. This may be applied in a static mode (knee motion not allowed) or dynamic mode (apply a posterior force to the femur and an anterior force to the tibia throughout the range of motion).

PCL braces may thus be used:

- Following an acute PCL tear, to allow the PCL to heal in a less elongated position. Bracing for 4 months (6 weeks static bracing in extension followed by free flexion) is often utilised.

- PCL braces may be also used post PCL reconstruction, to minimise stretching of the graft.
- In chronic PCL instability to:
  - Improve symptoms as a form of long term management.
  - Assess the potential benefit of subsequent PCL reconstruction; if brace use improves the patient's symptoms, this response to bracing may suggest that PCL reconstruction surgery may have a similar but more long lasting effect.

PCL bracing may be with:

- Static force brace—applies a constant anterior force to the tibia in relation to the femur
- Dynamic force brace– applies an anterior force on the tibia in relation to the femur which varies with knee flexion (higher force in deeper knee flexion- where the PCL is known to experience higher posterior forces)

10.1.4 Stretching Knee Braces

Stretching braces aim to stretch out the soft tissues of the knee to improve range of motion [18–21]. They may be applied to improve flexion, extension, or both, according to the motion deficit. Such bracing may be with:

- Static stretch brace—applies a constant stretch without motion. It works by applying a constant displacement at the end of achievable motion, by varying the applied force. The brace places the knee at the end of motion range, at which the stretch is then applied. This is usually applied for 15–30 min about 3 times a day. The force and duration of brace wear is gradually increased as tolerated by the patient.
- Dynamic stretch brace—applies stretching whilst allowing some motion. It works by applying a low force to achieve displacement at the joint. The patient often starts wearing the splint 1–2 h a day. The duration is gradually increased, aiming to reach overnight use (about 8 h a day).

For both types, the tension is increased, until slight discomfort is felt. There is some evidence to suggest that static progressive stretching may lead to faster restoration of motion as compared to dynamic stretch devices.

10.2 External Devices for the Ankle and Foot (Ankle/Foot Orthoses)

External devices applied across the ankle and foot [22–38] may be utilised to:

- Control range of motion
- Control the position of one bone in relation to another (such as at the subtalar/ankle joints) to:

  - Improve joint stability
  - Modify foot position in relation to the ground

- Improve neuromuscular control
  - Enhance proprioception
  - Supportive
- Modify weight distribution by altering the point of contact of the foot with the ground and hence:
  - Alter pressure distribution across the foot
  - Modify the magnitude/re-direct the adduction moment acting at the knee
- Stretching soft tissues to improve the range of motion in stiffness
  - Increase ankle mobility
- Compensate for leg length discrepancies—equalise leg length

Orthoses may be applied to the:

- Ankle in isolation
- Foot in isolation
- Combined ankle and foot

External devices applied to the foot may be described according to:

Point of force application to the foot

- Medial—to restore the medial arch and shift the weightbearing contact point of the foot medially. Utilised to improve knee pain in lateral compartment arthritis of the knee or to improve patellofemoral (PF) pain
- Lateral—to shift the weightbearing contact point of the foot laterally. Utilised to improve knee pain in medial compartment arthritis

The extent of application along the foot

- Heel cups/heel raise
- Full foot length
- Partial foot length—¾ length
- Part of foot (Hind-foot, mid-foot, fore-foot, hallux)

External device location in relation to the shoe

- In shoe
- Outside sole
- Incorporated in shoe's sole

External device shape

- Flat—uniform in thickness along its full length with no inbuilt arch support or wedging
- Arch shaped
- Wedges
- Heel raises

External device stiffness

- Soft
- Stiff

Insoles may exert their effects by:

- Shock absorption
- Enhancing proprioception
- Altering foot position and hence altering point of contact with the ground
- Altering dynamic foot motion—rear foot motion—subtalar and ankle joint
- Acting as space fillers—allowing full plantar contact and reducing muscle activity

Two situations in which foot insoles may be utilised are described in greater detail next.

1. Medial compartment degeneration [22–39]

    - Lateral wedge insoles

        - 5–10° (as tolerated)
        - Extending all the way along the foot are preferable—rather than limited to hind foot

    - They have been shown to reduce the adduction moment acting across the knee (by moving the point of foot contact with the ground more laterally), hence reducing loading of the medial compartment.

    It has been suggested that the variability in response to lateral foot wedges amongst patients may be due to variability in foot posture amongst patients (pes planus (flat foot) vs. pes cavus (high arched foot)). Lateral wedge use may lead to eversion of the ankle and subtalar joints, exacerbating a flat foot posture. Hatfield et al. [38] compared changes in knee and ankle/subtalar biomechanics when using lateral wedge orthotics with or without custom medial arch support in patients with knee osteoarthritis and flat feet. Lateral wedge support in isolation, and lateral wedge with medial arch support reduced the knee adduction moment. However, the lateral wedge resulted in a more everted foot position than lateral wedge plus arch support. Participants reported significantly more immediate comfort with lateral wedge plus arch support as compared to when using isolated lateral wedge support. Hence, the authors concluded that combined orthotics may be more preferable in those with medial knee osteoarthritis and flat feet.

    Medial wedge insoles may help symptoms in lateral compartment disease of the knee.

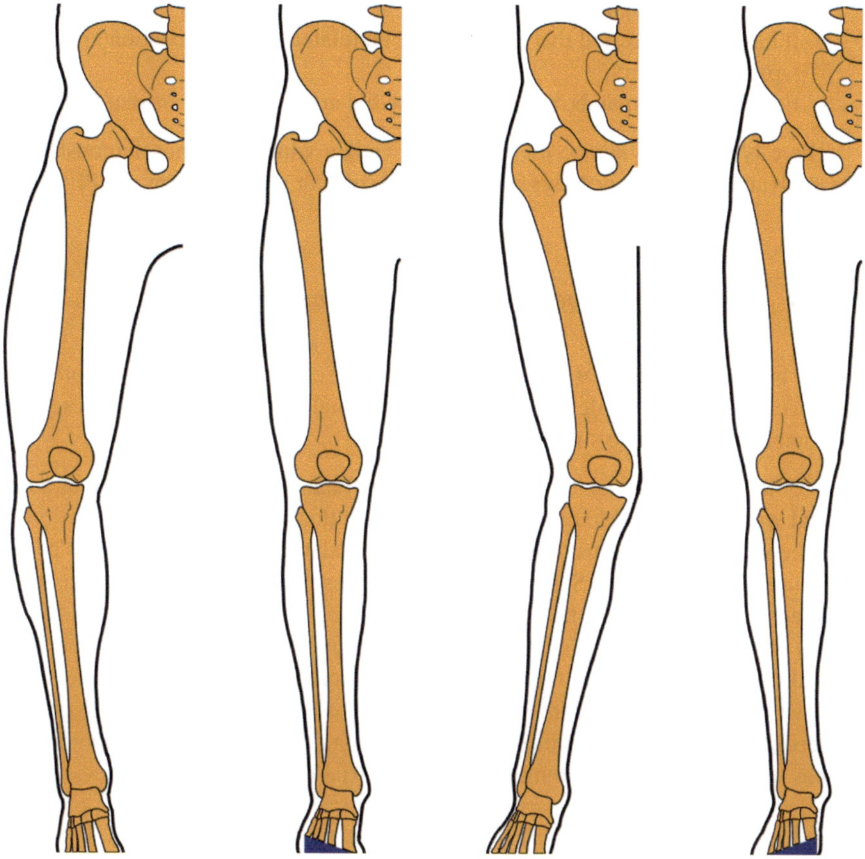

Lateral wedge insoles may be used in medial compartment arthritis and medial wedge insoles and medial arch supports in lateral compartment disease

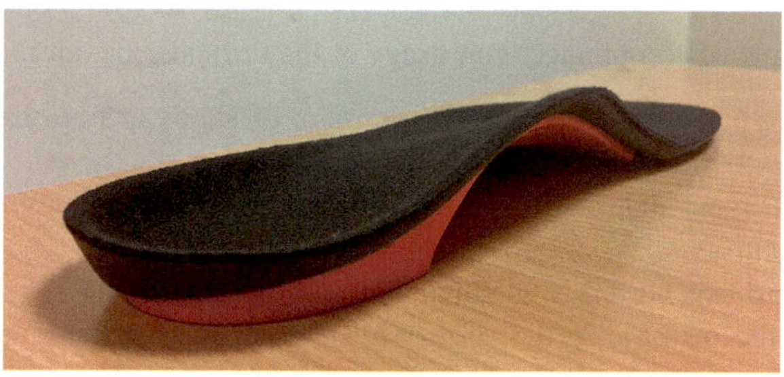

Medial arch support

2. PF pain in the presence of absence of PF degeneration [40–43]

- Medial arch support or medial wedge
- It has been suggested that PF pain may be related to foot pronation and a collapsed medial arch.
- Foot pronation may be reduced by a medial arch support or medial wedge

There is limited evidence for their effectiveness which does not demonstrate a clear advantage of foot orthoses over simple insoles or physiotherapy for PF pain.

10.2.1 Combining Foot with Ankle Orthosis [44–47]

It has been suggested that combining foot orthoses with an ankle support may enhance the effect of insoles by controlling the subtalar and ankle joints. These may be combined or separate structures such as:

- Foot lateral wedge insoles combined with subtalar joint strapping—use of a lateral wedge may lead to calcaneal eversion, but this may not lead to reduction in knee varus, due to varus of the talus at the subtalar joint (and hence varus of the tibia at the ankle joint). Subtalar strapping pushes the talus (and hence tibia, if the knee varus deformity is flexible) into valgus.
- An ankle foot orthosis that consists of a foot insole connected to a lever with a pad that applies a valgus force to the tibia (which reduces the varus angle of the knee). This moves the contact point of the foot laterally and hence the ground reaction force (GRF) closer to the knee, reducing the knee adduction moment. It has been shown in a randomised controlled trial (RCT) that such a device is as effective as a medial compartment unloading knee brace in improving pain and function.

10.2.2 Compliance in Foot Orthoses

In order to improve compliance with usage of the orthosis consider:

- Using an orthosis for each of multiple pairs of shoes or one that can be used across shoes (work, causal, sports)
- Choose the type and size of orthosis based on how spacious the shoe is to improve comfort
- Select an orthosis hardness which allows comfort
- Moulding the orthosis to the foot (whilst incorporating the changes that will allow it to exert its biomechanical effect) to improve comfort

Learning Pearls

- Both mechanical and non-mechanical braces have been shown to influence lower limb biomechanics. Hence, many braces may exert their effect by both a mechanical and a proprioceptive mode of action.
- Mechanical braces may be less favoured by patients as compared to non-mechanical devices as they may cause discomfort due to the pressure applied. Similarly, foot external devices may not be utilised as they limit the choice of foot wear. Hence, compliance with usage is an important factor to consider in assessing the effectiveness of external devices. A substantial proportion of patients (25% in one study [48]) may discontinue brace use within 3 months due to discomfort and perceived lack of evidence; this suggests that patient engagement is essential.
- A vast amount of previous work has examined the effectiveness of external devices in improving symptoms in knee arthritis. Examination of this work suggests that there is conflicting evidence as to their effectiveness. Furthermore, even when effective, the benefit of such devices is not uniform across patients.
- It has been shown that symptoms may worsen following application of an unloading knee brace, and that it may take 6–12 months for symptoms to improve above baseline. Hence, one may have to persevere with wearing the brace for several months before deciding whether it is effective or not. Lee et al. [9] assessed 63 consecutive patients with end-stage unicompartmental knee OA (lateral or medial) who were prescribed an unloading knee brace, whilst awaiting surgery. Surgical interventions were required for 38 patients, of whom 50% required total knee replacement, 37% had unicompartmental knee replacement and 13% had high tibial osteotomy. Medial compartmental osteoarthritis accounted for about 74% of unsuccessful patients. In this population, patients wore the brace for an average of 8 months (1–24), with about 41% stopping to wear the brace within 6 months. At 24 months, 25% of the patients were still wearing the unloader knee brace. A success was defined as a patient avoiding surgery by wearing the brace. Where patients wore the brace for 6 months rather than 3 months, the proportion of success doubled from 4% to 8%.
- Where an external device helps initially but then symptoms deteriorate, one needs to consider the possibility that this may be due to wear or stretching of the device. Regular renewal of the foot orthosis or brace may be necessary.
- In the future, gait analysis may be utilised at an individual level to determine individual gait characteristics that may then guide choice of brace and application [22].
- Tailoring patellar taping to individual needs (i.e. to control lateral tilt, glide and spin) may be important in order to optimise pain reduction.
- Assisting devices may be utilised in addition or instead of external devices. A walking stick held in the contralateral arm has been shown to reduce the adduction moment in the ipsilateral knee and improve symptoms [49–52].

References

1. Mistry DA, Chandratreya A, Lee PYF. An update on unloading knee braces in the treatment of unicompartmental knee osteoarthritis from the last 10 years: a literature review. Surg J (N Y). 2018;4(3):e110–8.
2. Lewis JL, Lew WD, Stulberg SD, Patrnchak CM, Shybut GT. A new concept in orthotics joint design—The Northwestern University knee orthosis system. Part II. Orthotics Prosthetics. 1984;38(1):13–28.
3. Montgomery DL, Koziris PL. The knee brace controversy. Sports Med. 1989;8:260–72.
4. Dessery Y, Belzile EL, Turmel S, Corbeil P. Comparison of three knee braces in the treatment of medial knee osteoarthritis. Knee. 2014;21(6):1107–14. 4 point systems
5. van Egmond N, van Grinsven S, van Loon CJ. Is there a difference in outcome between two types of valgus unloading braces? A randomized controlled trial. Acta Orthop Belg. 2017;83(4):690–9.
6. Hjartarson HF, Toksvig-Larsen S. The clinical effect of an unloader brace on patients with osteoarthritis of the knee, a randomized placebo controlled trial with one year follow up. BMC Musculoskelet Disord. 2018;19(1):341.
7. Mauricio E, Sliepen M, Rosenbaum D. Acute effects of different orthotic interventions on knee loading parameters in knee osteoarthritis patients with varus malalignment. Knee. 2018;25(5):825–33.
8. Thoumie P, Marty M, Avouac B, Pallez A, Vaumousse A, Pipet LPT, Monroche A, Graveleau N, Bonnin A, Amor CB, Coudeyre E. Effect of unloading brace treatment on pain and function in patients with symptomatic knee osteoarthritis: the ROTOR randomized clinical trial. Sci Rep. 2018;8(1):10519. https://doi.org/10.1038/s41598-018-28782-3.
9. Lee PY, Winfield TG, Harris SR, Storey E, Chandratreya A. Unloading knee brace is a cost-effective method to bridge and delay surgery in unicompartmental knee arthritis. BMJ Open Sport Exerc Med. 2017;2(1):e000195. https://doi.org/10.1136/bmjsem-2016-000195.
10. Minzlaff P, Saier T, Brucker PU, Haller B, Imhoff AB, Hinterwimmer S. Valgus bracing in symptomatic varus malalignment for testing the expectable "unloading effect" following valgus high tibial osteotomy. Knee Surg Sports Traumatol Arthrosc. 2015;23(7):1964–70.
11. Haladik JA, Vasileff WK, Peltz CD, Lock TR, Bey MJ. Bracing improves clinical outcomes but does not affect the medial knee joint space in osteoarthritic patients during gait. Knee Surg Sports Traumatol Arthrosc. 2014;22(11):2715–20.
12. Ramsey DK, Briem K, Axe MJ, Snyder-Mackler L. A mechanical theory for the effectiveness of bracing for medial compartment osteoarthritis of the knee. J Bone Joint Surg Am. 2007;89(11):2398–407.
13. Brandon SCE, Brown MJ, Clouthier AL, Campbell A, Richards JD, Deluzio KJ. Contributions of muscles and external forces to medial knee load reduction due to osteoarthritis braces. Knee. 2019;26(3):564–77.
14. LaPrade RF, Venderley MB, Dahl KD, Dornan GJ, Turnbull TL. Functional brace in ACL surgery: force quantification in an in vivo study. Orthop J Sports Med. 2017;5(7):2325967117714242. https://doi.org/10.1177/2325967117714242.
15. Smith SD, Laprade RF, Jansson KS, Arøen A, Wijdicks CA. Functional bracing of ACL injuries: current state and future directions. Knee Surg Sports Traumatol Arthrosc. 2014;22(5):1131–41.
16. LaPrade RF, Smith SD, Wilson KJ, Wijdicks CA. Quantification of functional brace forces for posterior cruciate ligament injuries on the knee joint: an in vivo investigation. Knee Surg Sports Traumatol Arthrosc. 2015;23(10):3070–6.
17. Jansson KS, Costello KE, O'Brien L, Wijdicks CA, Laprade RF. A historical perspective of PCL bracing. Knee Surg Sports Traumatol Arthrosc. 2013;21(5):1064–70.
18. Jansen CM, Windau JE, Bonutti PM, Brillhart MV. Treatment of a knee contracture using a knee orthosis incorporating stress-relaxation techniques. Phys Ther. 1996;76(2):182–6.
19. Bhave A, Sodhi N, Anis HK, Ehiorobo JO, Mont MA. Static progressive stretch orthosis-consensus modality to treat knee stiffness-rationale and literature review. Ann Transl Med. 2019;7(Suppl 7):S256. https://doi.org/10.21037/atm.2019.06.55.

20. Pierce TP, Cherian JJ, Mont MA. Static and dynamic bracing for loss of motion following total knee arthroplasty. J Long-Term Eff Med Implants. 2015;25(4):337–43.
21. Sodhi N, Yao B, Anis HK, Khlopas A, Sultan AA, Newman JM, Mont MA. Patient satisfaction and outcomes of static progressive stretch bracing: a 10-year prospective analysis. Ann Transl Med. 2019;7(4):67. https://doi.org/10.21037/atm.2018.08.31.
22. Felson DT, Parkes M, Carter S, Liu A, Callaghan MJ, Hodgson R, Bowes M, Jones RK. The efficacy of a lateral wedge insole for painful medial knee osteoarthritis after prescreening: a randomized clinical trial. Arthritis Rheumatol. 2019;71(6):908–15.
23. Mannisi M, Dell'Isola A, Andersen MS, Woodburn J. Effect of lateral wedged insoles on the knee internal contact forces in medial knee osteoarthritis. Gait Posture. 2019;68:443–8.
24. Dadabo J, Fram J, Jayabalan P. Noninterventional therapies for the management of knee osteoarthritis. J Knee Surg. 2019;32(1):46–54.
25. Petersen W, Ellermann A, Henning J, Nehrer S, Rembitzki IV, Fritz J, Becher C, Albasini A, Zinser W, Laute V, Ruhnau K, Stinus H, Liebau C. Non-operative treatment of unicompartmental osteoarthritis of the knee: a prospective randomized trial with two different braces-ankle-foot orthosis versus knee unloader brace. Arch Orthop Trauma Surg. 2019;139(2):155–66.
26. Zhang J, Wang Q, Zhang C. Ineffectiveness of lateral-wedge insoles on the improvement of pain and function for medial knee osteoarthritis: a meta-analysis of controlled randomized trials. Arch Orthop Trauma Surg. 2018;138(10):1453–62.
27. Fischer AG, Ulrich B, Hoffmann L, Jolles BM, Favre J. Effect of lateral wedge length on ambulatory knee kinetics. Gait Posture. 2018;63:114–8.
28. Sliepen M, Mauricio E, Rosenbaum D. Acute and mid-term (six-week) effects of an ankle-foot-orthosis on biomechanical parameters, clinical outcomes and physical activity in knee osteoarthritis patients with varus malalignment. Gait Posture. 2018;62:297–302.
29. Jafarnezhadgero AA, Oliveira AS, Mousavi SH, Madadi-Shad M. Combining valgus knee brace and lateral foot wedges reduces external forces and moments in osteoarthritis patients. Gait Posture. 2018;59:104–10.
30. Shaw KE, Charlton JM, Perry CKL, de Vries CM, Redekopp MJ, White JA, Hunt MA. The effects of shoe-worn insoles on gait biomechanics in people with knee osteoarthritis: a systematic review and meta-analysis. Br J Sports Med. 2018;52(4):238–53.
31. Sawada T, Tanimoto K, Tokuda K, Iwamoto Y, Ogata Y, Anan M, Takahashi M, Kito N, Shinkoda K. Rear foot kinematics when wearing lateral wedge insoles and foot alignment influence the effect of knee adduction moment for medial knee osteoarthritis. Gait Posture. 2017;57:177–81.
32. Hunt MA, Takacs J, Krowchuk NM, Hatfield GL, Hinman RS, Chang R. Lateral wedges with and without custom arch support for people with medial knee osteoarthritis and pronated feet: an exploratory randomized crossover study. J Foot Ankle Res. 2017;10:20. https://doi.org/10.1186/s13047-017-0201-x.
33. Yılmaz B, Kesikburun S, Köroğlu O, Yaşar E, Göktepe AS, Yazıcıoğlu K. Effects of two different degrees of lateral-wedge insoles on unilateral lower extremity load-bearing line in patients with medial knee osteoarthritis. Acta Orthop Traumatol Turc. 2016;50(4):405–8.
34. Menger B, Kannenberg A, Petersen W, Zantop T, Rembitzki I, Stinus H. Effects of a novel foot-ankle orthosis in the non-operative treatment of unicompartmental knee osteoarthritis. Arch Orthop Trauma Surg. 2016;136(9):1281–7.
35. Weinhandl JT, Sudheimer SE, Van Lunen BL, Stewart K, Hoch MC. Immediate and 1 week effects of laterally wedge insoles on gait biomechanics in healthy females. Gait Posture. 2016;45:164–9.
36. Arnold JB. Lateral wedge insoles for people with medial knee osteoarthritis: one size fits all, some or none? Osteoarthr Cartil. 2016;24(2):193–5.
37. Campos GC, Rezende MU, Pasqualin T, Frucchi R, Bolliger NR. Lateral wedge insole for knee osteoarthritis: randomized clinical trial. Sao Paulo Med J. 2015;133(1):13–9.
38. Hatfield GL, Cochrane CK, Takacs J, Krowchuk NM, Chang R, Hinman RS, Hunt MA. Knee and ankle biomechanics with lateral wedges with and without a custom arch support in those with medial knee osteoarthritis and flat feet. J Orthop Res. 2016;34(9):1597–605.

39. Sodhi N, Yao B, Khlopas A, Davidson IU, Sultan AA, Samuel LT, Lamaj S, Newman JM, Pivec R, Fisher KA, Gaal B, Mont MA. A case for the brace: a critical, comprehensive, and up-to-date review of static progressive stretch, dynamic, and turnbuckle braces for the management of elbow, knee, and shoulder pathology. Surg Technol Int. 2017;31:303–18.
40. Collins NJ, Hinman RS, Menz HB, Crossley KM. Immediate effects of foot orthoses on pain during functional tasks in people with patellofemoral osteoarthritis: A cross-over, proof-of-concept study. Knee. 2017;24(1):76–81.
41. Yosmaoğlu HB, Selfe J, Sonmezer E, Sahin İE, Duygu SÇ, Acar Ozkoslu M, Richards J, Janssen J. Targeted treatment protocol in patellofemoral pain: does treatment designed according to subgroups improve clinical outcomes in patients unresponsive to multimodal treatment? Sports Health. 2020;12(2):170–80.
42. Mølgaard CM, Rathleff MS, Andreasen J, Christensen M, Lundbye-Christensen S, Simonsen O, Kaalund S. Foot exercises and foot orthoses are more effective than knee focused exercises in individuals with patellofemoral pain. J Sci Med Sport. 2018;21(1):10–5.
43. Rodrigues P, Chang R, TenBroek T, Hamill J. Medially posted insoles consistently influence foot pronation in runners with and without anterior knee pain. Gait Posture. 2013;37(4):526–31.
44. Toda Y, Tsukimura N. A six-month followup of a randomized trial comparing the efficacy of a lateral-wedge insole with subtalar strapping and an in-shoe lateral-wedge insole in patients with varus deformity osteoarthritis of the knee. Arthritis Rheum. 2004;50(10):3129–36.
45. Toda Y, Tsukimura N, Segal N. An optimal duration of daily wear for an insole with subtalar strapping in patients with varus deformity osteoarthritis of the knee. Osteoarthr Cartil. 2005;13(4):353–60.
46. Toda Y, Tsukimura N, Kato A. The effects of different elevations of laterally wedged insoles with subtalar strapping on medial compartment osteoarthritis of the knee. Arch Phys Med Rehabil. 2004;85(4):673–7.
47. Toda Y, Segal N, Kato A, Yamamoto S, Irie M. Effect of a novel insole on the subtalar joint of patients with medial compartment osteoarthritis of the knee. J Rheumatol. 2001;28(12):2705–10.
48. Brouwer RW, van Raaij TM, Verhaar JA, Coene LN, Bierma-Zeinstra SM. Brace treatment for osteoarthritis of the knee: a prospective randomized multi-centre trial. Osteoarthr Cartil. 2006;14(8):777–83.
49. Moller F, Ortiz-Muñoz L, Irarrázaval S. Contralateral canes for knee osteoarthritis. Medwave. 2020;20(1):e7759. https://doi.org/10.5867/medwave.2020.01.7759.
50. Moe RH, Fernandes L, Osterås N. Daily use of a cane for two months reduced pain and improved function in patients with knee osteoarthritis. J Physiother. 2012;58(2):128. https://doi.org/10.1016/S1836-9553(12)70094-2.
51. Chan GN, Smith AW, Kirtley C, Tsang WW. Changes in knee moments with contralateral versus ipsilateral cane usage in females with knee osteoarthritis. Clin Biomech (Bristol, Avon). 2005;20(4):396–404.
52. Fang MA, Heiney C, Yentes JM, Harada ND, Masih S, Perell-Gerson KL. Effects of contralateral versus ipsilateral cane use on gait in people with knee osteoarthritis. PM R. 2015;7(4):400–6.

Chapter 11
Knee Injection and Needling Therapy

Injection or needling interventions are extensively used in the management of knee disorders. This chapter discusses injection therapy, including the types of injectates commonly utilised, their possible underlying mechanisms of action, as well as potential associated complications. Techniques commonly used in injecting the knee are also presented. In addition, reference is made to dry needling techniques in the management of tendon and muscle disorders, as well as to the use of barbotage in the treatment of calcific ligamentopathy or tendinopathy.

11.1 Injection Therapy

Several agents may be injected in the knee and these are described below. There is substantial controversy as to the extent of effectiveness of these injectates, and a wide variation is observed in the benefit obtained amongst patients. Patients need to be warned of the possibility that such injections may have no benefit, and that even when improvement in symptoms occurs, such improvement may be short lived. It is not possible to reliably predict at an individual level which patient will benefit the most from knee injections.

11.2 Types of Knee Injections

Commonly utilised knee injections include the following.

C. Panayiotou Charalambous, *The Knee Made Easy*,
https://doi.org/10.1007/978-3-030-54506-2_11

11.2.1 Steroid Injections [1–3]

Steroid injections are used for their anti-inflammatory effect to help:

- Improve pain
- Reduce soft tissue inflammation, oedema and joint stiffness

They may be injected into the:

- Knee joint—for capsulitis, synovitis, arthritis
- Around tendons/tendon insertion onto bone—knee tendinopathy, enthesopathy

Their effects are difficult to fully predict at an individual level with regards to:

- Obtaining any benefit at all
- Extent of any beneficial effect
- Duration of any beneficial effect

Evidence suggests that their effects may last up to 3 months.

They are usually administered mixed with a local anaesthetic, which increases the volume of fluid to be injected, and hence its distribution area.

There have been concerns with steroid injections in that:

- They may adversely affect cartilage and tendon cells [4–6] by:
  - Reducing cell proliferation
  - Causing cell degeneration
  - Reducing collagen formation impairing the ability of tendon cells to repair
- They may reduce local immune responses increasing the risk of infection in subsequent arthroplasty procedures [7–9]
- They may be systemically absorbed causing blood sugar elevation in patients with diabetes [7]
- They may lead to osteonecrosis [8]

11.2.2 Visco-supplementation-Hyaluronic Acid Injections

Hyaluronic acid and its derivatives are available in multiple commercial preparations. Their aim is to supplement the natural hyaluronic acid found in synovial fluid. Depending on the commercial preparation, they may be administered as a single injection or as a course of 3–5 weekly injections.

- A single injection has been shown to be as effective as a 3–5 injection course [9]
- Hyaluronic acid injections have also been shown to be equivalent to steroid injections in the treatment of osteoarthritic knee pain [10]
- Hyaluronic acid may be more effective in early stages of osteoarthritis, and its effects may be less in the presence of severe arthritis [11]

Hyaluronic acid aims to reduce pain and improve function and may exert its effects by [12, 13]:

- Limiting cell death, and hence protecting cartilage degeneration
- Reducing inflammation
- Reducing synovial fibrosis
- Reducing synovial new vessel formation

Hyaluronic acid may be injected into the knee joint for:

- Degenerative arthritis, chondral defects

11.2.3 Platelet Rich Plasma Injections

Whole blood is obtained from the patient by venepuncture and is centrifuged. This allows platelets and growth factors (such as TGF-b, PDGF, FGF) to be separated from the rest of the blood, and hence be delivered in a much higher concentration (three to five fold) [13–25].

Platelets and growth factors may:

- Stimulate tissue healing and regeneration
- Have an anti-inflammatory effect

Different preparations of PRP are described, according to their platelet concentration. They may also be described as leukocyte rich or poor (if they contain a higher or lower leukocyte concentration than baseline). Leukocyte rich PRP preparations may lead to a higher inflammatory reaction.

This platelet/growth factor concentrate is then injected at the area of interest such as:

- Into tendons/tendon insertion onto bone—for tendinopathy, enthesopathy
- Knee joint—for arthritis

PRP injections may be superior to hyaluronic acid and steroid injections in the treatment of knee arthritis with regards to pain improvement. There is also evidence that a single injection is as effective as multiple PRP injections (2 or 3) with regards to pain improvement at 6 months following injection.

11.2.4 Mesenchymal Stem Cells [26–30]

Mesenchymal stem cells may be obtained from:

- Autologous bone marrow aspirates
- Percutaneously obtained adipose tissue
- Allogenic umbilical cord/amniotic tissue

They may be administered without cell expansion, or following culture expansion in vitro.

They may exert their effects by the release of mediators that:

- Reduce inflammation
- Reduce cartilage breakdown
- Promote cartilage matrix synthesis

Mesenchymal cell injections are injected into the:

- Knee joint—for chondral damage and osteoarthritis
- Tendons/tendon insertion onto bone—for tendinopathy

11.2.5 *Ozone Injections* [31–33]

Ozone injections have been used in treating knee pain, but high quality evidence for their effectiveness is awaited.

11.2.6 *Local Anaesthetic Injections* [34–39]

- Local anaesthetic may be administered as a component of other injectates, to increase the volume of the administered solution, and hence the area into which it can be delivered.
- Local anaesthetic injections may be used in isolation as treatment of:
  - Myofascial trigger points
  - Peripheral nerve blockage to improve chronic pain
  - Peripheral nerve blockage in peripheral nerve dysfunction
- Sole local anaesthetic injections may also be used as diagnostic injections to help:
  - Determine if the pain a patient complains of originates from the area injected
  - Determine if muscle relaxation improves the patient's symptoms

There have been concerns about the effects of local anaesthetic injections [40, 41] including:

- Cytotoxicity to tenocytes and chondrocytes
- Impairment of the biomechanical properties of tendons
- Induction of tendon cell apoptosis

11.2.7 *Normal Saline Injections*

Normal saline may be injected into muscular/fascial tender spots, to help pain originating from such spots. Its effects may be mediated by a mechanical pressure mechanism.

Hydrodissection—this refers to injection of normal saline along with steroid around a nerve, to release peri-neural adhesions, to improve neurogenic pain.

11.3 Contraindications to Injection Therapy

The following are potential contraindications to injection therapy:

- Local or systemic infection
- Hypersensitivity to the injectate
- Uncontrolled diabetes (for steroid injections)
- Acute fracture at the site of the injection
- Anticoagulation therapy due to the risk of bleeding –current evidence however suggests that routine discontinuation is not necessary, as the risk of bleeding is very small [42, 43]

11.4 Potential Complications of Knee Injections

Several complications of injection therapy have been described [5, 8, 44–50]. Some are seen across injectates, and some are more injectate specific. These complications must be discussed with the patient prior to injecting the knee and include:

- Infection
- Bleeding (bruising, soft tissue haematoma, haemarthrosis)
- Nerve or vessel damage
- Hypersensitivity reactions
- Local reactions—pain and tenderness (post hyaluronic acid injections)
- Subcutaneous fat atrophy, thinning of the skin, pigmentation loss –post steroid injections (if adversely injected into subcutaneous fat tissue)
- Aggravation of pain—post steroid injections—usually self-limiting
- Menstrual bleeding—heavier, erratic, post-menopausal (post steroid injections)
- Blood sugar derangement—post steroid injections
- Aggravation of tendinopathy—post PRP injections
- Tendon tear (post steroid injections)

11.5 Knee Injection Techniques

Injections into the knee may be administered under radiological guidance such as image intensifier radiography or dynamic ultrasound, to help the accuracy of administration. Such guidance is preferable for injections administered into tight spaces, or near tubular tendons (into which injection is to be avoided), or near neurovascular structures. Radiological guidance is also preferable in administering nerve blocks around the knee. Hence, radiological guidance is preferable for injections into the:

- Pes anserinus—US
- Patellar tendon—US
- Genicular nerve blocks—US, plain radiography

Injections however may be also performed using palpable anatomical landmarks and the techniques for these are described below.

11.5.1 Knee Joint Intra-articular Injection

Patient is sitting or lying supine with the leg straight:

- Medial parapatellar approach
  - Palpate the interval (soft spot) between the under surface of the medial facet of the patella and the anterior surface of the femur. Moving the patella from medial to lateral and back can help identify this interval. Getting the patient to relax the extensor mechanism will facilitate the above
  - Insert the needle into this interval angled in a lateral and posterior direction
  - If the needle hits the patella or the femur, withdraw slightly, and change the angle as necessary before reinserting
- Lateral parapatellar approach
  - Palpate the interval (soft spot) between the undersurface of the lateral facet of the patella and the anterior surface of the femur. Moving the patella from medial to lateral and back can help identify this interval. Getting the patient to relax the extensor mechanism will facilitate the above
  - Insert the needle into this interval, angled in a medial and posterior direction
  - If the needle hits the patella or the femur, withdraw slightly and change the angle as necessary before reinserting
- Suprapatellar approach
  - Palpate the junction of the lateral and superior borders of the patella. Moving the patella from medial to lateral and back can help identify this interval. Getting the patient to relax their extensor mechanism will facilitate the above
  - Insert the needle from lateral, just superior to this junction, aiming in a medial and posterior direction towards the femur
  - If the needle hits the patella or the femur withdraw slightly and change the angle as necessary before reinserting

Patient is sitting or lying supine with the knee flexed:

- Anterolateral approach
  - Identify the soft spot just lateral to the patellar tendon and above the lateral part of the tibiofemoral joint

  - Insert the needle aiming medially towards the femoral notch
  - If the injectate cannot be injected easily, the tip of the needle may be in the fat pad, and may need to be repositioned
- Anteromedial approach
  - Identify the soft spot just medial to the patellar tendon and above the medial part of the tibiofemoral joint
  - Insert the needle aiming laterally towards the femoral notch
  - If the injectate cannot be injected easily, the tip of the needle may be in the fat pad, and may need to be repositioned

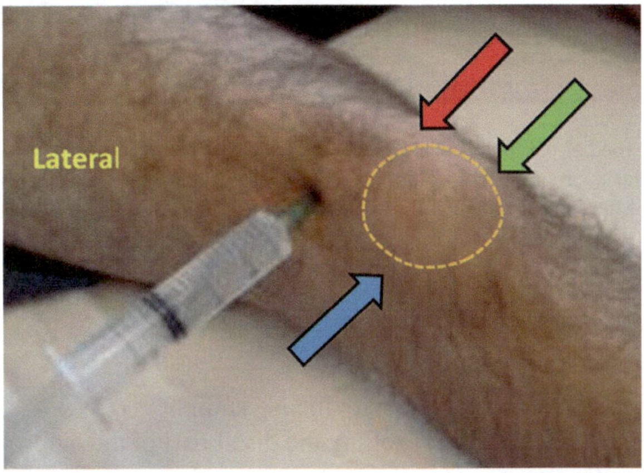

Approaches for intra-articular injection of the knee: Syringe—lateral suprapatellar. Red arrow—medial suprapatellar. Blue arrow—lateral parapatellar. Green arrow—medial parapatellar

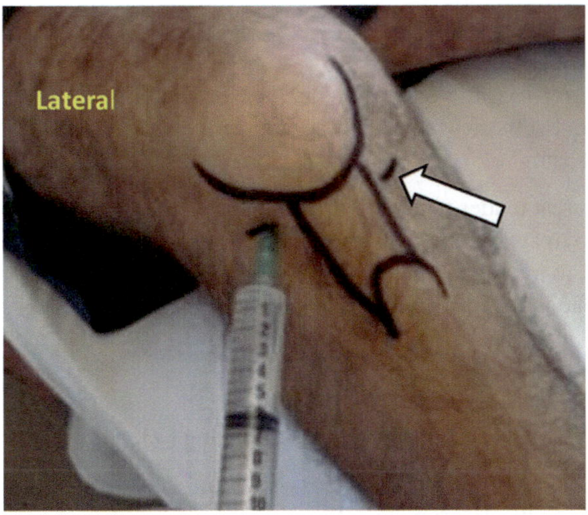

Approaches for intra-articular injection of the knee on either side of the patellar tendon. Syringe—anerolateral. White arrow—anteromedial

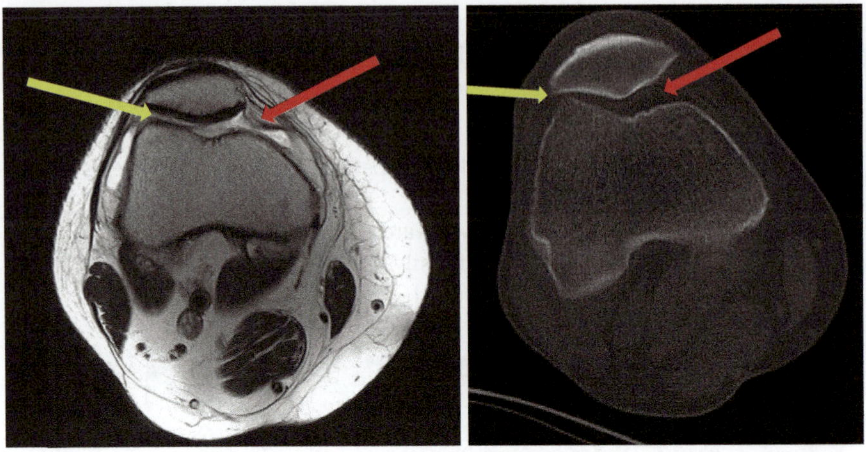

Injection via the medial parapatellar approach (red) may be technically easier as compared to the lateral parapatellar approach (yellow) due to more space at the medial part of the patellofemoral space (because of the shape of the patella and the lateral patellar tilting which is often encountered)

11.5.2 Pes Anserinus Injection

- Patient is sitting or lying supine with the leg straight
- Palpate the pes anserinus area, rolling the distal part of the hamstring tendons
- Insert the needle aiming medially, in the interval between the tendons and bone

11.6 Dry Needling

Dry needling involves the repetitive insertion of a solid needle to make multiple fenestrations in the tissue (rather than administering an injectate) [51, 52].

This may be in:

- Muscle, to treat tender points
- Tendons, to treat tendinopathy
- Ligaments, to treat ligamentopathy
- Tendon-bone insertion (enthesis)—to treat enthesopathy

Acupuncture also involves dry needling, but a description of that is beyond the scope of this chapter.

Dry needling may exert its effects by stimulating [53, 54]:

- Local blood flow (to increase local oxygenation)
- Fibroblast activity (to promote collagen formation and tissue regeneration)
- Activation of neural pathways that inhibit pain

- Mechanical pressure effect—to activate local reflexes that suppress pain

Technique for dry needling of tendon:

- The diseased area is identified using ultrasound
- An acupuncture needle is inserted through the skin into the tendon and multiple fenestrations are made in the tendon

Dry needling may be performed for various tendons around the knee, including distal quadriceps tendon tendinopathy, or patellar tendon tendinopathy.

11.7 Barbotage

Barbotage is a technique used to break down and remove calcific deposits in tendons or ligaments [55].

Technique

- Ultrasound is used to identify the calcification
- A needle is inserted percutaneously to puncture the calcific deposit. The calcific deposit is then irrigated with normal saline injected through the needle to break it down
- Once the calcific deposit is broken, the calcium may be aspirated through the same needle or through another (separately introduced) needle

Learning Pearls

- In assessing a patient who had a knee injection previously, it is useful to determine which specific area was injected (in particular whether this was an intra-articular or extra-articular injection).
- Injecting a steroid may be preferable for acutely inflamed tissues rather than for chronic non-inflammatory pain.
- The effectiveness of steroid injections may diminish with repeated injections– the first injection may be the one most likely to be effective.
- The effect of locally injected steroids may be mediated at least partly through systemic absorption—as, on occasion, patients report that the injection of one joint also improved pain in distant joints.

References

1. Saltychev M, Mattie R, McCormick Z, Laimi K. The magnitude and duration of the effect of intra-articular corticosteroid injections on pain severity in knee osteoarthritis—a systematic review and meta-analysis. Am J Phys Med Rehabil. 2020; https://doi.org/10.1097/PHM.0000000000001384.

2. Martin CL, Browne JA. Intra-articular corticosteroid injections for symptomatic knee osteoarthritis: what the orthopaedic provider needs to know. J Am Acad Orthop Surg. 2019;27(17):e758–66.
3. Lee JH, Lee JU, Yoo SW. Accuracy and efficacy of ultrasound-guided pes anserinus bursa injection. J Clin Ultrasound. 2019;47(2):77–82.
4. Dean BJ, Franklin SL, Murphy RJ, Javaid MK, Carr AJ. Glucocorticoids induce specific ion-channel-mediated toxicity in human rotator cuff tendon: a mechanism underpinning the ultimately deleterious effect of steroid injection in tendinopathy? Br J Sports Med. 2014;48(22):1620–6.
5. Poulsen RC, Watts AC, Murphy RJ, Snelling SJ, Carr AJ, Hulley PA. Glucocorticoids induce senescence in primary human tenocytes by inhibition of sirtuin 1 and activation of the p53/p21 pathway: in vivo and in vitro evidence. Ann Rheum Dis. 2014;73(7):1405–13.
6. Wernecke C, Braun HJ, Dragoo JL. The effect of intra-articular corticosteroids on articular cartilage: a systematic review. Orthop J Sports Med. 2015;3(5):2325967115581163.
7. Choudhry MN, Malik RA, Charalambous CP. Blood glucose levels following intra-articular steroid injections in patients with diabetes: a systematic review. JBJS Rev. 2016;4(3) pii: 01874474-201603000-00002 https://doi.org/10.2106/JBJS.RVW.O.00029.
8. Lee JH, Wang SI, Noh SJ, Ham DH, Kim KB. Osteonecrosis of the medial tibial plateau after intra-articular corticosteroid injection: a case report. Medicine (Baltimore). 2019;98(44):e17248. https://doi.org/10.1097/MD.0000000000017248.
9. Vincent P. Intra-articular hyaluronic acid in the symptomatic treatment of knee osteoarthritis: a meta-analysis of single-injection products. Curr Ther Res Clin Exp. 2019;90:39–51. https://doi.org/10.1016/j.curtheres.2019.02.003.
10. Ran J, Yang X, Ren Z, Wang J, Dong H. Comparison of intra-articular hyaluronic acid and methylprednisolone for pain management in knee osteoarthritis: A meta-analysis of randomized controlled trials. Int J Surg. 2018;53:103–10.
11. Nicholls M, Shaw P, Niazi F, Bhandari M, Bedi A. The impact of excluding patients with end-stage knee disease in intra-articular hyaluronic acid trials: a systematic review and meta-analysis. Adv Ther. 2019;36(1):147–61.
12. Gallorini M, Berardi AC, Berardocco M, Gissi C, Maffulli N, Cataldi A, Oliva F. Hyaluronic acid increases tendon derived cell viability and proliferation in vitro: comparative study of two different hyaluronic acid preparations by molecular weight. Muscles Ligaments Tendons J. 2017;7(2):208–14.
13. Ghosh P, Guidolin D. Potential mechanism of action of intra-articular hyaluronan therapy in osteoarthritis: are the effects molecular weight dependent? Semin Arthritis Rheum. 2002;32(1):10–37.
14. Wu PI, Diaz R, Borg-Stein J. Platelet-rich plasma. Phys Med Rehabil Clin N Am. 2016;27(4):825–53.
15. Mlynarek RA, Kuhn AW, Bedi A. Platelet-rich plasma (PRP) in orthopedic sports medicine. Am J Orthop (Belle Mead NJ). 2016;45(5):290–326.
16. Zhu Y, Yuan M, Meng HY, Wang AY, Guo QY, Wang Y, Peng J. Basic science and clinical application of platelet-rich plasma for cartilage defects and osteoarthritis: a review. Osteoarthr Cartil. 2013;21(11):1627–37.
17. Dupley L, Charalambous CP. Platelet-rich plasma injections as a treatment for refractory patellar tendinosis: a meta-analysis of randomised trials. Knee Surg Relat Res. 2017;29(3):165–71.
18. Vilchez-Cavazos F, Millán-Alanís JM, Blázquez-Saldaña J, Álvarez-Villalobos N, Peña-Martínez VM, Acosta-Olivo CA, Simental-Mendía M. Comparison of the clinical effectiveness of single versus multiple injections of platelet-rich plasma in the treatment of knee osteoarthritis: a systematic review and meta-analysis. Orthop J Sports Med. 2019;7(12):2325967119887116. https://doi.org/10.1177/2325967119887116.
19. Kenmochi M. Clinical outcomes following injections of leukocyte-rich platelet-rich plasma in osteoarthritis patients. J Orthop. 2019;18:143–9.
20. Le ADK, Enweze L, DeBaun MR, Dragoo JL. Current clinical recommendations for use of platelet-rich plasma. Curr Rev Musculoskelet Med. 2018;11(4):624–34.

21. Chen P, Huang L, Ma Y, Zhang D, Zhang X, Zhou J, Ruan A, Wang Q. Intra-articular platelet-rich plasma injection for knee osteoarthritis: a summary of meta-analyses. J Orthop Surg Res. 2019;14(1):385. https://doi.org/10.1186/s13018-019-1363-y.
22. Lin KY, Yang CC, Hsu CJ, Yeh ML, Renn JH. Intra-articular injection of platelet-rich plasma is superior to hyaluronic acid or saline solution in the treatment of mild to moderate knee osteoarthritis: a randomized, double-blind, triple-parallel, placebo-controlled clinical trial. Arthroscopy. 2019;35(1):106–17.
23. Huang Y, Liu X, Xu X, Liu J. Intra-articular injections of platelet-rich plasma, hyaluronic acid or corticosteroids for knee osteoarthritis: a prospective randomized controlled study. Orthopade. 2019;48(3):239–47.
24. Di Martino A, Di Matteo B, Papio T, Tentoni F, Selleri F, Cenacchi A, Kon E, Filardo G. Platelet-rich plasma versus hyaluronic acid injections for the treatment of knee osteoarthritis: results at 5 years of a double-blind, randomized controlled trial. Am J Sports Med. 2019;47(2):347–54.
25. Cole BJ, Karas V, Hussey K, Pilz K, Fortier LA. Hyaluronic acid versus platelet-rich plasma: a prospective, double-blind randomized controlled trial comparing clinical outcomes and effects on intra-articular biology for the treatment of knee osteoarthritis. Am J Sports Med. 2017;45(2):339–46.
26. Doyle EC, Wragg NM, Wilson SL. Intraarticular injection of bone marrow-derived mesenchymal stem cells enhances regeneration in knee osteoarthritis. Knee Surg Sports Traumatol Arthrosc. 2020; https://doi.org/10.1007/s00167-020-05859-z.
27. Garza JR, Campbell RE, Tjoumakaris FP, Freedman KB, Miller LS, Santa Maria D, Tucker BS. Clinical efficacy of intra-articular mesenchymal stromal cells for the treatment of knee osteoarthritis: a double-blinded prospective randomized controlled clinical trial. Am J Sports Med. 2020;48(3):588–98.
28. Dilogo IH, Canintika AF, Hanitya AL, Pawitan JA, Liem IK, Pandelaki J. Umbilical cord-derived mesenchymal stem cells for treating osteoarthritis of the knee: a single-arm, open-label study. Eur J Orthop Surg Traumatol. 2020; https://doi.org/10.1007/s00590-020-02630-5.
29. Kim SH, Djaja YP, Park YB, Park JG, Ko YB, Ha CW. Intra-articular injection of culture-expanded mesenchymal stem cells without adjuvant surgery in knee osteoarthritis: a systematic review and meta-analysis. Am J Sports Med. 2019;24:363546519892278. https://doi.org/10.1177/0363546519892278.
30. Usuelli FG, Grassi M, Maccario C, Vigano M, Lanfranchi L, Alfieri Montrasio U, de Girolamo L. Intratendinous adipose-derived stromal vascular fraction (SVF) injection provides a safe, efficacious treatment for Achilles tendinopathy: results of a randomized controlled clinical trial at a 6-month follow-up. Knee Surg Sports Traumatol Arthrosc. 2018;26(7):2000–10.
31. Sconza C, Respizzi S, Virelli L, Vandenbulcke F, Iacono F, Kon E, Di Matteo B. Oxygen-ozone therapy for the treatment of knee osteoarthritis: a systematic review of randomized controlled trials. Arthroscopy. 2020;36(1):277–86. https://doi.org/10.1016/j.arthro.2019.05.043.
32. Raeissadat SA, Tabibian E, Rayegani SM, Rahimi-Dehgolan S, Babaei-Ghazani A. An investigation into the efficacy of intra-articular ozone (O2-O3) injection in patients with knee osteoarthritis: a systematic review and meta-analysis. J Pain Res. 2018;11:2537–50.
33. Manoto SL. Editorial commentary: is medical ozone therapy beneficial in the treatment of knee osteoarthritis? Arthroscopy. 2020;36(1):287–8.
34. Kim DH, Yoon DM, Yoon KB. The effects of myofascial trigger point injections on nocturnal calf cramps. J Am Board Fam Med. 2015;28(1):21–7.
35. Frost FA, Jessen B, Siggaard-Andersen J. A control, double-blind comparison of mepivacaine injection versus saline injection for myofascial pain. Lancet. 1980;1(8167):499–500.
36. Baldry P. Management of myofascial trigger point pain. Acupunct Med. 2002;20(1):2–10.
37. Yilmaz V, Umay E, Gundogdu I, Aras B. The comparison of efficacy of single intraarticular steroid injection versus the combination of genicular nerve block and intraarticular steroid injection in patients with knee osteoarthritis: a randomised study. Musculoskelet Surg. 2019; https://doi.org/10.1007/s12306-019-00633-y.

38. Kim DH, Choi SS, Yoon SH, Lee SH, Seo DK, Lee IG, Choi WJ, Shin JW. Ultrasound-guided genicular nerve block for knee osteoarthritis: a double-blind, randomized controlled trial of local anesthetic alone or in combination with corticosteroid. Pain Physician. 2018;21(1):41–52.
39. Romanoff ME, Cory PC Jr, Kalenak A, Keyser GC, Marshall WK. Saphenous nerve entrapment at the adductor canal. Am J Sports Med. 1989;17(4):478–81.
40. Kreuz PC, Steinwachs M, Angele P. Single-dose local anesthetics exhibit a type-, dose-, and time-dependent chondrotoxic effect on chondrocytes and cartilage: a systematic review of the current literature. Knee Surg Sports Traumatol Arthrosc. 2018;26(3):819–30.
41. Honda H, Gotoh M, Kanazawa T, Nakamura H, Ohta K, Nakamura K, Shiba N. Effects of lidocaine on torn rotator cuff tendons. J Orthop Res. 2016;34(9):1620–7.
42. Yui JC, Preskill C, Greenlund LS. Arthrocentesis and joint injection in patients receiving direct oral anticoagulants. Mayo Clin Proc. 2017;92(8):1223–6.
43. Ahmed I, Gertner E. Safety of arthrocentesis and joint injection in patients receiving anticoagulation at therapeutic levels. Am J Med. 2012;125(3):265–9.
44. Charalambous CP, Prodromidis AD, Kwaees TA. Do intra-articular steroid injections increase infection rates in subsequent arthroplasty? A systematic review and meta-analysis of comparative studies. J Arthroplast. 2014;29(11):2175–80.
45. Werner BC, Cancienne JM, Browne JA. The timing of total hip arthroplasty after intraarticular hip injection affects postoperative infection risk. J Arthroplast. 2016;31(4):820–3.
46. Chambers AW, Lacy KW, Liow MHL, Manalo JPM, Freiberg AA, Kwon YM. Multiple hip intra-articular steroid injections increase risk of periprosthetic joint infection compared with single injections. J Arthroplast. 2017;32(6):1980–3.
47. Fawi HMT, Hossain M, Matthews TJW. The incidence of flare reaction and short-term outcome following steroid injection in the shoulder. Shoulder Elbow. 2017;9(3):188–94.
48. Charalambous CP, Tryfonidis M, Sadiq S, Hirst P, Paul A. Septic arthritis following intra-articular steroid injection of the knee—a survey of current practice regarding antiseptic technique used during intra-articular steroid injection of the knee. Clin Rheumatol. 2003;22(6):386–90.
49. Desmottes MC, Delorme L, Clay M, Troussier B, Leccia MT. Skin necrosis following intra-articular hyaluronic acid injection in the knee of a 63-year-old male. Joint Bone Spine. 2020. pii: S1297-319X(20)30002-6; https://doi.org/10.1016/j.jbspin.2020.01.002.
50. Richardson SS, Schairer WW, Sculco TP, Sculco PK. Comparison of infection risk with corticosteroid or hyaluronic acid injection prior to total knee arthroplasty. J Bone Joint Surg Am. 2019;101(2):112–8.
51. Stoychev V, Finestone AS, Kalichman L. Dry needling as a treatment modality for tendinopathy: a narrative review. Curr Rev Musculoskelet Med. 2020; https://doi.org/10.1007/s12178-020-09608-0.
52. Dunning J, Butts R, Mourad F, Young I, Flannagan S, Perreault T. Dry needling: a literature review with implications for clinical practice guidelines. Phys Ther Rev. 2014;19(4):252–65.
53. Riggin CN, Chen M, Gordon JA, Schultz SM, Soslowsky LJ, Khoury V. Ultrasound-guided dry needling of the healthy rat supraspinatus tendon elicits early healing without causing permanent damage. J Orthop Res. 2019;37(9):2035–42.
54. Nagraba Ł, Tuchalska J, Mitek T, Stolarczyk A, Deszczyński J. Dry needling as a method of tendinopathy treatment. Ortop Traumatol Rehabil. 2013;15(2):109–16.
55. Gatt DL, Charalambous CP. Ultrasound-guided barbotage for calcific tendonitis of the shoulder: a systematic review including 908 patients. Arthroscopy. 2014;30(9):1166–72.

Chapter 12
Knee Physiotherapy: A Surgeon's Perspective

Physiotherapy has an important role in reducing troublesome symptoms and improving function in disorders of the knee. Physiotherapy may be used in isolation in managing knee conditions or may compliment surgery (in optimising a patient for surgery or in enhancing recovery post-surgery).

This chapter aims to describe some of the principles of knee physiotherapy. It is not intended to be an in depth analysis of physiotherapy techniques but a basic explanation of terms and principles as perceived by an orthopaedic surgeon.

The principles described may help guide the surgeon in requesting specific physiotherapy input for a particular condition, and may also enhance the ability of the physiotherapist to appreciate the surgeon's aims and concerns when asking for such therapy. Clear and regular sharing of information is essential in such multidisciplinary care.

Initially some of the physiotherapy nomenclature is presented along with techniques that may be utilised in managing the troublesome knee. Approaches for improving knee stability, reducing joint stiffness, and rehabilitating the knee following an injury or surgical repair are also presented. The role of early versus late mobilisation and the role of early loading of the injured or surgically repaired site is also discussed. Furthermore, the concept of arthrogenic muscle inhibition of the knee and its management is described.

12.1 Physiotherapy Nomenclature

Some of the common terms used in physiotherapy [1–11] are presented here. Physiotherapy interventions may be described as:

- Passive—interventions applied to a patient
- Active—activities performed by the patient

Limb mobilisation may be described as:

C. Panayiotou Charalambous, *The Knee Made Easy*,
https://doi.org/10.1007/978-3-030-54506-2_12

- Passive—movement achieved by:
  - The patient using the opposite leg, arm, trunk
  - The therapist
- Active assisted—movement achieved through action of the limb itself assisted by:
  - The patient's opposite limb
  - The therapist
- Active—movement achieved solely through action of the limb in consideration

Mobilisation/strengthening exercises may be described as:

- Open kinetic chain active exercises—the distal part of the limb is free (for the lower limb the foot is free, as in straight leg raising)
- Closed kinetic chain exercises—the distal part of the limb is supported (for the lower limb the foot is supported, as in cycling, squatting). These may encourage more symmetric contraction of antagonist muscles and also provide more sensory feedback

Muscles contract in order to:

- Maintain a particular position/posture—such as when standing still
- Bring about motion—such as leg elevation, knee flexion/extension
- Oppose/decelerate a motion—such as allowing controlled flexion of the knee from full extension, preventing the fall of the elevated leg due to the effect of gravity upon straight leg raising, decelerate the limb as it comes from swing face to making contact with the ground and weightbearing

Several types of muscle contraction are described:

- Concentric contraction—contraction where the muscle shortens while generating a force overcoming an applied resistance—in straightening the knee the quadriceps muscle shortens
- Eccentric contraction—a contraction which occurs while the muscle lengthens. Essentially the muscle is trying to oppose an applied force but the applied force is greater than the tension generated by the muscle. This occurs when the straight knee is flexed towards the floor in a controlled fashion. The quadriceps tenses to oppose the force of the leg weight, to allow a slow controlled descend of the leg.
- Isometric contraction—an increase in muscle tension without a change in muscle length. Such contractions are used to maintain posture, such as the trunk and hip muscles. Knee isometric contractions may involve trying to initiate a movement against firm resistance that cannot be overcome (such as trying to extend the leg whilst pressing the knee against the couch). Isometric contractions may help maintain muscle bulk without moving the knee joint and hence stressing any surgical repair
- Isotonic contraction—contraction where the tension remains constant and leads to either muscle shortening or lengthening. It can either be concentric or

eccentric. Knee isotonic contractions may involve a movement against resistance (gravity or otherwise) that can be overcome.

Hence, muscle contractions may help preserve muscle bulk even when limb or joint motion is limited (such as in joint stiffness or when protecting a surgical repair).

Eccentric contractions have been shown to induce beneficial changes in tendon structure and be effective in improving pain and function in tendinopathies.

Muscles may be described as:

- Agonists—work in synergy
- Antagonists—work in opposition

12.2 Physiotherapy Techniques

Several techniques may be employed in physiotherapy and some of these are described below.

12.2.1 Local Treatment to Improve Pain

Physiotherapy may reduce pain in multiple ways as below:

1. Local passive treatment

   According to the gate control theory of pain, activation of sensory nerves that transmit touch may inhibit the transmission of pain signals in the dorsal horn of the spinal cord and hence reduce the perception of pain [12, 13]. This may explain why rubbing an area that hurts may improve pain. This is also the basis of several modalities used to improve local pain [14–17] such as:

   - TENS
   - Heat therapy—a rise in local temperature may lead to an increase in the local vascular response. Heat therapy can be applied in the form of:
     - Moist heat pack
     - Ultrasound
     - Diathermy—Megapulse is pulsed shortwave diathermy that can heat the deep tissue and increase collagen extensibility
   - Acupuncture—it is uncertain exactly how acupuncture exerts its effects, but it may stimulate the release of encephalin and endorphins as well as regulate prostaglandin synthesis, all of which may modulate pain perception. Application of localised mechanical pressure or electrical pulsing may exert a similar effect.

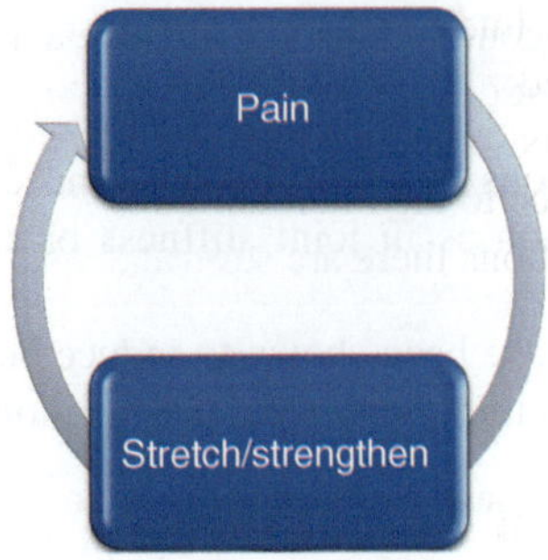

Two-way interaction between physiotherapy interventions and knee pain. Pain may limit the ability to strengthen or stretch the knee. Similarly anf attempt to strengthen or stretch the knee may aggravate pain

2. Improvement in knee biomechanics—this aims at reducing abnormal mechanics which may cause pain through uneven, erratic, raised, or unbalanced loading. This is achieved by establishing balanced joint control and motion, improving joint stability through:
   a. Posture control
   b. Proprioception enhancement
   c. Strengthening/rebalancing muscles
3. Stretching of:
   a. Contracted periarticular soft tissues, to reduce stiffness and improve range of motion—hence reducing the contraction of muscles trying to overcome such stiffness, and the resultant contact pressures from such muscle contractions
   b. Musculofascial tender spots

12.2.2 *Muscle Strengthening*

Muscle strengthening aims to increase:

- Maximum achievable load
- Endurance

In dealing with muscles the aims are to:

1. Reactivate and recruit previously inactive muscles
2. Strengthen muscles to compensate for a lost muscle (due to weakness or tendon tear) or compensate for a torn ligament

For example in anterior cruciate ligament (ACL) tear one may compensate for what has been lost by strengthening the hamstring muscles which can limit the anterior translation of the tibia on the femur, and hence have a similar effect to the ACL

[18–23]. This is analogous to a parachutist whose main parachute fails. Release of a reserve parachute may stop or slow the free fall and allow safe landing. The ability to activate and recruit such muscles may vary from individual to individual which may explain why some patients develop symptomatic instability after an ACL tear whilst others don't.

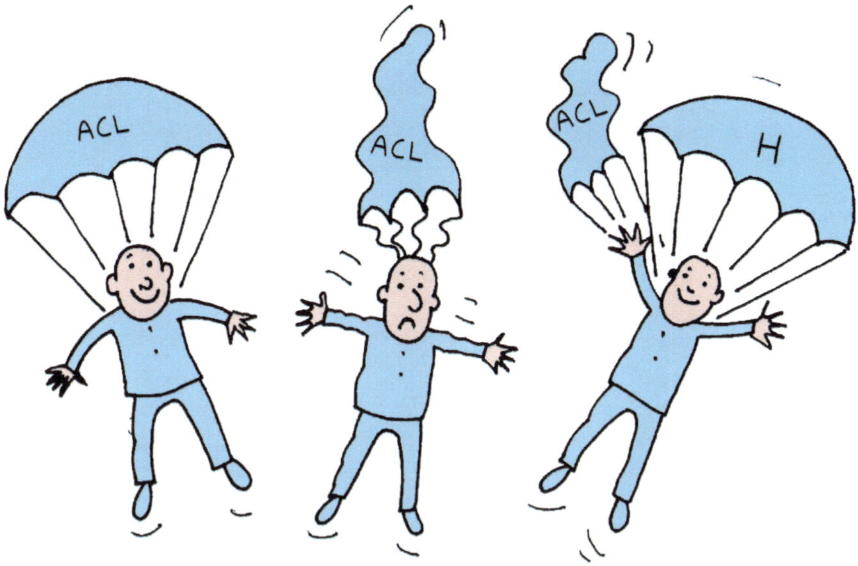

Compensation of an ACL tear by hamstring strengthening is analogous to a reserve parachute employed when the primary one fails

Muscle strengthening may involve:

- Electrical stimulation to recruit inactive muscles
- Isometric/isotonic exercises
- Concentric/eccentric exercises
- Gradual increase in the:
  - Amount of loading
  - Repetition (cycles) of loading
  - Frequency of loading

Some quadriceps and hamstring strengthening exercises are described below:

12.2.2.1 Quadriceps Strengthening

- Isometric—patient supine with leg straight. Small pillow under the knee. Patient presses foot down onto the couch.

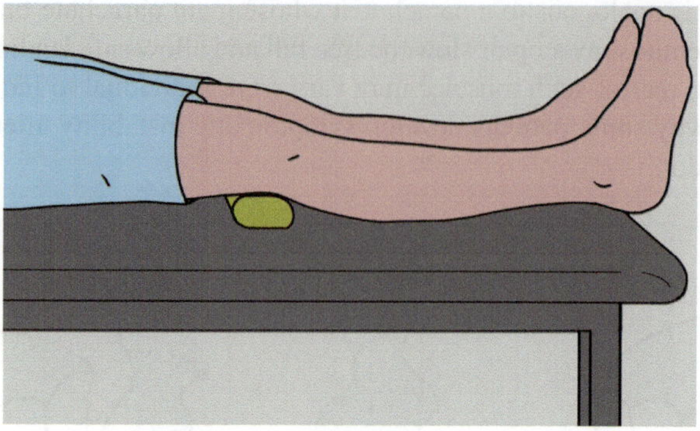

Isometric quadriceps strengthening

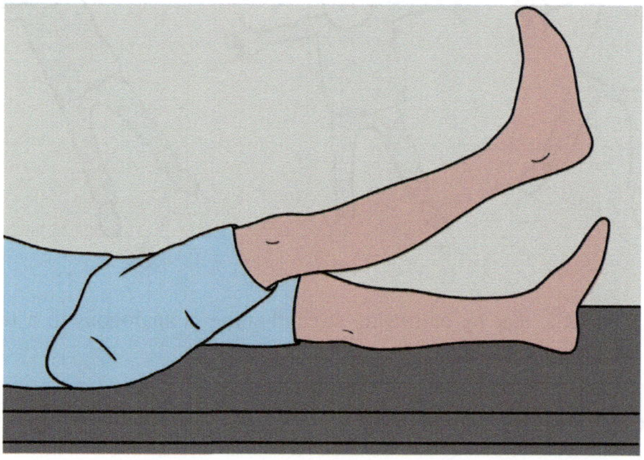

Straight leg raising

- Isotonic
  - Concentric
    - Straight leg raising—patient is laying supine, dorsiflexes the foot and elevates the lower leg straight, holds, and then returns to the starting position slowly
    - Knee extension- patient is seated with the knee flexed hanging from the side of a couch. The patient straightens the knee, holds, and returns to the starting position slowly

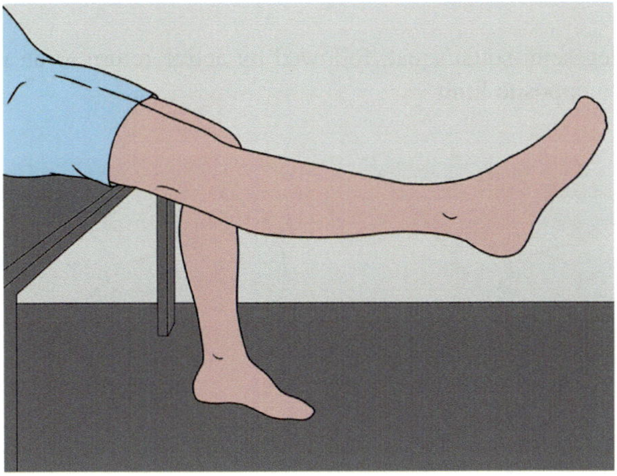

Knee extension

- Single leg semi-squat or squat, followed by active return to fully straight knee using the same limb—patient stands on exercise leg and holds onto a stable surface. The non-exercise leg is in 90° knee flexion. The patient then flexes the exercising knee to 30–45°, holds, and returns to extension.

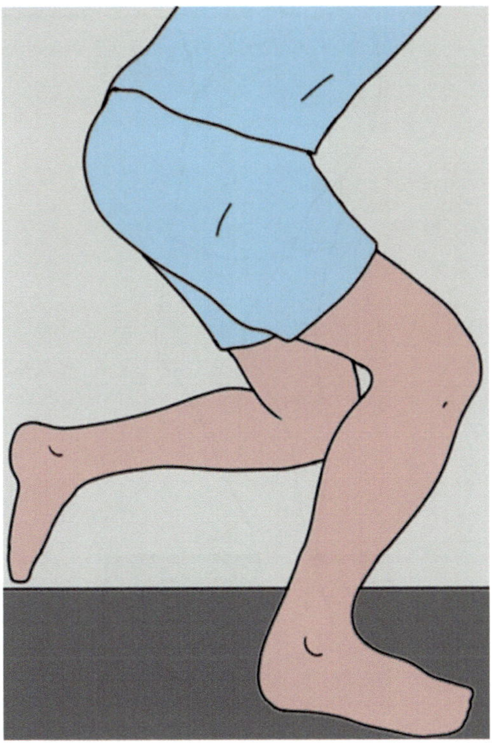

Single leg concentric semi squat

- Eccentric
  - Single leg semi-squat/squat, followed by active return to an initial position using the opposite limb

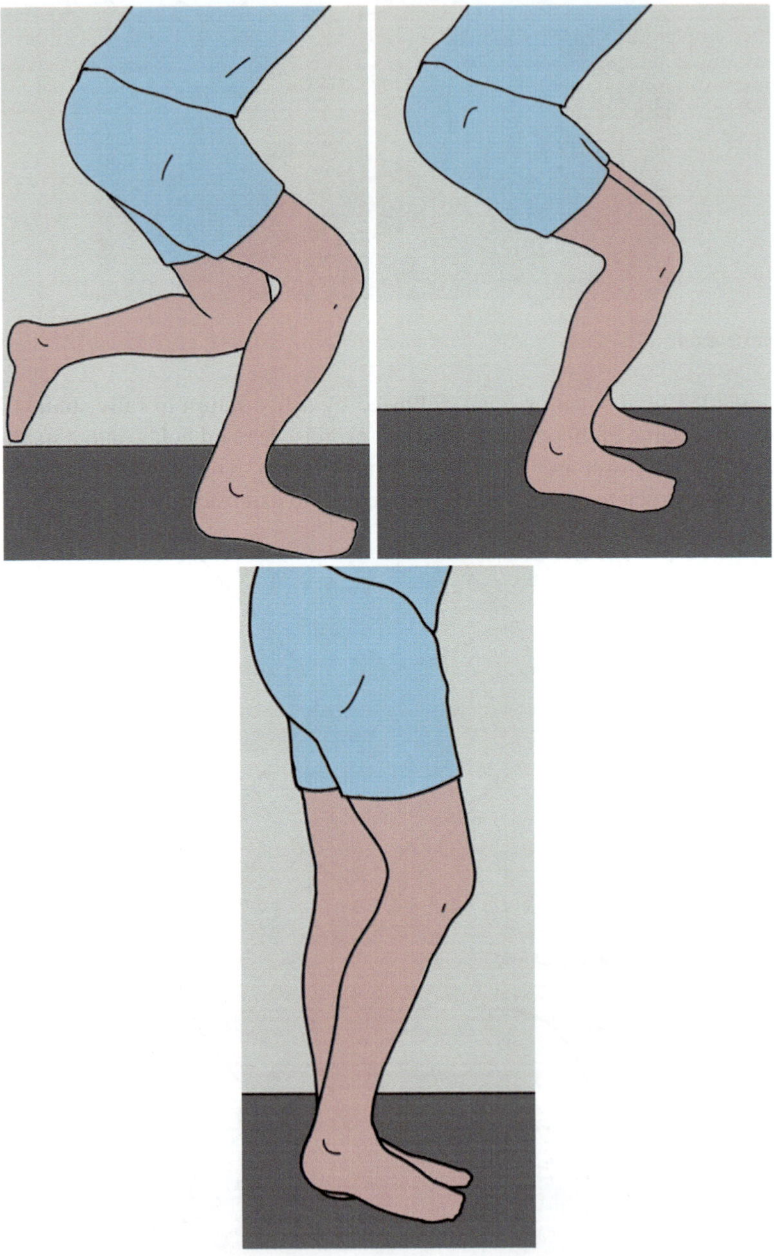

Single leg eccentric semi squat

12.2.2.2 Hamstring Strengthening

- Isometric—patient supine with the knee flexed to 90°. Patient presses foot down onto the couch.

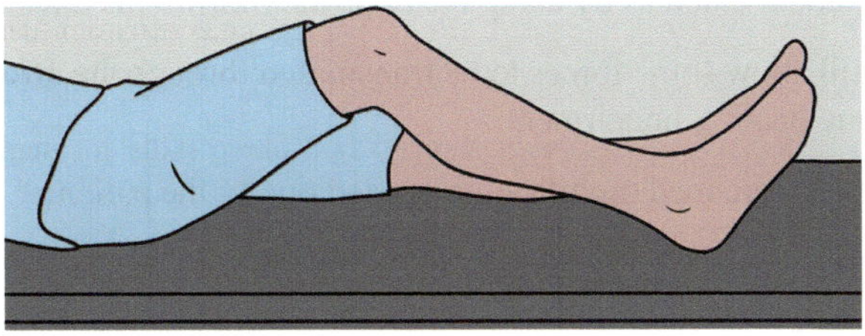

Isometric Hamstring strengthening

- Isotonic
  - Concentric—hamstring curls—laying prone, the patient actively flexes the knee, holds, and returns to initial position slowly

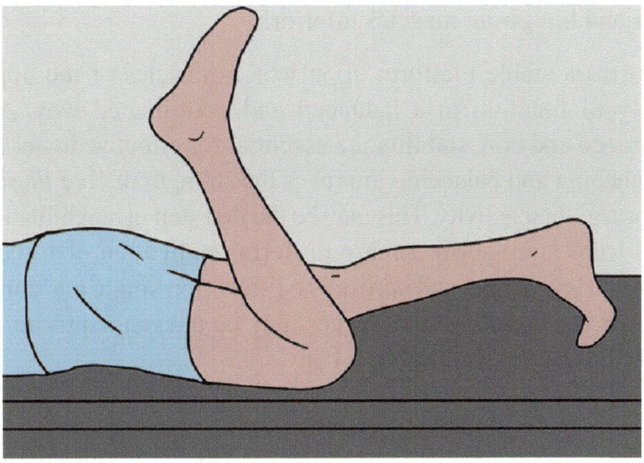

Concentric hamstring strengthening

- Eccentric—laying prone the patient uses a theraband or opposite leg to passively flex the knee, and then slowly controls the descent of the knee (under the influence of gravity) into extension

12.2.3 *Joint Mobilisation*

Joint mobilisation may be achieved by:

Passive motion—carried out by the therapist or patient (such as by using the opposite limb). This aims to:

- Reduce the forces transmitted through the affected knee and limit any disturbance to healing (soft tissue or bony) that such forces may impose.

Active assisted motion—performed partly by the patient, using the protected body part, and partly by assistance. Such assistance may be provided by the therapist or by the patient (such as by using the opposite limb). This aims to:

- Limit but still allow some forces to be transmitted through the affected knee and thus limit any healing impairment.

Active motion—unaided mobilisation carried out by the patient.

12.2.4 Core Strengthening and Balancing

The area around the lumbar spine is known as the core [24–26]. This includes the:

- Abdominal muscles anteriorly
- Paraspinal muscles and gluteus posteriorly
- Diaphragm superiorly
- Pelvic floor and hip girdle muscles inferiorly

The core forms a stable platform upon which muscles of the upper and lower extremities rely to function in a balanced and coordinated way. Adequate core strength, endurance and core stability are essential for effective lower limb function.

Core strengthening and balancing improves the strength of core muscles and facilitates coordination of their activity. This may be the first step in rehabilitation of the knee.

A balanced trunk may allow a more uniform application of forces across both limbs upon double leg stance, and across one limb upon single leg stance. If the core muscles are weak the distribution of forces may be uneven, equivalent to a weightlifter trying to lift unequal weights on a bar.

12.2.5 Soft Tissue Stretching

This refers to application of a force to elongate the soft tissues. Such force may be applied by:

- The therapist—passive manipulation
- The patient—manipulating own limb using the opposite limb or trunk—such as:
  - Using opposite leg to push ipsilateral knee into more flexion
  - Kneeling on a knee using the trunk weight to flex the knee further

Stretching acts on muscles, ligaments and other soft tissues.

- Initial stretching increases the muscle resting length (sarcomere and connective tissue)
- When a muscle is stretched its tone rises initially followed by relaxation; further stretching elongates the ligaments
- Stretching may also elongate or break intra-articular adhesions, or adhesions between soft tissue and bones, enhancing mobility

Hence, in stretching exercises a stretching force is usually applied for about 30 s to allow initial muscle relaxation followed by elongation of static soft tissue structures (ligaments) [27, 28].

12.2.6 Proprioception Training [29–45]

Proprioception is the ability to:

- Sense the positon of the body, joint or body segment in space (joint position sense/limb position sense)
- Sense any joint or body segment movement (kinaesthesia)
- Process at a central level the above sensory inputs to modulate motor output and maintain muscle control

Proprioception is the process that allows one to touch the heel of one foot to the toes of the other, touch a finger to the nose with eyes closed, stand still with eyes shut, or allow an acrobat to walk blindfolded on a tightrope. The brain processes the sensory input in a subconscious way which allows voluntary activity to concentrate on other specific actions. Proprioception is believed to play a role in the ability of muscles to coordinate their contraction to maintain joint stability, and allows body segments to maintain balance. Proprioception allows the body to react in a fast and subconscious way to any sudden changes in the environment. This influences the position or movement of the body or body components to reduce the risk of lower limb or knee injury.

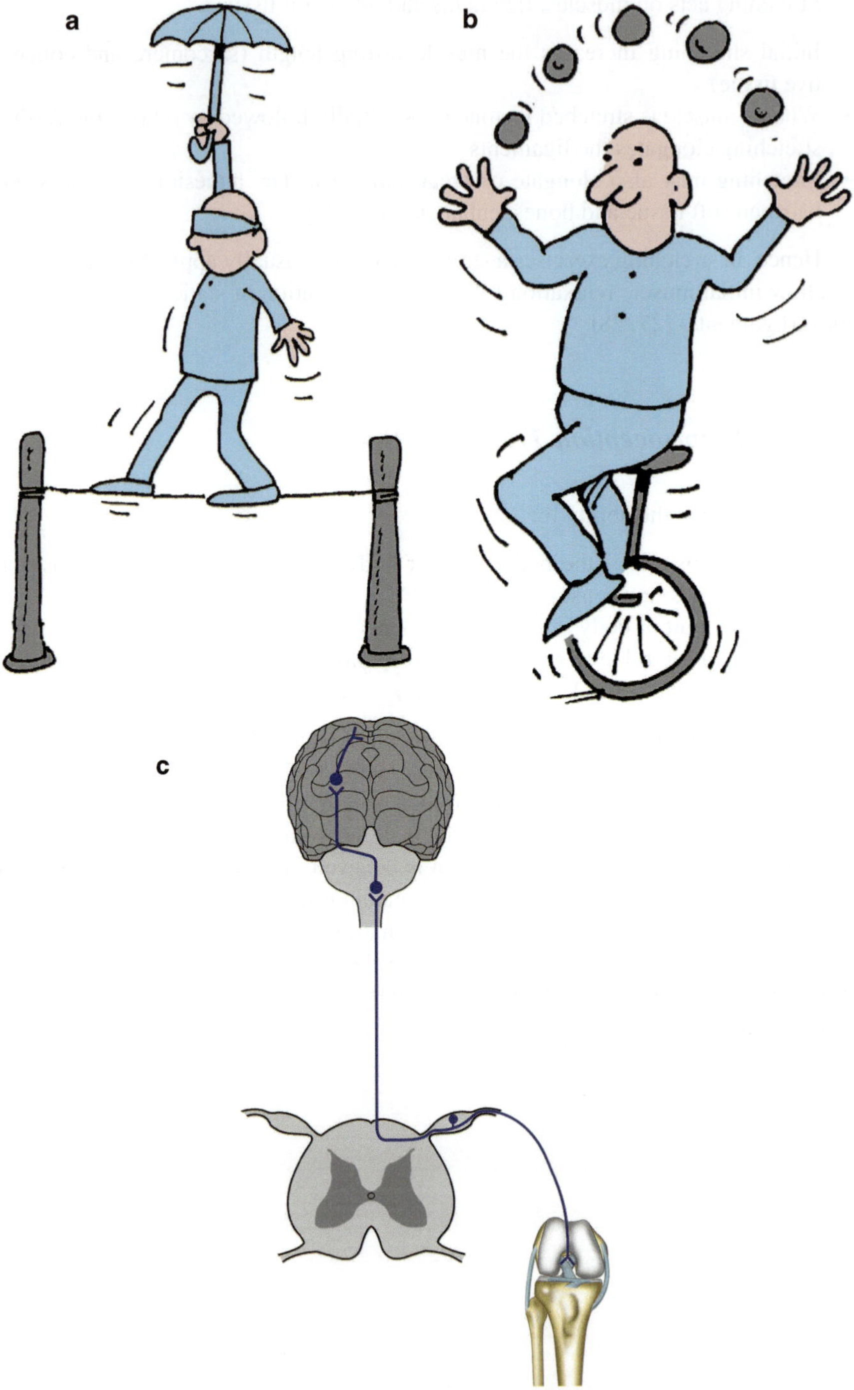

Balancing activities (**a**, **b**) rely on effective proprioception. Sensory pathway for proprioception from mechanoreceptors in the knee ligaments to the central across system (**c**)

Sensory input originates from receptors found in:

- Muscle (muscle spindle)
- Tendons
- Ligaments
- Joint capsule (Golgi body)

From these receptors, sensory fibres pass to the dorsal nerve roots and enter the dorsal horn of the spinal cord. Here they synapse with ascending neurons transmitting impulses to the brain (medulla, thalamus, somatosensory cortex).

Proprioception relies on adequate sensory input. This may be compromised by fatigue and also by ligament injuries. Proprioception may also be impaired in osteoarthritis and in patients with joint hypermobility.

In training for proprioception the following three levels may be considered:

1. Static balance activities
2. Dynamic balance activities
3. Coordination and activity training

Proprioceptive exercises for the knee may be tailored, based on whether the patient aims to achieve open or closed kinetic chain activities. Proprioceptive training exercises include:

- Mirroring movement of the lower extremity—patient tries to match movement of one leg with the other
- Duplicating the position of the lower extremity—one leg is placed in a certain position and the patient tries to put the opposite leg in same position
- Closed chain mobilisation exercises—patient presses on a trampoline ball rather than a rigid surface
- Balancing on a wobble board, exercise ball, trampoline

Proprioception may also be enhanced by the application of a sleeve or splint around the knee or leg that increases the cutaneous sensory input to the central nervous system.

12.2.7 *Biofeedback*

The patient is provided with feedback regarding lower limb or joint positioning, or with regards to muscle contraction, to facilitate muscle activation or to inhibit aberrant muscle activation—feedback may be provided by various means such as electronically on a screen [46–48].

12.2.8 Symptom Modification Techniques

Knee symptom modification techniques involve the application of a series of manual interventions to patients with knee symptoms to assess whether these reduce their symptoms [49, 50].

These interventions are applied whilst the patient carries out the leg or knee leg movement that most closely causes their symptoms. The ability of these procedures to improve symptoms is thus assessed. If a particular procedure does improve clinical symptoms, then it suggests that a rehabilitation programme could be helpful, and exercises that may achieve the same effect as the applied procedure can be utilised in a subsequent rehabilitation programme.

Such facilitation may be achieved by:

- Manual pressure exerted by the examiner
- Taping—to hold a structure (such as the patella) in place
- Placing a block/orthotic under the foot

If these facilitation procedures improve the patient's symptoms, they can form the basis for further physiotherapy exercises.

Knee symptom modification procedures may help reduce pain, improve movement or both and include:

1. Patellar facilitation—aims to influence the position of the patella in relation to the trochlea—if medial patellar gliding achieved by the therapist applying manual pressure during squatting improves the patient's symptoms, then strengthening of the vastus medialis or patellar taping may be employed in further rehabilitation.
2. Hip control facilitation—aims to improve hip control –the patient may try to activate the hip abductors or external rotators against resistance during a squat, and assess whether that improves patellofemoral (PF) pain.
3. Placing a block under the foot to improve foot pronation, to determine whether foot correction influences knee symptoms, and hence, whether foot muscle strengthening or rebalancing might achieve the same effect.

12.3 Physiotherapy to Improve Knee Stability

This may be achieved in several ways depending on the possible deficits including:

- Muscle strengthening to improve dynamic stabilisers
- Muscle rebalancing
- Proprioceptive training
- Core strengthening/balancing
- Pelvic and hip motion coordination
- Calf, ankle and foot strengthening/balancing/stretching

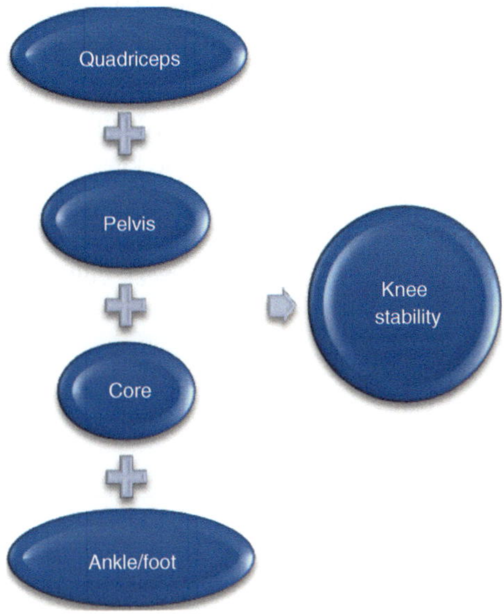

Knee stability may be improved by coordinating the activities of quadriceps, hip and core muscles, as well as the foot and ankle

12.4 Physiotherapy to Reduce Joint Stiffness

In trying to improve mobility of a stiff joint the aim is to:

- Elongate contracted structures
- Relax tense muscles
- Elongate/break down intra-articular adhesions/adhesions between extra-articular soft tissues and bone

  The following therapy principles may be utilised:

- The direction of stiffness is determined (knee flexion/extension/both)
- Specific exercises are applied for each direction in which there is stiffness, to elongate soft tissues
- The patella is mobilised along with stretching the tibiofemoral joint
- Stretching is applied by the patient or therapist
- Pain must be adequately controlled to minimise apprehension, guarding and opposition to the stretching force
- Muscles may be relaxed by:
  - Local massage
  - Chemical means: botulinum toxin injection, parenteral muscle relaxants

12.4.1 Stretching Exercises to Improve Extension

- Patient is seated with the hip flexed 90° and the foot resting on a stool, with no support behind the knee. The effect of gravity helps to stretch the knee into extension. Manual pressure on the front of the knee by the patient or therapist may also be applied.
- Patient lies prone with the thigh supported on the couch, and lower leg hanging freely. The effect of gravity helps to stretch the knee into extension.

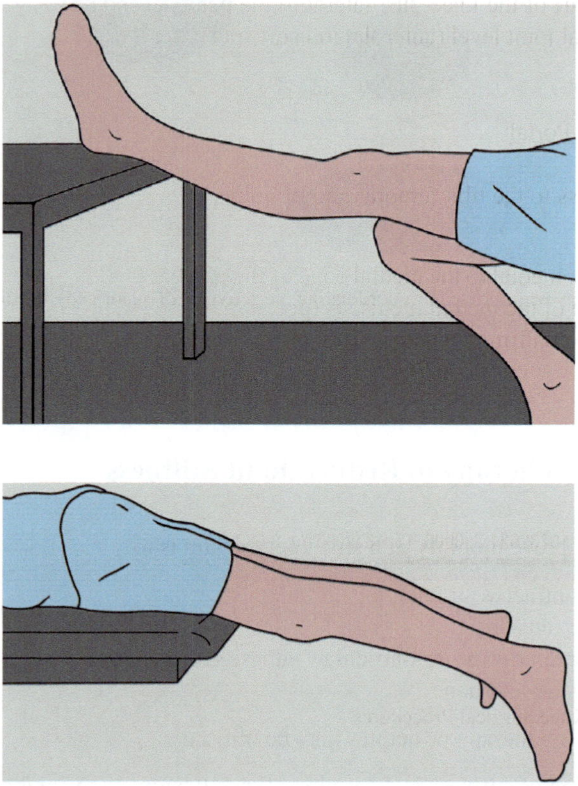

Extension stretching

12.4.2 Stretching Exercises to Improve Flexion

- Patient lies supine and actively flexes the knee. The opposite leg is used to apply a further flexion stretching force. A therapist may also apply a similar stretching force.

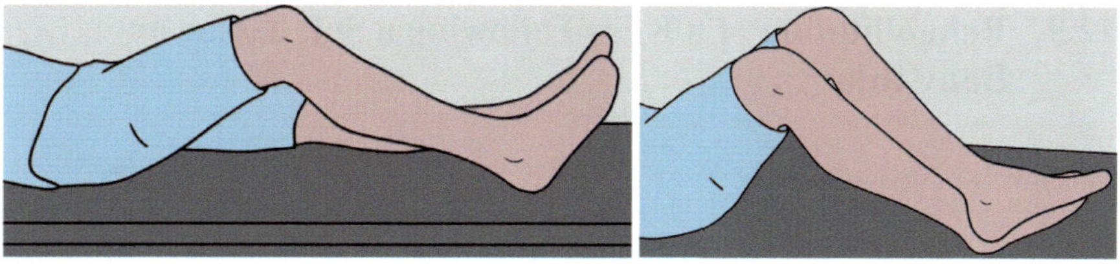

Flexion stretching

- Patient lies prone with the knee flexed. The effect of gravity helps to stretch the knee into further flexion. The opposite leg is used to apply a further flexion stretching force. Alternatively, a theraband is passed around the lower leg and used to apply a flexion stretching force. A therapist may also directly apply a similar stretching force in this position.
- The patient kneels on the lower leg applying a stretching force to the knee

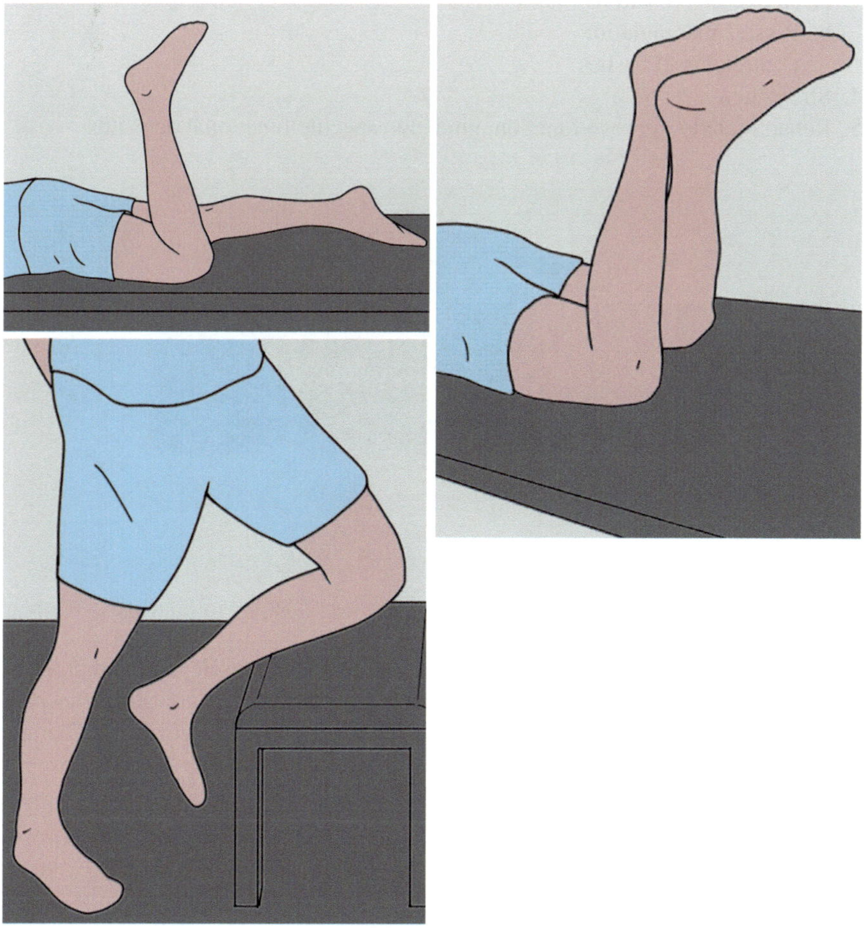

Flexion stretching

12.5 Rehabilitation of a Knee Following a Soft Tissue or Bony Injury

This involves several stages:

1. Rest, control pain, reduce inflammation
2. Protect the site of healing (by limiting motion and loading). This is achieved by utilising one of various levels of mobilisation whilst simultaneously enhancing proprioception and neuromuscular control:
   a. Immobilisation
   b. Passive mobilisation
   c. Active mobilisation
      i. Active assisted
      ii. Active
3. Regain motion
   a. Active mobilisation
   b. Passive manipulation
      i. Stretch soft tissues
4. Strengthen
5. Rehabilitate to improve function, guided to specific functional demands

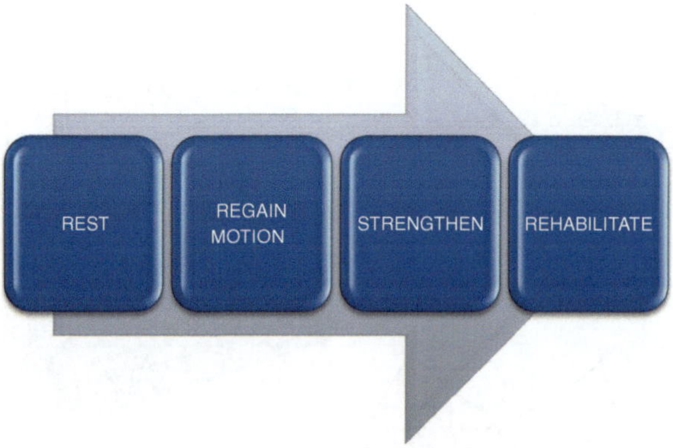

Steps in rehabilitating the knee following a soft tissue or bony injury

Throughout all stages, an attempt is made to maintain muscle bulk and proprioception. Any exercises applied should avoid substantially aggravating the pain which may inhibit motion and have a counterproductive effect on recovery. Therapy aims to avoid or break this vicious cycle. Hence, initially gentle exercises or exercises performed in a particular knee position (such as slight flexion) are prescribed, which are gradually increased guided by pain.

The protection period gives time for the injured site to heal, which for bone to bone is about 6–12 weeks and tendon or ligament to bone about 8–12 weeks [51, 52].

This protection period is followed by mobilisation to regain active motion, eliminate stiffness, and strengthen. This is followed by rehabilitation that aims to return the knee and patient to a desirable and achievable functional level. In this phase, goal orientated tasks and specific functional patterns of activity are introduced, which resemble the activities that the individual is likely to face in real life. Finally, the patient is exposed to real life training.

12.6 Rehabilitation Post-Surgical Soft Tissue or Bony Repair

The approach to rehabilitation may similarly be described in five stages following surgical repair:

1. Control pain and reduce inflammation
2. Protect the repair by limiting motion and loading. This is achieved by utilising various levels of mobilisation whilst simultaneously enhancing proprioception and neuromuscular control.
   a. Immobilisation
   b. Passive mobilisation
   c. Active mobilisation—in a controlled way to avoid uneven force application across the knee, avoid abnormal translation of one articular surface over another and hence abnormal forces on a repair or on reconstructed soft tissue
      i. Active assisted
      ii. Active
3. Regain motion
   a. Active mobilisation
   b. Passive manipulation
      i. Stretch soft tissues
4. Strengthen
5. Rehabilitate to improve function, guided to specific functional demands

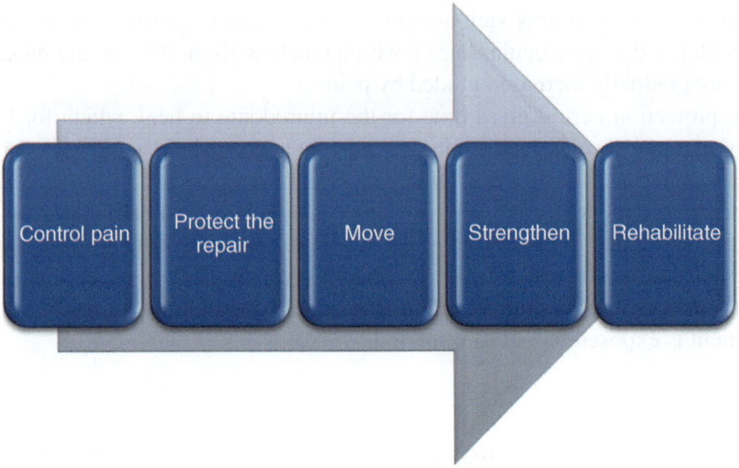

Steps in rehabilitating the knee following a soft tissue or bony surgical repair

12.7 Early vs. Delayed Mobilisation and Loading in Soft Tissue Injuries or Surgery

Following a:

- Soft tissue or bony injury of the knee where natural repair is taking place
- Soft tissue or bony surgical repair of the knee or reconstruction with a graft

the amount of mobilisation and loading of the area under consideration may be limited until adequate healing has taken place.

There is concern that excessive mobilisation or excessive loads may lead to:

- Gap formation or translation between the apposed tissues at the injured or repaired site (such as soft tissue on a bony surface or a soft tissue graft in a bone tunnel)
- Dysfunction or failure of the repair
- Stretching of a newly applied graft which has yet to mature

It has been shown that in tendon tears [53–60]:

- Delayed mobilisation may lead to higher strength than early mobilisation
- Low level loading may lead to higher strength than complete unloading

- Tendon cells (fibroblasts) are capable of mechanotransduction—they can respond to force application by altering collagen, extracellular matrix and growth factor production. Mechanical loading can thus alter tissue biology.
- Forces applied along the line of tendon action may enhance optimal collagen fibre alignment and maturation.

Early mobilisation is usually preferable to avoid or minimise stiffness due to:

- Contracture of soft tissues
- Formation of intra-articular or peri-articular adhesions

There is evidence that although early mobilisation following tendon or ligamentous injuries and surgery may speed recovery at early follow up post-injury or post-surgery, at longer follow up (one year or longer) the amount of stiffness and functional outcomes may not differ between early and delayed mobilisation groups [61, 62].

The above suggest that:

- An initial period of absolute immobilisation or unloading may not be essential
- Early mobilisation may be:
  - Performed with passive or active assisted exercises
  - Allowed in a range that does not unduly load the injured or repaired site. In surgical repairs this “safe “range of motion may be determined intraoperatively and communicated to the therapist (such as how much knee flexion is possible before applying too much tension on a repaired quadriceps tendon tear)
- Early loading may be applied using:
  - Isometric exercises
- Mobilisation and loading may be guided by:
  - The possibility of compromising a natural or surgical repair site
  - The strength of a surgical repair and need to offload such repair

rather than by an arbitrary push to achieve early mobilisation.

12.8 Rehabilitation of Articular Cartilage Injuries/Repair

A special situation in knee physiotherapy is rehabilitation of articular cartilage. This may be following articular cartilage repair or resurfacing, or following articular cartilage injuries (isolate chondral or intra-articular fractures) [63]. The aim is to allow early mobilisation.

The approach to rehabilitation may similarly be described in five stages:

1. Control pain, reduce inflammation
2. Protect the damaged or repaired area by limiting loading and motion to control compressive and shear forces whilst simultaneously enhancing proprioception and neuromuscular control

   This is achieved by utilising various levels of mobilisation:

   a. Immobilisation
   b. Passive mobilisation (for the patella—the patient or therapist holds the patella and moves it side to side and proximal to distal)
   c. Active mobilisation—in a controlled, balanced way
      i. Active assisted
      ii. Active

3. Regain motion

   d. Active mobilisation
   e. Passive manipulation
      i. Stretch soft tissues

4. Strengthen
5. Rehabilitate to improve function, guided to specific functional demands

Early mobilisation is warranted is articular injuries due to the deleterious effects that immobilisation may have on articular cartilage (softening, degeneration, matrix disruption, chondrocyte apoptosis) [64–67].

The range of motion may be such as to limit excessive forces on the part of the articular cartilage involved (such as limit knee flexion to 30° in patellar chondral injuries).

Aquatic exercises and cycling minimise compressive loads at the tibiofemoral articulation but may provide stimulus for healing, hence they have a role to play in articular cartilage rehabilitation.

12.9 Milestones of Rehabilitation [68, 69]

In knee rehabilitation the following factors need consideration and communication to the therapist:

- Range of allowed motion (whilst considering its effects on the tibiofemoral and PF articulations)
- Planes of allowed motion—straight, turning/twisting
- Level of weightbearing
- Closed vs. open chain strengthening
- Generic vs. task specific activities
- Non-contact vs. contact activities

12.9.1 *Weightbearing*

- Weightbearing is gradually increased to the level required for functional activities

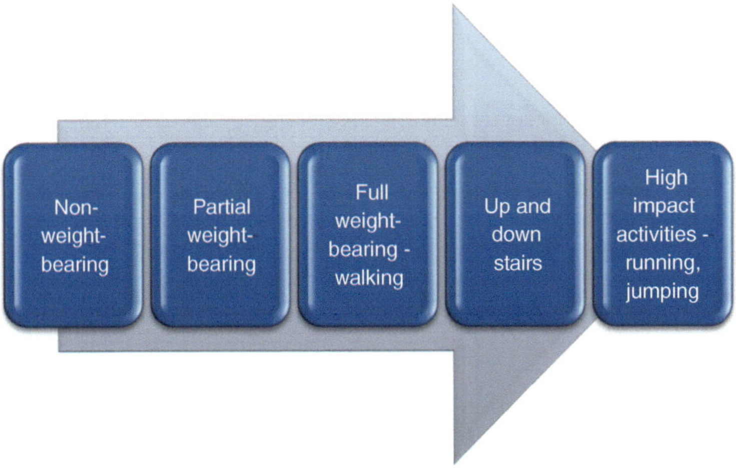

Milestones of weight bearing

12.9.2 *Progressing in Activity*

- When deciding when to progress to a more active level of rehabilitation, it is necessary to consider what is happening to the injured, repaired, or reconstructed site, and whether it needs to be protected. However, it is also essential to consider the overall improvement of the knee, core, rest of lower limb as well as the patient overall (cardiorespiratory state, apprehension, confidence). Some of the knee factors that may guide progression to the next level include:
- Painless knee range of motion
- Absent or minimal effusion
- Adequate knee muscle strength
- Adequate knee control

12.10 Arthrogenic Muscle Inhibition

This describes inhibition of voluntary activation of quadriceps leading to weakness along with atrophy of the muscle [70–78]. This is observed following injury or surgery to the knee and is also encountered in degenerative or inflammatory conditions of the knee. Quadriceps wasting can appear dramatic.

Such inhibition may:

1. Persist for a long time (even years) following the cessation of the event leading to its onset
2. Occur secondary to intra- or extra-articular pathology

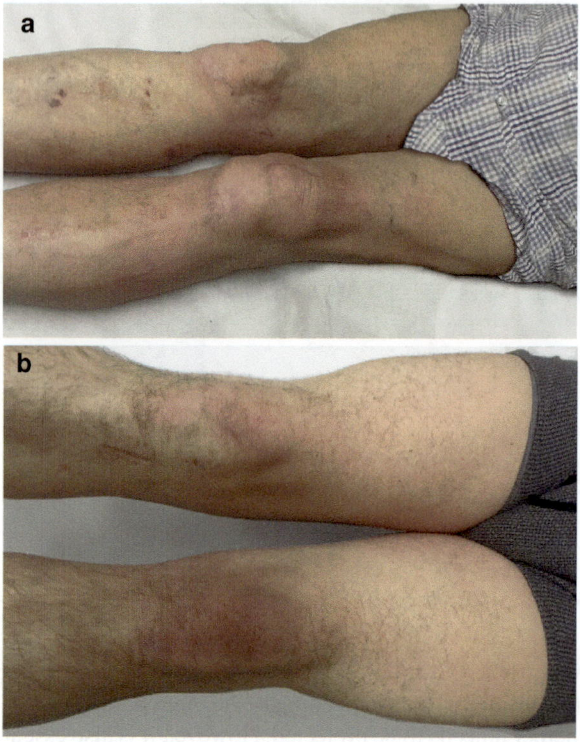

Quadriceps wasting associated with knee arthritis (**a**) and following ACL reconstruction (**b**)

Its pathogenesis is not fully defined but it has been suggested that afferent sensory signals from the knee (from pain receptors, inflammation receptors or mechanoreceptors) may lead to inhibition of spinal motor neurones innervating the quadriceps. Modulation of the frontal motor cortex and corticospinal tracts has also been proposed. Such neural changes result into decreased activation output for the knee extensor muscles. Hence, the following have been suggested as potential causes:

- Knee pain
- Knee inflammation
- Knee effusion—causing stretching of the capsule
- Tight suturing of the knee capsule following surgery

Following an injury, inhibition of voluntary quadriceps activation may act as a protective mechanism to prevent further injury. However, it may become a chronic issue if uncontrolled.

In a substantial proportion of patients it involves the ipsilateral (to a knee insult) quadriceps, but also the contralateral quadriceps. It may also affect the hamstring tendons.

12.10.1 Investigations

- MRI lumbosacral spine to exclude a more proximal neurological cause
- Nerve conduction studies/Electromyography (EMG) to exclude a neurological cause

12.10.2 Management

Several modalities have been described including:

- Recognising and explaining to the patient the problem—reassuring of the lack of a sinister underlying neurological condition
- Reducing sensory input that may facilitate quadriceps inhibition—control pain, minimise knee effusion
- Physiotherapy—restoring voluntary quadriceps activation (through disinhibition) is the first step in improving quadriceps strength. This may be achieved with:
  - Cryotherapy
  - TENS
  - Quadriceps strengthening exercises– both in flexion and extension

TENS applies low intensity stimulus to target sensory nerve fibres, to influence the presynaptic reflex inhibitory mechanism that leads to quadriceps dysfunction.

Learning Pearls

- Communication between surgeon and therapist is essential for mutual understanding as to what therapy aims to achieve, and the extent or pace at which therapy is applied.
- Pain control is essential in allowing patients to perform physiotherapy. Pain control should be an initial and integral part of therapy. Central as well as peripheral pain processing must be considered. Pharmacological and psychological input may be needed in controlling chronic knee pain.

- Closed chain exercises following ACL reconstruction allow synergistic contraction between the quadriceps and hamstring muscles. This helps to provide an even application of forces across the knee, avoiding abnormal translation of the tibia in relation to the femur, and hence minimising abnormal forces on a newly reconstructed graft. In contrast, open chain exercises of the quadriceps may apply excessive and unopposed anterior translation forces on the tibia in relation to the femur, and may stretch a newly reconstructed ACL.
- Renstrom et al. [79] showed that isometric hamstring activity in isolation reduces the ACL strain, hence isometric hamstring exercises can be initiated early following ACL reconstruction. Quadriceps activation increased the ACL strain between 0 and 45° of flexion.
- Torry et al. [80] showed that different patterns of adaptive gait may exist in the ACL deficient knee. In their study, some patients exhibited a hip strategy with increased hip extensor output and decreased knee extensor output, which allowed normal knee kinematics. Some patients demonstrated a knee strategy which resulted in increased knee stiffness and used a flexed knee gait. Shabani et al. [81] showed that ACL deficient knees show a higher flexion gait during stance and excessive internal tibial rotation during walking as an adaptation to prevent excessive anterior tibial translation. They suggested that ACL deficient knees may adopt to prevent excessive anteroposterior translation, but not rotational instability.
- Escamilla et al. [82] assessed knee forces and muscle activity in closed chain (squat and leg press) and open chain (knee extension) exercises. Overall, the squat generated approximately twice as much hamstring activity as the leg press and knee extension. Quadriceps muscle activity was greatest in open chain when the knee was near full extension. Tension in the ACL was present only in open chain exercises, and occurred near full extension. PF compressive force was greatest in closed chain near full flexion and in the midrange of the knee during open chain extension.
- Stensdotter et al. [83] examined whether the components of the quadriceps muscle are activated differently in open versus closed chain tasks. In closed chain knee extension, the onset of EMG activity of the four different muscle components of the quadriceps was more simultaneous than in the open chain. In open chain, rectus femoris had the earliest EMG onset whilst vastus medialis obliquus was activated last and with smaller amplitude as compared to closed chain. They suggested that closed chain exercises promote more balanced initial quadriceps activation than open chain exercises. This may be of importance in choosing training exercises for improving PF joint control.

References

1. Uhl TL, Muir TA, Lawson L. Electromyographical assessment of passive, active assistive, and active shoulder rehabilitation exercises. PM R. 2010;2(2):132–41.
2. Gowitzke BA, Milner M. Scientific bases of human movement. Baltimore, MD: Williams and Wilkins; 1988.
3. Padulo J, Laffaye G, Chamari K, Concu A. Concentric and eccentric: muscle contraction or exercise? Sports Health. 2013;5(4):306. https://doi.org/10.1177/1941738113491386.
4. Perriman A, Leahy E, Semciw AI. The effect of open- versus closed-kinetic-chain exercises on anterior tibial laxity, strength, and function following anterior cruciate ligament reconstruction: a systematic review and meta-analysis. J Orthop Sports Phys Ther. 2018;48(7):552–66.
5. Jewiss D, Ostman C, Smart N. Open versus Closed Kinetic Chain Exercises following an Anterior Cruciate Ligament Reconstruction: A Systematic Review and Meta-Analysis. J Sports Med (Hindawi Publ Corp). 2017;(2017):4721548.
6. Witvrouw E, Danneels L, Van Tiggelen D, Willems TM, Cambier D. Open versus closed kinetic chain exercises in patellofemoral pain: a 5-year prospective randomized study. Am J Sports Med. 2004;32(5):1122–30.
7. Kvist J, Gillquist J. Sagittal plane knee translation and electromyographic activity during closed and open kinetic chain exercises in anterior cruciate ligament-deficient patients and control subjects. Am J Sports Med. 2001;29(1):72–82.
8. Wilk KE, Escamilla RF, Fleisig GS, Barrentine SW, Andrews JR, Boyd ML. A comparison of tibiofemoral joint forces and electromyographic activity during open and closed kinetic chain exercises. Am J Sports Med. 1996;24(4):518–27.
9. Witvrouw E, Lysens R, Bellemans J, Peers K, Vanderstraeten G. Open versus closed kinetic chain exercises for patellofemoral pain. A prospective, randomized study. Am J Sports Med. 2000;28(5):687–94.
10. Bynum EB, Barrack RL, Alexander AH. Open versus closed chain kinetic exercises after anterior cruciate ligament reconstruction. A prospective randomized study. Am J Sports Med. 1995;23(4):401–6.
11. Yack HJ, Collins CE, Whieldon TJ. Comparison of closed and open kinetic chain exercise in the anterior cruciate ligament-deficient knee. Am J Sports Med. 1993;21(1):49–54.
12. Melzack R, Wall PD. Pain mechanisms: a new theory. Science. 1965;150(3699):971–9.
13. Katz J, Rosenbloom BN. The golden anniversary of Melzack and Wall's gate control theory of pain: Celebrating 50 years of pain research and management. Pain Res Manag. 2015;20(6):285–6.
14. Sluka KA, Walsh D. Transcutaneous electrical nerve stimulation: basic science mechanisms and clinical effectiveness. J Pain. 2003;4(3):109–21.
15. Rawe IM. The case for over-the-counter shortwave therapy: safe and effective devices for pain management. Pain Manag. 2014;4(1):37–43.
16. Goats GC. Pulsed electromagnetic (short-wave) energy therapy. Br J Sports Med. 1989;23(4):213–6.
17. Ondrejkovicova A, Petrovics G, Svitkova K, Bajtekova B, Bangha O. Why acupuncture in pain treatment? Neuro Endocrinol Lett. 2016;37(3):163–8.
18. Guelich DR, Xu D, Koh JL, Nuber GW, Zhang LQ. Different roles of the medial and lateral hamstrings in unloading the anterior cruciate ligament. Knee. 2016;23(1):97–101.
19. Tibone JE, Antich TJ. Electromyographic analysis of the anterior cruciate ligament-deficient knee. Clin Orthop Relat Res. 1993;288:35–9.
20. Liu W, Maitland ME. The effect of hamstring muscle compensation for anterior laxity in the ACL-deficient knee during gait. J Biomech. 2000;33(7):871–9.
21. Boerboom AL, Hof AL, Halbertsma JP, van Raaij JJ, Schenk W, Diercks RL, van Horn JR. Atypical hamstrings electromyographic activity as a compensatory mechanism in anterior cruciate ligament deficiency. Knee Surg Sports Traumatol Arthrosc. 2001;9(4):211–6.

22. Tsepis E, Vagenas G, Giakas G, Georgoulis A. Hamstring weakness as an indicator of poor knee function in ACL-deficient patients. Knee Surg Sports Traumatol Arthrosc. 2004;12(1):22–9.
23. Shiavi R, Limbird T, Borra H, Edmondstone MA. Electromyography profiles of knee joint musculature during pivoting: changes induced by anterior cruciate ligament deficiency. J Electromyogr Kinesiol. 1991;1(1):49–57.
24. Huxel Bliven KC, Anderson BE. Core stability training for injury prevention. Sports Health. 2013;5(6):514–22.
25. Willson JD, Dougherty CP, Ireland ML, Davis IM. Core stability and its relationship to lower extremity function and injury. J Am Acad Orthop Surg. 2005;13(5):316–25.
26. Kibler WB, Press J, Sciascia A. The role of core stability in athletic function. Sports Med. 2006;36(3):189–98.
27. Magnusson SP. Passive properties of human skeletal muscle during stretch maneuvers. A review. Scand J Med Sci Sports. 1998;8(2):65–77.
28. Bandy WD, Irion JM. The effect of time on static stretch on the flexibility of the hamstring muscles. Phys Ther. 1994;74(9):845–50.
29. Jerosch J, Prymka M. Proprioception and joint stability. Knee Surg Sports Traumatol Arthrosc. 1996;4(3):171–9.
30. Hogervorst T, Brand RA. Mechanoreceptors in joint function. J Bone Joint Surg Am. 1998;80(9):1365–78.
31. Johansson H, Sjölander P, Sojka P. A sensory role for the cruciate ligaments. Clin Orthop Relat Res. 1991;268:161–78.
32. Johansson H. Role of knee ligaments in proprioception and regulation of muscle stiffness. J Electromyogr Kinesiol. 1991;1(3):158–79.
33. Lattanzio PJ, Petrella RJ. Knee proprioception: a review of mechanisms, measurements, and implications of muscular fatigue. Orthopedics. 1998;21(4):463–70.
34. Jeong HS, Lee SC, Jee H, Song JB, Chang HS, Lee SY. Proprioceptive training and outcomes of patients with knee osteoarthritis: a meta-analysis of randomized controlled trials. J Athl Train. 2019;54(4):418–28.
35. Dargo L, Robinson KJ, Games KE. Prevention of Knee and Anterior Cruciate Ligament Injuries Through the Use of Neuromuscular and Proprioceptive Training: An Evidence-Based Review. J Athl Train. 2017;52(12):1171–2.
36. Relph N, Herrington L, Tyson S. The effects of ACL injury on knee proprioception: a meta-analysis. Physiotherapy. 2014;100(3):187–95.
37. Hewett TE, Paterno MV, Myer GD. Strategies for enhancing proprioception and neuromuscular control of the knee. Clin Orthop Relat Res. 2002;402:76–94.
38. Ageberg E. Consequences of a ligament injury on neuromuscular function and relevance to rehabilitation—using the anterior cruciate ligament-injured knee as model. J Electromyogr Kinesiol. 2002;12(3):205–12.
39. Hiemstra LA, Lo IK, Fowler PJ. Effect of fatigue on knee proprioception: implications for dynamic stabilization. J Orthop Sports Phys Ther. 2001;31(10):598–605.
40. Smith TO, Jerman E, Easton V, Bacon H, Armon K, Poland F, Macgregor AJ. Do people with benign joint hypermobility syndrome (BJHS) have reduced joint proprioception? A systematic review and meta-analysis. Rheumatol Int. 2013;33(11):2709–16.
41. Caraffa A, Cerulli G, Projetti M, Aisa G, Rizzo A. Prevention of anterior cruciate ligament injuries in soccer. A prospective controlled study of proprioceptive training. Knee Surg Sports Traumatol Arthrosc. 1996;4(1):19–21.
42. Silva PB, Mrachacz-Kersting N, Oliveira AS, Kersting UG. Effect of wobble board training on movement strategies to maintain equilibrium on unstable surfaces. Hum Mov Sci. 2018;58:231–8.
43. Birmingham TB, Kramer JF, Inglis JT, Mooney CA, Murray LJ, Fowler PJ, Kirkley S. Effect of a neoprene sleeve on knee joint position sense during sitting open kinetic chain and supine closed kinetic chain tests. Am J Sports Med. 1998;26(4):562–6.
44. Beynnon BD, Good L, Risberg MA. The effect of bracing on proprioception of knees with anterior cruciate ligament injury. J Orthop Sports Phys Ther. 2002;32(1):11–5.

45. Wu GK, Ng GY, Mak AF. Effects of knee bracing on the sensorimotor function of subjects with anterior cruciate ligament reconstruction. Am J Sports Med. 2001;29(5):641–5.
46. Marshall AN, Hertel J, Hart JM, Russell S, Saliba SA. Visual biofeedback and changes in lower extremity kinematics in individuals with medial knee displacement. J Athl Train. 2020; https://doi.org/10.4085/1062-6050-383-18.
47. Christanell F, Hoser C, Huber R, Fink C, Luomajoki H. The influence of electromyographic biofeedback therapy on knee extension following anterior cruciate ligament reconstruction: a randomized controlled trial. Sports Med Arthrosc Rehabil Ther Technol. 2012;4(1):41. https://doi.org/10.1186/1758-2555-4-41.
48. Teran-Yengle P, Birkhofer R, Weber MA, Patton K, Thatcher E, Yack HJ. Efficacy of gait training with real-time biofeedback in correcting knee hyperextension patterns in young women. J Orthop Sports Phys Ther. 2011;41(12):948–52.
49. Chaconas E, Gray S, Kempfert D. Mobilization with movement symptom modification procedure for a 38 year old male with patella femoral pain syndrome. Man Ther. 2016;25:e63–4. https://doi.org/10.1016/j.math.2016.05.096.
50. Lehman GJ. The role and value of symptom-modification approaches in musculoskeletal practice. J Orthop Sports Phys Ther. 2018;48(6):430–5.
51. Rodeo SA, Arnoczky SP, Torzilli PA, Hidaka C, Warren RF. Tendon-healing in a bone tunnel. A biomechanical and histological study in the dog. J Bone Joint Surg Am. 1993;75(12): 1795–803.
52. St Pierre P, Olson EJ, Elliott JJ, O'Hair KC, McKinney LA, Ryan J. Tendon-healing to cortical bone compared with healing to a cancellous trough. A biomechanical and histological evaluation in goats. J Bone Joint Surg Am. 1995;77(12):1858–66.
53. Lee BG, Cho NS, Rhee YG. Effect of two rehabilitation protocols on range of motion and healing rates after arthroscopic rotator cuff repair: aggressive versus limited early passive exercises. Arthroscopy. 2012;28(1):34–42.
54. Eliasson P, Andersson T, Aspenberg P. Achilles tendon healing in rats is improved by intermittent mechanical loading during the inflammatory phase. J Orthop Res. 2012;30(2):274–9.
55. Eliasson P, Andersson T, Aspenberg P. Rat Achilles tendon healing: mechanical loading and gene expression. J Appl Physiol (1985). 2009;107(2):399–407.
56. Andersson T, Eliasson P, Aspenberg P. Tissue memory in healing tendons: short loading episodes stimulate healing. J Appl Physiol (1985). 2009;107(2):417–21.
57. Hettrich CM, Gasinu S, Beamer BS, Stasiak M, Fox A, Birmingham P, Ying O, Deng XH, Rodeo SA. The effect of mechanical load on tendon-to-bone healing in a rat model. Am J Sports Med. 2014;42(5):1233–41.
58. Killian ML, Cavinatto L, Galatz LM, Thomopoulos S. The role of mechanobiology in tendon healing. J Shoulder Elb Surg. 2012;21(2):228–37.
59. Galatz LM, Charlton N, Das R, Kim HM, Havlioglu N, Thomopoulos S. Complete removal of load is detrimental to rotator cuff healing. J Shoulder Elb Surg. 2009;18(5):669–75.
60. Galloway MT, Lalley AL, Shearn JT. The role of mechanical loading in tendon development, maintenance, injury, and repair. J Bone Joint Surg Am. 2013;95(17):1620–8.
61. Serino J, Mohamadi A, Orman S, McCormick B, Hanna P, Weaver MJ, Harris MB, Nazarian A, von Keudell A. Comparison of adverse events and postoperative mobilization following knee extensor mechanism rupture repair: a systematic review and network meta-analysis. Injury. 2017;48(12):2793–9.
62. Langenhan R, Baumann M, Ricart P, Hak D, Probst A, Badke A, Trobisch P. ostoperative functional rehabilitation after repair of quadriceps tendon ruptures: a comparison of two different protocols. Knee Surg Sports Traumatol Arthrosc. 2012;20(11):2275–8.
63. Irrgang JJ, Pezzullo D. Rehabilitation following surgical procedures to address articular cartilage lesions in the knee. J Orthop Sports Phys Ther. 1998;28(4):232–40.
64. Hagiwara Y, Ando A, Chimoto E, Saijo Y, Ohmori-Matsuda K, Itoi E. Changes of articular cartilage after immobilization in a rat knee contracture model. J Orthop Res. 2009;27(2):236–42.
65. Hall MC. Articular changes in the knee of the adult rat after prolonged immobilization in extension. Clin Orthop Relat Res. 1964;34:184–95.

66. Troyer H. The effect of short-term immobilization on the rabbit knee joint cartilage. A histochemical study. Clin Orthop Relat Res. 1975;107:249–57.
67. Mutsuzaki H, Nakajima H, Wadano Y, Furuhata S, Sakane M. Influence of knee immobilization on chondrocyte apoptosis and histological features of the anterior cruciate ligament insertion and articular cartilage in rabbits. Int J Mol Sci. 2017;18(2):pii: E253. https://doi.org/10.3390/ijms18020253.
68. Wilk KE, Briem K, Reinold MM, Devine KM, Dugas J, Andrews JR. Rehabilitation of articular lesions in the athlete's knee. J Orthop Sports Phys Ther. 2006;36(10):815–27.
69. Mithoefer K, Hambly K, Logerstedt D, Ricci M, Silvers H, Della VS. Current concepts for rehabilitation and return to sport after knee articular cartilage repair in the athlete. J Orthop Sports Phys Ther. 2012;42(3):254–73. milestones rehabilitation knee
70. Sonnery-Cottet B, Saithna A, Quelard B, Daggett M, Borade A, Ouanezar H, Thaunat M, Blakeney WG. Arthrogenic muscle inhibition after ACL reconstruction: a scoping review of the efficacy of interventions. Br J Sports Med. 2019;53(5):289–98.
71. Hart JM, Kuenze CM, Diduch DR, Ingersoll CD. Quadriceps muscle function after rehabilitation with cryotherapy in patients with anterior cruciate ligament reconstruction. J Athl Train. 2014;49(6):733–9.
72. Harkey MS, Gribble PA, Pietrosimone BG. Disinhibitory interventions and voluntary quadriceps activation: a systematic review. J Athl Train. 2014;49(3):411–21.
73. Rice DA, McNair PJ. Quadriceps arthrogenic muscle inhibition: neural mechanisms and treatment perspectives. Semin Arthritis Rheum. 2010;40(3):250–66.
74. Palmieri-Smith RM, Kreinbrink J, Ashton-Miller JA, Wojtys EM. Quadriceps inhibition induced by an experimental knee joint effusion affects knee joint mechanics during a single-legged drop landing. Am J Sports Med. 2007;35(8):1269–75.
75. Palmieri RM, Tom JA, Edwards JE, Weltman A, Saliba EN, Mistry DJ, Ingersoll CD. Arthrogenic muscle response induced by an experimental knee joint effusion is mediated by pre- and post-synaptic spinal mechanisms. J Electromyogr Kinesiol. 2004;14(6):631–40.
76. Hopkins J, Ingersoll CD, Edwards J, Klootwyk TE. Cryotherapy and Transcutaneous Electric Neuromuscular Stimulation Decrease Arthrogenic Muscle Inhibition of the Vastus Medialis After Knee Joint Effusion. J Athl Train. 2002;37(1):25–31.
77. Hurley MV, Jones DW, Newham DJ. Arthrogenic quadriceps inhibition and rehabilitation of patients with extensive traumatic knee injuries. Clin Sci (Lond). 1994;86(3):305–10.
78. Gabler C, Kitzman PH, Mattacola CG. Targeting quadriceps inhibition with electromyographic biofeedback: a neuroplastic approach. Crit Rev Biomed Eng. 2013;41(2):125–35.
79. Renström P, Arms SW, Stanwyck TS, Johnson RJ, Pope MH. Strain within the anterior cruciate ligament during hamstring and quadriceps activity. Am J Sports Med. 1986;14(1):83–7.
80. Torry MR, Decker MJ, Ellis HB, Shelburne KB, Sterett WI, Steadman JR. Mechanisms of compensating for anterior cruciate ligament deficiency during gait. Med Sci Sports Exerc. 2004;36(8):1403–12.
81. Shabani B, Bytyqi D, Lustig S, Cheze L, Bytyqi C, Neyret P. Gait changes of the ACL-deficient knee 3D kinematic assessment. Knee Surg Sports Traumatol Arthrosc. 2015;23(11):3259–65.
82. Escamilla RF, Fleisig GS, Zheng N, Barrentine SW, Wilk KE, Andrews JR. Biomechanics of the knee during closed kinetic chain and open kinetic chain exercises. Med Sci Sports Exerc. 1998;30(4):556–69.
83. Stensdotter AK, Hodges PW, Mellor R, Sundelin G, Häger-Ross C. Quadriceps activation in closed and in open kinetic chain exercise. Med Sci Sports Exerc. 2003;35(12):2043–7.

Chapter 13
Knee Pain

Pain may be considered the commonest symptom patients present with. Pain may be an isolated complaint, or present along with other symptoms (including weakness, swelling, locking, paraesthesia, stiffness or instability).

This chapter discusses some of the potential sources of knee pain and gives guidance as to the principles used in identifying the origin of pain. These include, amongst others, pain's location, nature, onset, and clinical examination findings. Furthermore, this chapter describes the principles of investigating and managing the painful knee.

Pain is a clinical symptom which often responds to treatment in a non-predictable way (unlike stiffness or mechanical symptoms). This is because the underlying cause, mediation, perception of pain, and peripheral, as well as central reaction to pain may be difficult to fully characterise at an individual level.

13.1 Sources of Knee Pain

Several sources of knee pain are recognised [1–18]. These are described according to the anatomical structure or area giving rise to pain. These sources of pain are presented below:

C. Panayiotou Charalambous, *The Knee Made Easy*,
https://doi.org/10.1007/978-3-030-54506-2_13

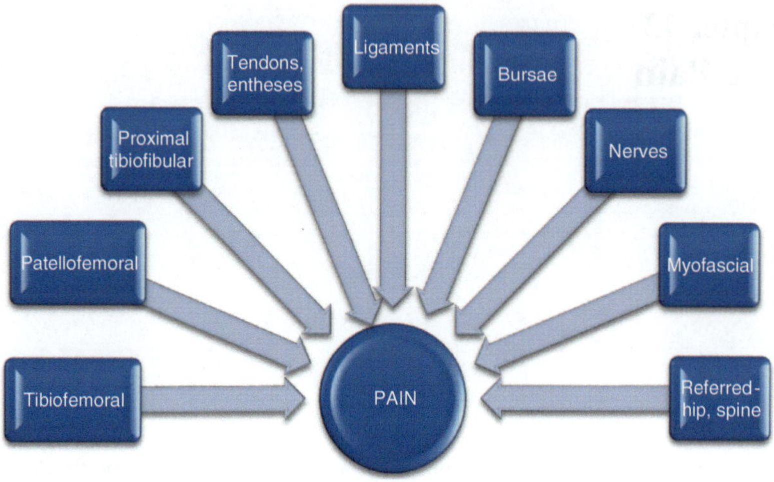

Potential sources of knee pain

13.1.1 Tibiofemoral Joint Pain

This is deep seated pain, felt within the knee joint. It may be diffuse in cases of arthritis or specifically localised (such as to the posteromedial or posterolateral part of the joint) in meniscal tears.

Causes of tibiofemoral joint pain include:

- Arthritis
- Osteonecrosis
- Chondral dysfunction
- Meniscal dysfunction, degeneration or tears
- Fat pad dysfunction
- Synovial dysfunction
- Instability
- Intermittent mechanical block

Pain due to degenerative or inflammatory causes may be diffuse, constant and dull in nature, aggravated by knee motion and by loading the tibiofemoral joint.

Pain due to a meniscal tear in the absence of other knee degeneration tends to be well localised with the patient being able to point with a finger to the painful area. It may be worsened by rotating or twisting the leg, hypeflexing the knee, or by straightening the knee from a hyperflexed position. It may be accompanied by clicking.

Pain due to knee instability may be constant, vague, dull or burning. Alternatively, it may be intermittent, sharp pain, associated with episodes of subluxation of the joint.

Sudden, diffuse, sharp pain may also be due to mechanical locking such as due to an unstable meniscal tear or loose body.

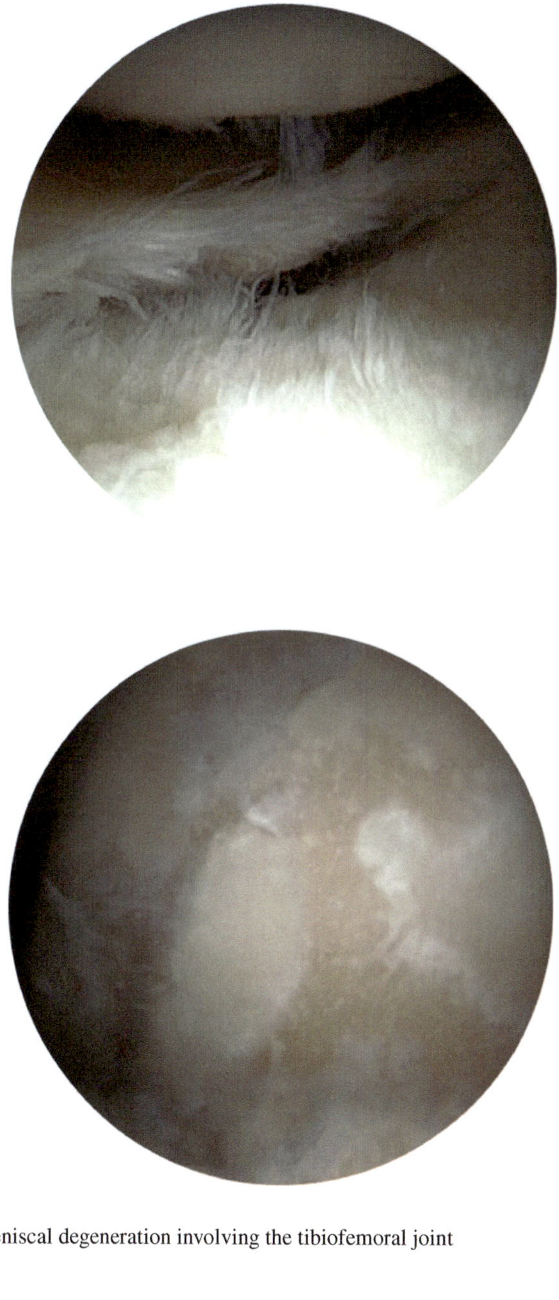

Chondral and meniscal degeneration involving the tibiofemoral joint

13.1.2 Patellofemoral Joint Pain

Patellofemoral (PF) joint pain is felt in front of the knee. It tends to be diffuse with the patient often holding the whole front of the knee with their palm. Interestingly, PF pain is also often felt at the back of the knee.

PF pain may be aggravated by hyperflexion activities such as squatting, prolonged sitting (car driving, movie watching), and going up or down stairs.

Pain from the PF joint may be associated with audible or palpable crepitus in the front of the knee, as well as a feeling of knee stiffness following prolonged hyperfexion. Such stiffness may be described by the patient as "locking" although this is not true mechanical locking (but "pseudolocking").

PF pain may also be transient, sharp and intermittent, related to episodes of patellar instability (subluxation or transient dislocation).

PF pain may be associated with the leg giving way, often the result of transient inhibition of the quadriceps muscle rather than true mechanical instability.

Causes of PF pain include:

- Post-traumatic
- Joint overloading
- Arthritis/degeneration/chondral dysfunction
- PF instability
- Synovial dysfunction, Plica dysfunction
- Bi-partite patella

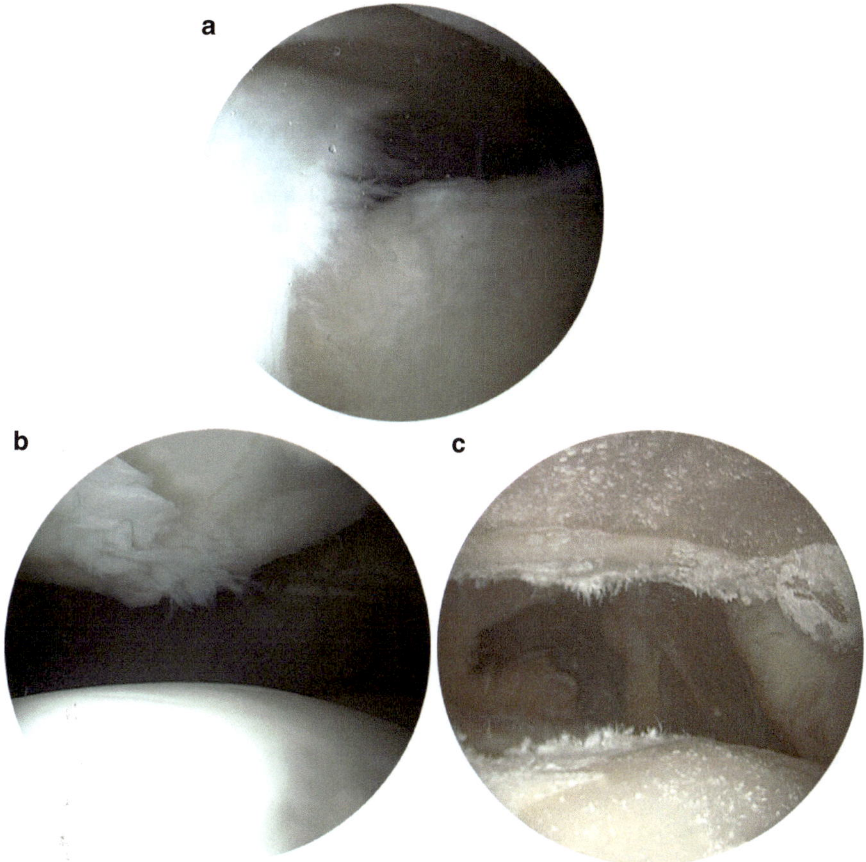

Thickened medial plica (**a**), chondral damage (**b**) and arthritis (**c**) are some of the causes of patellofemoral joint pain

13.1.3 Proximal Tibiofibular Joint Pain

This is pain felt at the posterolateral aspect of the knee, over the proximal tibiofibular joint. It tends to be well localised with the patient being able to point with a finger to the painful area.

Pain may be aggravated by stressing the joint such as during rotation activities of the lower leg with the knee in flexion. Causes of proximal tibiofibular joint pain include:

- Arthritis
- Post-traumatic sprain
- Instability
- Synovial dysfunction

13.1.4 Periarticular Tendon Pain

This is pain felt in the area of one or more periarticular tendons or their bone insertion (enthesis). It is often well localised, but also radiating along the muscle's belly (such as posteromedial or posterolateral aspect of the knee along the medial or lateral hamstring tendons, radiating proximally along the hamstring muscles' bellies).

Tendon pain may be dull, burning or cramp like. Alternatively, it may be sharp and severe, worsened by:

- Activation of the muscles involved (for hamstring tendons—knee flexion, lower leg rotation)
- Stretching of the tendons involved

Tendon pain may be due to several underlying pathologies including:

- Tenosynovitis
- Tendinopathy
- Enthesopathy
- Tendon subluxation/dislocation (snapping tendon)

13.1.5 Ligamentous Pain

This is pain felt in the area of one or more knee ligaments. It may be:

- Localised at the ligament's
  - Origin
  - Mid-substance
  - Insertion
- Diffuse along the ligament's course

Ligamentous pain may be dull or sharp. It may be worsened by stretching of the ligament.

Ligamentous pain may be due to several underlying pathologies including:

- Traumatic sprain, tear
- Degeneration
- Calcification

13.1.6 Periarticular Bursal Pain

This is pain in the area of a periarticular bursa. It may be accompanied by:

- Bursal swelling
- Signs of acute inflammation—redness, warmth or tenderness

Bursal pain may be due to:

- Distension of the bursa
- Secondary pressure effects of the bursa on adjacent structures, such as tendons and nerves

Bursal pain may be dull, burning or cramp like in chronic disorders. It may be sharp and severe in acute inflammatory conditions. It may be worsened by knee motion that stretches or compresses the bursa.

Bursitis may be classified according to the underlying bursal pathology causing pain:

- Inflammatory
- Reactive
- Haemorrhagic
- Infective
- Neoplastic

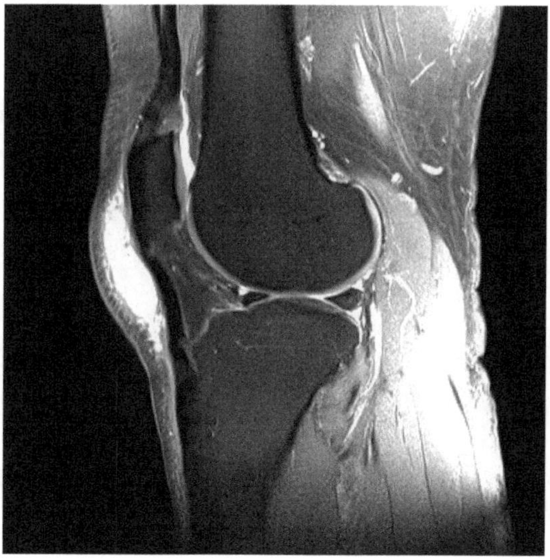

Prepatellar/infrapatellar bursitis

13.1.7 Pain Referred from a Distal Site

This is pain felt over the knee but originates from a distant site:

- Lumbosacral spine
- Hip

Hence, when dealing with knee pathology these areas must be thorough clinically assessed and examined. On some occasions knee pathology may coexist with a distant pathology with each accounting for part of the knee pain (double crush).

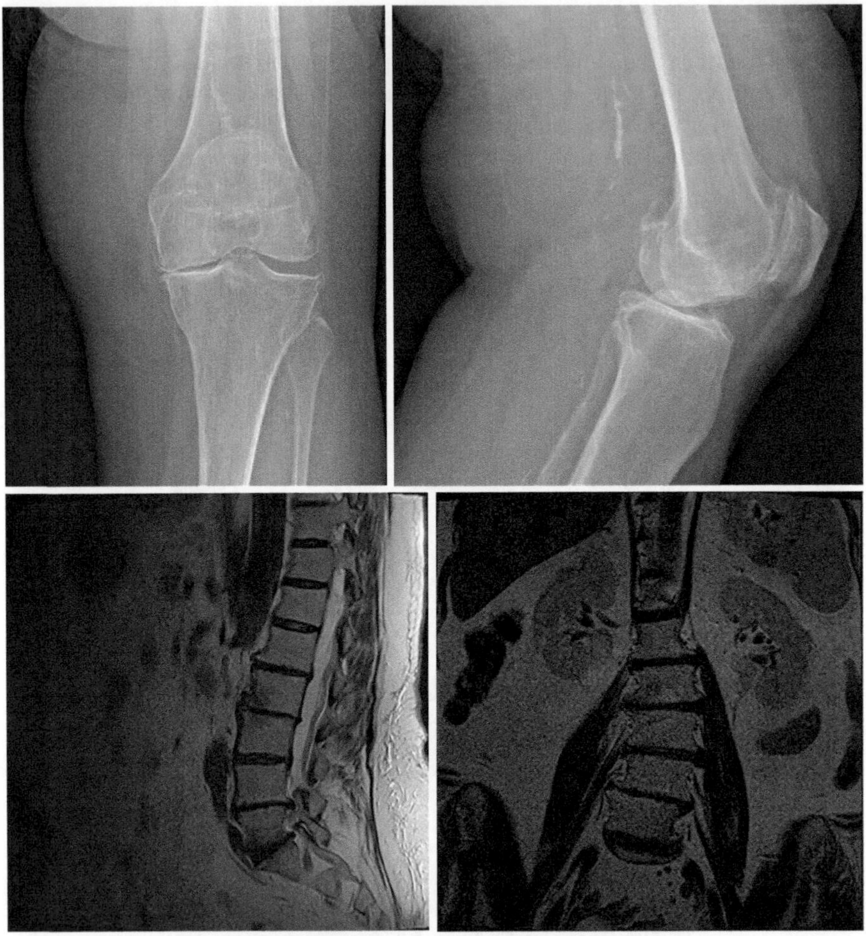

Knee osteoarthritis and lumbosacral spine foraminal stenosis

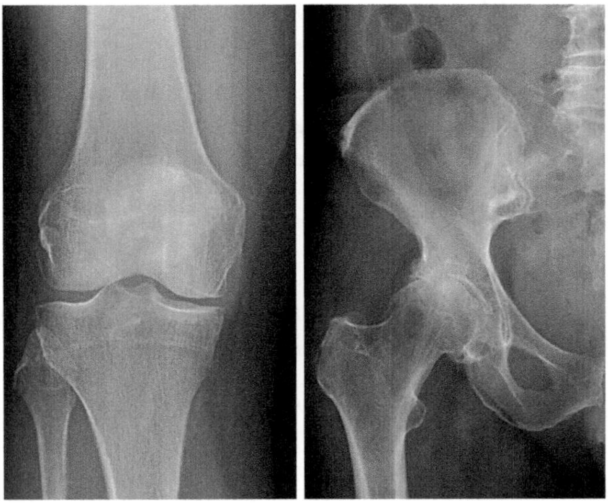

Right knee early OA with associated right hip severe osteoarthritis, in a patient presenting with substantial knee pain

13.1.7.1 Lumbosacral Spine Origin Pain

Lumbosacral spine pain may have two sources of origin occurring together or in isolation:

1. Mechanical pain—this is pain originating from the bones, articulations, discs or ligamentous structures of the lumbosacral spine. Such pain is usually felt in line with the lumbosacral spine and referred to the paraspinal, gluteal and thigh muscles above the level of the knee. Causes of mechanical lumbosacral spine pain include degeneration, arthritis or any other congenital or acquired disturbance of spinal anatomy and function.
2. Neurogenic pain—this is pain experienced due to lumbosacral nerve root compression or irritation, and may be felt anywhere in the area of innervation of that nerve root. Such pain tends to be burning or sharp, associated with paraesthesia, and may radiate down the leg all the way to the foot, in the area of distribution of the nerve root involved (dermatome). Causes of neurogenic lumbosacral spine pain include—spinal foraminal stenosis, disc prolapse, lumbosacral spine degeneration, or any other lesion that compresses or irritates the lumbosacral nerve roots (infection, neoplasia). Hirabayashi et al. [19] reported on 17 cases with L3 radiculopathy (lumbar canal stenosis, extraforaminal stenosis, lumbar disk herniation, and degenerative scoliosis). Of these, 12 reported thigh pain and five reported knee or hip pain.

13.1.7.2 Hip Origin Pain

Pain from the ipsilateral hip may be felt in the knee. Hence, hip examination is essential when evaluating the painful knee.

13.1.8 Peripheral Nerve—Neurogenic Pain

Dysfunction of the nerves innervating the knee may cause pain. Such pain is often dull, burning or non-specific, felt in the area of cutaneous sensory innervation or deep distribution of that nerve. Alternatively, it may sharp and severe. Some of the nerves which must be considered are:

- Femoral
- Cutaneous nerve of the thigh
- Saphenous
- Infrapatellar
- Sciatic
- Tibial
- Common peroneal nerve

Dysfunction of these nerves may occur at the level of the lumbosacral or sciatic plexuses or more peripherally.

13.1.9 Myofascial Pain

This is pain that originates from the knee, thigh, hip or paraspinal muscles or fascia. This is usually felt in the muscle/fascia affected and is worsened by movement, muscle stretching, or certain body postures. Causes include:

- Muscle spasm—due to overcompensating for dysfunction of other muscles, abnormal knee tendons' function or position
- Muscle contracture

This may affect:

- A large part of the muscle/fascia
- Isolated trigger points

13.2 Identifying the Origin of Knee Pain

Clinical history and examination are used to determine the origin of pain and hence guide appropriate investigations and management. The following characteristics of pain may help point towards a likely diagnosis:

13.2.1 Pain Location

The area where pain is felt may point to its possible origin, and certain patterns are recognised. However, the knee region is densely innervated, with substantial overlap in nerve territories, and hence overlap in the area whereby pain from such territories is experienced.

In line with this, Bennell et al. [20] examined the distribution of pain following the experimental injection of hypertonic saline into the fat pad of healthy individuals. Pain was felt in the area of the fat pad, mainly medial to the patellar tendon in most, yet some experienced pain radiating proximally in the thigh as far as the groin.

In addition, determining the area or structure of pain origin is not the full answer, as various pathologies affecting a structure may present with pain and must thus be considered in the differential diagnosis.

Nevertheless, the following suggests how the location of knee pain may guide to its source:

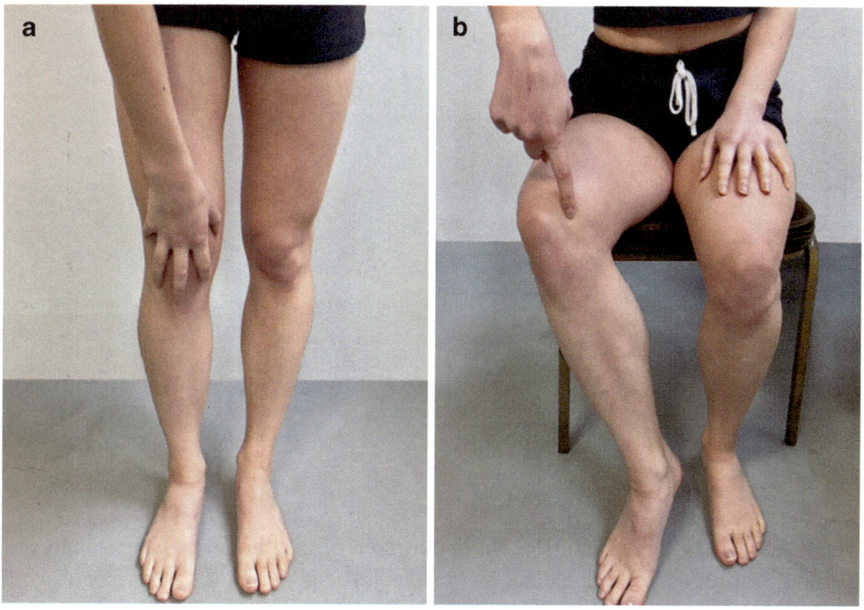

Patellofemoral joint pain is often felt diffusely anteriorly (**a**) whereas medial menisal tear pain is localised to the posteromedial part of the knee (**b**)

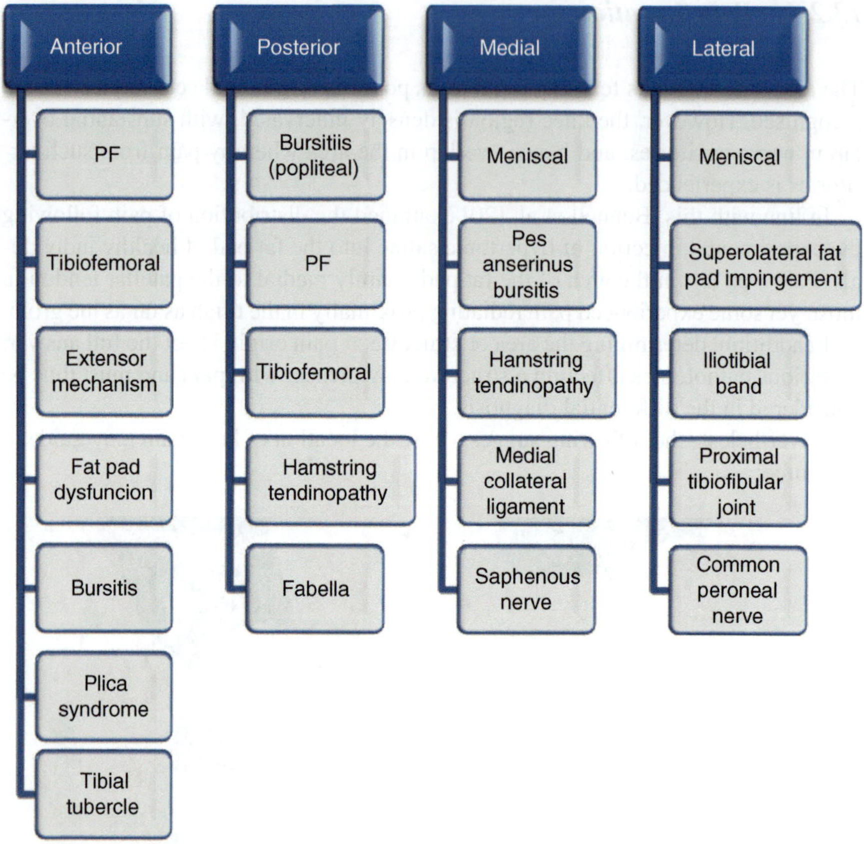

The location of where knee pain is felt may guide as to the area or disorder of origin

13.2.2 Pain Onset

The onset of pain may point to a particular area of origin and possible diagnosis. Certain conditions in the knee are associated with sudden onset, severe pain, with no precipitating event and include:

1. Inflammatory arthritis (crystal arthropathy- gout, pseudogout)
2. Infection–septic arthritis, osteomyelitis
3. Bursitis
4. Calcific tendinopathy of tendons or periarticular ligaments

13.2.3 Patient's Age

The patient's age may point towards a likely cause for the pain, with some painful conditions being more common in certain age groups. However, substantial overlap between the age groups exists. Some conditions that are associated with certain age ranges are considered below, although this is not exhaustive or exclusive.

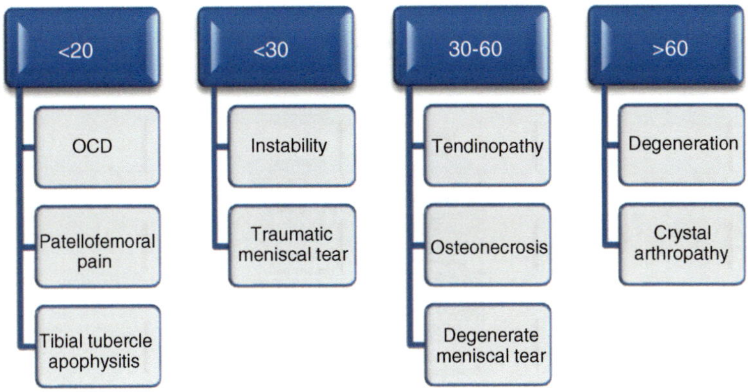

The patient's age may guide as to the potential cause of knee pain. OCD = osteochondritis dissecans

13.2.4 *Symptoms Associated with Knee Pain*

Pain is often accompanied by other knee symptoms, the presence of which may help determine the underlying knee disorder. Some such associations are described below.

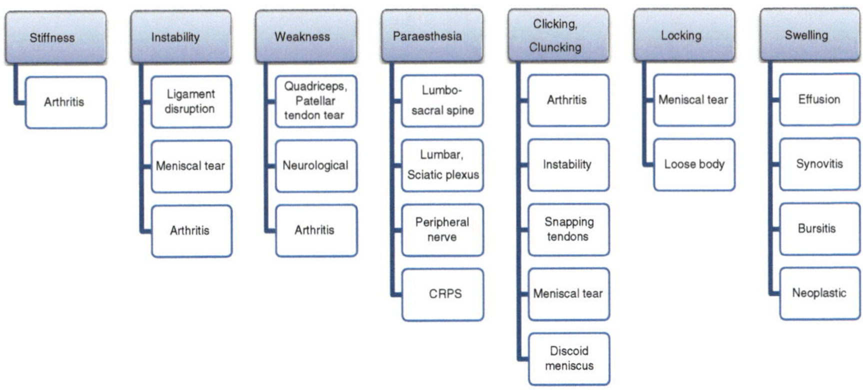

The presence of other clinical symptoms in addition to pain, may guide as to the source of knee pain

13.2.5 *Palpable Knee Tenderness*

During clinical examination the knee is palpated for tenderness. The area of tenderness may guide to the source of pain. Some of the conditions that may be suggested by localised tenderness are described next.

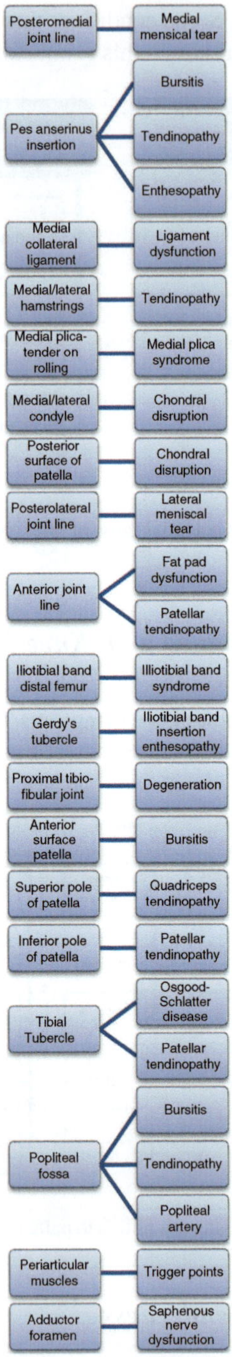

Potential sources of knee pain guided by the area of palpable tenderness

13.2.6 Knee Pain Provoking Clinical Tests

Certain clinical special tests [21], when positive, may point towards a particular origin of pain.

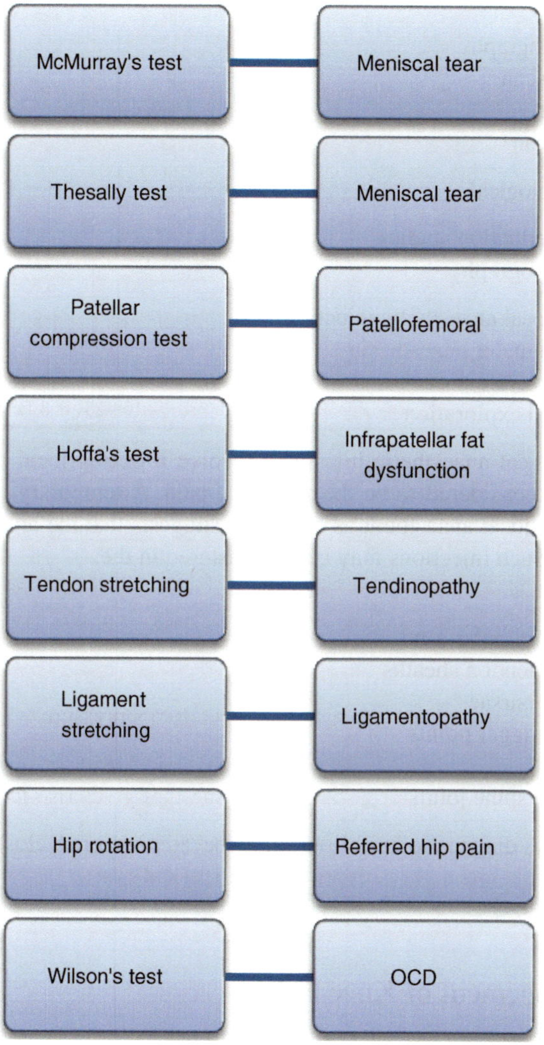

Potential sources of knee pain guided by positive pain provoking clinical tests

13.3 Investigations for Knee Pain

Investigations for the painful knee are directed towards confirming the working diagnosis and excluding alternative diagnoses. These include:

- Radiological
  - Plain radiographs
  - MRI/CT scan
  - Bone scan
  - SPECT scan
- Neurophysiological
  - Nerve conduction studies
  - Electromyography
- Diagnostic local anaesthetic injections
- Examination under anaesthesia
- Arthroscopic evaluation
- Open surgical exploration

Diagnostic local anaesthetic injections involve injecting local anaesthetic into the area that is considered to be the source of pain. A temporary improvement in pain (whilst the local anaesthetic is effective) suggests that the area injected is the origin of pain. Such injections may be administered in the:

- Knee joint
- Proximal tibiofibular joint
- Periarticular tendon sheaths
- Periarticular bursae
- Myofascial trigger points
- Hip joint
- Lumbosacral spine joints

Alternatively, diagnostic injections may be administered close to periarticular nerves.

13.4 Management of Knee Pain

Management of knee pain involves:

- Symptomatic pain control
- Tackling the underlying condition causing the pain

The exact management may be influenced by the working diagnosis but the management ladder [22] may guide as to the approach utilised, although on occasions initial steps may be bypassed.

Surgical procedures for the painful knee may involve:

- Soft tissue procedures
  - Repair
  - Excision
  - Release
  - Reconstruction
  - Transfer
  - Decompression
- Bony procedures
  - Excision
  - Reconstruction
  - Decompression
- Arthroplasty procedures
  - Realignment
  - Replacement
  - Excision
  - Interposition
  - Fusion

Surgical interventions for pain are directed towards the underlying cause. It must be considered that in some instances we may not be exactly sure as to the origin of pain, or as to which part of a surgical intervention actually improves the pain.

If one looks at arthroscopic knee surgery for a degenerative meniscal tear in the presence of associated degenerative changes of the tibiofemoral joint, the following may be performed as part of the procedure:

- Washout of the tibiofemoral joint
- Debridement of any associated knee synovitis
- Debridement of any articular cartilage fibrillations or flaps
- Excision of the torn part of the meniscus (partial meniscectomy)
- Decompression of a para-meniscal cyst that may be found in relation to some meniscal tears

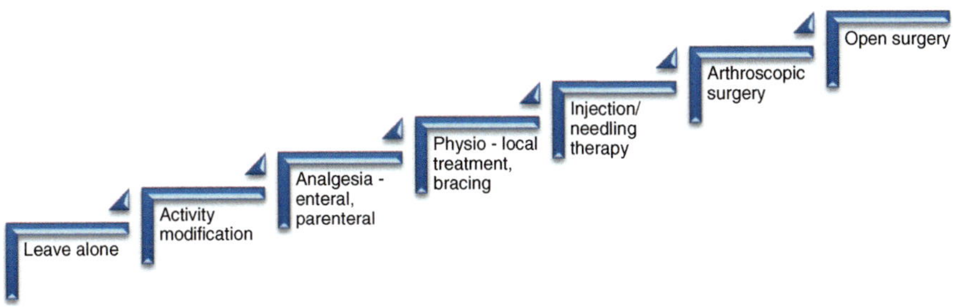

Management ladder for knee pain

Similarly, if one looks at knee arthroplasty for tibiofemoral pain due to arthritis, the following may be performed as part of the procedure:

- Resection of the worn articular surfaces and underlying subchondral bone
- Curettage or decompression of small subchondral cysts
- Excision of part of the synovium
- Excision of part or all of the knee fat pads
- Division of articular nerves in performing the surgical approach to the joint or in deliberately denervating part of the joint (such as the patella)
- Excision of periarticular osteophytes
- Release of periarticular ligaments to improve knee alignment, hence altering weight distribution across the joint and reducing the forces exerted on periarticular tendons and muscles

There is controversy as to which of the above surgical procedure components, or if any at all, are important in alleviating pain; a multicentre randomised trial compared arthroscopic partial meniscectomy with sham surgery (arthroscopic evaluation) in the management of degenerative meniscal tears. It was shown that arthroscopic partial meniscectomy offered no substantial benefit over sole skin incision, suggesting that the benefit of surgery may be at least partly mediated by a placebo effect [23].

Learning Pearls

- Various pathological conditions may cause similar clinical symptoms and clinical examination signs:
  - Medial meniscal tear and medial tibiofemoral compartment articular cartilage degeneration may cause medial joint line pain.

  Hence, it may be very difficult or impossible to distinguish between various potential pathologies that cause pain solely based on clinical grounds. Radiological and other investigations are thus often needed to determine the exact diagnosis.

- Several pathologies may coexist and it is often not possible to determine their individual contribution to a patient's symptoms.
- A particular pathology may give rise to various patterns of pain location. Medial compartment osteoarthritis has been shown to cause diffuse (41%), isolated medial (16%), anteromedial (12%), and posteromedial (11%) pain [7]. Preoperative pain location (localised medial pain) has been shown to be a poor predictor of outcome after medial unicompartmental knee replacement arthroplasty, with equivalent outcomes observed between those with pure medial knee pain, pure anterior knee pain or combined (generalised) knee pain [12]. Similarly, lack of correlation has been shown between location of pain (medial, lateral, posterior) and the arthroscopic findings of a meniscal tear [8].
- Diabetes may be associated with higher pain severity in patients with knee arthritis [6]

References

1. Hong E, Kraft MC. Evaluating anterior knee pain. Med Clin North Am. 2014;98(4):697–717.
2. Slotkin S, Thome A, Ricketts C, Georgiadis A, Cruz AI Jr, Seeley M. Anterior knee pain in children and adolescents: overview and management. J Knee Surg. 2018;31(5):392–8.
3. Flores DV, Mejía Gómez C, Pathria MN. Layered approach to the anterior knee: normal anatomy and disorders associated with anterior knee pain. Radiographics. 2018;38(7):2069–101.
4. English S, Perret D. Posterior knee pain. Curr Rev Musculoskelet Med. 2010;3(1-4):3–10.
5. Muché JA, Lento PH. Posterior knee pain and its causes: a clinician's guide to expediting diagnosis. Phys Sportsmed. 2004;32(3):23–30.
6. Alenazi AM, Alshehri MM, Alothman S, Alqahtani BA, Rucker J, Sharma N, Segal NA, Bindawas SM, Kluding PM. The association of diabetes with knee pain severity and distribution in people with knee osteoarthritis using data from the osteoarthritis initiative. Sci Rep. 2020;10(1):3985. https://doi.org/10.1038/s41598-020-60989-1.
7. Van Ginckel A, Bennell KL, Campbell PK, Wrigley TV, Hunter DJ, Hinman RS. Location of knee pain in medial knee osteoarthritis: patterns and associations with self-reported clinical symptoms. Osteoarthr Cartil. 2016;24(7):1135–42.
8. Campbell J, Harte A, Kerr DP, Murray P. The location of knee pain and pathology in patients with a presumed meniscus tear: preoperative symptoms compared to arthroscopic findings. Ir J Med Sci. 2014;183(1):23–31.
9. Thompson LR, Boudreau R, Hannon MJ, Newman AB, Chu CR, Jansen M, Nevitt MC, Kwoh CK, Osteoarthritis Initiative Investigators. The knee pain map: reliability of a method to identify knee pain location and pattern. Arthritis Rheum. 2009;61(6):725–31.
10. Wood LR, Peat G, Thomas E, Duncan R. Knee osteoarthritis in community-dwelling older adults: are there characteristic patterns of pain location? Osteoarthr Cartil. 2007;15(6):615–23.
11. Cotofana S, Wyman BT, Benichou O, Dreher D, Nevitt M, Gardiner J, Wirth W, Hitzl W, Kwoh CK, Eckstein F, Frobell RB. OAI Investigators Group. Relationship between knee pain and the presence, location, size and phenotype of femorotibial denuded areas of subchondral bone as visualized by MRI. Osteoarthr Cartil. 2013;21(9):1214–22.
12. Liddle AD, Pandit H, Jenkins C, Price AJ, Dodd CA, Gill HS, Murray DW. Preoperative pain location is a poor predictor of outcome after Oxford unicompartmental knee arthroplasty at 1 and 5 years. Knee Surg Sports Traumatol Arthrosc. 2013;21(11):2421–6.
13. Baum J. Joint pain. It isn't always arthritis. Postgrad Med. 1989;85(1):311–3. 316, 321
14. Sakamoto J, Manabe Y, Oyamada J, Kataoka H, Nakano J, Saiki K, Okamoto K, Tsurumoto T, Okita M. Anatomical study of the articular branches innervated the hip and knee joint with reference to mechanism of referral pain in hip joint disease patients. Clin Anat. 2018;31(5):705–9.
15. Lesher JM, Dreyfuss P, Hager N, Kaplan M, Furman M. Hip joint pain referral patterns: a descriptive study. Pain Med. 2008;9(1):22–5.
16. Dibra FF, Prieto HA, Gray CF, Parvataneni HK. Don't forget the hip! Hip arthritis masquerading as knee pain. Arthroplast Today. 2017;4(1):118–24.
17. Al-Hadithy N, Rozati H, Sewell MD, Dodds AL, Brooks P, Chatoo M. Causes of a painful total knee arthroplasty. Are patients still receiving total knee arthroplasty for extrinsic pathologies? Int Orthop. 2012;36(6):1185–9.
18. Sánchez-Romero EA, Pecos-Martín D, Calvo-Lobo C, García-Jiménez D, Ochoa-Sáez V, Burgos-Caballero V, Fernández-Carnero J. Clinical features and myofascial pain syndrome in older adults with knee osteoarthritis by sex and age distribution: a cross-sectional study. Knee. 2019;26(1):165–73.
19. Hirabayashi H, Takahashi J, Hashidate H, Ogihara N, Tashiro A, Misawa H, Ebara S, Mitsui K, Wakabayashi S, Kato H. Characteristics of L3 nerve root radiculopathy. Surg Neurol. 2009;72(1):36–40.
20. Bennell K, Hodges P, Mellor R, Bexander C, Souvlis T. The nature of anterior knee pain following injection of hypertonic saline into the infrapatellar fat pad. J Orthop Res. 2004;22(1):116–21.

21. Charalambos CP. Clinical examination. In: The knee made easy: Springer; 2017.
22. Charalambous CP. Professionalism in surgery. In: Career skills for surgeons: Springer; 2017. p. 5–46.
23. Sihvonen R, Paavola M, Malmivaara A, Itälä A, Joukainen A, Nurmi H, Kalske J, Järvinen TL, Finnish Degenerative Meniscal Lesion Study (FIDELITY) Group. Arthroscopic partial meniscectomy versus sham surgery for a degenerative meniscal tear. N Engl J Med. 2013;369(26):2515–24.

Chapter 14
Knee Stiffness

Stiffness is a condition whereby there is loss of passive joint motion. This may be painless or painfull. This chapter discusses the concepts of true and apparent knee stiffness, and discusses potential causes, investigations and management.

14.1 True Versus Apparent Knee Stiffness

In dealing with knee stiffness it is essential to distinguish between true and apparent stiffness [1].

Apparent limitation of motion may be due to:

- Pain
- Weakness

Patients may be reluctant to move their knee as that would cause pain and may refer to this as "stiffness". Similarly, they may be unable to move the knee due to weakness but describe this loss of motion as "stiffness". Hence, it is essential to determine whether one is dealing with true stiffness, where there is true loss of passive motion.

14.2 Passive Versus Active Knee Motion

In describing active and passive movements of the knee one may consider the analogy to driving a car. Car motion requires the driver pressing the gas pedal and creating electric signals, which are then communicated by electrical circuits to the engine. Fuel is then burnt creating energy, with the generated force transmitted to the wheels for motion. Car motion also needs a good set of wheels and tyres and a smooth surface to move along.

C. Panayiotou Charalambous, *The Knee Made Easy*,
https://doi.org/10.1007/978-3-030-54506-2_14

If the gas pedal is faulty and the signal can not be initiated, or if the electric circuits fall apart, or if the fuel runs out, then the car will not actively move. Nevertheless, the driver can still get out and pull the car along, as long as there is no mechanical obstruction, and the tyres and road surface are smooth (this is analogous to passive motion).

Similarly, active knee motion needs an effective neuromuscular system, from brain stimulation to muscle contraction and force transmission via tendons to bones. Knee motion also requires smooth articular surfaces that can easily move relative to each other, and a soft tissue envelop (ligaments, muscles, tendons) that have some slack, allowing motion to occur before they become taut. If these neuromuscular and musculotendinous systems are disrupted, active motion may not be feasible, and the patient may not be able to actively move the knee. Nevertheless, the examiner will still be able to hold and move the patient's knee (passive motion).

However, in the case of the car, if the tyres are clamped or if the wheels fall in deep road holes, no matter how hard the driver presses the gas pedal, and no matter how much force the engine creates, the car is unlikely to move (loss of active motion). Similarly, no matter how hard the driver pulls on the rope the car is also unlikely to move along (loss of passive motion).

Along similar lines, if the soft tissues around the tibiofemoral joint (capsule, ligaments, tendons, muscles) contract and shorten, swell and thicken, and lose their slack, or if the articulating surfaces are worn, becoming irregular, with bumps or projecting osteophytes, no matter how hard the muscles contract, or how much effort the patient makes, the knee is unlikely to move (loss of active motion). This loss of motion will be observed even when the examiner holds the patient's knee and tries to move it (loss of passive motion) [1].

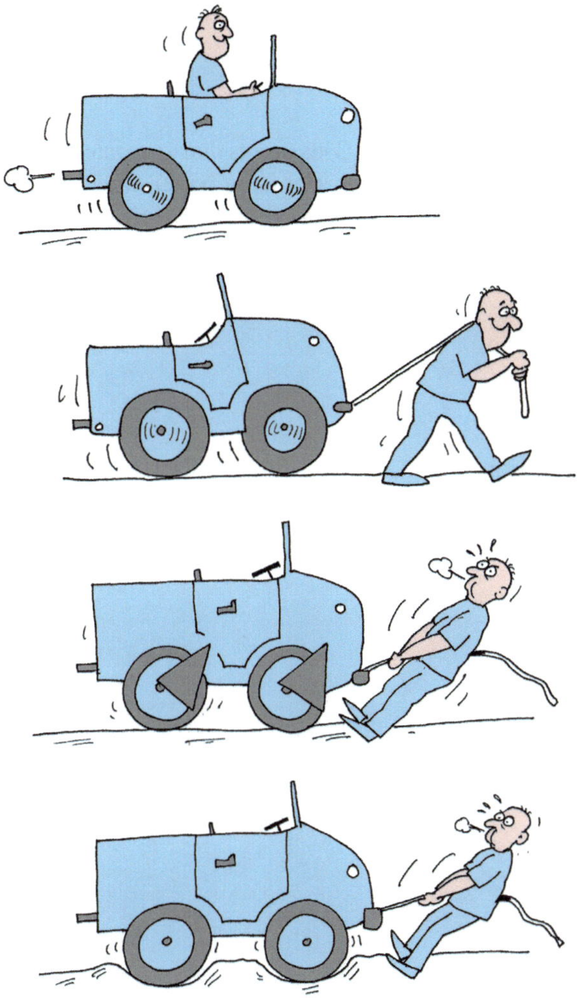

A car with no fuel can still be pulled passively along. But if its wheels are clamped or if they fall in deep potholes, the car can move neither actively not passively

Knee stiffness may be described in various ways including:

1. Direction of Knee Motion Loss

The direction of motion loss may be:

- Global—affecting all directions
- In one direction (flexion or extension)

The direction of motion loss may be influenced by the underlying pathology. In tibiofemoral degeneration there is often loss of extension and flexion. In quadriceps contracture there may be loss of flexion but extension is affected less.

2. Duration of Knee Motion Loss

- Intermittent
- Constant

Intermitted motion loss may be due to locking. This occurs due to an intermittent mechanical block (such as an unstable meniscal tear or loose body), whereas constant stiffness may be more due to persistent mechanical reasons (soft tissue contractures or bony/cartilaginous/foreign body/surgical device mechanical block).

3. Cause of Knee Stiffness

This may be:

- Congenital
- Acquired
  - Traumatic (including surgery)
    - Dislocation, fracture malunion, adhesions, capsular contracture, metalwork
  - Degenerative
  - Inflammatory
  - Infective—Septic arthritis

4. Structure Limiting Knee Motion

The structure limiting motion may be:

- Soft Tissue
  - Capsule
  - Muscle-Tendon
  - Ligaments
  - Adhesions
    - Intra-articular
    - Periarticular
    - Extra-articular
- Cartilaginous
  - Meniscal
  - Loose body
- Bony
  - Intra-articular
  - Periarticular
  - Extra-articular
- Foreign body/surgical device
  - Intra-articular

- Periarticular
- Extra-articular

The structure causing stiffness may guide its management.

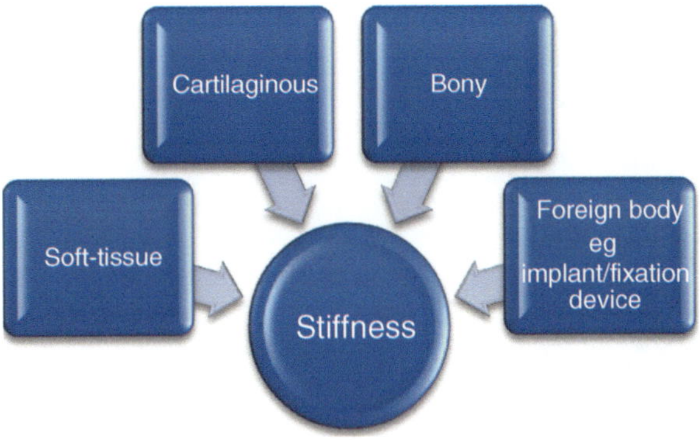

Knee stiffness may be described according to the structure limiting motion

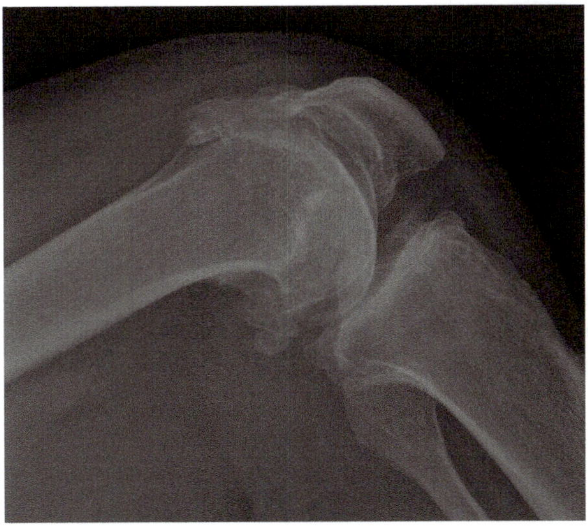

Large posterior osteophytes, account for motion loss in knee osteoarthritis

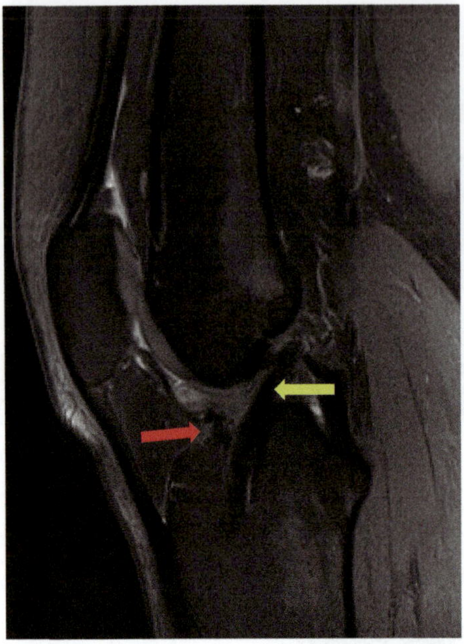

Cyclops lesion (red arrow), post ACL reconstruction (yellow arrow) surgery, may limit full extension

14.3 Differential Diagnosis of Knee Stiffness

Some of the most common causes of tibiofemoral joint stiffness encountered in clinical practise, and which must be considered in the differential diagnosis are:

- Knee arthritis
  - Degenerative
  - Inflammatory
- Post-traumatic stiffness—surgery, fracture malunion, adhesions, soft tissue contractures, joint dislocation
- Osteonecrosis of the knee
- Loose bodies, meniscal tears
- Septic arthritis

A thorough clinical history will usually identify the most likely cause. Patient's age may also guide as to the likely diagnosis accounting for the observed stiffness, but this is not absolute.

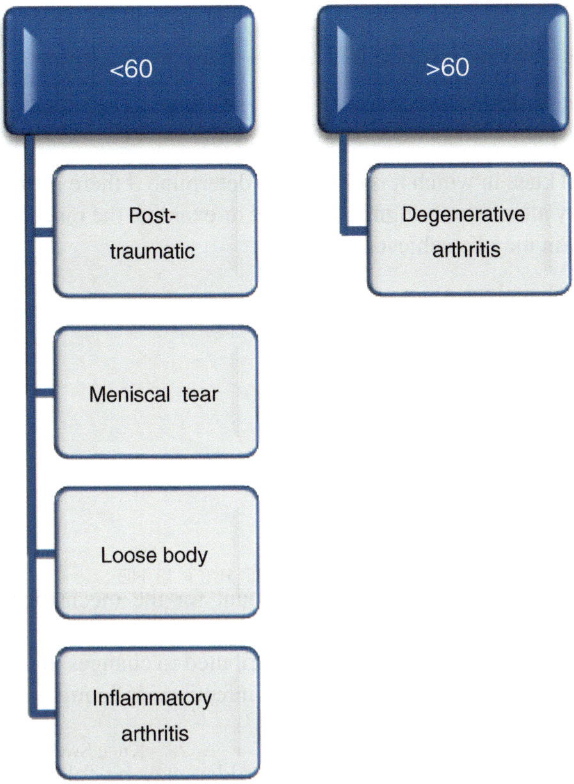

The patient's age may guide as to the potential cause of knee stiffness

14.4 Investigations for Knee Stiffness

Investigations for the stiff knee aim to confirm the working diagnosis (as to the presence of true stiffness) and its likely cause, and exclude any possible alternative diagnoses. These include:

- Radiological
  - Plain radiographs
  - MRI/CT Scan
  - Bone scan
- Neurophysiological
  - Nerve conduction studies
  - Electromyography

- Haematological
  - Inflammatory markers
- Examination under anaesthesia
- Arthroscopic evaluation

When faced with a painful knee in which it is difficult to determine if there is true or apparent stiffness, one may attempt to minimise pain and re-examine the range of motion. Such reduction in pain may be achieved by:

- Adequate oral or parenteral analgesia
- Knee local anaesthetic injections
- Examination under regional or general anaesthesia

14.5 Management of Knee Stiffness

Management of stiffness [2–9] involves:

- Tackling the structures (soft tissue or bony) that account for the mechanical block to motion
- Tackling the underlying condition which may have contributed to changes in the properties of these structures (including underlying infection, inflammatory arthritis)

In tackling the deranged structures the management ladder may be followed although on occasions initial steps may be bypassed.

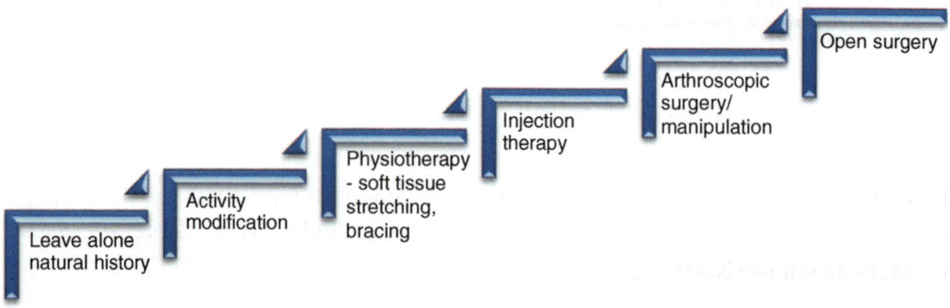

Management ladder for knee stiffness

In some cases of stiffness, the underlying process has a natural history of improvement; stiffness following knee arthroplasty has been shown to improve in most patients over a period of 1–2 years [10, 11]. Some patients may not experience much trouble from their stiffness as their day to day activities do not require full knee motion; or may be able to adjust their activities and thus manage to cope with some loss of knee motion. Hence, there is a good argument in many cases for leaving things alone.

- Non-surgical management
  - Physiotherapy aims to stretch the soft tissue structures contributing to stiffness.
  - Steroid injections may reduce knee inflammation helping to improve pain and also reduce any inflammatory related changes in the soft tissues that contribute to stiffness.
- Surgical management

This is directed towards the structures contributing to loss of motion and may include:

- Soft tissue
  a. Stretching (manipulation)
  b. Release (arthroscopic or open division)
  c. Lengthening (of contracted tendons or muscles)
- Bony
  a. Reposition (reducing a dislocated joint)
  b. Realignment (osteotomy)
  c. Resection/removal (meniscal tear, loose body, surgical devices)
  d. Joint arthroplasty

Learning Pearls

- Patients may function well in performing activities of daily living with ranges of motion well below the maximum range of knee motion that is achievable in a healthy joint.
- In stretching the painful stiff knee, thorough pain control is necessary. Inadequate pain control may cause patient apprehension or muscle spasm, hindering the ability to perform sufficient stretching of the soft tissues. Pain control may be achieved with oral or parenteral analgesia, with intra-articular steroid injections, or with local anaesthetic nerve blocks.
- Distinction between stiffness and locking is essential. Intermittent locking due to a mechanical block causes loss of active and passive motion for the duration of locking but motion usually returns once the mechanical block is removed (spontaneously or surgically). However, if locking persists, the soft tissues around the knee may contract, leading to persistent stiffness even when the mechanical block is removed. Hence, determining the duration of loss of knee motion is important when obtaining a clinical history for the troublesome knee.

References

1. Charalambos CP. Shoulder stiffness. In: The shoulder made easy: Springer; 2019. p. 225–34.
2. Charalambous CP. Professionalism in surgery. In: Career skills for surgeons: Springer; 2017. p. 5–46.
3. Ekhtiari S, Horner NS, de Sa D, Simunovic N, Hirschmann MT, Ogilvie R, Berardelli RL, Whelan DB, Ayeni OR. Arthrofibrosis after ACL reconstruction is best treated in a step-wise approach with early recognition and intervention: a systematic review. Knee Surg Sports Traumatol Arthrosc. 2017;25(12):3929–37.
4. Pierce TP, Cherian JJ, Mont MA. Static and dynamic bracing for loss of motion following total knee arthroplasty. J Long-Term Eff Med Implants. 2015;25(4):337–43.
5. Bhave A, Sodhi N, Anis HK, Ehiorobo JO, Mont MA. Static progressive stretch orthosis-consensus modality to treat knee stiffness-rationale and literature review. Ann Transl Med. 2019;7(Suppl 7):S256. https://doi.org/10.21037/atm.2019.06.55.
6. Saini P, Trikha V. Manipulation under anesthesia for post traumatic stiff knee-pearls, pitfalls and risk factors for failure. Injury. 2016;47(10):2315–9.
7. Pujol N, Boisrenoult P, Beaufils P. Post-traumatic knee stiffness: surgical techniques. Orthop Traumatol Surg Res. 2015;101(1 Suppl):S179–86.
8. Chen MR, Dragoo JL. Arthroscopic releases for arthrofibrosis of the knee. J Am Acad Orthop Surg. 2011;19(11):709–16.
9. Tardy N, Thaunat M, Sonnery-Cottet B, Murphy C, Chambat P, Fayard JM. Extension deficit after ACL reconstruction: Is open posterior release a safe and efficient procedure? Knee. 2016;23(3):465–71.
10. Quah C, Swamy G, Lewis J, Kendrew J, Badhe N. Fixed flexion deformity following total knee arthroplasty. A prospective study of the natural history. Knee. 2012;19(5):519–21.
11. Aderinto J, Brenkel IJ, Chan P. Natural history of fixed flexion deformity following total knee replacement: a prospective five-year study. J Bone Joint Surg Br. 2005;87(7):934–6.

Chapter 15
Knee Locking

Locking of the knee is a condition whereby the knee gets stuck in one position and can not actively or passively move further. In plain terms "locking" refers to rigid fixation in one position, but in orthopaedics terms "locking" often refers to inability to fully extend the knee actively or passively (but flexion being possible). Although the latter description of the term is utilised in this chapter, it should not be considered as absolute, and it is possible for both extension and flexion to be limited in some cases of locking.

Locking may be painless or associated with pain. This chapter discusses the concepts of true locking and apparent locking (pseudolocking). In addition it discusses the causes of knee locking, its investigation and management.

15.1 True Knee Locking Versus Apparent Knee Locking (Pseudolocking)

In dealing with knee locking it is essential to distinguish between true locking and pseudolocking [1–3].

- True locking refers to the situation whereby a mechanical block is stopping the knee from extending further. If pain, or apprehension were to be abolished, the knee would still not be able to move
- Apparent locking refers to the situation whereby the patient perceives that the knee cannot extend further, but there is not a true mechanical cause accounting for this
- Apparent locking may be due to:
  - Pain
  - Apprehension
  - Weakness
  - Stiffness

C. Panayiotou Charalambous, *The Knee Made Easy*,
https://doi.org/10.1007/978-3-030-54506-2_15

If the above were to be abolished, motion of the knee is possible. In many cases, apparent locking cannot be distinguished from true locking simply based on clinical grounds (clinical history and examination) and it is diagnosed in retrospect after relevant investigations or surgical exploration of the knee.

Patients may be reluctant to move their knee as that would cause pain and they may refer to this as "locking", or "jamming". Hence, it is essential to determine whether one is dealing with true locking, where there is loss of passive extension.

Resistance to knee extension may also be due to hamstring tendon spasm in response to knee pain.

True and apparent locking may be differentiated by considering the following:

1. Onset of Locking

The onset of locking may be:

- Sudden
- Gradual

The onset may also be:

- Associated with an audible sound/or felt snap
- Not associated with an audible/felt snap
- Associated with audible/felt gentle grinding

The patient may complain that the knee locks suddenly, and cannot further extend the knee (true locking). Alternatively, the patient may describe that after keeping the knee in a certain position for a prolonged period of time (e.g. sitting, kneeling) it is difficult for the knee to start moving and extend normally (apparent locking).

The patient may complain that onset of locking was associated with an audible/felt sound/snap (true locking). Alternatively, the patient may describe that no sound/snap was experienced, or that the onset of locking was associated with an audible/felt gentle grinding upon attempted knee motion (apparent locking).

2. Duration of Locking

- Intermittent
- Constant

Locking may be intermittent, coming and going, with normal motion regained in between, or may be constant—started and is ongoing by the time the physician meets the patient.

True locking is more likely to be constant, but is also frequently intermittent.

3. Termination of Locking

The end of locking may be:

- Sudden
- Gradual

The patient may report that the knee unlocks suddenly (often with a snap), suggestive of true locking. Alternatively, the patient may describe that after slowly trying to move the knee, the knee starts going with range of motion increasing slowly, consistent with apparent locking. Apparent locking is not followed by sudden unlocking.

4. Associated with Joint Effusion/Synovitis

True locking may be followed by swelling of the knee joint due to underlying synovitis or effusion, as a result of the underlying pathology causing the locking. Apparent locking is not usually followed by synovitis in the knee joint [3].

15.2 Clinical Symptoms of True Knee Locking

- Inability to fully straighten the knee (although flexion is usually possible)
- “Clicking”, “clunking”, “popping”, “grating”, “snapping”
- May occur in isolation or be associated with other symptoms including:
  - Pain
  - Instability
  - Weakness
  - Stiffness
  - Knee swelling

15.3 Clinical Signs of True Knee Locking

- Inability to fully straighten the knee actively or passively (although flexion is usually possible)
- Signs consistent with underlying disorder causing locking
  - Tibiofemoral joint line tenderness
  - Effusion

15.4 Sources of True Knee Locking

True locking may be due to any mechanical block (intra-articular or extra-articular) that limits knee extension. Multiple such mechanical factors have been described including the below [4–15]:

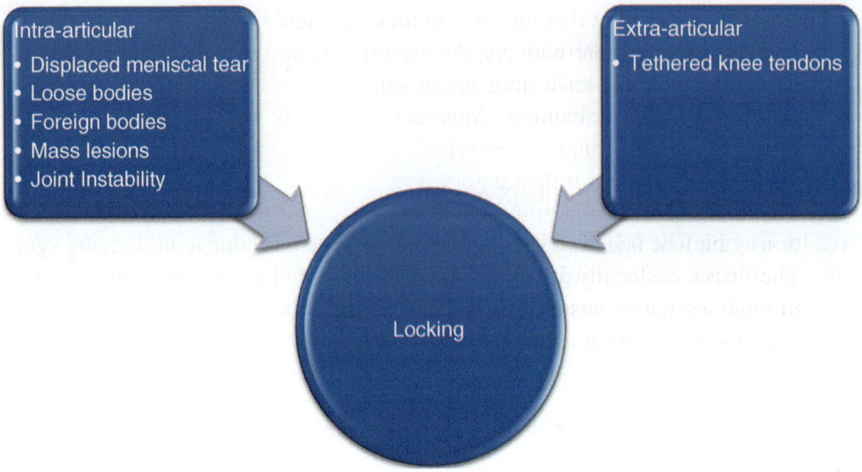

Potential causes of knee locking

Potential pathologies affecting parts of the knee that can give rise to true locking are shown next.

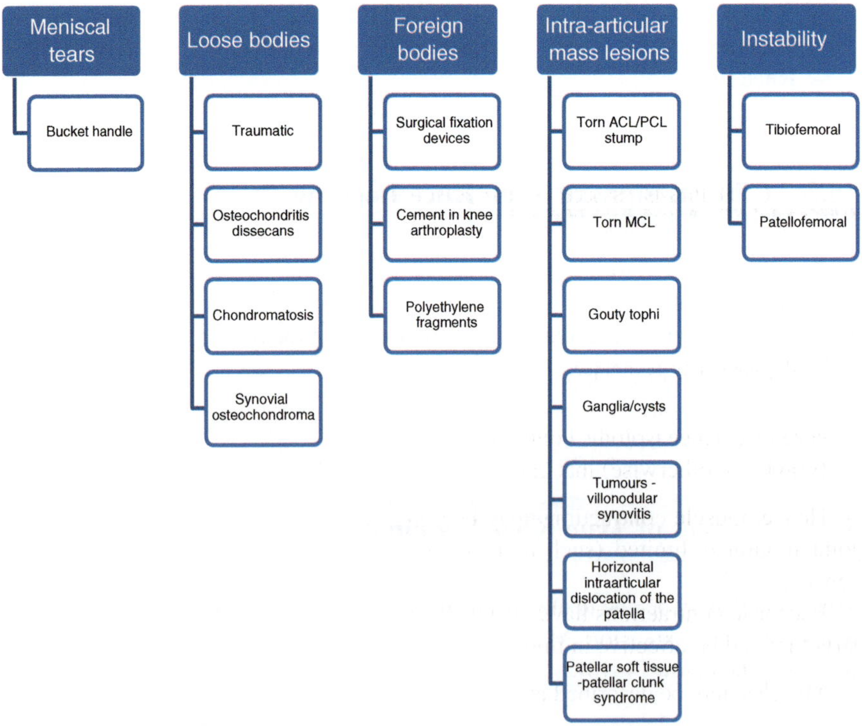

Potential articular and pathologies causing knee locking

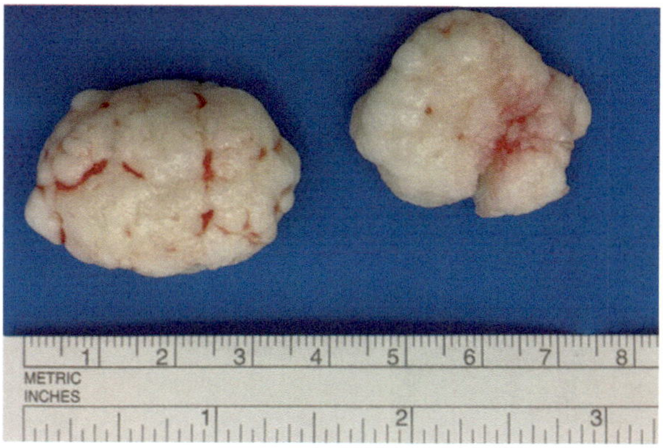

Osteochondral loose bodies causing knee locking

15.5 Investigations for Knee Locking

- Radiological
  - Plain radiographs
  - MRI [16–18]
  - CT Scan

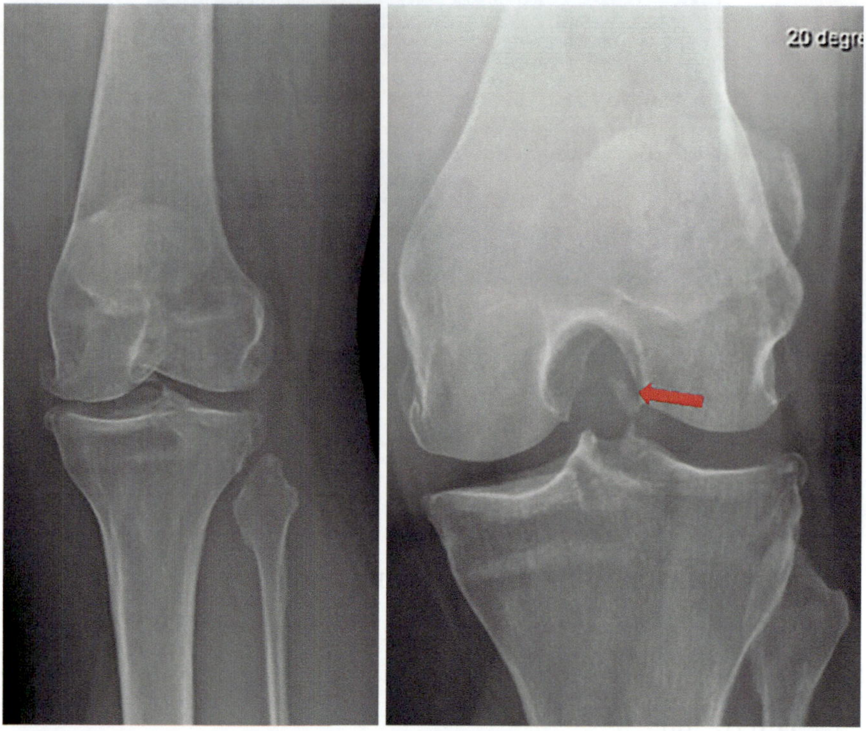

Loose body or osteophyte (red arrow) in femoral notch (AP and notch views)

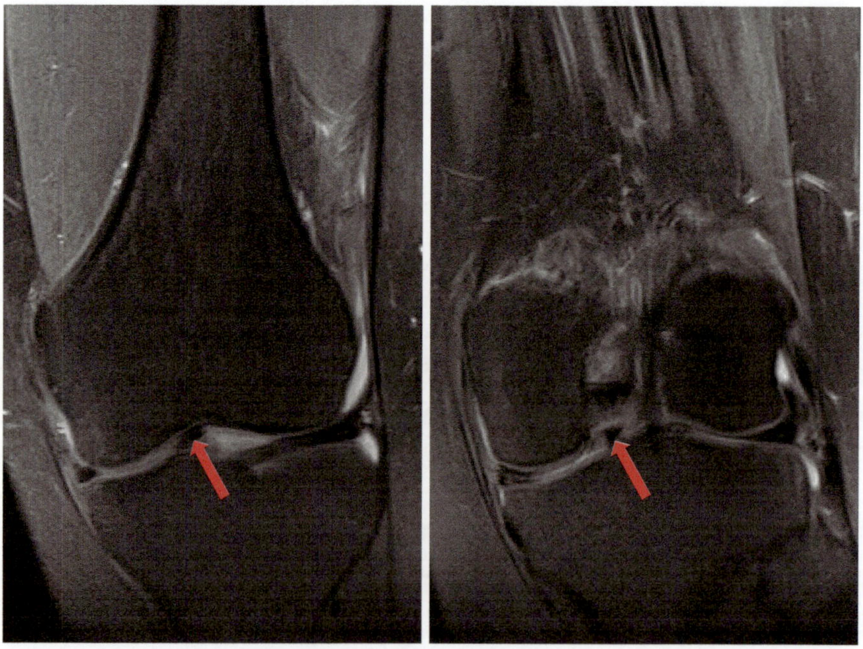

Bucket handle tear with fragment displaced in the femoral notch

- Arthroscopic evaluation

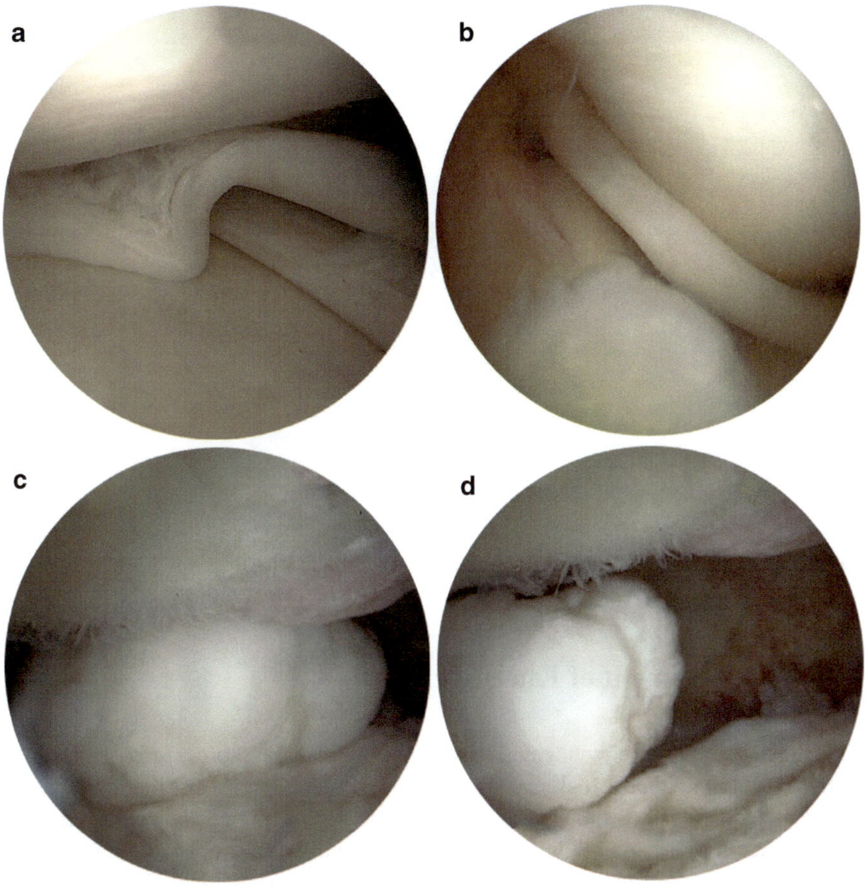

Potential causes of knee locking: (**a**) Displaced bucket handle meniscal tear located in the tibio-femoral articulation. (**b**) Displaced bucket handle meniscal tear located in the femoral notch. (**c**, **d**) Loose osteochondral body

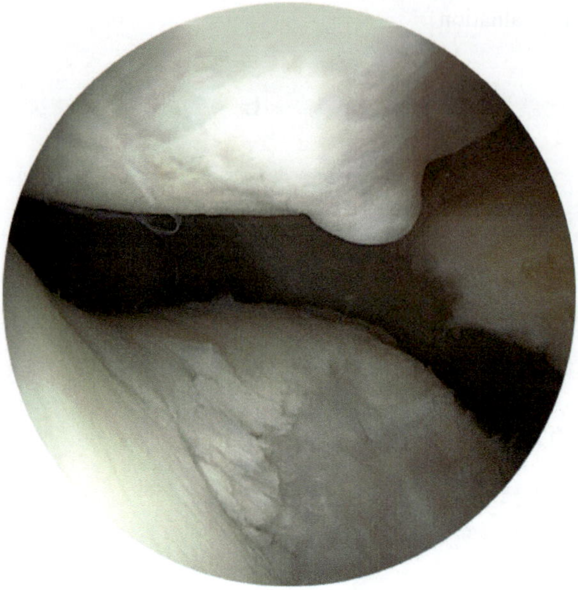

Patellofemoral chondral degeneration may present as knee pseudolocking

15.6 Management of Knee Locking

This depends on the frequency and severity of clinical symptoms. Infrequent intermittent locking may be left alone. Acute locking is dealt with according to the management ladder [19], although on occasions initial steps may be bypassed. The locked knee may be manipulated to restore motion. Arthroscopic or open surgery aims at removing or repairing the structure causing the mechanical obstruction.

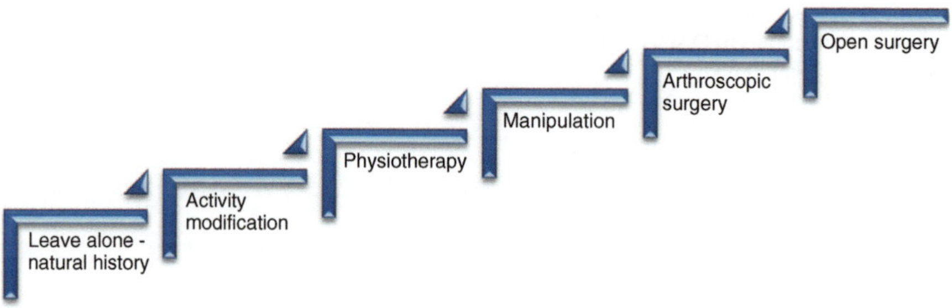

Management ladder for knee locking

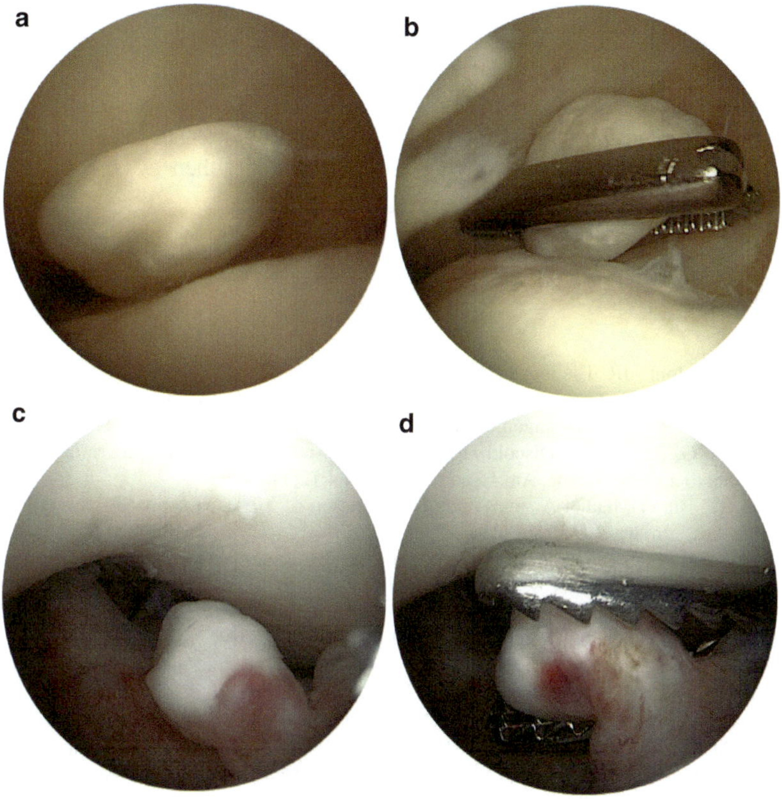

Arthroscopic removal of loose body (**a**, **b**) and partially attached body (**c**, **d**) for intermittent knee locking

Learning Pearls

- Intermitted motion loss may be due to locking (due to an unstable meniscal tear or loose body), whereas constant stiffness may be more due to persistent mechanical reasons (soft tissue contractures or bony mechanical block)
- In distinguishing between true and apparent locking it is essential to get the patient to relax the knee muscles which may oppose extension (hamstrings). Palpation of these whilst attempting to extend the knee may help determine whether they are tense (and hence opposing motion) or relaxed (and hence unlikely to be opposing motion)
- The presence of an intra-articular lesion does not necessarily imply the development of locking—a displaced bucket handle meniscal tear may not cause locking
- It is important to recognise and address a locked knee, as, if it persists, it may lead to soft tissue contracture and stiffness (which may be residual even if the mechanical block to extension is removed)

- Locking may also be observed following knee arthroplasty, but the potential causes often vary from those encountered in the native knee
- If locking is felt by the patient to be occurring at a constant spot in the knee, a meniscal tear is likely to be the underlying cause. In contrast, if something is felt to be moving around the knee, then a loose body is more likely

References

1. Allum RL, Jones JR. The locked knee. Injury. 1986;17(4):256–8.
2. Bansal P, Deehan DJ, Gregory RJ. Diagnosing the acutely locked knee. Injury. 2002;33(6):495–8.
3. McMurray TP. Internal derangements of the knee joint. Ann R Coll Surg Engl. 1948;3(4):210–9.
4. Hermann G, Berson BL. Discoid medial meniscus: two cases of tears presenting as locked knee due to athletic trauma. Am J Sports Med. 1984;12(1):74–6.
5. Joshi RP, Butler-Manuel A. Intra-articular migration of a broken screw tip presenting as a locked knee. Injury. 1997;28(9-10):707–8.
6. MacDonald PB. Combined tear of the posterior cruciate and medial collateral ligaments resulting in a locked knee. Arthroscopy. 1997;13(5):639–40.
7. Shelbourne KD, Johnson GE. Locked bucket-handle meniscal tears in knees with chronic anterior cruciate ligament deficiency. Am J Sports Med. 1993;21(6):779–82.
8. Brinsden MD, Parsons SW, Peace PK. Intra-articular migration of anterior cruciate ligament graft fixation presenting as a locked knee. Injury. 2003;34(5):383–4.
9. Swenning TA, Prohaska DJ. Isolated posterior cruciate ligament rupture presenting as a locked knee. Arthroscopy. 2004;20(4):429–31.
10. Seki K, Mine T, Tanaka H, Isida Y, Taguchi T. Locked knee caused by intraarticular ganglion. Knee Surg Sports Traumatol Arthrosc. 2006;14(9):859–61.
11. Espejo-Baena A, Coretti SM, Fernandez JM, Garcia-Herrera JM, Del Pino JR. Knee locking due to a single gouty tophus. J Rheumatol. 2006;33(1):193–5.
12. Krappel FA, Bauer E, Harland U. The migration of a BioScrew as a differential diagnosis of knee pain, locking after ACL reconstruction: a report of two cases. Arch Orthop Trauma Surg. 2006;126(9):615–20.
13. Hirano K, Deguchi M, Kanamono T. Intra-articular synovial lipoma of the knee joint (located in the lateral recess): a case report and review of the literature. Knee. 2007;14(1):63–7.
14. Appelt A, Baier M. Recurrent locking of knee joint caused by intraarticular migration of bioabsorbable tibial interference screw after arthroscopic ACL reconstruction. Knee Surg Sports Traumatol Arthrosc. 2007;15(4):378–80.
15. Jandhyala R, Wilson A, Bhagat S, Lavelle J. An unusual cause of locking. Knee Surg Sports Traumatol Arthrosc. 2007;15(5):682–4.
16. Elliott JM, Tirman PF, Grainger AJ, Brown DH, Campbell RS, Genant HK. MR appearances of the locked knee. Br J Radiol. 2000;73(874):1120–6.
17. McNally EG, Nasser KN, Dawson S, Goh LA. Role of magnetic resonance imaging in the clinical management of the acutely locked knee. Skelet Radiol. 2002;31(10):570–3.
18. Helmark IC, Neergaard K, Krogsgaard MR. Traumatic knee extension deficit (the locked knee): can MRI reduce the need for arthroscopy? Knee Surg Sports Traumatol Arthrosc. 2007;15(7):863–8.
19. Charalambous CP. Professionalism in surgery. In: Carrer skills for surgeons. Springer, cham. 2017.

Chapter 16
Knee Instability

This is a condition where there is symptomatic translation of one articulating surface in relation to another. The patient may experience pain, discomfort or apprehension, along with a feeling of the joint slipping out of place, or the knee giving way.

Knee instability may involve the tibiofemoral, patellofemoral (PF) or proximal tibiofibular joint.

This chapter discusses the principles in diagnosing, describing, classifying, investigating and managing instability around the knee. The need to differentiate between instability and laxity is also discussed.

16.1 Describing Knee Instability

Knee instability may be described in various ways and some of these are presented below.

According to the Joint Involved
One or more joints may be simultaneously affected by instability.

C. Panayiotou Charalambous, *The Knee Made Easy*,
https://doi.org/10.1007/978-3-030-54506-2_16

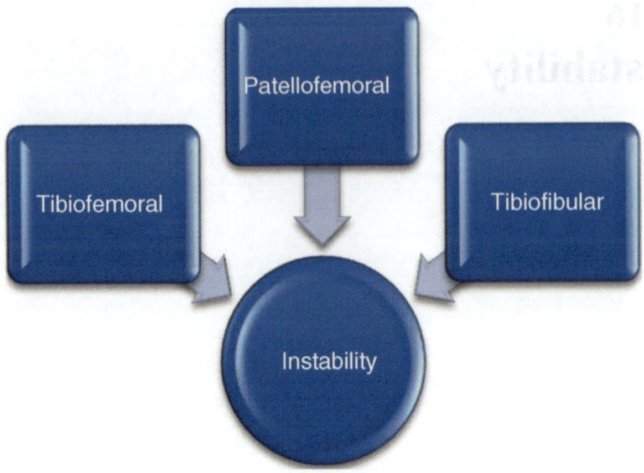

Instability may be described according to which articulation of the knee is involved

Number of Instability Episodes
- First time instability—refers to the first episode of instability
- Recurrent instability—refers to more than one episode of instability

Degree of Translation
- Subluxation
- Dislocation

One articulating surface may sublux (displace but still remain in partial contact with the opposite articulating surface). Alternatively, a joint may dislocate (with loss of all articular contact).

Reducibility
- Spontaneously reducible
- Spontaneously irreducible

Following dislocation the articulating surfaces may either spontaneously relocate or be locked in a dislocated position and need to be reduced medically by closed or open means.

According to the Direction of Translation of one Articulating Surface to the Other
- PF joint—translation of the patella in relation to the femoral trochlea
  - Lateral
  - Medial

- Tibiofemoral joint—translation of the tibia in relation to the femur
  - Sagittal—Anterior/posterior
  - Rotational
  - Coronal
  - Varus
  - Valgus
  - Multi directional—instability occurs in two or more directions
- Proximal tibiofibular—translation of the proximal fibula in relation to the tibia
  - Antero-lateral
  - Postero-medial
  - Superior

The direction of instability can be determined by:

- Clinical history—identifying the position that reproduces instability symptoms
- Clinical examination
  - Visual inspection
  - Palpation
  - Instability provocation tests
- Radiographs or other radiological investigations
  - If there is intermittent instability there is a need to review any radiological investigations obtained at the time of dislocation or subluxation
  - The patient may be asked to take a photograph of the knee at the time the event occurs (such as with the patella in a dislocated position)

According to the Initiating Event

- Congenital
- Acquired
  - Traumatic—as a result of specific, substantial trauma
  - Atraumatic—occurring with no precipitating substantial trauma
  - Microtraumatic—as a result of repetitive soft tissue injury

According to the Frequency of Instability

- First time—the first episode of instability
- Recurrent—the second or subsequent episode of instability
- Permanent—present all time
- Intermittent—alternating instability with stability
- Habitual—occurring with each flexion/extension cycle of the knee

According to the Presence of Volition

- Voluntary—the patient may dislocate a joint by influencing muscle contraction or by placing the knee in a particular position (such as tibiofemoral subluxation in young children, or patellar dislocation by flexing the knee and contracting vastus lateralis) [1, 2]

Involuntary—the patient cannot achieve the above

16.2 Causes of Knee Instability

Instability may be due to disruption or inefficiency of dynamic or static stabilisers:

Static

- Detached
- Torn
- Stretched

Dynamic

- Weak
- Uncoordinated
- Lack of stable platform to act upon

Abnormal muscle activation—muscles may be weak and not provide the necessary contraction to maintain stability. Alternatively, there may be uncoordinated contraction of the muscles acting across the knee. Under normal conditions such muscles contract in a coordinated way to achieve stability. However, imbalance may occur if the activity of one muscle is substantially reduced [3–5]. If one of the muscles contracts less intensely than it should, it may be overcome by the force of the opposing muscles, causing subluxation or dislocation. Muscle imbalance may also occur if a muscle contracts more intensely than it should. Muscle imbalance (vastus medialis vs. vastus lateralis) may be seen in patellar instability.

Defective proprioception—for muscles to contract in a balanced way, the brain must receive necessary proprioceptive feedback, with regards the position of the knee, lower limb and overall body in space [6–9].

Excessive joint laxity—the capsule and knee ligaments contribute to joint stability. However, if these are lax their contributory stabilising effect diminishes. This may also be associated with defective proprioception and altered muscle strength. Excessive knee joint laxity may predispose to knee instability, and confer poorer results following stabilisation surgery [10–14].

Insufficient core control—knee stability is partially achieved by the coordinated contraction of muscles acting across the joint. Many of these muscles have attachments all the way up to the pelvis. Hence, motion of the pelvis and core may influence knee stability. The underlying core on which some movement occurs needs to be steady and balanced [15–17]. Poor core control may be considered analogous to trying to lift a weight which is unbalanced (huge on one site and small on the other).

Insufficient hip control—dysfunctional hip biomechanics may alter knee control and loading, predisposing to ligamentous tears or functional knee instability. Weakness of hip abductors, external rotators and extensors may predispose to dynamic valgus of the knee upon landing from jumping, increasing the strain on the ACL and predisposing to ACL tears [18–20].

Insufficient Ankle and Foot Control—Ankle control has been related to altered knee biomechanics and instability. Ankle instability may be related to decreased ankle dorsiflexion during landing activities, which in turn may place the knee in less flexion, predisposing to ACL tears [21, 22].

Insufficient ankle and foot control, is analogous to a weight lifter trying to lift a heavy weight bar whilst trying to balance on a wobbly ball.

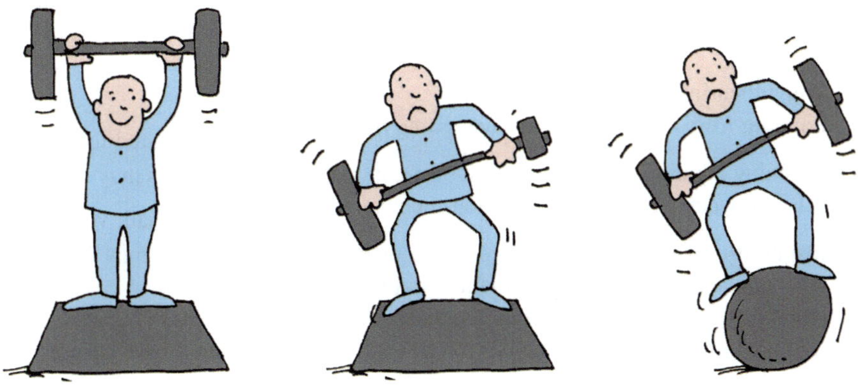

Poor core control is analogous to a weghtlifter trying to lift an unbalanced weight. Insufficient ankle and foot control, is analogous to a weightlifter trying to lift a heavy weight bar whilst balancing on a wobbly ball

16.3 Clinical Symptoms of Knee Instability

- Feeling of abnormal displacement—this may range from:
  - Feeling "wobbly" to
  - "Popping in and out" to
  - "Popping out and can't go back", "coming out to the edge" to
  - "Coming out fully"
- Knee giving way, locking
- Pain, vague, leg heaviness
- Clicking, clunking
- Dead leg syndrome, paraesthesia
- Dislocation—where a joint comes out of joint. In some cases the patient may be able to reduce the dislocated joint, or the joint may spontaneously reduce. Alternatively, the patient may need to attend hospital to have a reduction under sedation or general anaesthesia.
- Subluxation—where a knee joint almost comes out with a particular movement but then spontaneously reduces.
- Apprehension—fear of placing the leg in a particular position because the joint may slip out.

Symptoms may be aggravated by leg or knee position or motion:

- Rotational instability—as when turning or twisting
- Posterior instability—as when decelerating in a straight line, descending stairs
- PF instability—straightening the knee from full flexion, flexing knee from full extension
- Weightbearing vs. non-weightbearing
- Landing from a jump with the knee going into valgus

Questioning about the activities which bring on instability symptoms may help distinguish between a mechanical and non-mechanical cause.

- Instability on knee motion or upon the onset of weightbearing may signify a mechanical cause (such as ligament disruption)
- Instability occurring at rest, with the individual standing still, may signify a neurological/muscular cause (such as a reflex inhibition associated with knee pain)

Similarly, in mechanical instability, questioning about the leg/knee motion that brings on instability may guide as to the structures involved:

- Rotational instability may indicate anterior cruciate ligament (ACL) disruption
- Instability upon descending stairs may indicate posterior cruciate ligament (PCL) disruption
- Instability upon the stance phase of gait may indicate collateral ligament disruption

16.4 Clinical Signs of Knee Instability

These aim to assess:

- Apprehension, subluxation, dislocation and relocation of the examined joint
- Direction of instability
- Laxity of the tibiofemoral, PF, and proximal tibiofibular joints
- Generalised joint laxity
- Abnormal muscle activation
- Core weakness/imbalance

16.5 Investigations for Knee Instability

Investigations of the unstable knee aim to confirm the presence of instability, determine its likely cause, and identify any structural lesions that may be amenable to surgical intervention. These include:

- Radiological
  - Plain radiographs—including stress views (flexion kneeling lateral view for posterior tibiofemoral instability)
  - MRI/MRI arthrogram/CT Scan
- Neurophysiological
  - Nerve conduction studies
  - Electromyography
- Examination under general anaesthesia—joint translation and laxity is assessed with the patient under general anaesthesia to abolish pain and allow muscle relaxation
- Arthroscopic evaluation

16.6 Management of Knee Instability

Management depends on:

- Symptoms—severity, frequency
- Underlying cause
- Direction of instability
- Functional impairment—effect on day to day function, recreational or other activities

Management aims to relocate the joint (if dislocated) and improve joint stability to minimise the risk of further subluxations or dislocations. Interventions may thus help to improve associated functional loss, apprehension, or pain.

16.6.1 Non-surgical

- Activity modification, avoiding unstable leg/knee positions
- External devices—taping, bracing, ankle foot orthotics
- Physiotherapy to address deficits in:
  - Core imbalance—core strengthening
  - Poor pelvic control—strengthening of pelvic muscles
  - Poor hip control –weakness of abductors, extensors, external rotators
  - Foot and ankle control/position
  - Proprioception—proprioceptive training
  - Abnormal muscle patterning—biofeedback, inhibit overactive and enhance underactive muscles, improve neuromuscular control
  - Quadriceps and hamstring weakness- muscle strengthening, balance

It should be noted that non-surgical management does not specifically address any damaged or stretched static joint restraints, but aims to improve stability by enhancing the function of dynamic stabilisers (through strengthening, better control and coordination). A torn ligament (such as the ACL or medial patellofemoral ligament (MPFL)) will not be replaced by physiotherapy, but muscles may be strengthened to compensate for the torn ligament.

16.6.2 Surgical

If symptoms do not improve with non-surgical intervention and patient has structural lesions that are amenable to surgery, surgery may be considered. Structural derangements are corrected either directly or indirectly.

- Directly—correct the structural defect itself
- Indirectly—compensate for the structural defect

Surgical interventions for stability may be described according to the structures addressed as:

- Soft tissue procedure
- Bony procedure
- Combined soft-tissue/bony procedure

It is important to recognise that:

- Surgery addresses only structural defects, hence, other, non-structural contributors to instability may still need addressing with physiotherapy
- Correcting structural defects may facilitate the correction of other contributors such as:
  - Proprioception
  - Abnormal muscle patterning

16.7 Special Situations of Knee Instability

Certain considerations must be made in some specific instability scenarios and these are described below.

16.7.1 Initial Presentation after an ACL Tear

It is recognised that a substantial proportion of patients with an ACL tear continue to be symptomatic with their knee giving way, either in day to day activities or upon higher demand activities. In contrast, a substantial proportion of patients continue to function well in day to day and recreational activities even though their ACL is torn.

Hence, when faced with a patient after an ACL tear, one needs to decide as to whether to administer physiotherapy and then assess how the knee behaves, reserving surgery only for those who return with symptomatic knee instability. The alternative is to offer surgery to all or to a targeted group of individuals (based on parameters that may predispose them to on-going instability), once the acute inflammation of the knee settles and full extension is achieved.

There is currently insufficient evidence to answer this question. It is recognised that a delay in ACL reconstruction may be associated with an increased risk of further meniscal injuries or chondral damage. Hence, there is an argument for offering early surgery to young individuals who are planning to return to high demand activities, or activities that require rotational control (turning or twisting). This is the option favoured by the author as it avoids the two extremes [23, 24].

16.7.2 First time Patellar Dislocator

It is recognised that an initial lateral dislocation of the patella (traumatic or with minimal trauma) is associated with an increased risk of subsequent instability, especially in young individuals [25–30]. When faced with a first time patellar dislocator the consideration is to either:

- Reduce the patella and also intervene surgically to stabilise the PF joint to minimise the risk of subsequent dislocations (with MPFL repair or reconstruction), especially in subgroups of patients who have certain factors that may predispose them to increased risk of recurrent instability.
- Reduce the patella, observe and rehabilitate, and only consider intervening if further (recurrent) dislocations occur.

At the moment there is no high quality evidence supporting one approach over the other, hence the second option is favoured by the author as that is the least invasive approach.

16.7.3 Non-Compliant Patients

Certain patient groups may be less likely to comply with medical guidance following surgical intervention such as soft tissue stabilisation surgery. Such patients may be those with learning difficulties, history of alcohol or substance abuse. Options for this group of patients include:

- Symptomatic treatment avoiding surgical intervention
- Surgical intervention with more robust bracing/plastering post-surgery

16.7.4 Posterolateral Corner Injury

Posterolateral corner (PLC) injuries are often associated with other ligamentous injuries (ACL, PCL) and hence may be overlooked in the acute presentation. Such injuries may involve avulsion of the PLC stabilisers from their point of insertion, which may be amenable to reattachment if identified early. If initially overlooked, and only recognised at a later stage (more than 3 weeks), reattachment of such avulsed ligaments may not be possible and reconstruction surgery (which is more extensive surgery) may become essential. Hence, it is vital to examine for PLC injuries in the acutely injured knee. Even when extensive knee swelling, pain and tenderness are present, it is usually possible to perform the dial test to assess the PLC [31, 32].

16.7.5 Instability vs. Hyperlaxity

Laxity is a physiological condition that is different to instability but may predispose to the development of knee instability.

Lax joints may have longer and more stretchable ligaments which permit greater translation of their articular surfaces, and thus greater range of motion. Most patients with hyperlaxity do not have instability as they can maintain their joints in situ through dynamic control, despite having substantially more joint motion than the average norm. Hence, they do not have symptomatic abnormal joint translation [33].

Excessive joint translation does not equate to instability. Similarly, it is possible to have knee instability without hyperlaxity. Hyperlaxity, however, may increase the risk of knee instability.

Some causes of hyperlaxity are described below:

Congenital

- Benign joint hypermobility syndrome (may affect up to 20% of the population, more common in women, Asians and Africans) [34, 35]
- Connective tissue disorders
  - Marfan's syndrome
  - Ehlers-Danlos syndrome
  - Osteogenesis imperfecta

Acquired

- Repetitive microtrauma causing stretching of the capsule and ligaments—in athletes such as ballet dancers or gymnasts [36, 37]

Generalized joint laxity per se does not require any treatment and is usually asymptomatic. It may be apparent on clinical examination as:

- Hyperextension or hyperflexion of the tibiofemoral articulation
- Excessive medial or lateral translation of the tibia in relation to the femur upon varus or valgus loading
- Excessive lateral translation of the patella at the PF joint

Such constitutional laxity is usually bilateral, hence comparison with the opposite knee is essential.

16.7.6 Knee Instability in Osteoarthritis [38–40]

Patients with degenerative changes of the knee may complain of instability, with the knee giving way or buckling. This may be due to a true mechanical cause such as intermittent locking due a loose body or meniscal tear, or due to ligament dysfunction. However, subjective reports of instability often do not correlate with objective findings upon clinical examination. It may be that instability in the arthritic knee is related to defective proprioception or altered muscle control.

Learning Pearls

Muscles are the main dynamic stabilisers of the knee joint. They allow the knee to maintain stability in high demand activities, even when the ligaments are disrupted (such as going back to sports with an ACL deficient knee). This important role of knee muscles may be appreciated by noting that the legs are feeling wobbly after a period of intense exercise (even though all the knee ligaments and other static stabilisers are intact).

References

1. Robinson D, Halperin N. Active knee joint subluxation: its influence on the prognosis of ligament reconstruction. Acta Orthop Scand. 1991;62(3):264–5.
2. Parikh SN, Lykissas MG. Classification of lateral patellar instability in children and adolescents. Orthop Clin North Am. 2016;47(1):145–52.
3. Hortobágyi T, Westerkamp L, Beam S, Moody J, Garry J, Holbert D, DeVita P. Altered hamstring-quadriceps muscle balance in patients with knee osteoarthritis. Clin Biomech (Bristol, Avon). 2005;20(1):97–104.
4. Tsepis E, Vagenas G, Giakas G, Georgoulis A. Hamstring weakness as an indicator of poor knee function in ACL-deficient patients. Knee Surg Sports Traumatol Arthrosc. 2004;12(1):22–9.
5. Horlings CG, Küng UM, van Engelen BG, Voermans NC, Hengstman GJ, van der Kooi AJ, Bloem BR, Allum JH. Balance control in patients with distal versus proximal muscle weakness. Neuroscience. 2009;164(4):1876–86.
6. McCaughan D, Booth A, Jackson C, Lalor S, Ramdharry G, O'Connor RJ, Phillips M, Bowers R, McDaid C. Orthotic management of instability of the knee related to neuromuscular and central nervous system disorders: qualitative interview study of patient perspectives. BMJ Open. 2019;9(10):e029313. https://doi.org/10.1136/bmjopen-2019-029313.
7. Kim HJ, Lee JH, Lee DH. Proprioception in patients with anterior cruciate ligament tears: a meta-analysis comparing injured and uninjured limbs. Am J Sports Med. 2017;45(12):2916–22.
8. van der Esch M, van der Leeden M, Roorda LD, Lems WF, Dekker J. Predictors of self-reported knee instability among patients with knee osteoarthritis: results of the Amsterdam osteoarthritis cohort. Clin Rheumatol. 2016;35(12):3007–13.
9. Chang AH, Lee SJ, Zhao H, Ren Y, Zhang LQ. Impaired varus-valgus proprioception and neuromuscular stabilization in medial knee osteoarthritis. J Biomech. 2014;47(2):360–6.
10. Nomura E, Inoue M, Kobayashi S. Generalized joint laxity and contralateral patellar hypermobility in unilateral recurrent patellar dislocators. Arthroscopy. 2006;22(8):861–5.
11. Smith TO, Jerman E, Easton V, Bacon H, Armon K, Poland F, Macgregor AJ. Do people with benign joint hypermobility syndrome (BJHS) have reduced joint proprioception? A systematic review and meta-analysis. Rheumatol Int. 2013;33(11):2709–16.
12. Lee HM, Cheng CK, Liau JJ. Correlation between proprioception, muscle strength, knee laxity, and dynamic standing balance in patients with chronic anterior cruciate ligament deficiency. Knee. 2009;16(5):387–91.
13. Larson CM, Bedi A, Dietrich ME, Swaringen JC, Wulf CA, Rowley DM, Giveans MR. Generalized hypermobility, knee hyperextension, and outcomes after anterior cruciate ligament reconstruction: prospective, case-control study with mean 6 years follow-up. Arthroscopy. 2017;33(10):1852–8.
14. Howells NR, Eldridge JD. Medial patellofemoral ligament reconstruction for patellar instability in patients with hypermobility: a case control study. J Bone Joint Surg Br. 2012;94(12):1655–9.

15. Zazulak BT, Hewett TE, Reeves NP, Goldberg B, Cholewicki J. Deficits in neuromuscular control of the trunk predict knee injury risk: a prospective biomechanical-epidemiologic study. Am J Sports Med. 2007;35(7):1123–30.
16. Zazulak BT, Hewett TE, Reeves NP, Goldberg B, Cholewicki J. The effects of core proprioception on knee injury: a prospective biomechanical-epidemiological study. Am J Sports Med. 2007;35(3):368–73.
17. Hewett TE, Myer GD. The mechanistic connection between the trunk, knee, and anterior cruciate ligament injury. Exerc Sport Sci Rev. 2011;39(4):161–6.
18. Hewett TE, Torg JS, Boden BP. Video analysis of trunk and knee motion during non-contact anterior cruciate ligament injury in female athletes: lateral trunk and knee abduction motion are combined components of the injury mechanism. Br J Sports Med. 2009;43(6):417–22.
19. Cashman GE. The effect of weak hip abductors or external rotators on knee valgus kinematics in healthy subjects: a systematic review. J Sport Rehabil. 2012;21(3):273–84.
20. Jacobs CA, Uhl TL, Mattacola CG, Shapiro R, Rayens WS. Hip abductor function and lower extremity landing kinematics: sex differences. J Athl Train. 2007;42(1):76–83.
21. Hoch MC, Farwell KE, Gaven SL, Weinhandl JT. Weight-bearing dorsiflexion range of motion and landing biomechanics in individuals with chronic ankle instability. J Athl Train. 2015;50(8):833–9.
22. Theisen A, Day J. Chronic ankle instability leads to lower extremity kinematic changes during landing tasks: a systematic review. Int J Exerc Sci. 2019;12(1):24–33.
23. Ferguson D, Palmer A, Khan S, Oduoza U, Atkinson H. Early or delayed anterior cruciate ligament reconstruction: Is one superior? A systematic review and meta-analysis. Eur J Orthop Surg Traumatol. 2019;29(6):1277–89.
24. Deabate L, Previtali D, Grassi A, Filardo G, Candrian C, Delcogliano M. Anterior cruciate ligament reconstruction within 3 weeks does not increase stiffness and complications compared with delayed reconstruction: a meta-analysis of randomized controlled trials. Am J Sports Med. 2019;5:363546519862294. https://doi.org/10.1177/0363546519862294.
25. Parikh SN, Lykissas MG, Gkiatas I. Predicting risk of recurrent patellar dislocation. Curr Rev Musculoskelet Med. 2018;11(2):253–60.
26. Lewallen L, McIntosh A, Dahm D. First-time patellofemoral dislocation: risk factors for recurrent instability. J Knee Surg. 2015;28(4):303–9.
27. Christensen TC, Sanders TL, Pareek A, Mohan R, Dahm DL, Krych AJ. Risk factors and time to recurrent ipsilateral and contralateral patellar dislocations. Am J Sports Med. 2017;45(9):2105–10.
28. Huntington LS, Webster KE, Devitt BM, Scanlon JP, Feller JA. Factors associated with an increased risk of recurrence after a first-time patellar dislocation: a systematic review and meta-analysis. Am J Sports Med. 2019;11:363546519888467. https://doi.org/10.1177/0363546519888467.
29. Martin RK, Leland DP, Krych AJ, Dahm DL. Treatment of first-time patellar dislocations and evaluation of risk factors for recurrent patellar instability. Sports Med Arthrosc Rev. 2019;27(4):130–5.
30. Smith TO, Donell S, Song F, Hing CB. Surgical versus non-surgical interventions for treating patellar dislocation. Cochrane Database Syst Rev. 2015;(2):CD008106. https://doi.org/10.1002/14651858.CD008106.pub3.
31. Pacheco RJ, Ayre CA, Bollen SR. Posterolateral corner injuries of the knee: a serious injury commonly missed. J Bone Joint Surg Br. 2011;93(2):194–7.
32. LaPrade RF, Wentorf FA, Fritts H, Gundry C, Hightower CD. A prospective magnetic resonance imaging study of the incidence of posterolateral and multiple ligament injuries in acute knee injuries presenting with a hemarthrosis. Arthroscopy. 2007;23(12):1341–7.
33. Maffulli N. Laxity versus instability. Orthopedics. 1998;21(8):837. 842
34. Hakim A, Grahame R. Joint hypermobility. Best Pract Res Clin Rheumatol. 2003;17(6):989–1004.

35. Jessee EF, Owen DS Jr, Sagar KB. The benign hypermobile joint syndrome. Arthritis Rheum. 1980;23(9):1053–6.
36. Rehmani R, Endo Y, Bauman P, Hamilton W, Potter H, Adler R. Lower extremity injury patterns in elite ballet dancers: ultrasound/MRI imaging features and an institutional overview of therapeutic ultrasound guided percutaneous interventions. HSS J. 2015;11(3):258–77.
37. Miller EH, Schneider HJ, Bronson JL, McLain D. A new consideration in athletic injuries. The classical ballet dancer. Clin Orthop Relat Res. 1975;111:181–91.
38. Chaudhari AMW, Schmitt LC, Freisinger GM, Lewis JM, Hutter EE, Pan X, Siston RA. Perceived instability is associated with strength and pain, not frontal knee laxity, in patients with advanced knee osteoarthritis. J Orthop Sports Phys Ther. 2019;49(7):513–7.
39. Wallace DT, Riches PE, Picard F. The assessment of instability in the osteoarthritic knee. EFORT Open Rev. 2019;4(3):70–6.
40. Freisinger GM, Hutter EE, Lewis J, Granger JF, Glassman AH, Beal MD, Pan X, Schmitt LC, Siston RA, Chaudhari AMW. Relationships between varus-valgus laxity of the severely osteoarthritic knee and gait, instability, clinical performance, and function. J Orthop Res. 2017;35(8):1644–52.

Chapter 17
Knee Weakness

Knee weakness may be defined as loss of strength or power of knee motion due to inability to create an adequate force. This may be painless or painful. This chapter discusses the concepts of true and apparent weakness and discusses the causes of true knee weakness, its investigation and management.

17.1 True Versus Apparent Knee Weakness

In dealing with knee weakness it is essential to distinguish between true and apparent weakness.

Apparent weakness may be due to:

- Pain
- Instability

Apparent weakness may be due to the patient being reluctant to move the knee, or exert a strong force across the knee, as that would cause pain and the patient may refer to this reduction of knee motion as weakness. Apparent weakness may also be seen in underlying knee instability, whereby the patient avoids a particular knee movement because that may lead to subluxation or dislocation. Hence, it is necessary to determine whether one is dealing with apparent weakness or true weakness where there is loss of active motion due to inability to create sufficient force strength across a joint.

C. Panayiotou Charalambous, *The Knee Made Easy*,
https://doi.org/10.1007/978-3-030-54506-2_17

True weakness may manifest in inability to perform day to day activities or more strenuous activities. It may present as inability to generate an adequate sudden force or as reduction of endurance.

When examining for weakness it is essential to minimise pain (with parenteral analgesia or with an injection of local anaesthetic into the painful area) to allow the examiner to assess strength.

17.2 Causes of Knee Weakness [1]

In evaluating the cause of weakness one must consider normal motor control. Control of motion begins in the primary motor cortex of the brain's frontal lobe. Like other parts of the body the knee is represented in the primary motor cortex. Upper motor neurons in the primary motor cortex give rise to nerve fibres that descend through the brain stem, where most of them cross to the opposite side of the body and form the corticospinal tract that descends through the spine. These nerve fibres terminate at the appropriate spinal level where they synapse and transmit messages to lower motor neurons, the cell bodies of which are located in the ventral horn of the grey matter of the spinal cord. Ventral horn lower motor neurons transmit nerve signals through the ventral roots and then through peripheral roots to muscles. Transmission occurs from the nerve to muscle at the neuro-muscular junction. This leads to muscle fibre activation and contraction. Contraction allows a muscle to act via its tendon and the tendon's insertion onto the bone to apply a force and adjust movement. In addition to the above neural pathway, neurons originate in the brain stem (basal ganglia) and influence other aspects of motion such as coordination [2–5]. Hence, knee weakness may be the result of a deficit occurring anywhere in a pathway that starts in the brain and finishes at the tendon-bone junction, as described below.

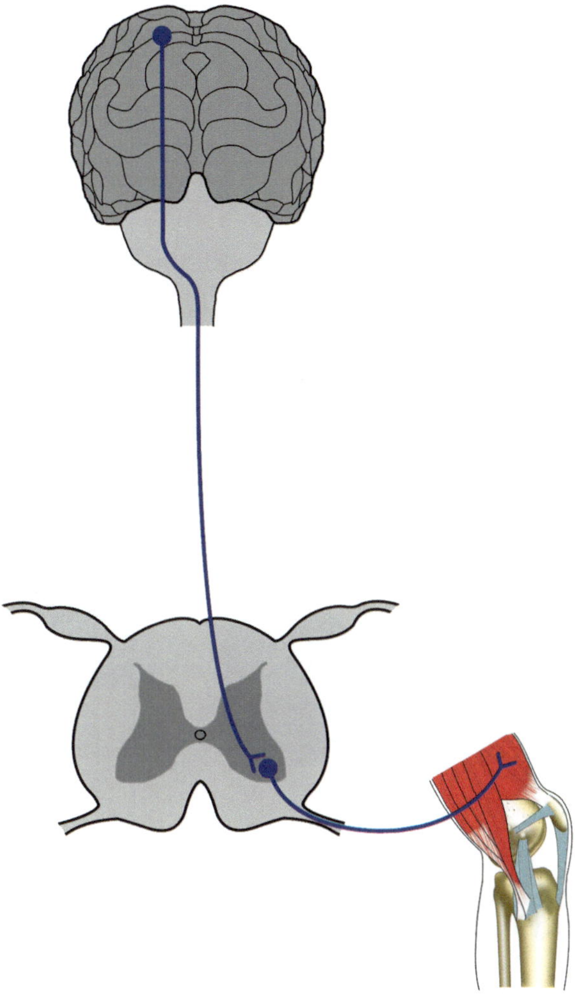

Motor pathways from brain to knee muscles

- Neurological causes of weakness
  - Upper neurone lesion
    - Brain
    - Spinal cord
  - Lower motor neurone lesion
    - Spinal cord
    - Peripheral nerve
  - Neuromuscular junction

- Muscular causes of weakness
  - Myopathies
  - Muscular tears
- Tendinous causes of weakness
  - Tear
  - Avulsion from insertion onto bone
- Bony causes -that impairs the ability of muscles and tendons to exert their normal function
  - Joint instability
  - Malalignment (e.g. post-traumatic)

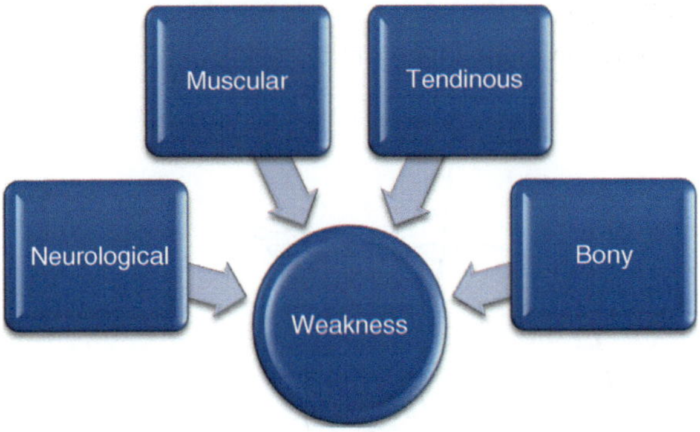

Sources of knee weakness

17.3 Identifying the Cause of Knee Weakness

In trying to determine the cause of knee weakness some of the factors to consider in the clinical history and clinical examination are:

- Painful or painless?
- Involves one or more muscles?
- Isolated knee or multiple joint weakness?
- Unilateral or bilateral weakness?
- Gradual or sudden onset?
- Onset related to precipitating factor (such as trauma)?
- Fluctuating, constant or deteriorating weakness?
- Associated sensory symptoms?
- Family history of neuromuscular conditions?
- History of exposure to muscle or nerve toxic agents or conditions?

- Exposure to muscle or nerve toxic medicines?
- Weak muscles innervated by one or multiple nerves?
- Does the weakness follow a peripheral nerve pattern, spinal root or central nervous system (spinal cord or brain) pattern?
- Lower or upper motor neurone symptoms and signs?
- Loss of muscle bulk (muscle wasting)?
- Associated rigidity or lack of coordination?
- Nerve and muscle activity may be affected by various conditions that are sought of in the clinical history and include:
  - Inflammatory disorders (e.g. rheumatological disorders)
  - Endocrine disorders (e.g. thyroid dysfunction)
  - Metabolic conditions (e.g. diabetes mellitus)
  - Neoplasia (e.g. paraneoplastic syndromes, direct infiltration)
  - Infection
  - Alcohol
  - Medicines
- *Painful weakness* may be due to:
  - Inflammation—following an injury and tendon tear
  - Mechanical factors

    Quadriceps tendon tears

  - Nerve dysfunction—nerve irritation, compression, intrinsic neuritis
- *Upper motor neuron lesions* may lead to:
  - Minimal muscle atrophy (some atrophy may develop due to disuse)
  - Absent fasciculations
  - Increased spasticity
  - Exaggerated reflexes
- *Lower motor neuron lesions* may lead to:
  - Reduced muscle tone
  - Reduced reflex responses
  - Muscle atrophy
  - Fasciculations
- *Associated sensory symptoms* may suggest a neurological rather than an intrinsic muscular cause
- *Fluctuating strength* may be seen in:
  - Myopathy such as myasthenia gravis
  - Central disorders such as transient ischaemic attacks

- *Onset of weakness*
  - Sudden—traumatic—may suggest structural failure such as tendon tear
  - Sudden non-traumatic—may suggest a neurological cause such as neuritis or central nerve system dysfunction
  - Gradual onset—may suggest degenerative tendon tear, or neurological cause
- *Distribution of weakness*
  - Neuromuscular conditions (neuropathies, myopathies) tend to affect multiple joints or body parts rather than just the knee
  - Myopathies tend to be proximal and bilateral
- *Tone and coordination*
  - Rigidity or lack of coordination (e.g. in Parkinson's disease) may present as weakness because of difficulty in performing motor activities.
- *Family history*
  - Some neuropathies or myopathies are hereditary with positive family history

Frequently encountered causes of knee weakness include:

- Apparent weakness related to knee pain
- True weakness related to:
  - Extensor mechanism disruption (quadriceps or patellar tendon tear)
  - Lumbosacral spondylosis causing nerve root impingement

17.3.1 Investigations for Knee Weakness

Investigations of the weak knee aim to confirm the presence of true weakness and its likely cause, and exclude any possible alternative diagnoses. These include:

- Radiological
  - Plain radiographs
  - MRI/CT Scan
- Neurophysiological
  - Nerve conduction studies
  - Electromyography
- Haematological—Inflammatory screen, glucose control, thyroid function tests
- Diagnostic local anaesthetic injections
- Arthroscopic evaluation
- Examination under anaesthesia

17.4 Management of Knee Weakness

Management of weakness involves:

- Addressing deficiencies in the neuromuscular control of motion
- Addressing the underlying condition which may have led to neuromuscular dysfunction (diabetes, thyroid disorders, inflammatory arthritis)
- Addressing the structures the discontinuity of which may account for the mechanical loss of motion (such as a torn tendon)
- Strengthening alternative muscles to take over and compensate for what is lost [6, 7]
- Strengthening muscles to compensate for lost ligaments contributing to apparent weakness due to instability [8–11]—such as:
  - Strengthening the hamstring muscles to compensate for a torn anterior cruciate ligament (ACL)
  - Strengthening quadriceps to compensate for a torn posterior cruciate ligament (PCL)

In tackling the deficient structures the management ladder [12] is followed although on occasion initial steps may be bypassed.

- Non-surgical management
  - Physiotherapy aims to strengthen weak muscles, or strengthen alternative ones to compensate for weak ones
  - Bracing aims to compensate for weak muscles and aid joint stability and thus mobilisation
  - Steroid injections may:

    Reduce neural pressure due to perineural inflammation or mass lesions to improve nerve function
    Improve knee pain to aid muscle strengthening exercises

- Surgical management [13–26]
  This is directed towards the structures contributing to weakness and may include:
  Soft tissue

  a. Nerve dysfunction may be addressed:
     i. Directly by nerve surgery
     ii. Indirectly by tendon transfers

  b. Tendon tears may be addressed by:
     i. Primary repair +/− augmentation/bridging
     ii. Tendon transfers or reconstruction

- Bony

  a. Reposition (reducing a dislocated joint)
  b. Realignment (osteotomy)- to improve apparent weakness due to pain or instability, improve efficiency of the muscle-tendon-bone functional unit
  c. Resection/removal (lesions causing nerve pressure or altering muscle biomechanics)
  d. Arthroplasty

     i. Constrained replacement arthroplasty—to improve joint stability to compensate for weak muscles
     ii. Fusion arthroplasty—to improve joint stability to compensate for weak muscles

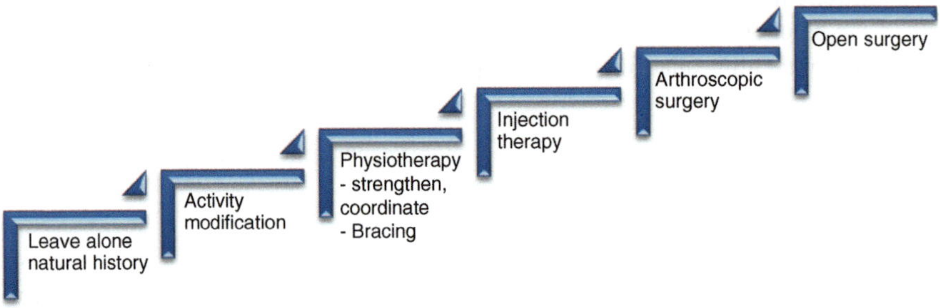

Management ladder for knee weakness

Learning Pearls

The presence of weakness may be:

- Objective, based on clinical examination findings
- Subjective, based on how the patient perceives their leg strength compared to their usual strength, or compared to their good leg strength

Even if the examiner is not be able to elicit the weakness that the patient describes, the possibility they true weakness exists should be considered and investigated further.

References

1. Charalambos CP. Shoulder weakness. In: The shoulder made easy: Springer; 2019. p. 217–23.
2. Benjamin-Cummings Publishing Company. In: Martini FH, Nath JL, Bartholomew EF, editors. Fundamentals of Anatomy & Physiology: Benjamin-Cummings Publishing Company; 2011.
3. Elsevier Inc. In: Rea P, editor. Essential clinical anatomy of the nervous system: Elsevier Inc; 2015.

4. Imperial Company Printers. In: Reeves AG, editor. Disorders of the nervous system: a primer. 3rd ed: Imperial Company Printers; 1995.
5. Garg N, Park SB, Vucic S, Yiannikas C, Spies J, Howells J, Huynh W, Matamala JM, Krishnan AV, Pollard JD, Cornblath DR, Reilly MM, Kiernan MC. Differentiating lower motor neuron syndromes. J Neurol Neurosurg Psychiatry. 2017;88(6):474–83.
6. van der Krogt MM, Delp SL, Schwartz MH. How robust is human gait to muscle weakness? Gait Posture. 2012;36(1):113–9.
7. Thompson JA, Chaudhari AM, Schmitt LC, Best TM, Siston RA. Gluteus maximus and soleus compensate for simulated quadriceps atrophy and activation failure during walking. J Biomech. 2013;46(13):2165–72.
8. Fowler PJ, Regan WD. The patient with symptomatic chronic anterior cruciate ligament insufficiency. Results of minimal arthroscopic surgery and rehabilitation. Am J Sports Med. 1987;15(4):321–5.
9. Pattee GA, Fox JM, Del Pizzo W, Friedman MJ. Four to ten year followup of unreconstructed anterior cruciate ligament tears. Am J Sports Med. 1989;17(3):430–5.
10. Cosgarea AJ, Jay PR. Posterior cruciate ligament injuries: evaluation and management. J Am Acad Orthop Surg. 2001;9(5):297–307.
11. Toritsuka Y, Horibe S, Hiro-Oka A, Mitsuoka T, Nakamura N. Conservative treatment for rugby football players with an acute isolated posterior cruciate ligament injury. Knee Surg Sports Traumatol Arthrosc. 2004;12(2):110–4.
12. Charalambous CP. Professionalism in surgery. In: Career skills for surgeons: Springer; 2017. p. 5–46.
13. Aydin A, Ozkan T, Aydin HU, Topalan M, Erer M, Ozkan S, Yildirim ZH. The results of surgical repair of sciatic nerve injuries. Acta Orthop Traumatol Turc. 2010;44(1):48–53.
14. Abou-Al-Shaar H, Yoon N, Mahan MA. Surgical repair of sciatic nerve traumatic rupture: technical considerations and approaches. Neurosurg Focus. 2018;44(VideoSuppl1):V3. https://doi.org/10.3171/2018.1.FocusVid.17568.
15. O'Malley MP, Pareek A, Reardon P, Krych A, Stuart MJ, Levy BA. Treatment of peroneal nerve injuries in the multiligament injured/dislocated knee. J Knee Surg. 2016;29(4):287–92.
16. Doi K, Sem SH, Hattori Y, Sakamoto S, Hayashi K, Maruyama A. Contralateral obturator nerve to femoral nerve transfer for restoration of knee extension after acute flaccid myelitis: a case report. JBJS Case Connect. 2019;9(4):e0073. https://doi.org/10.2106/JBJS.CC.19.00073.
17. Patwa JJ, Bhatt HR, Chouksey S, Patel K. Hamstring transfer for quadriceps paralysis in post polio residual paralysis. Indian J Orthop. 2012;46(5):575–80.
18. Saito H, Shimada Y, Yamamura T, Yamada S, Sato T, Nozaka K, Kijima H, Saito K. Arthroscopic quadriceps tendon repair: two case reports. Case Rep Orthop. 2015;2015:937581. https://doi.org/10.1155/2015/937581.
19. Severyns M, Renard G, Guillou R, Odri GA, Labrada-Blanco O, Rouvillain JL. Arthroscopic suture repair of acute quadriceps tendon ruptures. Orthop Traumatol Surg Res. 2017;103(3):377–80.
20. Chahla J, DePhillipo NN, Cinque ME, Kennedy NI, Lebus GF, Familiari F, Moatshe G, LaPrade RF. Open repair of quadriceps tendon with suture anchors and semitendinosus tendon allograft augmentation. Arthrosc Tech. 2017;6(6):e2071–7.
21. Lamberti A, Loconte F, Spinarelli A, Baldini A. Bilateral extensor mechanism allograft reconstruction for chronic spontaneous rupture: a case report and review of the literature. JBJS Case Connect. 2019;9(2):e0058. https://doi.org/10.2106/JBJS.CC.18.00058.
22. Mascarenhas R, Mcrae S, MacDonald PB. Semitendinosus allograft reconstruction of chronic biceps femoris rupture at the knee. J Knee Surg. 2009;22(4):381–4.
23. Prasad A, Donovan R, Ramachandran M, Dawson-Bowling S, Millington S, Bhumbra R, Achan P, Hanna SA. Outcome of total knee arthroplasty in patients with poliomyelitis: a systematic review. EFORT Open Rev. 2018;3(6):358–62.

24. Rahman J, Hanna SA, Kayani B, Miles J, Pollock RC, Skinner JA, Briggs TW, Carrington RW. Custom rotating hinge total knee arthroplasty in patients with poliomyelitis affected limbs. Int Orthop. 2015;39(5):833–8.
25. Anderson LA, Culp BM, Della Valle CJ, Gililland JM, Meneghini RM, Browne JA, Springer BD. High failure rates of concomitant periprosthetic joint infection and extensor mechanism disruption. J Arthroplast. 2018;33(6):1879–83.
26. Rao MC, Richards O, Meyer C, Jones RS. Knee stabilisation following infected knee arthroplasty with bone loss and extensor mechanism impairment using a modular cemented nail. Knee. 2009;16(6):489–93.

Chapter 18
Knee Paraesthesia

Paraesthesia refers to altered or reduced sensation. It may involve the knee or be more extensive involving other parts of the lower limb. Paraesthesia may be associated with other knee symptoms or occur in isolation. This chapter discusses potential sources of knee and lower leg paraesthesia as well as principles in its diagnosis, investigation, and management.

18.1 Sensory Pathways [1]

In evaluating the cause of paraesthesia consideration is made to the normal control of sensation (touch, temperature or pain).

Crude touch, pain and temperature are perceived by tactile, pain, and temperature receptors in the skin and soft tissues. These stimulate nerves, the cell bodies of which are in the dorsal root ganglia of the spinal cord, at the corresponding level. These nerves synapse with, and transmit messages to upper neurones, the cell bodies of which are in the dorsal horn of the spinal cord. The fibres of these upper neurons cross to the opposite site of the body and ascend through the spinal cord as the spinothalamic tracts to the thalamus. From the thalamus further neurones transmit signals to the primary sensory cortex in the brain's frontal lobe.

Specific touch is perceived by tactile receptors in the skin and soft tissues which stimulate nerves, the cell bodies of which are located in the dorsal root ganglia of the spinal cord at the corresponding level. These nerves ascend through the posterior columns of the spinal cord to the medulla. At the medulla they synapse with neurones that cross to the opposite site of the body, and pass to the thalamus where they further synapse with neurones that pass to the primary sensory cortex in the frontal lobe [2–4].

Like other parts of the body the knee and lower limb are represented in the primary sensory cortex.

C. Panayiotou Charalambous, *The Knee Made Easy*,
https://doi.org/10.1007/978-3-030-54506-2_18

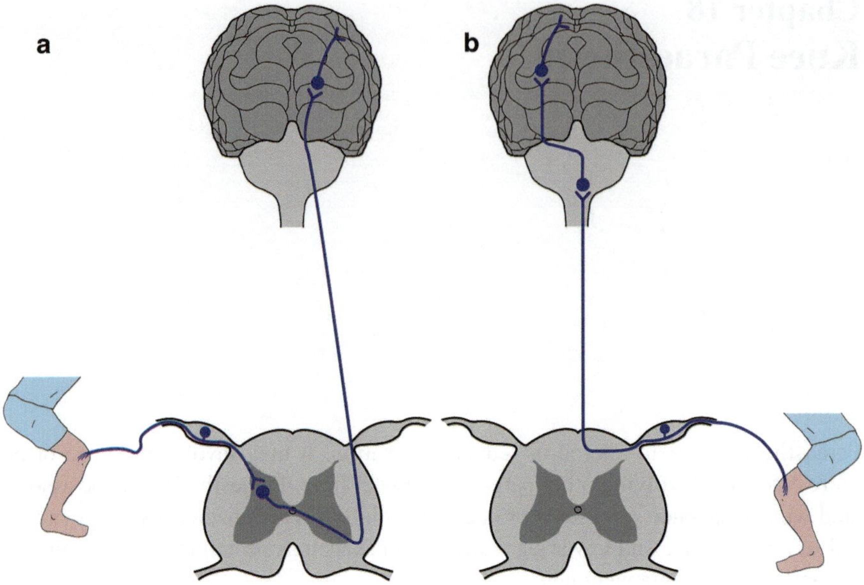

(**a**) Sensory pathways for pain and crude touch. (**b**) Sensory pathways for specific touch

18.2 Sites of Neurological Dysfunction

As demonstrated by the above neural pathways, paraesthesia may be the result of a deficit occurring anywhere between peripheral soft tissue receptors and brain. These include:

- Peripheral nerve
- Lumbar or sacral plexus
- Lumbosacral spine nerve roots
- Spinal cord
- Brain

18.3 Causes of Neurological Dysfunction

Nerve fibre activity may be impaired by [5–7]:

- Ischaemia
- Demyelination—leading to a decrease in conduction velocity
- Axonal degeneration—loss of nerve fibres

Nerve fibre activity may be affected by:

- Extrinsic lesions that impair nerve perfusion, metabolism, or structure such as:
  - Compression
  - Traction
  - Discontinuity—nerve laceration
- Intrinsic lesions—that impair nerve perfusion, metabolism, structure or function:
  - Inflammatory conditions (e.g. rheumatological)
  - Endocrine disorders (e.g. thyroid dysfunction)
  - Metabolic conditions (e.g. diabetes mellitus)
  - Neoplasia—paraneoplastic syndromes
  - Infection
  - Vitamin deficiency
  - Toxins
    - Alcohol
    - Medicines

The above principles may be applied to all neural levels (of the central or peripheral nervous system).

Nerve compression may lead to:

- Perineural oedema
- Demyelination
- Degeneration of distal axons
- Nerve sprout formation
- Regeneration of nerve fibres
- Remyelination

The duration and severity of paraesthesia may be related to the amount and duration of nerve compression:

- Intermittent paraesthesia may be due to intermittent compression that leads to intermittent interruption of the neural microcirculation by oedema.
- Constant paraesthesia may signify more severe prolonged compression that may lead to demyelination; symptoms recover once compression is relieved but this recovery can take a lot of time.
- Constant sensory loss may be due to severe compression leading to axon degeneration; symptoms fail to recover fully when compression is relieved.

Nerve traction (stretching) may have detrimental effects on nerve function similar to compression by:

- Increasing intraneural pressure
- Impairing nerve blood flow

Limitation of nerve gliding may lead to local nerve stretching with limb motion. Sudden application of substantial nerve traction may also lead to nerve discontinuity.

18.4 Conditions Leading to Knee Paraesthesia

Some of the common conditions causing knee paraesthesia are:

- Lumbosacral spondylosis causing nerve root impingement
- Surgical incisions of the knee or dissection during such incisions [8–11]
- Complex regional pain syndrome (CRPS) (Reflex Sympathetic Dystrophy) [12, 13]
  - Type 1—in the absence of specific nerve damage
  - Type 2—associated with major nerve damage

CRPS is characterised by hyperalgesia in response to light palpation, autonomic changes, trophic changes (dry and scaly skin), oedema, functional loss, stiffness, weakness, hyperhidrosis, pain out of proportion in relation to the severity of the insult and out of proportion in relation to the timing of the insult, being persistent for long time). Pain is regional (not in a particular nerve distribution) and has sensory, motor, and vasomotor changes. CRPS may reflect an exaggeration of normal physiological responses, involving multiple areas of the PNS and CNS resulting in excessive sympathetic output. Diagnosis of CRPS is clinical. It is often encountered following surgery or trauma. Treatment involves desensitization therapy (sensory stimulation using various textures), TENS, and graded gentle mobilisation to avoid permanent stiffness. It can be disabling to the patient, affecting activities of daily leaving and quality of life.

Other clinical conditions to consider include:

- Spina bifida
- Cerebrovascular accident
- Multiple sclerosis

18.5 Clinical Symptoms in Knee Paraesthesia

Patients may complain of:

- Altered sensation
- Pins and needles
- Reduced sensation
- Tingling
- Numbness
- Dead leg
- Associated knee symptoms—pain, instability, weakness, stiffness
- Hyperalgesia—pain on light touch e.g. by clothes, bed sheet

18.6 Clinical Examination in Knee Paraesthesia [14, 15]

- Assess overall posture
- Knee examination looking for evidence of:
  - Previous surgery or trauma
- A full neurological examination is carried out including:
  - Objective sensory assessment—light touch, pain, temperature, joint position
  - Mapping sensory deficit—in some cases symptoms may not be accompanied by objective demonstration of neurological dysfunction
  - Muscle activity:
    - Strength
    - Wasting
  - Reflexes
  - Tests for lumbosacral spine nerve root dysfunction
  - Tests for peripheral nerve lesion (Tinel's)
  - Lower limb strength, coordination, clonus
  - Signs of CRPS—hyperalgesia in response to light palpation, autonomic changes, trophic changes (dry and scaly skin), stiffness, weakness.

18.7 Identifying the Cause of Paraesthesia

In trying to determine the cause of paraesthesia factors to consider are:

- *Painful vs. painless*
  - Associated pain may suggest:
    - A lesion stimulating nociceptors and also impairing nerve function
    - An extrinsic lesion irritating the nerve
  - An intrinsic lesion causing nerve dysfunction—neuritis
  - CRPS
- *Distribution*
  - Nerve
    - Single peripheral nerve involvement
    - Multiple peripheral nerve involvement
    - Dermatomal
  - Unilateral or bilateral?
    - If bilateral, consider higher lesion—spinal cord, brain

- *Associated weakness or muscle atrophy*
  - This may signify a substantial disruption of nerve function (including its motor component) rather than intermittent nerve fibre ischaemia
  - An upper motor neuron lesion is associated with:
    - Minimal atrophy (some atrophy may develop because of disuse)
    - Absent fasciculations
    - Increased spasticity
    - Exaggerated stretch reflexes
  - A lower motor neuron lesion leads to:
    - Reduced muscle tone
    - Reduced reflex reactions
    - Atrophy
    - Fasciculations
- *Gradual vs. sudden onset*
  - Sudden –traumatic/surgical—may suggest structural nerve failure
  - Sudden non-traumatic—may suggest an intrinsic nerve cause such as neuritis or central nerve system dysfunction
  - Gradual onset—may suggest gradual onset compression as in lumbosacral spine spondylosis
- *Precipitating factor*
  - None
  - Trauma
    - Knee
    - Spine
    - Lower limb
  - Surgery
    - Arthroscopic or open knee surgery
    - Spine
    - Lower limb
- *Intermittent vs. constant*
- *Family history of neurological conditions*
  - Certain neuropathies are hereditary
- *Aggravating factors*
  - Posture
    - Standing upright worse—leaning forwards better –suggestive of spinal stenosis
- *Worse at night*

18.8 Investigations for Knee Paraesthesia

Investigations of paraesthesia aim to confirm the working diagnosis and determine underlying causes. These include:

- Radiological imaging of the nerve pathways and related bony and soft tissue structures to look for any mass lesions or other causes of external compression
  - Plain radiographs
  - Ultrasound/MRI/CT Scan
- Neurophysiological
  - Nerve conduction studies
  - Electromyography (EMG) studies
- Blood tests to exclude systemic causes of nerve dysfunction including:
  - Inflammatory markers
  - B12 levels
  - Urea, electrolytes, calcium
  - HgA1c

18.9 Management of Knee Paraesthesia

Management of paraesthesia [15–24] involves:

- Leave alone
- Symptomatic control of paraesthesia especially if painful:
  - Simple analgesia
    - Non-steroidal anti-inflammatories
  - Neuropathic analgesia
    - Gabapentin
    - Pregabalin
    - Low dose amitriptyline
    - Local anaesthetic nerve blocks
  - Local massage
  - Acupuncture
  - Sensory reeducation
    - Touching objects of different textures
    - Identifying different temperatures
    - Identifying different pressures
    - Determining joint/limb position

- Addressing the underlying condition that may have led to impairment of nerve function (such as underlying infection, inflammatory arthritis, vasculitis, diabetes)
- Addressing extrinsic causes of nerve dysfunction

18.10 Management of Extrinsic Causes of Nerve Dysfunction

In dealing with extrinsic causes of nerve dysfunction the following management ladder [25] may be considered, although on occasions initial steps may be bypassed.

- Leave alone
- Activity modification:
  - Avoid exacerbating factors, limb positions, repetitive activities
- Physiotherapy
  - Improve lumbosacral spine, knee and lower limb biomechanics
- Reduce nerve traction by posture control
  - Improve core control
  - Reduce compression:
    - Relax tense muscles
    - Stretch tense hypertrophied muscles
    - Lumbosacral spine traction
  - Mobilise nerves
    - Stretch
    - Local massage
- Injection therapy– reduce compression
  - Steroid injections around nerves to reduce perineural inflammation
  - Local anaesthetic injections to reduce muscle spasm
  - Botulinum toxin injections to reduce muscle spasm
- Arthroscopic surgery
  - Decompress lesions (such as meniscal cysts or a bursa) causing nerve compression
- Open surgery
  - Decompress nerves
  - Repair nerves

Learning Pearls

- Objective clinical neurological findings may be absent despite the patient complaining of paraesthesia. This may be due to intermittent nerve compression or traction which may be positional or posture related, or due to some internal pathology such as tight muscles, or impinging structures. This may be considered analogous to leg numbness that one may experience when lying in an awkward position for too long, but which quickly resolves once that posture is corrected. Absence of objective neurological findings should not cast doubt on the validity of clinical symptoms.
- Hypersensitivity to pain on light palpation should raise the possibility of CRPS [12, 13]
- Lower limb paraesthesia following arthroscopic or open surgery to the knee may be related to multiple factors. These include:
  - Lumbosacral spine nerve compression due to changes in lumbosacral biomechanics (by altered gait, alterations in leg length)
  - Peripheral nerve blocks
  - Thigh nerve compression by tourniquet use
  - Division of subcutaneous nerve branches or nerves by skin incising or deeper dissection
  - Traction by surgical retractors
  - Pressure compression during surgery or post-surgery by cast application (such as compression of the common peroneal nerve at the fibular head)
  - CRPS as a reaction to the insult of surgery

References

1. Charalambos CP. Shoulder paraesthesia. In: The shoulder made easy: Springer; 2019. p. 245–55.
2. Elsevier Inc. In: Rea P, editor. Essential clinical anatomy of the nervous system: Elsevier Inc; 2015.
3. Reeves AG, editor. Disorders of the nervous system: a primer. 3rd ed: Imperial Company Printers; 1995.
4. Gilman S, Newman SW. Manter and Gatz's essentials of clinical neuroanatomy and neurophysiology. 8th ed. Philadelphia, PA: FA Davis; 1992.
5. Mackinnon SE. Pathophysiology of nerve compression. Hand Clin. 2002;18(2):231–41.
6. Burnett MG, Zager EL. Pathophysiology of peripheral nerve injury: a brief review. Neurosurg Focus. 2004;16(5):E1.
7. Rempel D, Dahlin L, Lundborg G. Pathophysiology of nerve compression syndromes: response of peripheral nerves to loading. J Bone Joint Surg Am. 1999;81(11):1600–10.
8. Cohen SB, Flato R, Wascher J, Watson R, Salminen M, O'Brien D, Tjoumakaris F, Ciccotti M. Incidence and characterization of hypoesthesia in the distribution of the infrapatellar branch of the saphenous nerve after anterior cruciate ligament reconstruction: a prospective study of patient-reported numbness. J Knee Surg. 2018;31(6):585–90.

9. Subramanian S, Lateef H, Massraf A. Cutaneous sensory loss following primary total knee arthroplasty. A two years follow-up study. Acta Orthop Belg. 2009;75(5):649–53.
10. Tsukada S, Kurosaka K, Nishino M, Hirasawa N. Cutaneous hypesthesia and kneeling ability after total knee arthroplasty: a randomized controlled trial comparing anterolateral and anteromedial skin incision. J Arthroplast. 2018;33(10):3174–80.
11. Kim KI, Juh HS, Kim GB, Lee SH. Lateral numbness in the lower leg: an underestimated complication following medial open-wedge high tibial osteotomy. Knee. 2019;26(5):1041–8.
12. van Bussel CM, Stronks DL, Huygen FJ. Complex regional pain syndrome type I of the knee: a systematic literature review. Eur J Pain. 2014;18(6):766–73.
13. Dowd GS, Hussein R, Khanduja V, Ordman AJ. Complex regional pain syndrome with special emphasis on the knee. J Bone Joint Surg Br. 2007;89(3):285–90.
14. McKnight JT, Adcock BB. Paresthesias: a practical diagnostic approach. Am Fam Physician. 1997;56(9):2253–60.
15. Deli G, Bosnyak E, Pusch G, Komoly S, Feher G. Diabetic neuropathies: diagnosis and management. Neuroendocrinology. 2013;98(4):267–80.
16. Moore RA, Derry S, Aldington D, Cole P, Wiffen PJ. Amitriptyline for neuropathic pain in adults. Cochrane Database Syst Rev. 2015;7:CD008242. https://doi.org/10.1002/14651858.CD008242.
17. Li S, Xie P, Liang Z, Huang W, Huang Z, Ou J, Lin Z, Chai S. Efficacy comparison of five different acupuncture methods on pain, stiffness, and function in osteoarthritis of the knee: a network meta-analysis. Evid Based Complement Alternat Med. 2018;2018:1638904. https://doi.org/10.1155/2018/1638904.
18. Gandor F, Tisch S, Grabs AJ, Delaney AJ, Bester L, Darveniza P. Botulinum toxin A in functional popliteal entrapment syndrome: a new approach to a difficult diagnosis. J Neural Transm (Vienna). 2014;121(10):1297–301.
19. Cass SP. Piriformis syndrome: a cause of nondiscogenic sciatica. Curr Sports Med Rep. 2015;14(1):41–4.
20. Ji JH, Shafi M, Kim WY, Park SH, Cheon JO. Compressive neuropathy of the tibial nerve and peroneal nerve by a Baker's cyst: case report. Knee. 2007;14(3):249–52.
21. Widmer F, Gerster JC. Medial meniscal cyst imitating a tumor, with compression of the saphenous nerve. Rev Rhum Engl Ed. 1998;65(2):149–52.
22. Valdivia Valdivia JM, Weinand M, Maloney CT Jr, Blount AL, Dellon AL. Surgical treatment of superimposed, lower extremity, peripheral nerve entrapments with diabetic and idiopathic neuropathy. Ann Plast Surg. 2013;70(6):675–9.
23. Abou-Al-Shaar H, Yoon N, Mahan MA. Surgical repair of sciatic nerve traumatic rupture: technical considerations and approaches. Neurosurg Focus. 2018;44, V3(VideoSuppl1) https://doi.org/10.3171/2018.1.FocusVid.17568.
24. O'Malley MP, Pareek A, Reardon P, Krych A, Stuart MJ, Levy BA. Treatment of peroneal nerve injuries in the multiligament injured/dislocated knee. J Knee Surg. 2016;29(4):287–92.
25. Charalambous CP. Professionalism in surgery. In: Career skills for surgeons: Springer; 2017. p. 5–46.

Chapter 19
Knee Noise

Symptoms of knee noise including crepitus, clicking, clunking, popping or grinding are often described around the knee, either in isolation or accompanying other complaints such as those of pain or instability. This chapter discusses some of the causes of such symptoms, along with the investigation and management of their underlying causative disorders.

19.1 Sources of Abnormal Knee Noise

Abnormal knee noise may originate from several areas, but sometimes it is difficult to determine its exact origin. On occasions it may be challenging for the clinician and patient to fully agree as to where the abnormal noise is coming from.

C. Panayiotou Charalambous, *The Knee Made Easy*,
https://doi.org/10.1007/978-3-030-54506-2_19

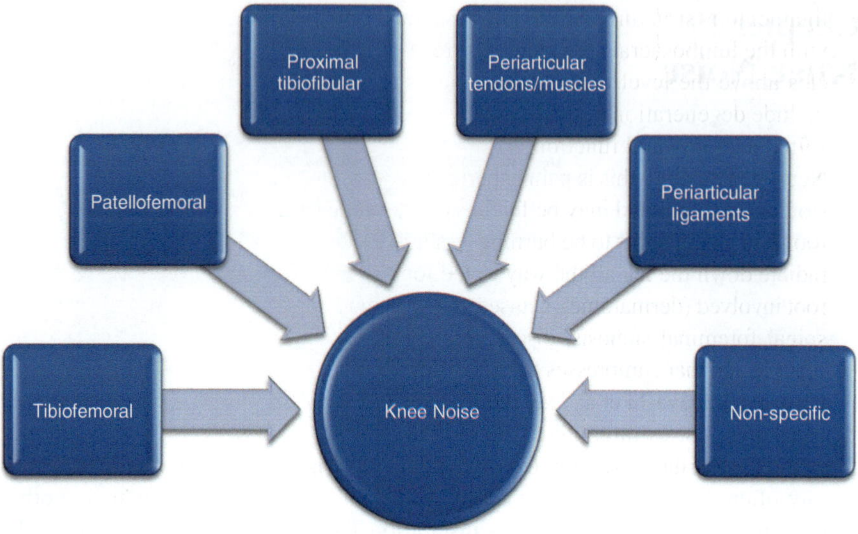

Potential sources of knee noise

Potential pathologies affecting parts of the knee that can give rise to abnormal knee noise are shown next. These noises may be physiological or may reflect a mechanical event such as abnormal translation or abnormal mechanical contact between two surfaces [1–11]. Some of these are described below.

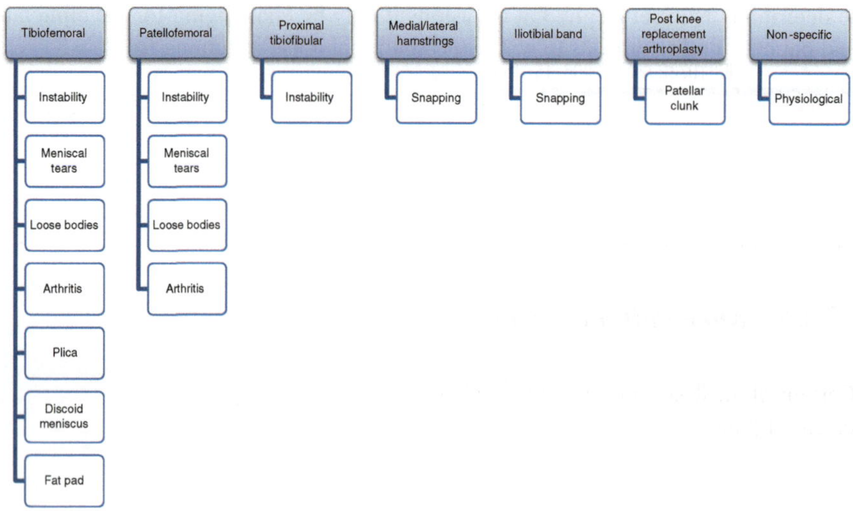

Potential pathologies leading to knee noise

19.1.1 Physiological Noise

Physiological noise may be due to:

- Buildup of air in the joint—changes in pressure lead to the formation of tiny bubbles of gas, which may make a popping noise. Cracking is associated with bubble (clear space-void) formation within the synovial fluid, rather than collapse of a preexisting bubble. When two surfaces in close contact are pulled apart the surfaces resist separation until a critical point is reached at which they separate rapidly. Distraction forces result in a drop in the pressure in the synovial fluid so that dissolved gas comes out of solution forming a bubble.
- Friction between anatomical structures (tendons, ligaments, articular surfaces).

Physiological noise is often unpredictable as to when it occurs, but it is quite common. Simple reassurance is sufficient in such cases.

19.1.2 Knee Noise following Knee Replacement Arthroplasty

Knee noise is common following knee replacement arthroplasty, and its presence may be associated with poorer satisfaction and functional outcomes. Counselling patients prior to surgery about the possibility of such noise may help manage expectations.

Its causes include

- Physiological—due to friction between anatomical structures (tendons, ligaments, patella) and the prosthesis
- Tendon/ligament snapping
- Patellar clunk
- Edge loading of hard surfaces

Nam et al. [11] evaluated patient perceived noise following total knee replacement arthroplasty (TKR) or unicompartmental knee replacement arthroplasty (UKR) in about 2000 patients who had one of various types of knee implants. They reported that:

- Overall, 27% of all patients undergoing knee arthroplasty reported hearing grinding, popping, or clicking from their operative knee in the preceding month
- Men and younger patients were more likely to report knee noise
- Knee noise was more common after TKR (29%) than UKR (21%)
- Amongst TKR designs, the likelihood of knee noise was higher in posterior-stabilized (41%), rotating platform (45%), and gender specific (36%) designs than in cruciate retaining (23%) knees
- Patient perceived noise generation was associated with more ongoing symptoms from their replaced knee, including difficulty getting in and out of a chair, limp, swelling, and stiffness compared with those who did not report noise post TKR.

19.1.3 Knee Noise following Anterior Cruciate Ligament Reconstruction Surgery

This may be due to:

- Ongoing instability
- Patellofemoral maltracking
- ACL graft impingement/snapping
- Residual tibiofemoral instability
- Degenerative changes
- Impingement of soft tissues on graft fixation devices

19.2 Clinical Symptoms of Knee Noise

- Audible knee noise on leg motion
- Soft or loud
- Clicking, clunking, popping, grating, snapping
- May occur in isolation or be associated with other symptoms including:
  - Pain
  - Instability
  - Locking/jamming
  - Reduced leg motion
  - Weakness
  - Knee swellings

19.3 Clinical Signs of Knee Noise

- Audible knee noise
- Palpable crepitus
- Signs consistent with underlying disorder causing noise

19.4 Investigations for Knee Noise

- Radiological
  - Plain radiographs
  - Dynamic Ultrasound/MRI/MRI arthrogram/CT Scan

- Neurophysiological—(if associated neuropathic sensory symptoms or if muscles weakness considered as cause of joint instability causing knee noise)
  - Nerve conduction studies
  - Electromyography
- Examination under anaesthesia
- Arthroscopic evaluation

19.5 Management of Knee Noise

This depends on clinical symptoms. If there are no substantial associated symptoms such as pain or instability, symptoms of clunking or clinking may be left alone, whilst reassuring the patient. However, in the presence of associated symptoms or if noise is very troublesome then management is directed at the underlying cause. The management ladder may be followed, although on occasions initial steps may be bypassed.

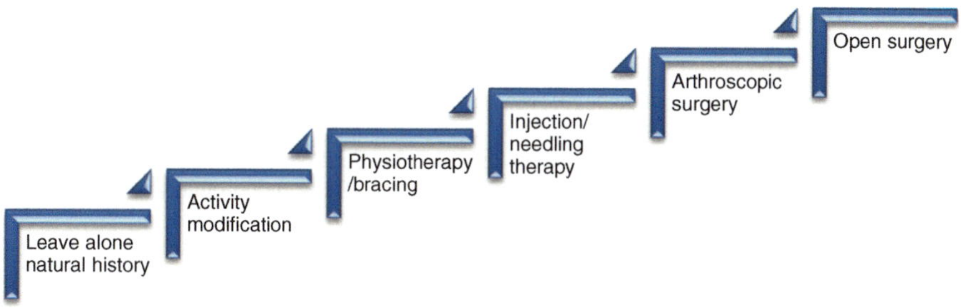

Management ladder for knee noise

> **Learning Pearls**
> - The examiner may not be able to hear the noise the patient describes, but may be able to feel it on palpation
> - Noise may suggest an underlying pathological cause if associated with:
>   - Joint swelling
>   - Pain
>   - Locking
>   - Instability

- Knee crepitus has been shown to be an early indication of patellofemoral lesions, but not tibiofemoral lesions.
- Chronic repetitive noise needs to be distinguished from a sudden noise reported by the patient as occurring at the time of injury. In the absence of a fracture, the report of a "popping noise" at injury may be suggestive of:
  - Cruciate ligament tear
  - Collateral ligament tear
  - Meniscal tear

References

1. Song SJ, Park CH, Liang H, Kim SJ. Noise around the knee. Clin Orthop Surg. 2018;10(1):1–8.
2. Neely LA, Kernohan WG, Barr DA, Mee CH, Mollan RA. Optical measurements of physiological patellofemoral crepitus. Clin Phys Physiol Meas. 1991;12(3):219–26.
3. Protopapas MG, Cymet TC. Joint cracking and popping: understanding noises that accompany articular release. J Am Osteopath Assoc. 2002;102(5):283–7.
4. Kawchuk GN, Fryer J, Jaremko JL, Zeng H, Rowe L, Thompson R. Real-time visualization of joint cavitation. PLoS One. 2015;10(4):e0119470.
5. Addison OL. Two cases of partial subluxation of knee-joints, with voluntary production of noise during flexion and extension. Proc R Soc Med. 1912;5(Sect Study Dis Child):9–10.
6. Zarah J, Chaudhry ZS, Freedman KB, Marchetto P, Hammoud S. Knee Squeaking Secondary to Intra-articular Nonabsorbable Suture: a Report of 2 Cases. Orthop J Sports Med. 2017;5(7):2325967117716386. https://doi.org/10.1177/2325967117716386.
7. Singh VK, Shah G, Singh PK, Saran D. Extraskeletal ossifying chondroma in Hoffa's fat pad: an unusual cause of anterior knee pain. Singap Med J. 2009;50(5):e189–92.
8. Wong JW, Yau PW, Chiu PK. Arthroscopic treatment of patellar symptoms in posterior stabilized total knee replacement. Int Orthop. 2002;26(4):250–2.
9. Duan G, Cai S, Lin W, Pan Y. Risk factors for patellar clunk or crepitation after primary total knee arthroplasty: a systematic review and meta-analysis. J Knee Surg. 2020; https://doi.org/10.1055/s-0040-1701515.
10. Sharkey PF, Miller AJ. Noise, numbness, and kneeling difficulties after total knee arthroplasty: is the outcome affected? J Arthroplast. 2011;26(8):1427–31.
11. Nam D, Barrack T, Nunley RM, Barrack RL. What is the frequency of noise generation in modern knee arthroplasty and is it associated with residual symptoms? Clin Orthop Relat Res. 2017;475(1):83–90.

Chapter 20
Knee Swellings

Patients may present with a visible or palpable swelling around the knee. This chapter focuses on how to describe such swellings and on the clinical symptoms and signs to be sought when dealing with these. Principles of investigating and managing knee swellings are also discussed.

20.1 Types of Knee Swellings

The spectrum of swellings that may be encountered around the knee is very broad [1–56]. Such swellings may be described in several ways including the ones described below:

According to the Aggressiveness of the Swelling

A swelling that is rapidly and constantly getting bigger is more worrying that one that fluctuates in size or is getting smaller.

Aggressive swellings may be painless but may also cause constant severe pain if complicated by:

C. Panayiotou Charalambous, *The Knee Made Easy*,
https://doi.org/10.1007/978-3-030-54506-2_20

- Local infiltration of surrounding tissues
- Pressure on nearby nerves
- Intrasubstance bleeding with a rise in the swelling's pressure

Benign swellings may cause pain due to pressure effect, or may be associated with pain originating from the underlying tissue that gives rise to the swelling as seen in:

- Horizontal meniscal tear leading to a parameniscal cyst

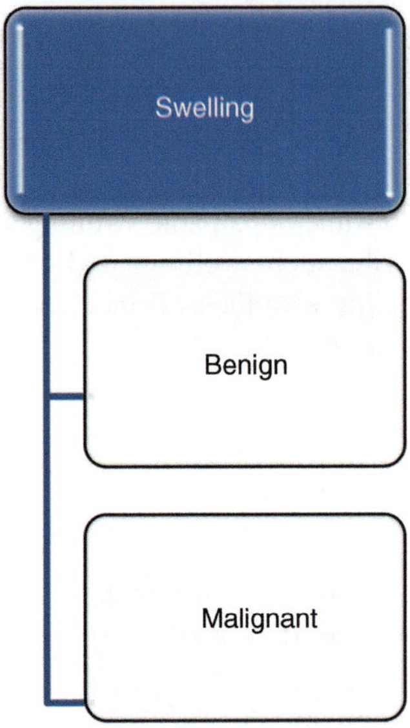

Knee swellings may be described according to their neoplastic potential

According to the Anatomical Origin of the Swelling

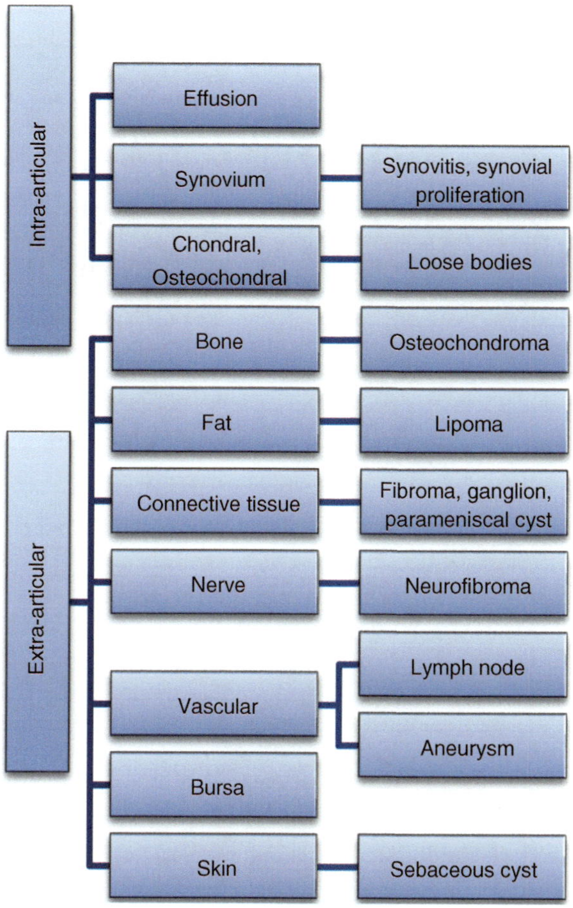

The origin of knee swellings may be intra-articular or extra-articular

A diffuse intra-articular swelling of the knee may be due to

- Effusion
- Synovitis

Effusion may be:

- Haemarthrosis (containing blood)
- Inflammatory
- Infective
- Reactive—sympathetic effusion—this is a non infective effusion, not exhibiting an inflammatory component (has low white cell count). Patients may present with pain, swelling, warmth and erythema. It may be seen in association with inflammation or infection in an adjacent anatomical structure, deep venous thrombosis, nearby trauma, or hip pathology.

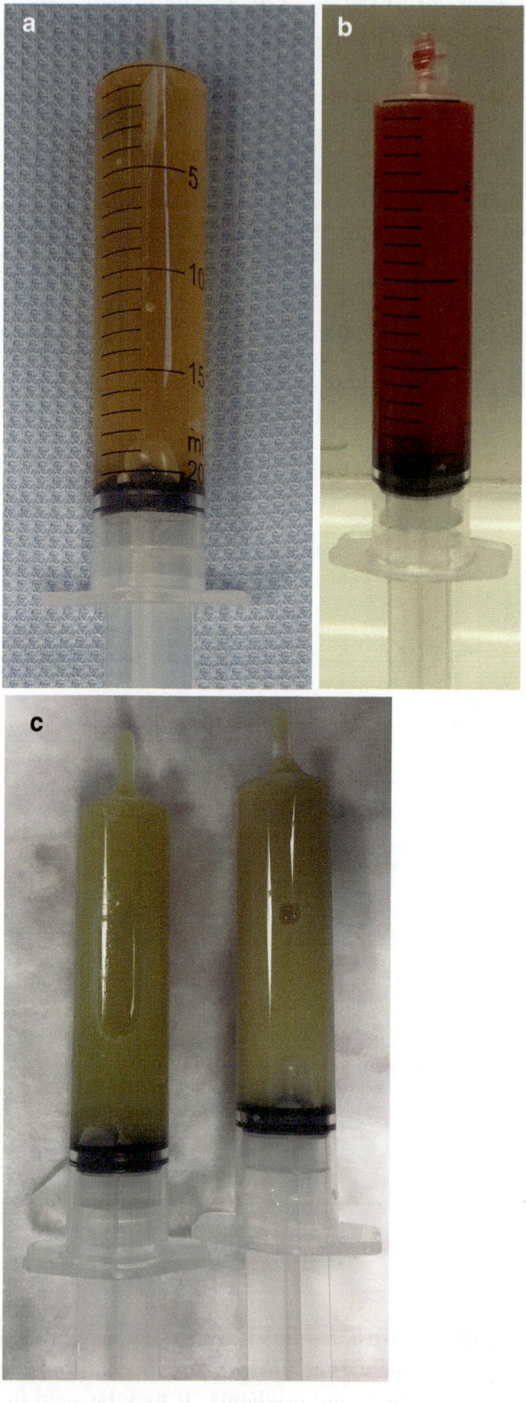

The appearance of an aspirated effusion may guide as to its underlying cause: (**a**) Inflammatory; (**b**) Haemorrhagic; (**c**) Infective

Causes for Haemarthrosis

- Cruciate ligament tear
- Peripheral meniscal tear (capsular detachment, red on red tear)
- Intra-articular fracture (femur, tibia, patella)
- Haematological condition
  - Haemophilia
- Medications—warfarin

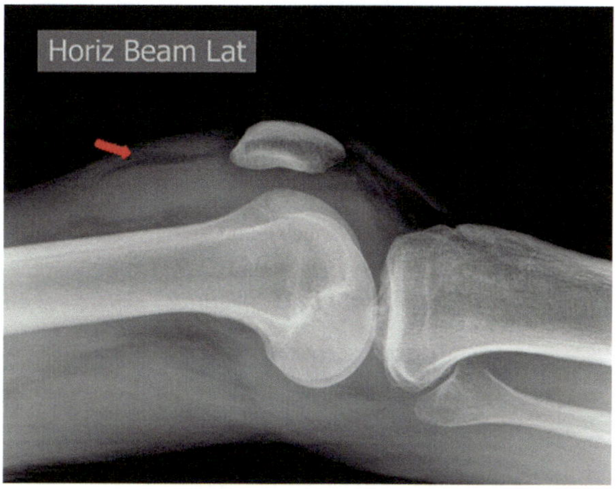

When presenting with diffuse knee swelling due to an effusion following an acute knee injury, the presence of a radiological lipohaemarthrosis (red arrow) should raise the possibility of an intra-articular knee fracture (horizontal lateral plain radiograph)

According to the Location of the Swelling

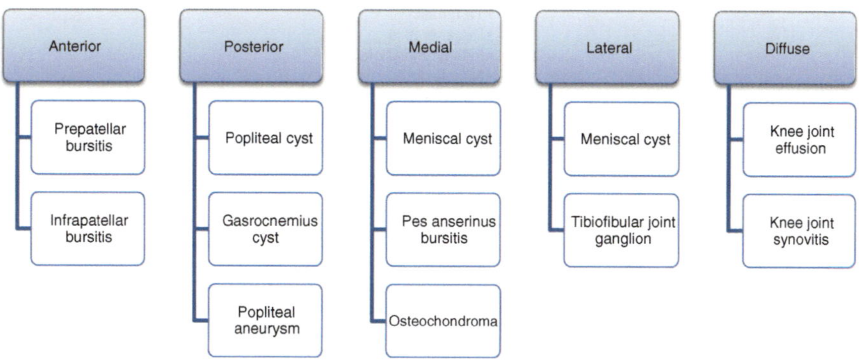

The location of a knee swelling may guide as to its origin

According to Swelling Composition

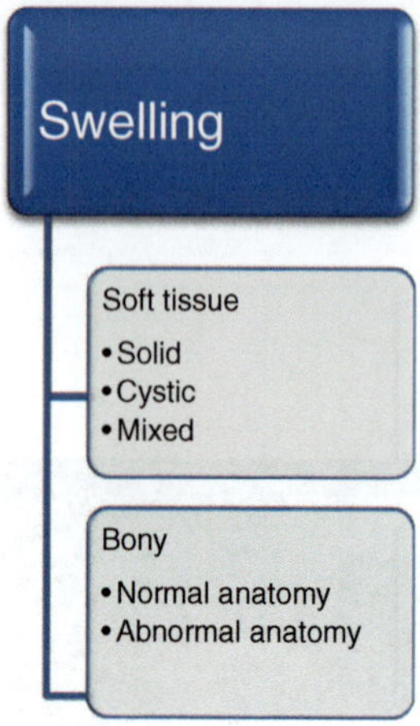

Knee swellings may be described according to their composition

According to the Precipitating Cause of the Swelling

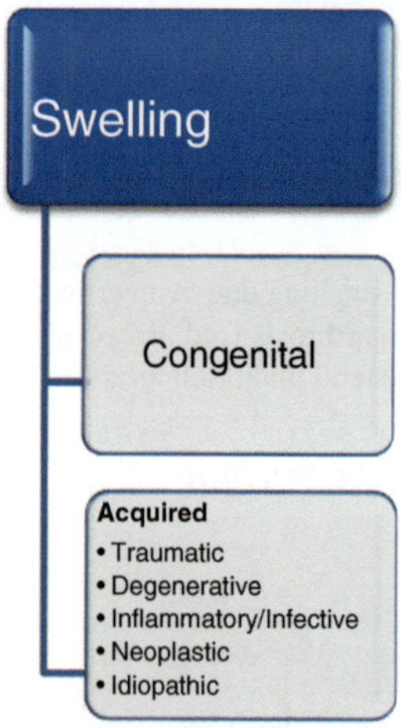

Knee swellings may be described according to their precipitating cause

20.2 Clinical Symptoms of Knee Swellings

- Complaint of: "lump", "swelling", "prominence", "deformity", "asymmetry" between sides, "something out of place", "something sticking out", noticed by patient or brought to the patient's attention by others.
- Getting bigger/smaller/fluctuating in size
- Onset—sudden/gradual, precipitating factor such as trauma, no precipitating event
- Speed of change
- Constant size and shape or changing with knee motion or time
- Associated symptoms—pain, paraesthesia, clicking/clucking, instability

20.3 Clinical Examination for Knee Swellings

- Location
- Shape
- Size
- Origin—tracing its base—localised to skin, subcutaneous tissue, muscle, bone
- Consistency –firm, soft, fluctuant
- Mobility –freely mobile, tethered to underlying tissues, reduced by muscle contraction
- Specials tests:
  - Pulsatile
  - Translumination
  - Tinel's sign

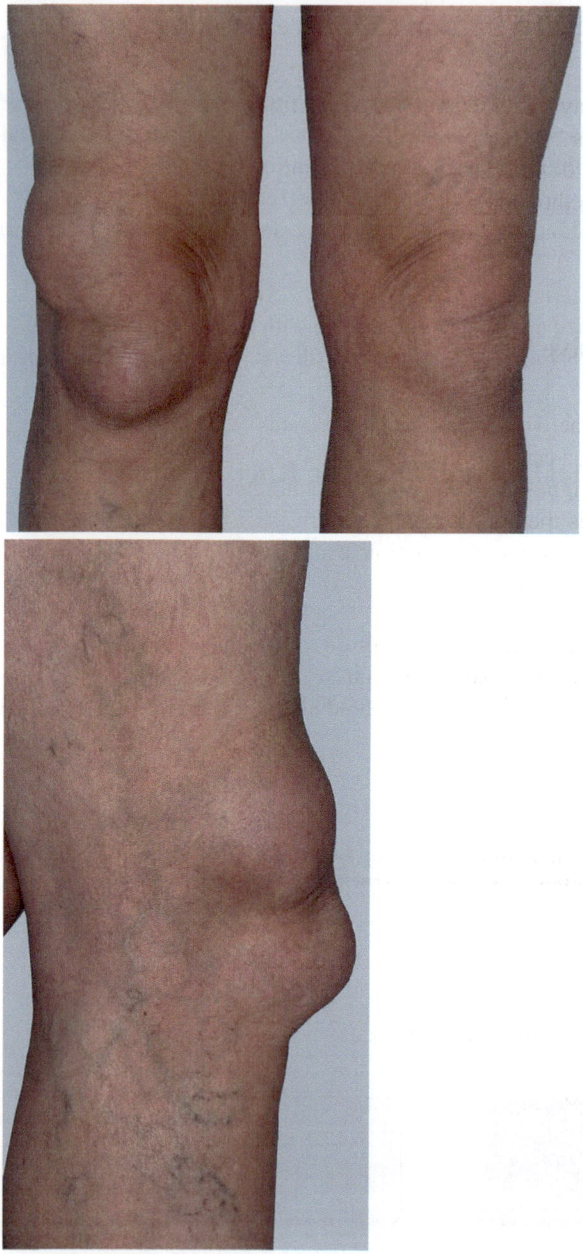

Prepatellar and infrapatellar bursitis

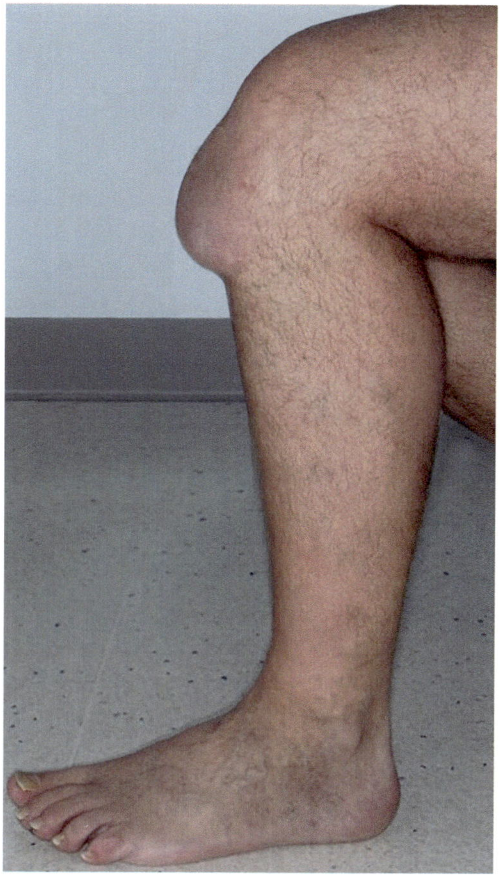

Infrapatellar bursitis

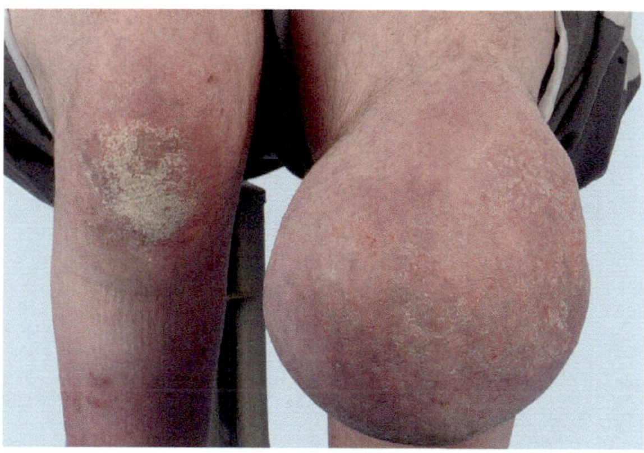

Chronic neglected infrapatellar bursitis presenting as as massive swelling

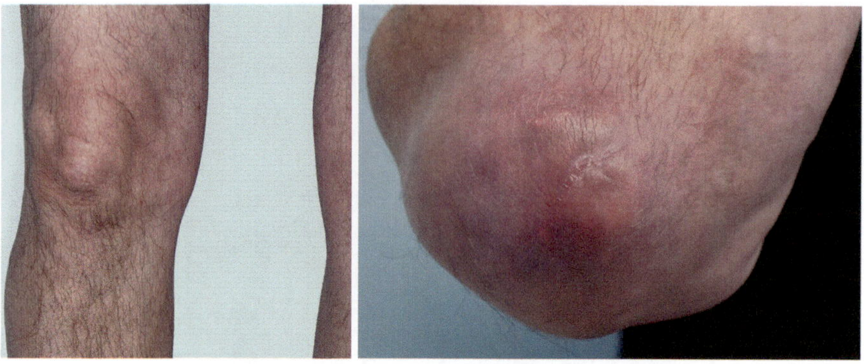

Gouty tophi involving the knee and elbows

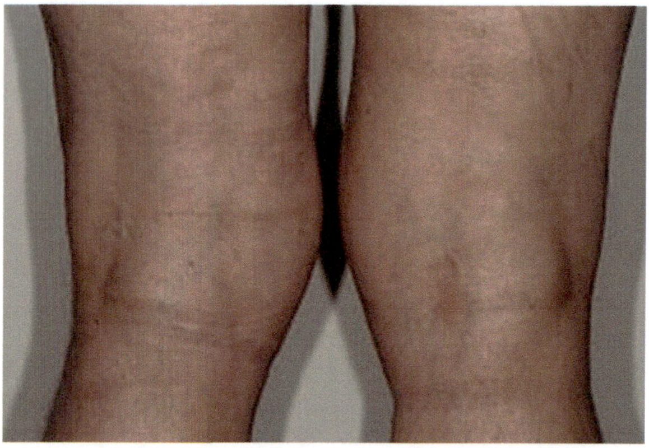

Popliteal bursa right knee

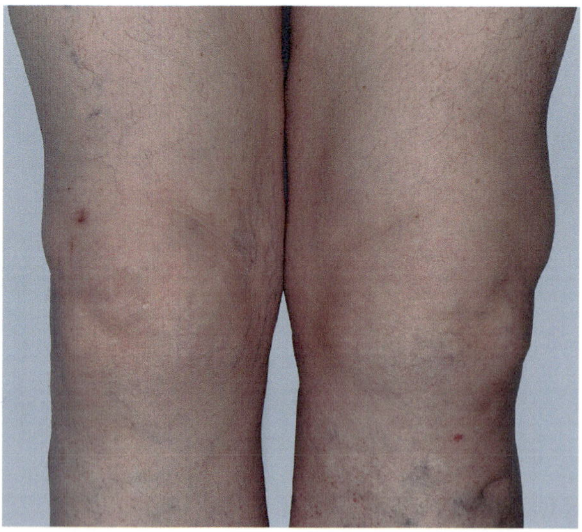

Diffuse knee swelling -efffusion

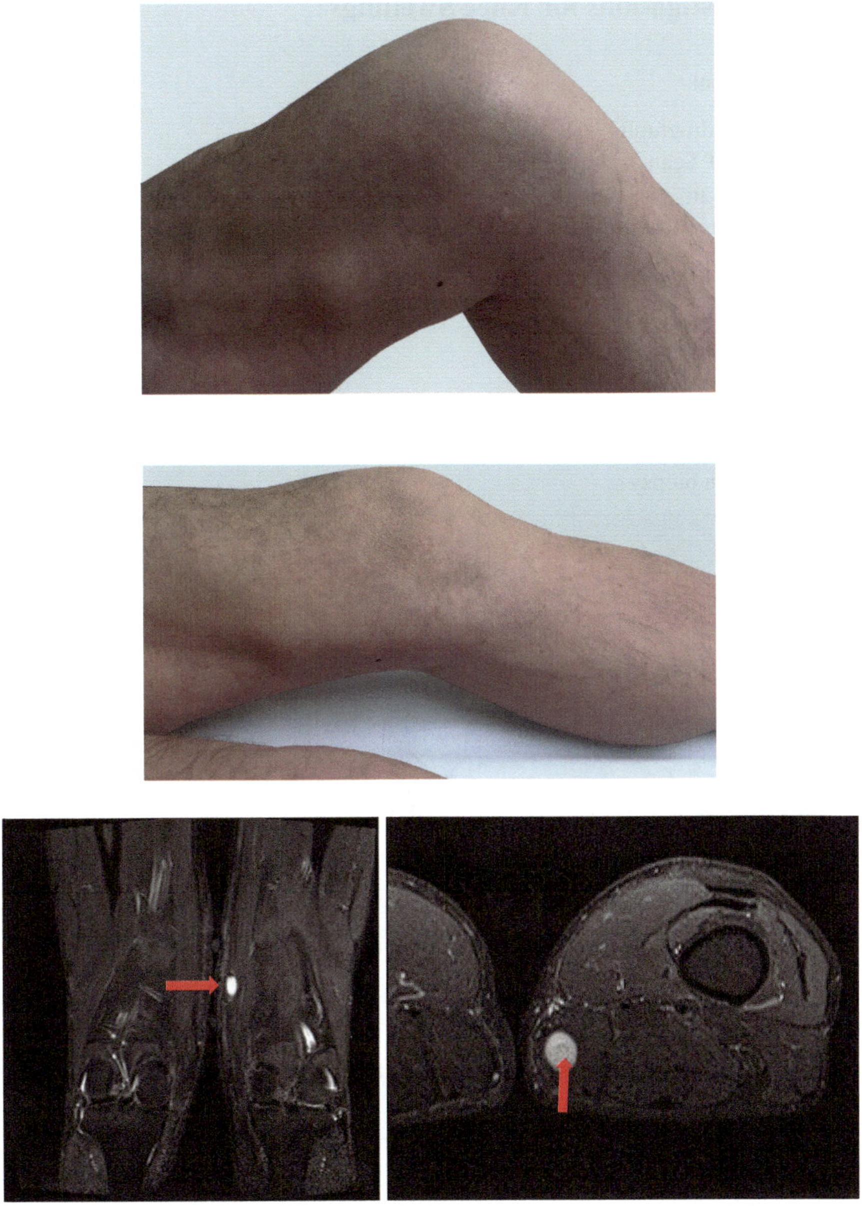

Soft tissue swelling (red arrow) related to Sartorius, in a patient presenting with anterior knee pain numbness due to saphenous nerve schwannoma (MRI)

20.4 Investigations for Knee Swellings

- Radiological
  - Plain radiographs
  - MRI/CT Scan
  - Bone scan
  - Dynamic ultrasound—for masses that alter with knee motion
- Neurophysiological
  - Nerve conduction studies
  - Electromyography
- Arthroscopic/open evaluation
  - Sample biopsy
  - Excision biopsy

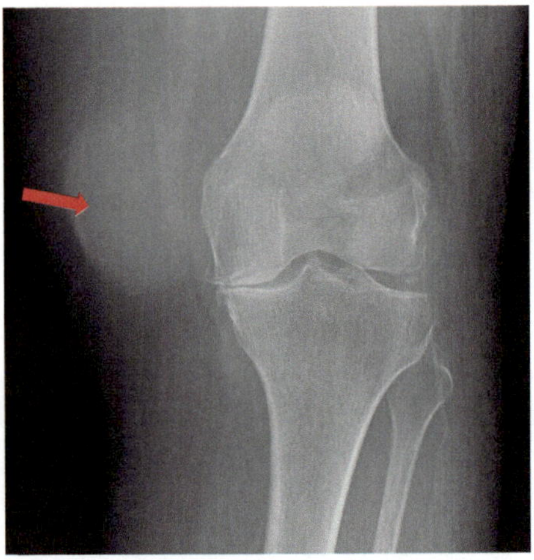

Large soft tissue swelling (even evident on the soft tissue component of a plain radiograph-red arrow). Clinically it was shown to be a lipoma

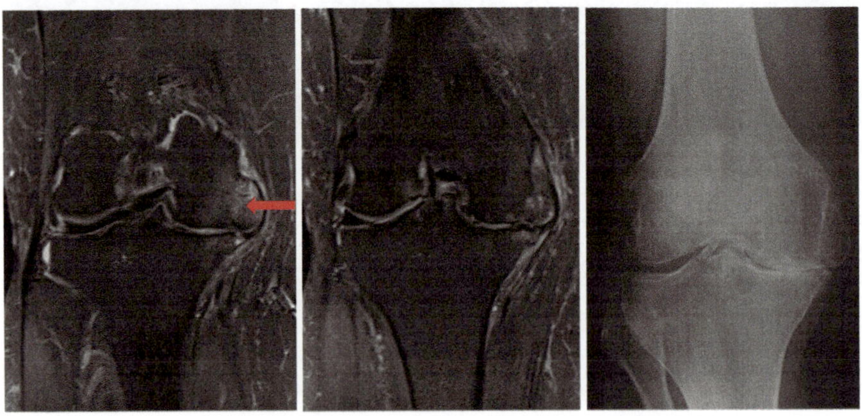

Large medial femoral osteophyte(red arrow), causing MCL elongation and felt as as prominent medial swelling

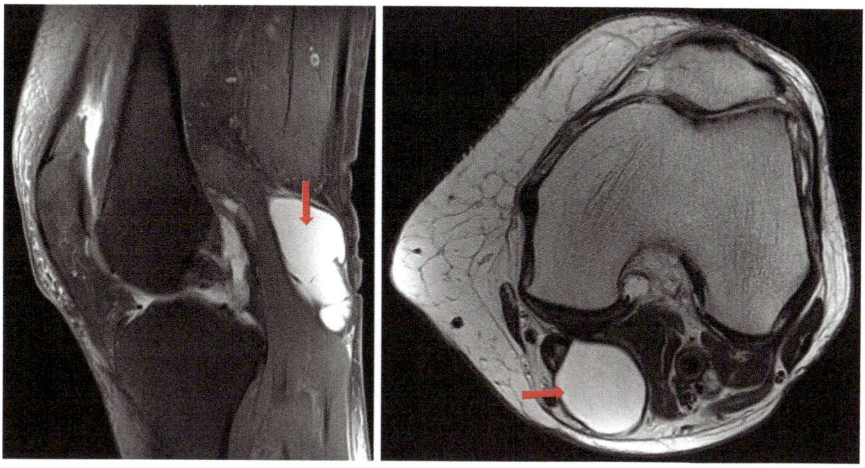

Large popliteal bursa

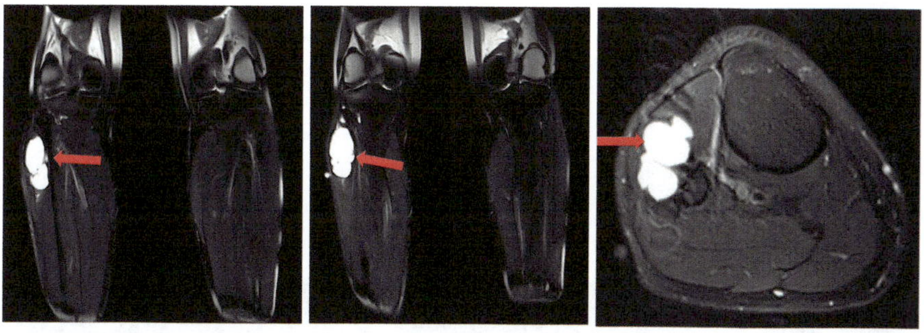

Multi-loculated cyst arising from the proximal tibio-fibular joint (MRI)

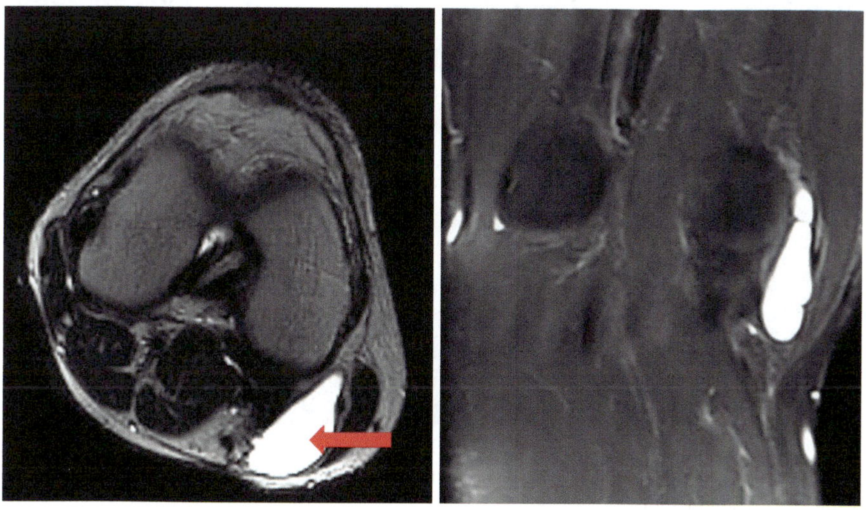

Large cystic lesion (ganglion) (red arrow) beneath sartorius, posteromedially

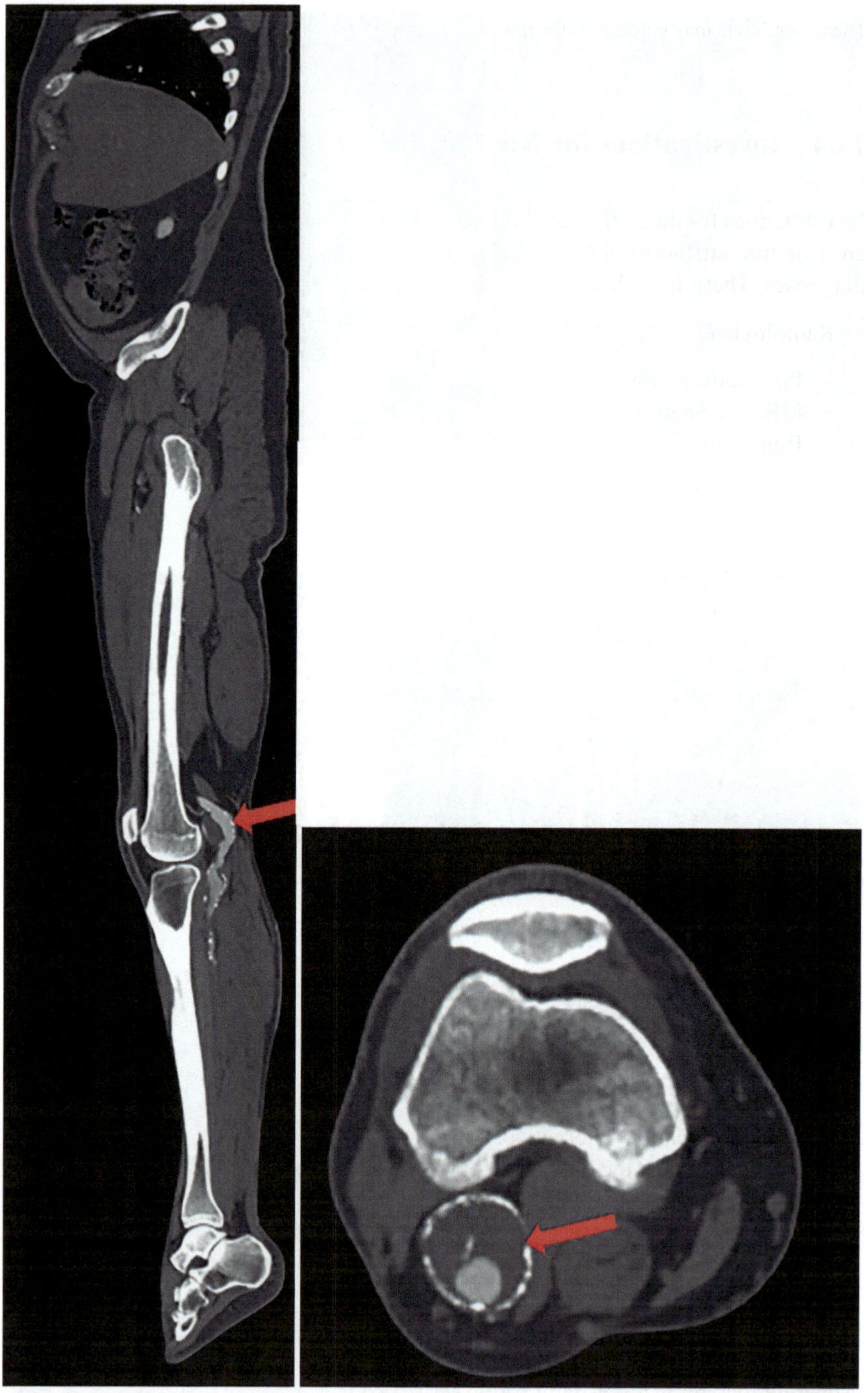

Pulsatile swelling in the popliteal fossa shown to be a partially thrombosed popliteal aneurysm (red arrow) on CT angiogram

20.5 Management of Knee Swellings

This will depend on symptoms, nature and aggressiveness of the swelling. Asymptomatic swellings may be left alone with reassurance. If symptomatic, then management may involve:

- Addressing the swelling
- Addressing the underlying condition that may have led to the swelling

The management ladder [57] may be followed, although on occasions initial steps may be bypassed.

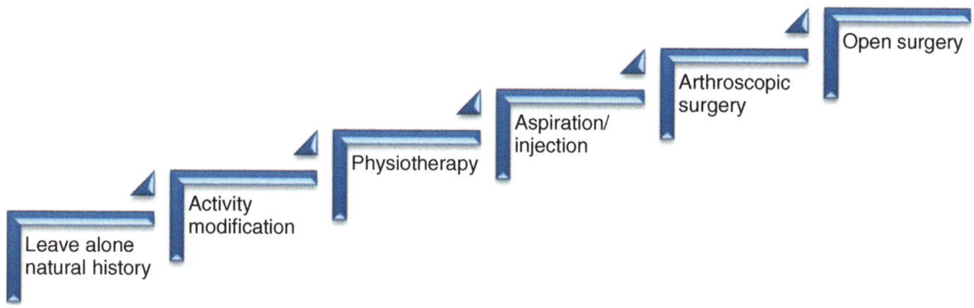

Learning Pearls

- Worrying features of soft tissue swellings include:
  - Recent enlargement
  - Location deep to the subcutaneous fascia
  - Limited mobility relative to deep tissues
  - Larger than 4 cm
  - Indeterminate nature on imaging
- The nature of such swellings may need verification by biopsy. This is better done at a centre that is capable of extensive swelling excision if this is found to be malignant. Hence, early referral to a regional soft tissue tumour unit is recommended.
- Defects in the patellar retinaculum may allow the herniation of intra-articular structures which present as knee masses (herniation of the infrapatellar fat pad through a focal defect in the lateral patella retinaculum presenting as an anterolateral mass, visible in flexion but disappearing in knee extension)

- *Lipoma arborescens* is an intra-articular mass lesion that may lead to impingement and degeneration. It is most often encountered in the supra-patellar pouch of the knee but can occur anywhere in the knee joint. It may present as knee swelling, due to its mass effect and also due to associated effusion. MRI may show a "tree-like" appearance, and macroscopic examination reveals a yellow-brown villous appearance—a "baked- bean" appearance. It is a benign condition, whereby adipose tissue replaces the subsynovial layer leading to villous hypertrophy of the synovium. It may be associated with osteoarthritis but may also occur in relation to chronic mechanical irritation (such as trauma). It may cause mechanical impingement or entrapment with knee motion, leading to effusion. It may be left alone, but if causing substantial symptoms, surgical management (arthroscopic or open synovectomy) may be utilised. Local recurrence is very rare.
- The synovium may act as a site of malignant metastasis from other sites (such a lung carcinoma), a differential diagnosis to be considered when encountering synovial swellings of uncertain aetiology.

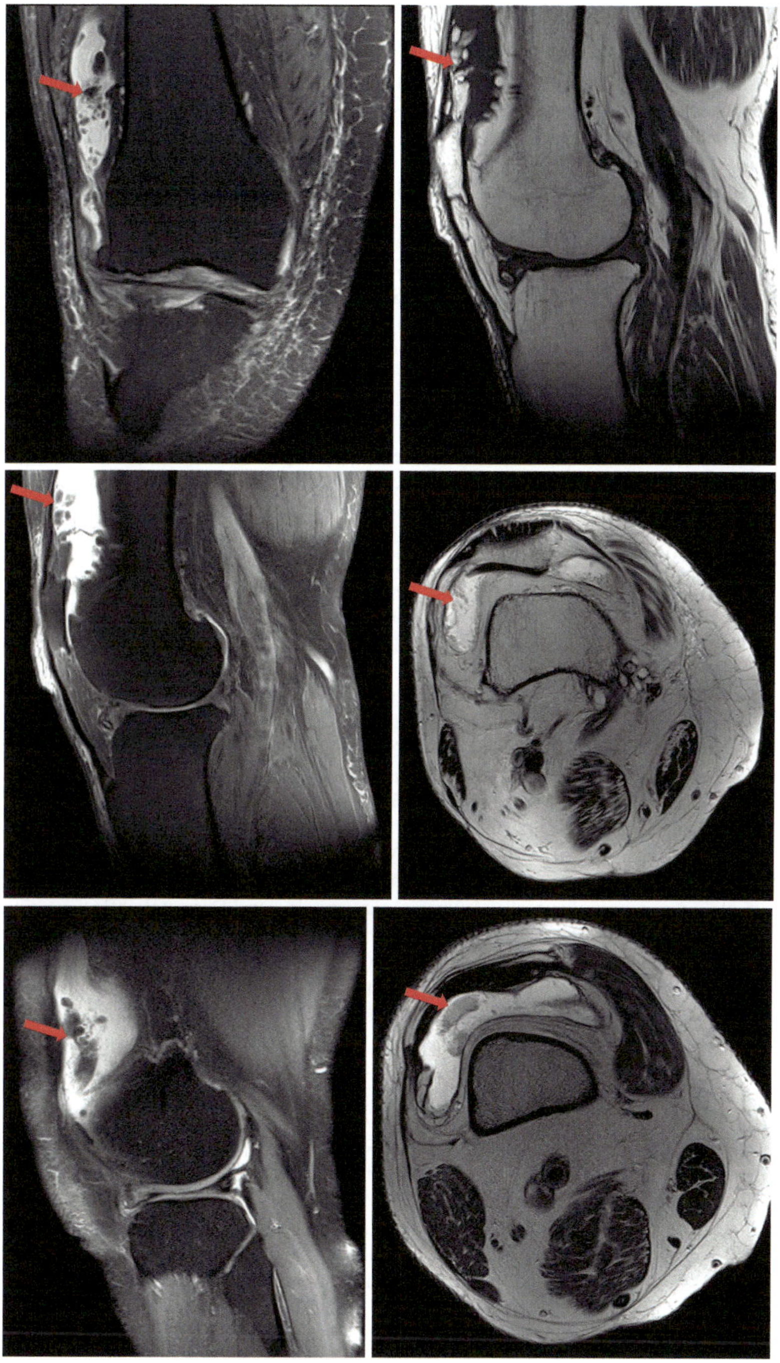

Lipoma-arborescens showing villous appearance and associated with large effusion

References

1. Westhovens R, Dequeker J. Musculoskeletal manifestations of benign and malignant tumors of bone. Curr Opin Rheumatol. 2003;15(1):70–5.
2. Damron TA, Beauchamp CP, Rougraff BT, Ward WG Sr. Soft-tissue lumps and bumps. Instr Course Lect. 2004;53:625–37.
3. Frassica FJ, McCarthy EF, Bluemke DA. Soft-tissue masses: when and how to biopsy. Instr Course Lect. 2000;49:437–42.
4. Dagur G, Gandhi J, Smith N, Khan SA. Anatomical approach to clinical problems of popliteal fossa. Curr Rheumatol Rev. 2017;13(2):126–38.
5. Schmidt-Rohlfing B, Tietze L, Siebert CH, Staatz G. Deep soft-tissue leiomyoma of the popliteal fossa in a 14-year-old girl. Arch Orthop Trauma Surg. 2001;121(10):604–6.
6. Griffiths HT, Elston CW, Colton CL, Swannell AJ. Popliteal masses masquerading as popliteal cysts. Ann Rheum Dis. 1984;43(1):60–2.
7. Shah A, James SL, Davies AM, Botchu R. A diagnostic approach to popliteal fossa masses. Clin Radiol. 2017;72(4):323–37.
8. Sabnis BM, Barrett D. Baked beans in the knee? An odd-looking synovial swelling in the knee joint. BMJ Case Rep. 2012;2012:pii: bcr-2012-007399. https://doi.org/10.1136/bcr-2012-007399.
9. Chadha M, Singh AP. Unusual knee swelling: a diagnostic dilemma. Arch Orthop Trauma Surg. 2007;127(7):593–6.
10. Barker AE, Remarks ON. Bursal swellings about the knee-joint. Br Med J. 1911;1(2631):1302–4.
11. Kester C, Wallace MT, Jelinek J, Aboulafia A. Gouty involvement of the patella and extensor mechanism of the knee mimicking aggressive neoplasm. A case series. Skelet Radiol. 2018;47(6):865–9.
12. Moraux A, Bianchi S, Le Corroller T. Soft tissue masses of the knee related to a focal defect of the lateral patellar retinaculum. J Ultrasound Med. 2018;37(7):1821–5.
13. Tsifountoudis I, Kapoutsis D, Tzavellas AN, Kalaitzoglou I, Tsikes A, Gkouvas G. Lipoma Arborescens of the knee: report of three cases and review of the literature. Case Rep Med. 2017;2017:3569512. https://doi.org/10.1155/2017/3569512.
14. İlyas G, Turgut A, Ayaz D, Kalenderer Ö. Intraarticular giant size angiolipoma of the knee causing lateral patellar dislocation. Balkan Med J. 2016;33(6):691–4.
15. Namazi N, Ghassemipour M, Rakhshan A, Abbasi A. Primary cutaneous synovial sarcoma: an extremely rare report of superficial synovial sarcoma. Indian J Dermatol. 2016;61(6):701.
16. Ghnaimat M, Alodat M, Aljazazi M, Al-Zaben R, Alshwabkah J. Giant cell tumor of tendon sheath in the knee. Electron Physician. 2016;8(8):2807–9.
17. Shallop B, Abraham JA. Synovial chondromatosis of pes anserine bursa secondary to osteochondroma. Orthopedics. 2014;37(8):e735–8.
18. Jabour P, Masrouha K, Gailey M, El-Khoury GY. Masses in the extensor mechanism of the knee: an unusual presentation of gout. J Med Liban. 2013;61(3):183–6.
19. Stein D, Cantlon M, Mackay B, Hoelscher C. Cysts about the knee: evaluation and management. J Am Acad Orthop Surg. 2013;21(8):469–79.
20. Yamashita H, Endo K, Enokida M, Teshima R. Multifocal localized pigmented villonodular synovitis arising separately from intra- and extra-articular knee joint: case report and literature review. Eur J Orthop Surg Traumatol. 2013;23(Suppl 2):S273–7.
21. Mayo M, Werner J, Joshi B, Abramovici L, Strauss EJ. An epidermal inclusion cyst mimicking chronic prepatellar bursitis: a case report. J Knee Surg. 2013;26(Suppl 1):S103–6.
22. Jose J, O'Donnell K, Lesniak B. Symptomatic intratendinous ganglion cyst of the patellar tendon. Orthopedics. 2011;34(2):135.
23. Tyler WK, Vidal AF, Williams RJ, Healey JH. Pigmented villonodular synovitis. J Am Acad Orthop Surg. 2006;14(6):376–85.
24. Zhang XS, Wang ZG. Primary leiomyosarcoma of the great saphenous vein: case report. Eur J Vasc Endovasc Surg. 2006;32(2):222–5.

25. Virkus WW. Evaluation of masses around the knee. J Knee Surg. 2005;18(4):292–7.
26. Yu WD, Shapiro MS. Cysts and other masses about the knee: identifying and treating common and rare lesions. Phys Sportsmed. 1999;27(7):59–68.
27. Yilmaz E, Karakurt L, Ozercan I, Ozdemir H. A ganglion cyst that developed from the infrapatellar fat pad of the knee. Arthroscopy. 2004;20(7):e65–8.
28. Akahane T, Isobe K, Shimizu T. Bilateral solid parameniscal masses in the knees. Arthroscopy. 2003;19(10):E14–8.
29. Dicaprio MR, Jokl P. Vascular leiomyoma presenting as medial joint line pain of the knee. Arthroscopy. 2003;19(3):E24.
30. Lombardi AV Jr, Mallory TH, Staab M, Herrington SM. Particulate debris presenting as radiographic dense masses following total knee arthroplasty. J Arthroplast. 1998;13(3):351–5.
31. Sevilla CA. Ganglion of the anterior cruciate ligament presented as a knee mass. Am J Orthop (Belle Mead NJ). 1996;25(1):46–8.
32. Shikhare SN, See PLP, Chou H, Al-Riyami AM, Peh WCG. Magnetic resonance imaging of cysts, cystlike lesions, and their mimickers around the knee joint. Can Assoc Radiol J. 2018;69(2):197–214.
33. Cowden CH 3rd, Barber FA. Meniscal cysts: treatment options and algorithm. J Knee Surg. 2014;27(2):105–11.
34. Damron TA, Sim FH. Soft-tissue tumors about the knee. J Am Acad Orthop Surg. 1997;5(3):141–52.
35. Damron TA, Rock MG. Unusual manifestations of proximal tibiofibular joint synovial cysts. Orthopedics. 1997;20(3):225–30.
36. Mason RJ, Friedman SJ, Frassica FJ. Medial meniscal cyst of the knee simulating a solitary bone lesion. A case report and review of the literature. Clin Orthop Relat Res. 1994;304:190–4.
37. Herman AM, Marzo JM. Popliteal cysts: a current review. Orthopedics. 2014;37(8):e678–84.
38. Frush TJ, Noyes FR. Baker's cyst: diagnostic and surgical considerations. Sports Health. 2015;7(4):359–65.
39. Tan IJ, Barlow JL. Sympathetic joint effusion in an urban hospital. ACR Open Rheumatol. 2019;1(1):37–42.
40. Ruangchaijatuporn T, Chang EY, Chung CB. Solitary subcutaneous sarcoidosis with massive chronic prepatellar bursal involvement. Skelet Radiol. 2016;45(12):1741–5.
41. Huang YC, Yeh WL. Endoscopic treatment of prepatellar bursitis. Int Orthop. 2011;35(3):355–8.
42. Stahnke M, Mangham DC, Davies AM. Calcific haemorrhagic bursitis anterior to the knee mimicking a soft tissue sarcoma: report of two cases. Skelet Radiol. 2004;33(6):363–6.
43. Bhat AK, Bhaskaranand K. Massive prepatellar bursitis in post-polio residual paralysis: a case report. J Orthop Surg (Hong Kong). 2001;9(1):71–3.
44. Karkos CD, Sampath SA, Bury R, Mohandas P, Forrest L. Arteriovenous fistula of the lateral superior and inferior geniculate arteries. A unique cause of a "recurrent prepatellar bursa". Int Angiol. 2002;21(3):280–3.
45. Donahue F, Turkel D, Mnaymneh W, Ghandur-Mnaymneh L. Hemorrhagic prepatellar bursitis. Skelet Radiol. 1996;25(3):298–301.
46. Kivimäki J. Occupationally related ultrasonic findings in carpet and floor layers' knees. Scand J Work Environ Health. 1992;18(6):400–2.
47. Roland GC, Beagley MJ, Cawley PW. Conservative treatment of inflamed knee bursae. Phys Sportsmed. 1992;20(2):66–77.
48. Sebaldt RJ, Tenenbaum J. Sympathetic synovial effusion associated with septic prepatellar bursitis: synovial fluid analysis with therapeutic implications. J Rheumatol. 1984;11(4):555–6.
49. Le Manac'h AP, Ha C, Descatha A, Imbernon E, Roquelaure Y. Prevalence of knee bursitis in the workforce. Occup Med (Lond). 2012;62(8):658–60.
50. Aydingoz U, Oguz B, Aydingoz O, Comert RB, Akgun I. The deep infrapatellar bursa: prevalence and morphology on routine magnetic resonance imaging of the knee. J Comput Assist Tomogr. 2004;28(4):557–61.
51. Klein W. Endoscopy of the deep infrapatellar bursa. Arthroscopy. 1996;12(1):127–31.

52. Taylor PW. Inflammation of the deep infrapatellar bursa of the knee. Arthritis Rheum. 1989;32(10):1312–4.
53. Song SJ, Bae DK, Park CH. Snapping knee due to a femoral osteochondroma after total knee arthroplasty. Knee Surg Relat Res. 2019;31(2):147–50.
54. Marrero Barrera PA, Marrero Ortiz PV. Ewing sarcoma superimposed on a previous osteochondroma in multiple osteochondromatosis. Orthopedics. 2014;37(4):e403–6.
55. Bugelli G, Dell'Osso G, Bottai V, Celli F, Loggini B, Guido G, Giannotti S. Giant Schwannoma of the saphenous nerve in the distal thigh: a case report. Surg Technol Int. 2016;28:285–8.
56. Abreu E, Aubert S, Wavreille G, Gheno R, Canella C, Cotten A. Peripheral tumor and tumor-like neurogenic lesions. Eur J Radiol. 2013;82(1):38–50.
57. Charalambous CP. Professionalism in surgery. In: career skills for surgeons. Springer, Cham; 2017. p. 5–46.

Chapter 21
Knee Tendon Disease

Knee tendon disease may be considered as a spectrum of disorders ranging from tenosynovitis to tendinopathy, to partial tears or total tear [1–8].

- Tenosynovitis—synovial inflammation, increased vascularity and fluid around the tendon, adhesions to the tendon
- Tendinopathy—acute tendon inflammation or chronic degeneration

Tears may be:

(a) Partial
(b) Complete

21.1 Knee Tendinopathy

Knee tendinopathy may be considered a spectrum of disorders ranging from acute inflammation to chronic degeneration. Tendinopathy may eventually lead to tendon tear. Tendinopathy may also be associated with calcium deposits within the tendon.

Tendinopathy may exhibit:

1. Oedema and haemorrhage of the tendon and surrounding synovium
2. Inflammation and fibrosis
3. Partial or full thickness tears

Tendinopathy may involve:

- The tendon substance
- The tendon's bony insertion—enthesis
- Both

Degeneration may involve the tendon's:

- Outer surface (superficial or deep)

C. Panayiotou Charalambous, *The Knee Made Easy*,
https://doi.org/10.1007/978-3-030-54506-2_21

- Internal substance
- Combined (outer surface and internal substance)

An acutely inflamed tendon may look macroscopically swollen (oedematous), with increased vascularity. A degenerate tendon may look macroscopically frayed or delaminated (with its various layers separated). Tendinopathy involving the internal substance of the tendon may not be easily identifiable as the outer surface of the tendon may look normal on visual inspection.

In tendinopathy the tendon may appear macroscopically:

- Normal/smooth or degenerate, frayed, delaminated
- Tubular or flattened and thickened

In tendinopathy the tendon may microscopically show various changes including [1–23]

- Infiltration by inflammatory cells—acute or chronic, mast cells
- Degenerative changes—tenocytes enlarged, increased in numbers, myxoid changes
- Increased apoptosis of tendon cells, leading to reduced tenocyte numbers in advanced degeneration
- Collagen fibres—thinner and disorganised
- Extracellular matrix—decreased matrix, mucoid degeneration, fibrocartilaginous metaplasia
- Increased concentration of matrix metalloproteinase and reduced tissue inhibitors of matrix metalloproteinases with resultant break down of extracellular matrix
- Neo-vascularisation—new vessel formation
- Neo-innervation—new sympathetic nerve formation accompanying the blood vessels and paratendinous tissue

21.2 Causes of Knee Tendinopathy

- Extrinsic

- These are external forces acting on the tendon:
  - Tensile overload—excessive force application (acute trauma or repetitive use)—low mechanical stretching has been shown to stimulate tendon stem cell proliferation and differentiation into tenocytes. However, large levels of stretching may lead to differentiation of stem cells into non-tenocytes (adipocytes, chondrocytes, osteocytes). Hence, although low levels of loading are beneficial for tendon homeostasis, overload may lead to tendon degeneration, and ectopic calcification [24, 25]
  - Impingement—compression and rubbing of the tendon by surrounding structures (osteophytes, exostoses, surgical fixation devices)

- Intrinsic
- These are changes originating within the tendon itself due to:
  - Aging
  - Inflammation
  - Hypoperfusion
  - Calcium deposition
  - Metabolic/inflammatory/endocrine/iatrogenic conditions including [26–37]:
    - Chronic renal failure -dialysis
    - Fluoroquinolone use (such as ciprofloxacin, levofloxacin)
    - Diabetes mellitus
    - Hyperparathyroidism
    - Gout
    - Rheumatoid arthritis
    - Systemic steroid use
    - Steroid injections into the tendon
    - Anabolic steroids
    - Obesity
- Combination of intrinsic and extrinsic causes

21.3 Clinical Symptoms of Knee Tendinopathy

- Pain
- Weakness
- Stiffness

21.4 Clinical Signs of Knee Tendinopathy

Positive pain provocation tests

- Local tenderness
- Stressing the tendon—by getting its muscle to contract against resistance
- Stretching the tendon—moving the limb or joint in such a way as to stretch the tendon in question

21.5 Investigations for Knee Tendinopathy

- Plain radiographs to look for:
  - Calcific deposits in tendon
  - Spurs at the entheses
  - Potential impinging lesions such as exostoses, loose bodies

- MRI scan
  - High signal areas indicating tendinopathy
  - Partial thickness tears - fluid signal with thinning of the tendon or an incomplete gap in the tendon
- Haematological—to assess metabolic conditions associated with tendinopathy

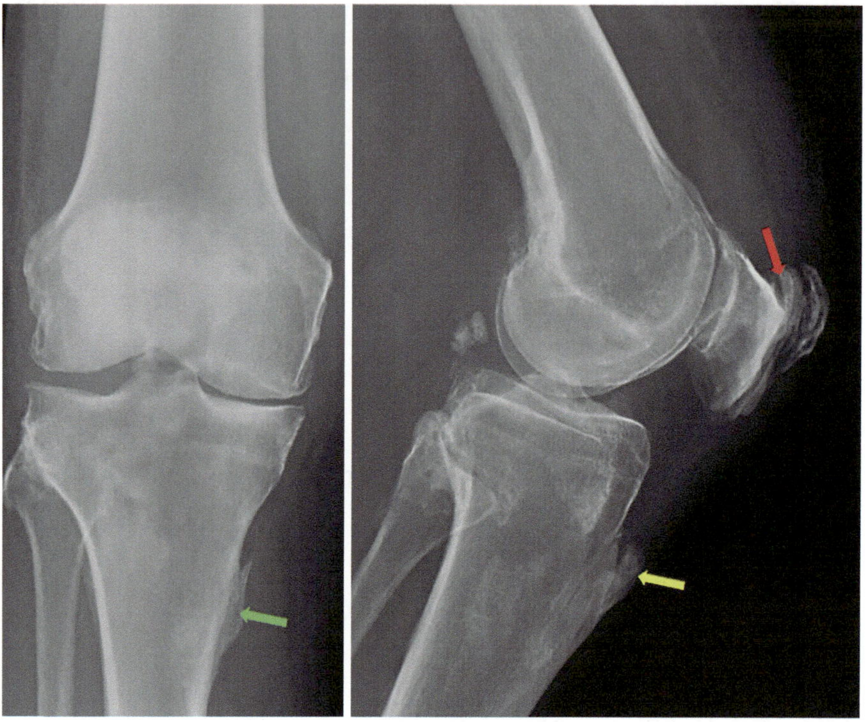

Enthesopathy of the patella and proximal tibia with multiple spurs at the quadriceps (red arrow), pes anserinus (green arrow) and patellar tendon (yellow arrow) insertions

The subsequent chapters discuss tendinopathy of the quadriceps, patellar and hamstring tendons, as they are commonly encountered around the knee. Nevertheless, the same principles may be applied to any tendon around the knee. Tendinopathy associated with calcium deposits is also described.

References

1. Christian RA, Rossy WH, Sherman OH. Patellar tendinopathy—recent developments toward treatment. Bull Hosp Jt Dis (2013). 2014;72(3):217–24.
2. Rosso F, Bonasia DE, Cottino U, Dettoni F, Bruzzone M, Rossi R. Patellar tendon: from tendinopathy to rupture. Asia Pac J Sports Med Arthrosc Rehabil Technol. 2015;2(4):99–107.

3. Millar NL, Hueber AJ, Reilly JH, Xu Y, Fazzi UG, Murrell GA, McInnes IB. Inflammation is present in early human tendinopathy. Am J Sports Med. 2010;38(10):2085–91.
4. Rees JD, Stride M, Scott A. Tendons—time to revisit inflammation. Br J Sports Med. 2014;48(21):1553–7.
5. De Giorgi S, Saracino M, Castagna A. Degenerative disease in rotator cuff tears: what are the biochemical and histological changes? Joints. 2014;2(1):26–8.
6. Neviaser A, Andarawis-Puri N, Flatow E. Basic mechanisms of tendon fatigue damage. J Shoulder Elbow Surg. 2012;21(2):158–63.
7. Seitz AL, McClure PW, Finucane S, Boardman ND 3rd, Michener LA. Mechanisms of rotator cuff tendinopathy: intrinsic, extrinsic, or both? Clin Biomech (Bristol, Avon). 2011;26(1):1–12.
8. Mehta S, Gimbel JA, Soslowsky LJ. Etiologic and pathogenetic factors for rotator cuff tendinopathy. Clin Sports Med. 2003;22(4):791–812.
9. Scott A, Lian Ø, Roberts CR, Cook JL, Handley CJ, Bahr R, Samiric T, Ilic MZ, Parkinson J, Hart DA, Duronio V, Khan KM. Increased versican content is associated with tendinosis pathology in the patellar tendon of athletes with jumper's knee. Scand J Med Sci Sports. 2008;18(4):427–35.
10. Xu Y, Murrell GA. The basic science of tendinopathy. Clin Orthop Relat Res. 2008;466(7):1528–38.
11. Samiric T, Parkinson J, Ilic MZ, Cook J, Feller JA, Handley CJ. Changes in the composition of the extracellular matrix in patellar tendinopathy. Matrix Biol. 2009;28(4):230–6.
12. Backman LJ, Fong G, Andersson G, Scott A, Danielson P. Substance P is a mechanoresponsive, autocrine regulator of human tenocyte proliferation. PLoS One. 2011;6(11):e27209. https://doi.org/10.1371/journal.pone.0027209.
13. Andersson G, Forsgren S, Scott A, Gaida JE, Stjernfeldt JE, Lorentzon R, Alfredson H, Backman C, Danielson P. Tenocyte hypercellularity and vascular proliferation in a rabbit model of tendinopathy: contralateral effects suggest the involvement of central neuronal mechanisms. Br J Sports Med. 2011;45(5):399–406.
14. Lundgreen K, Lian OB, Engebretsen L, Scott A. Tenocyte apoptosis in the torn rotator cuff: a primary or secondary pathological event? Br J Sports Med. 2011;45(13):1035–9.
15. Battery L, Maffulli N. Inflammation in overuse tendon injuries. Sports Med Arthrosc Rev. 2011;19(3):213–7.
16. Cook JL, Feller JA, Bonar SF, Khan KM. Abnormal tenocyte morphology is more prevalent than collagen disruption in asymptomatic athletes' patellar tendons. J Orthop Res. 2004;22(2):334–8.
17. Lian Ø, Scott A, Engebretsen L, Bahr R, Duronio V, Khan K. Excessive apoptosis in patellar tendinopathy in athletes. Am J Sports Med. 2007;35(4):605–11.
18. Scott A, Lian Ø, Bahr R, Hart DA, Duronio V, Khan KM. Increased mast cell numbers in human patellar tendinosis: correlation with symptom duration and vascular hyperplasia. Br J Sports Med. 2008;42(9):753–7.
19. Fu SC, Chan BP, Wang W, Pau HM, Chan KM, Rolf CG. Increased expression of matrix metalloproteinase 1 (MMP1) in 11 patients with patellar tendinosis. Acta Orthop Scand. 2002;73(6):658–62.
20. Hoksrud A, Ohberg L, Alfredson H, Bahr R. Color Doppler ultrasound findings in patellar tendinopathy (jumper's knee). Am J Sports Med. 2008;36(9):1813–20.
21. Jewson JL, Lambert GW, Storr M, Gaida JE. The sympathetic nervous system and tendinopathy: a systematic review. Sports Med. 2015;45(5):727–43.
22. Danielson P, Alfredson H, Forsgren S. Studies on the importance of sympathetic innervation, adrenergic receptors, and a possible local catecholamine production in the development of patellar tendinopathy (tendinosis) in man. Microsc Res Tech. 2007;70(4):310–24.
23. Rui YF, Lui PP, Rolf CG, Wong YM, Lee YW, Chan KM. Expression of chondro-osteogenic BMPs in clinical samples of patellar tendinopathy. Knee Surg Sports Traumatol Arthrosc. 2012;20(7):1409–17.
24. Zhang J, Wang JH. Mechanobiological response of tendon stem cells: implications of tendon homeostasis and pathogenesis of tendinopathy. J Orthop Res. 2010;28(5):639–43.

25. Rui YF, Lui PP, Ni M, Chan LS, Lee YW, Chan KM. Mechanical loading increased BMP-2 expression which promoted osteogenic differentiation of tendon-derived stem cells. J Orthop Res. 2011;29(3):390–6.
26. Chua SY, Chang HC. Bilateral spontaneous rupture of the quadriceps tendon as an initial presentation of alkaptonuria—a case report. Knee. 2006;13(5):408–10.
27. Kannus P, Józsa L. Histopathological changes preceding spontaneous rupture of a tendon. A controlled study of 891 patients. J Bone Joint Surg Am. 1991;73(10):1507–25.
28. Karistinos A, Paulos LE. "Ciprofloxacin-induced" bilateral rectus femoris tendon rupture. Clin J Sport Med. 2007;17(5):406–7.
29. Khaliq Y, Zhanel GG. Fluoroquinolone-associated tendinopathy: a critical review of the literature. Clin Infect Dis. 2003;36(11):1404–10.
30. Maddox PA, Garth WP Jr. Tendinitis of the patellar ligament and quadriceps (jumper's knee) as an initial presentation of hyperparathyroidism. A case report. J Bone Joint Surg Am. 1986;68(2):288–92.
31. Ranger TA, Wong AM, Cook JL, Gaida JE. Is there an association between tendinopathy and diabetes mellitus? A systematic review with meta-analysis. Br J Sports Med. 2016;50(16):982–9.
32. Song Y, Wu J, Chen J. Spontaneous multiple tendon rupture in a hemodialysis patient. Intern Med. 2014;53(14):1583.
33. Muzi F, Gravante G, Tati E, Tati G. Fluoroquinolones-induced tendinitis and tendon rupture in kidney transplant recipients: 2 cases and a review of the literature. Transplant Proc. 2007;39(5):1673–5.
34. Franceschi F, Papalia R, Paciotti M, Franceschetti E, Di Martino A, Maffulli N, Denaro V. Obesity as a risk factor for tendinopathy: a systematic review. Int J Endocrinol. 2014;2014:10. https://doi.org/10.1155/2014/670262.
35. Varghese B, Radcliffe GS, Groves C. Calcific tendonitis of the quadriceps. Br J Sports Med. 2006;40(7):652–4.
36. Kwan CK, Fu SC, Yung PS. A high glucose level stimulate inflammation and weaken pro-resolving response in tendon cells—a possible factor contributing to tendinopathy in diabetic patients. Asia Pac J Sports Med Arthrosc Rehabil Technol. 2019;19:1–6.
37. Wu K, Bauer E, Myung G, Fang MA. Musculoskeletal manifestations of alkaptonuria: a case report and literature review. Eur J Rheumatol. 2018;6(2):98–101.

Chapter 22
Quadriceps Tendinopathy

This is a condition whereby there is tendinopathy of the quadriceps tendon. This usually affects the distal part of the tendon or its point of attachment to the patella. It often precedes quadriceps tendon tears, particularly those tears occurring with minimal or no trauma.

Quadriceps tendinopathy may be due to multiple factors [1–18] including:

- Overload
- Muscle imbalance (core, lower limb)
- Inadequate warm-up/stretching when engaging in sports
- Knee extension deficit—fixed flexion deformity
- External impingement—such as by a prominent femoral component following knee replacement arthroplasty
- Malunited distal femoral fracture altering the line of quadriceps pull
- Mass lesion—loose bodies in synovial chondromatosis
- Metabolic/inflammatory/endocrine/iatrogenic conditions including:
  - Chronic renal failure—haemodialysis, renal transplant recipients
  - Fluoroquinolones (such as ciprofloxacin, levofloxacin)—effect amplified in renal deficiency patients
  - Diabetes mellitus
  - Hyperparathyroidism
  - Gout
  - Alkaptonuria
  - Rheumatoid arthritis
  - Systemic steroid use
  - Steroid injections into the tendon
  - Anabolic steroids
  - Obesity

C. Panayiotou Charalambous, *The Knee Made Easy*,
https://doi.org/10.1007/978-3-030-54506-2_22

22.1 Clinical Symptoms of Quadriceps Tendinopathy

- Pain at the anterior aspect of the knee, over the proximal part of the patella
- Pain worse on bending the knee
- Pain worse on actively extending the knee—straight leg raising
- Quadriceps weakness
- Knee stiffness

22.2 Clinical Signs of Quadriceps Tendinopathy

- Tenderness
  - Over the quadriceps tendon
  - Over the quadriceps insertion to the superior pole of the patella
- Pain aggravated by knee flexion or extension against resistance
- Quadriceps weakness (true or apparent)
- Knee stiffness (true or apparent)

22.3 Investigations for Quadriceps Tendinopathy

- Plain radiographs—look for spurs at the superior pole of the patella, prominent flange of femoral component
- MRI—look for quadriceps tendinopathy or tears, or impinging mass lesions
- CT scan—assess distal femoral morphology, exostoses
- Haematological—to assess metabolic conditions associated with tendinopathy

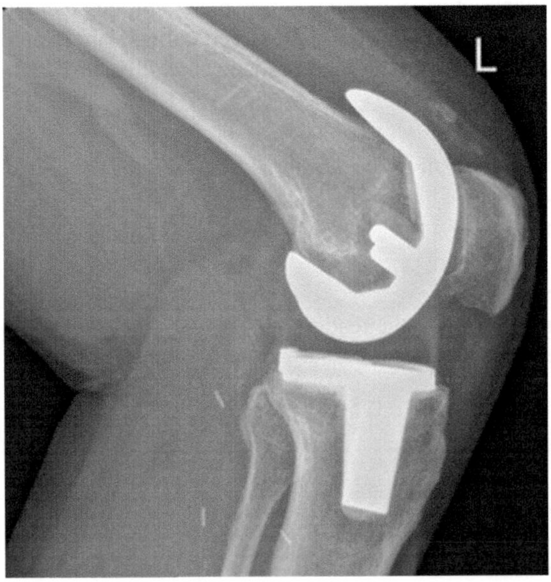

Prominent anterior flange of femoral component in TKR associated with quadriceps tendinopathy

22.4 Management of Quadriceps Tendinopathy

This is influenced by the underlying cause of the tendinopathy and may be non-surgical or surgical. The ladder of interventions may be utilised.

22.4.1 Non-surgical Interventions [19–21]

- Rest, activity modification, local passive therapy
- Posture improvement
- Eccentric exercises of the quadriceps
- Strengthening of knee stabilisers
- Posterior knee capsule stretching to address extension deficits
- Local injections:
  - PRP injections
  - Hyaluronic acid injections
- Quadriceps tendon percutaneous needling

22.4.2 Surgical Interventions [22, 23]

Surgical interventions aim to remove any inflammatory tissue, stimulate regeneration and excise any impinging lesions. These include:

- Debridement of the degenerate tendon, excision of calcific deposits
- Debridement of the tendon insertion site on the patella, excision of a patellar spur, drilling of the bone insertion site, +/− re-attachment of the tendon to the patella
- Excision of any impinging lesions

References

1. Andia I, Abate M. Hyperuricemia in tendons. Adv Exp Med Biol. 2016;920:123–32.
2. Deren ME, Klinge SA, Mukand NH, Mukand JA. Tendinopathy and tendon rupture associated with statins. JBJS Rev. 2016;4(5).
3. Lim CH, Landon KJ, Chan GM. Bilateral quadriceps Femoris tendon rupture in a patient with chronic renal insufficiency: a case report. J Emerg Med. 2016;51(4):e85–7.
4. Ventura-Ríos L, Sánchez-Bringas G, Pineda C, Hernández-Díaz C, Reginato A, Alva M, Audisio M, Bertoli A, Cazenave T, Gutiérrez M, Mora C, Py G, Sedano O, Solano C, de Miguel E. Tendon involvement in patients with gout: an ultrasound study of prevalence. Clin Rheumatol. 2016;35(8):2039–44.
5. Pfirrmann CW, Jost B, Pirkl C, Aitzetmüller G, Lajtai G. Quadriceps tendinosis and patellar tendinosis in professional beach volleyball players: sonographic findings in correlation with clinical symptoms. Eur Radiol. 2008;18(8):1703–9.

6. Franceschi F, Papalia R, Paciotti M, Franceschetti E, Di Martino A, Maffulli N, Denaro V. Obesity as a risk factor for tendinopathy: a systematic review. Int J Endocrinol. 2014;2014:10. https://doi.org/10.1155/2014/670262.
7. Varghese B, Radcliffe GS, Groves C. Calcific tendonitis of the quadriceps. Br J Sports Med. 2006;40(7):652–4.
8. Abram SG, Sharma AD, Arvind C. Atraumatic quadriceps tendon tear associated with calcific tendonitis. BMJ Case Rep. 2012;2012:bcr2012007031. https://doi.org/10.1136/bcr-2012-007031.
9. Maffulli N, Del Buono A, Spiezia F, Longo UG, Denaro V. Light microscopic histology of quadriceps tendon ruptures. Int Orthop. 2012;36(11):2367–71.
10. Arumilli B, Adeyemo F, Samarji R. Bilateral simultaneous complete quadriceps rupture following chronic symptomatic tendinopathy: a case report. J Med Case Rep. 2009;3:9031. https://doi.org/10.4076/1752-1947-3-9031.
11. Chua SY, Chang HC. Bilateral spontaneous rupture of the quadriceps tendon as an initial presentation of alkaptonuria—a case report. Knee. 2006;13(5):408–10.
12. Kannus P, Józsa L. Histopathological changes preceding spontaneous rupture of a tendon. A controlled study of 891 patients. J Bone Joint Surg Am. 1991;73(10):1507–25.
13. Karistinos A, Paulos LE. "Ciprofloxacin-induced" bilateral rectus femoris tendon rupture. Clin J Sport Med. 2007;17(5):406–7.
14. Khaliq Y, Zhanel GG. Fluoroquinolone-associated tendinopathy: a critical review of the literature. Clin Infect Dis. 2003;36(11):1404–10.
15. Maddox PA, Garth WP Jr. Tendinitis of the patellar ligament and quadriceps (jumper's knee) as an initial presentation of hyperparathyroidism. A case report. J Bone Joint Surg Am. 1986;68(2):288–92.
16. Ranger TA, Wong AM, Cook JL, Gaida JE. Is there an association between tendinopathy and diabetes mellitus? A systematic review with meta-analysis. Br J Sports Med. 2016;50(16):982–9.
17. Song Y, Wu J, Chen J. Spontaneous multiple tendon rupture in a hemodialysis patient. Intern Med. 2014;53(14):1583.
18. Muzi F, Gravante G, Tati E, Tati G. Fluoroquinolones-induced tendinitis and tendon rupture in kidney transplant recipients: 2 cases and a review of the literature. Transplant Proc. 2007;39(5):1673–5.
19. Couppé C, Svensson RB, Silbernagel KG, Langberg H, Magnusson SP. Eccentric or concentric exercises for the treatment of tendinopathies? J Orthop Sports Phys Ther. 2015;45(11):853–63.
20. Frizziero A, Vittadini F, Fusco A, Giombini A, Masiero S. Efficacy of eccentric exercise in lower limb tendinopathies in athletes. J Sports Med Phys Fitness. 2016;56(11):1352–8.
21. Yang SM, Chen WS. Conservative treatment of tendon injuries. Am J Phys Med Rehabil. 2020;99(6):550–7. https://doi.org/10.1097/PHM.0000000000001345.
22. Peng X, Feng Y, Chen G, Yang L. Arthroscopic treatment of chronically painful calcific tendinitis of the rectus femoris. Eur J Med Res. 2013;18:49.
23. Webb SA, Hopper MA, Chitnavis J. Calcific tendonitis of the quadriceps tendon. J Surg Case Rep. 2018;2018(4):rjy053. https://doi.org/10.1093/jscr/rjy053.

Chapter 23
Patellar Tendon Tendinopathy

This is a condition whereby there is tendinopathy of the patellar tendon. This usually affects the proximal point of attachment of the tendon to the patella or its distal insertion onto the tibial tubercle, but may also affect any site of the tendon substance.

Patellar tendon tendinopathy may be in principle due to multiple factors [1–15] including:

- Overload
- Muscle imbalance (core, lower limb)
- Inadequate warm-up/stretching when engaging in sports
- Knee extension deficit—fixed flexion deformity
- External impingement by lesions including:
  - The lateral femoral condyle in patellar tendon friction syndrome (in the presence of patella alta)
  - A prominent tibial component following knee replacement arthroplasty
  - Prominent tibial tubercle
  - Ossicles from tibial tubercle
  - Malunited proximal tibial fracture
  - Mass lesion—infrapatellar fat pad fibroma

23.1 Pathogenesis

Theories for the pathogenesis of patellar tendinopathy include:

- Inflammatory component
- Collagen breakdown and disorganisation
- Mechanical impingement
- High or inappropriate patellar tendon loading

C. Panayiotou Charalambous, *The Knee Made Easy*,
https://doi.org/10.1007/978-3-030-54506-2_23

23.2 Risk Factors for Patellar Tendinopathy

There is some evidence that the following risk factors may be related to patellar tendon tendinopathy:

- Activities that involve jumping or landing from a jump—basketball, volleyball, football
- High weight body mass index (BMI)
- Leg length discrepancy
- Reduced:
  - Quadriceps flexibility
  - Hamstring flexibility
  - Quadriceps strength
- Poor vertical jump performance
- Landing with stiff landing pattern
- Hip and foot/ankle impairments—weakness of hip extensors, reduced ankle dorsiflexion

23.3 Clinical Symptoms of Patellar Tendon Tendinopathy

- Pain
  - At the anteroinferior part of the knee
  - Over the patellar tendon
- Pain aggravated by:
  - Knee flexion
  - Loading the extensor mechanism of the knee
    - Active knee extension against resistance
- Knee weakness
- Knee stiffness

23.4 Clinical Signs of Patellar Tendon Tendinopathy

- Tenderness over the patellar tendon
- Tenderness over the distal pole of the patella or tibial tubercle
- Quadriceps weakness (true or apparent)
- Knee stiffness (true or apparent)

23.5 Investigations for Patellar Tendon Tendinopathy

- Plain radiographs—to look for:

  - Inferior pole of patella spurs
  - Tibial tuberosity prominence or fragmentation
  - Anterior prominence of the tibial component in knee replacement arthroplasty
  - Calcific deposits
- MRI—look for patellar tendon tendinopathy or tears, evaluate underlying fat pad and associated bursae
- CT scan—assess proximal tibia and tibial tuberosity morphology (this investigation is utilised rarely, in complex cases)

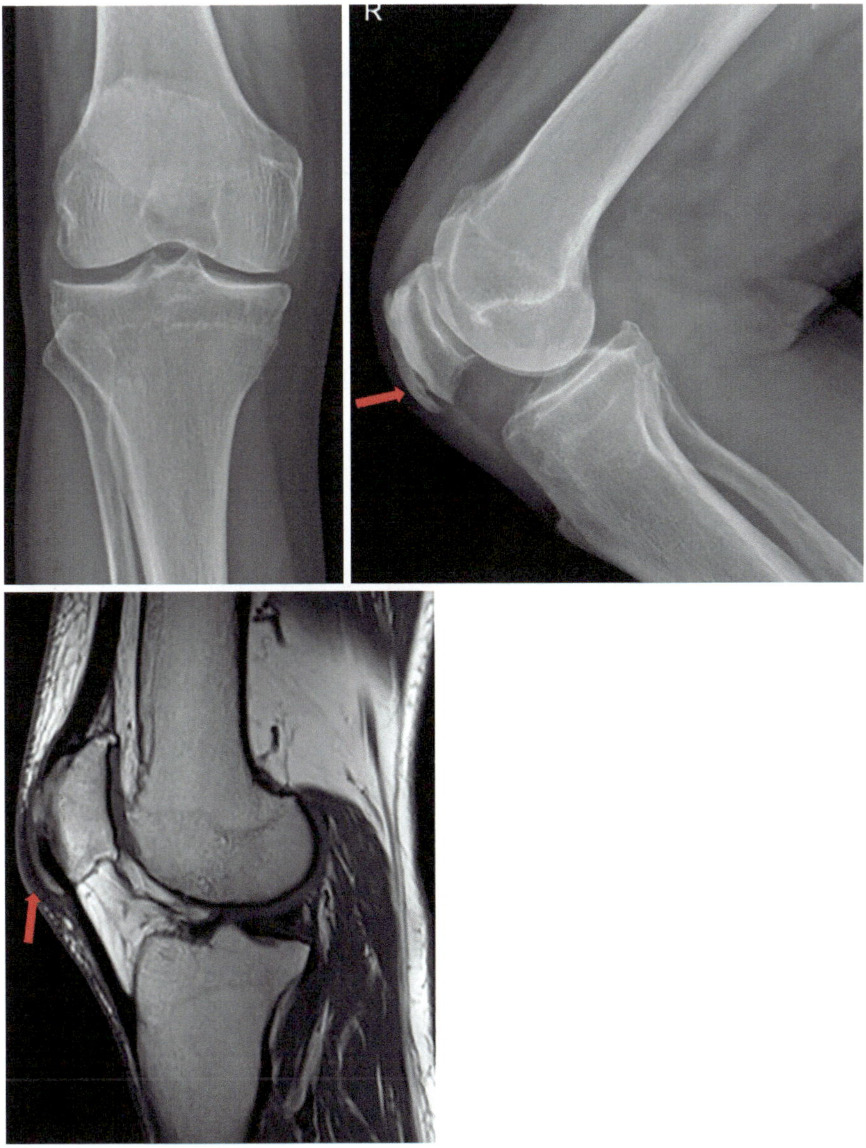

Patellar enthesopathy (red arrow)

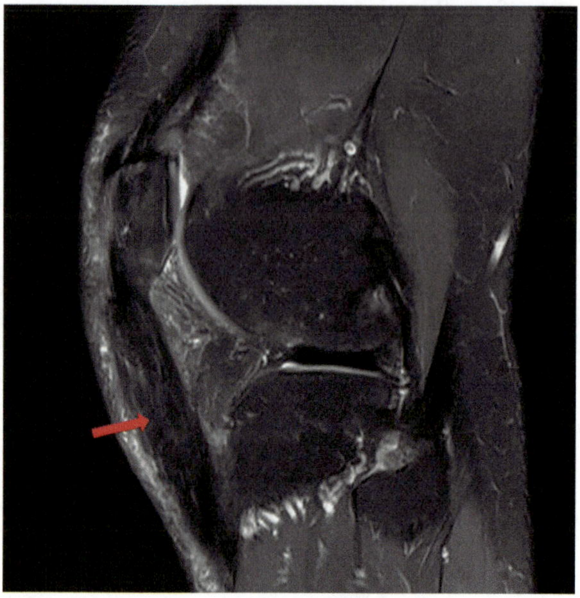

Thickened patellar tendon (red arrow) in patellar tendinopathy

23.6 Management of Patellar Tendon Tendinopathy

This is influenced by the underlying cause of the tendinopathy and may be non-surgical or surgical. The ladder of interventions may be utilised.

23.6.1 Non-surgical Interventions [16–25]

- Rest, activity modification, local passive therapy
- Posture improvement
- Landing pattern training—trunk flexion landing
- Eccentric exercises of the patellar tendon (eccentric squats on decline board)—more helpful for long term pain relief
- Isometric exercises may help during competitive periods for short term pain relief to avoid an athlete having to take time off sports until symptoms improve
- Body weight reduction
- Quadriceps and hamstring stretching to increase flexibility
- Stretching to improve stiffness- in posterior capsular contracture
- Increase quadriceps strength
- Patellar tendon strap which aims to:

  - Reduce quadriceps pre-landing activation, to reduce the tensile load on the patellar tendon
  - Improve proprioception
- Extracorporeal shock wave (ESW) therapy
- Local injections:
  - PRP injections
  - Hyaluronic acid injections
- Patellar tendon percutaneous needling

23.6.2 Surgical Interventions [26–32]

Surgical interventions aim to remove inflammatory tissue, stimulate regeneration and excise any impinging lesions. These include:

- Debridement of the degenerate tendon
- Debridement of the tendon insertion site on the patella, drilling of the bone insertion site (inferior pole of the patella-osteoplasty), debridement of the associated fat pad, +/– reattachment of the tendon to the patella
- Excision of any impinging lesions (loose ossicles, prominent tibial tubercle), drilling of the insertion site on the tibial tubercle +/– reattachment of the tendon to the tibial tubercle
- Osteotomy and reposition of a malunited fracture
- Correct patella alta—distalization of the tibial tubercle

The effect of treatment for patellar tendon tendinopathy is highly heterogeneous. This may be related to the observed diversity of the pathology of the underlying disease. Hence, it is not possible to predict reliably at an individual level who will benefit from non-surgical or surgical intervention.

Learning Pearls

- Non-surgical management is usually tried for about 6 months before considering surgery.
- There is lack of well-designed studies, with a long-term follow-up, and a large number of patients, upon which to draw strong conclusions with regards superiority of one treatment over the rest.
- Mass lesions of the patellar tendon (including gouty tophus) have been described and must be considered in the clinical evaluation of patellar tendinopathy.

References

1. Figueroa D, Figueroa F, Calvo R. Patellar tendinopathy: diagnosis and treatment. J Am Acad Orthop Surg. 2016;24(12):e184–92.
2. Van der Worp H, de Poel HJ, Diercks RL, van den Akker-Scheek I, Zwerver J. Jumper's knee or lander's knee? A systematic review of the relation between jump biomechanics and patellar tendinopathy. Int J Sports Med. 2014;35(8):714–22.
3. Sprague AL, Smith AH, Knox P, Pohlig RT, Grävare Silbernagel K. Modifiable risk factors for patellar tendinopathy in athletes: a systematic review and meta-analysis. Br J Sports Med. 2018;52(24):1575–85.
4. Morton S, Williams S, Valle X, Diaz-Cueli D, Malliaras P, Morrissey D. Patellar tendinopathy and potential risk factors: an international database of cases and controls. Clin J Sport Med. 2017;27(5):468–74.
5. Scattone Silva R, Nakagawa TH, Ferreira AL, Garcia LC, Santos JE, Serrão FV. Lower limb strength and flexibility in athletes with and without patellar tendinopathy. Phys Ther Sport. 2016;20:19–25.
6. Scattone Silva R, Purdam CR, Fearon AM, Spratford WA, Kenneally-Dabrowski C, Preston P, Serrão FV, Gaida JE. Effects of altering trunk position during landings on patellar tendon force and pain. Med Sci Sports Exerc. 2017;49(12):2517–27.
7. Lian Ø, Refsnes PE, Engebretsen L, Bahr R. Performance characteristics of volleyball players with patellar tendinopathy. Am J Sports Med. 2003;31(3):408–13.
8. Schmid MR, Hodler J, Cathrein P, Duewell S, Jacob HA, Romero J. Is impingement the cause of jumper's knee? Dynamic and static magnetic resonance imaging of patellar tendinitis in an open-configuration system. Am J Sports Med. 2002;30(3):388–95.
9. Chung CB, Skaf A, Roger B, Campos J, Stump X, Resnick D. Patellar tendon-lateral femoral condyle friction syndrome: MR imaging in 42 patients. Skelet Radiol. 2001;30(12):694–7.
10. Touraine S, Lagadec M, Petrover D, Genah I, Parlier-Cuau C, Bousson V, Laredo JD. A ganglion of the patellar tendon in patellar tendon-lateral femoral condyle friction syndrome. Skelet Radiol. 2013;42(9):1323–7.
11. O'Connell L, Memon AR, Foran P, Leen E, Kenny PJ. Synovial chondroma in Hoffa's fat pad: case report and literature review of a rare disorder. Int J Surg Case Rep. 2017;32:80–2.
12. Mendonça LD, Ocarino JM, Bittencourt NFN, Macedo LG, Fonseca ST. Association of hip and foot factors with patellar tendinopathy (Jumper's knee) in athletes. J Orthop Sports Phys Ther. 2018;48(9):676–84.
13. Golman M, Wright ML, Wong TT, Lynch TS, Ahmad CS, Thomopoulos S, Popkin CA. Rethinking patellar tendinopathy and partial patellar tendon tears: a novel classification system. Am J Sports Med. 2020;48(2):359–69.
14. Foley J, Elhelali R, Moiloa D. Spontaneous simultaneous bilateral patellar tendon rupture. BMJ Case Rep. 2019;12(2). pii: e227931. https://doi.org/10.1136/bcr-2018-227931.
15. Moura DL, Marques JP, Lucas FM, Fonseca FP. Simultaneous bilateral patellar tendon rupture. Rev Bras Ortop. 2016;52(1):111–4.
16. Chen PC, Wu KT, Chou WY, Huang YC, Wang LY, Yang TH, Siu KK, Tu YK. Comparative effectiveness of different nonsurgical treatments for patellar tendinopathy: a systematic review and network meta-analysis. Arthroscopy. 2019;35(11):3117–31.
17. Nuhmani S. Injection therapies for patellar tendinopathy. Phys Sportsmed. 2020;48(2):125–30.
18. van Ark M, Cook JL, Docking SI, Zwerver J, Gaida JE, van den Akker-Scheek I, Rio E. Do isometric and isotonic exercise programs reduce pain in athletes with patellar tendinopathy in-season? A randomised clinical trial. J Sci Med Sport. 2016;19(9):702–6.
19. Everhart JS, Cole D, Sojka JH, Higgins JD, Magnussen RA, Schmitt LC, Flanigan DC. Treatment options for patellar tendinopathy: a systematic review. Arthroscopy. 2017;33(4):861–72.
20. Rio E, Purdam C, Girdwood M, Cook J. Isometric exercise to reduce pain in patellar tendinopathy in-season; is it effective "on the road?". Clin J Sport Med. 2019;29:188–92. https://doi.org/10.1097/JSM.0000000000000549.

21. Dar G, Mei-Dan E. Immediate effect of infrapatellar strap on pain and jump height in patellar tendinopathy among young athletes. Prosthet Orthot Int. 2019;43(1):21–7.
22. Rio E, van Ark M, Docking S, Moseley GL, Kidgell D, Gaida JE, van den Akker-Scheek I, Zwerver J, Cook J. Isometric contractions are more analgesic than isotonic contractions for patellar tendon pain: an in-season randomized clinical trial. Clin J Sport Med. 2017;27(3):253–9.
23. Rosen AB, Ko J, Simpson KJ, Brown CN. Patellar tendon straps decrease pre-landing quadriceps activation in males with patellar tendinopathy. Phys Ther Sport. 2017;24:13–9.
24. Torres R, Ferreira J, Silva D, Rodrigues E, Bessa IM, Ribeiro F. Impact of patellar tendinopathy on knee proprioception: a cross-sectional study. Clin J Sport Med. 2017;27(1):31–6.
25. de Vries AJ, van den Akker-Scheek I, Haak SL, Diercks RL, van der Worp H, Zwerver J. Effect of a patellar strap on the joint position sense of the symptomatic knee in athletes with patellar tendinopathy. J Sci Med Sport. 2017;20(11):986–91.
26. Dan M, Phillips A, Johnston RV, Harris IA. Surgery for patellar tendinopathy (jumper's knee). Cochrane Database Syst Rev. 2019;9:CD013034. https://doi.org/10.1002/14651858.CD013034.pub2.
27. Lee DW, Kim JG, Kim TM, Kim DH. Refractory patellar tendinopathy treated by arthroscopic decortication of the inferior patellar pole in athletes: mid-term outcomes. Knee. 2018;25(3):499–506.
28. Pestka JM, Lang G, Maier D, Südkamp NP, Ogon P, Izadpanah K. Arthroscopic patellar release allows timely return to performance in professional and amateur athletes with chronic patellar tendinopathy. Knee Surg Sports Traumatol Arthrosc. 2018;26(12):3553–9.
29. Alaseirlis DA, Konstantinidis GA, Malliaropoulos N, Nakou LS, Korompilias A, Maffulli N. Arthroscopic treatment of chronic patellar tendinopathy in high-level athletes. Muscles Ligaments Tendons J. 2013;2(4):267–72.
30. Kruckeberg BM, Chahla J, Ferrari MB, Sanchez G, Moatshe G, LaPrade RF. Open patellar tendon tenotomy, debridement, and repair technique augmented with platelet-rich plasma for recalcitrant patellar tendinopathy. Arthrosc Tech. 2017;6(2):e447–53.
31. Khan WS, Smart A. Outcome of surgery for chronic patellar tendinopathy: a systematic review. Acta Orthop Belg. 2016;82(3):610–326.
32. Zhang B, Qu TB, Pan J, Wang ZW, Zhang XD, Ren SX, Wen L, Chen T, Ma DS, Lin Y, Cheng CK. Open patellar tendon tenotomy and debridement combined with suture-bridging double-row technique for severe patellar tendinopathy. Orthop Surg. 2016;8(1):51–9.

Chapter 24
Hamstring Tendon Tendinopathy

This is a condition whereby there is tendinopathy of one or more of the distal hamstring tendons. This usually affects the distal part of the tendon or its point of attachment to the proximal tibia or fibula.

Hamstring tendon tendinopathy may be due to multiple factors [1–9] including:

- Overload/overuse
  - High duration/frequency of activities
  - Participation in sports which require turning/twisting/direction change (football, basketball)
  - Muscle imbalance (core, lower limb)
  - Inadequate warm-up/stretching when engaging in sports
  - Inadequate technique of squatting, jumping, landing
- Friction with anatomically closely related structures—such as medial femoral condyle, posterior capsule in semimembranosus (SM) tendinopathy
- External impingement/friction such as by:
  - Exostoses
  - Osteophytes
  - Prominent femoral or tibial components following knee replacement arthroplasty
  - Malunited distal femoral or proximal tibial fracture
- Tendon snapping
- Mass lesion
- Knee valgus or varus malalignment, stretching the medial or lateral hamstring tendons respectively
- Foot overpronation or oversupination leading to knee malalignment and sretching of the hamstring tendons

C. Panayiotou Charalambous, *The Knee Made Easy*,
https://doi.org/10.1007/978-3-030-54506-2_24

24.1 Clinical Symptoms of Hamstring Tendon Tendinopathy

- Pain
  - Over the hamstring tendons or over their bony insertion
  - Radiating up the thigh (including up to the hip or pelvis) in line with the tendon or its muscle
- Swelling over the course of the tendons or their bony insertion due to associated synovitis/bursitis
- Pain aggravated by activity, especially repetitive knee motion
  - Activating the involved tendon—knee flexion
  - Stretching the involved tendon—knee extension
- Pain may be vary from low grade to intense/severe
- Hamstring weakness
- Knee stiffness

24.2 Clinical Signs of Hamstring Tendon Tendinopathy

- Tendon substance or insertion tenderness
- Apparent joint stiffness—due to pain
- Aggravated pain on:
  - Stressing the tendon—by getting its muscle to contract against resistance
  - Stretching the tendon—moving the limb or joint in such a way as to stretch the tendon examined
- Swelling:
  - Associated synovitis/bursitis
  - Impinging mass lesion
- Malalignment—knee, foot
- Muscle weakness/imbalance: core/hip/knee/foot
- Knee stiffness

24.3 Investigations for Hamstring Tendon Tendinopathy

- Plain radiographs—look for calcific deposits, enthesis spurs, impinging lesions
- MRI—look for hamstring tendon tendinopathy, tendon thickening, partial tears, synovitis, bursitis, impinging mass lesions
- Ultrasound—may allow more localised examination of the painful/tender area
- CT scan—assess distal femoral and proximal tibial morphology, impinging lesions
- Diagnostic local anaesthetic injection

24.4 Management of Hamstring Tendon Tendinopathy

This is influenced by the underlying cause of the tendinopathy and may be non-surgical or surgical. The ladder of interventions may be utilised.

24.4.1 Non-surgical Interventions

- Rest, activity modification, local passive therapy
- Posture improvement
- Eccentric exercises of the hamstring tendons
- Stretching of the involved tendon
- Strengthening of the involved muscles and knee stabilisers
- Extracorporeal shockwave therapy (ECSW)
- External devices knee/foot to correct alignment deformities
- Local injections:
  - PRP injections (tendon/insertion site)
  - Hyaluronic acid
  - Steroid (at insertion sites)
- Hamstring tendon percutaneous needling

24.4.2 Surgical Interventions [2, 10]

Surgical interventions aim to remove any inflammatory tissue, simulate regeneration and excise any impinging lesions. These include:

- Debridement of the degenerate tendon
- Debridement +/– drilling of the tendon insertion site
- Excision of any impinging lesions
- Tendon division—in low demand patients
- Tendon transfer—tendon division, rerouting and reinsertion onto the bone
  - In cases of chronic irritation of the SM tendon at the posteromedial corner of the knee, a SM rerouting procedure that places the SM tendon adjacent to the posterior border of the medial collateral ligament has been described [2].

Learning Pearls

- Patients presenting with tendinopathy related pain should be questioned about a recent increase in duration/frequency or intensity of activity related to the onset of symptoms
- Rest and reduction in activity may be essential in order to break the pain cycle and reduce the chance of progressing to chronic non-resolving pain

References

1. Bylund WE, de Weber K. Semimembranosus tendinopathy: one cause of chronic posteromedial knee pain. Sports Health. 2010;2(5):380–4.
2. Ray JM, Clancy WG Jr, Lemon RA. Semimembranosus tendinitis: an overlooked cause of medial knee pain. Am J Sports Med. 1988;16(4):347–51.
3. Reid L, Mofidi A. Bilateral snapping biceps femoris tendon: a case report and review of the literature. Eur J Orthop Surg Traumatol. 2019;29(5):1081–7.
4. Matar HE, Farrar NG. Snapping biceps femoris: clinical demonstration and operative technique. Ann R Coll Surg Engl. 2018;100(3):e59–61.
5. Chan W, Chase HE, Cahir JG, Walton NP. Calcific tendinitis of biceps femoris: an unusual site and cause for lateral knee pain. BMJ Case Rep. 2016;2016:bcr2016215745.
6. Karataglis D, Papadopoulos P, Fotiadou A, Christodoulou AG. Snapping knee syndrome in an athlete caused by the semitendinosus and gracilis tendons. A case report. Knee. 2008;15(2):151–4.
7. Bollen SR, Arvinite D. Snapping pes syndrome: a report of four cases. J Bone Joint Surg Br. 2008;90:334–5.
8. Hendel D, Weisbort M, Garti A. Semimembranosus tendonitis after total knee arthroplasty: good outcome after surgery in 6 patients. Acta Orthop Scand. 2003;74(4):429–30.
9. Weiser H. Semimembranosus insertion syndrome: a treatable and frequent cause of persistent knee pain. Arch Phys Med Rehabil. 1979;60:317–9.
10. Halperin N, Oren Y, Hendel D, Nathan N. Semimembranosus tenosynovitis: operative results. Arch Orthop Trauma Surg. 1987;106:281–4.

Chapter 25
Calcific Tendinopathy/Ligamentopathy

This is a condition whereby calcium is deposited in one or more tendons or ligaments around the knee. The calcific deposits consist of carbonate apatite [1–8]. Although calcific tendinopathy/ligamentopathy around the knee is well described, it is much less common as compared to calcific tendinopathy of the shoulder.

Involvement of the following tendons/ligaments has been previously described [9–20], but in principle any such structure could be affected:

- Quadriceps tendon
- Patellar tendon
- Popliteus tendon
- Lateral collateral ligament
- Medial collateral ligament (MCL)
- Anterior cruciate ligament
- Biceps femoris
- Medial plica

25.1 Pathophysiology of Calcific Tendinopathy

This remains uncertain but several theories have been proposed [6–8]:

1. Passive—calcium is deposited in degenerate tissue (tendon or ligament) where there is cell necrosis
2. Active—cell mediated calcification, followed by phagocyte resorption. In the shoulder it has been suggested that calcium deposition may signify an attempt of tendons, which are weak and have reduced stiffness, to increase their stiffness.

Calcium deposition may also be due to an underlying associated crystallisation disorder—phytate inhibits crystallisation and its urinary levels have been shown to be reduced in patients with calcific tendinopathy.

C. Panayiotou Charalambous, *The Knee Made Easy*,
https://doi.org/10.1007/978-3-030-54506-2_25

Three phases of calcific deposition have been described:

1. Pre-calcific—tendon/ligament undergoes metaplasia into cartilage
2. Calcific—calcium forms, is deposited, broken down and removed by macrophages and phagocytes
3. Post-calcific—fibroblasts lay down new collagen

The calcium deposits may be

- Toothpaste like fluid
- Sand like particles
- Small round bodies

The calcium deposits may be:

- Diffuse, infiltrating the tendon substance
- Distinct, shelled out lesions

25.2 Clinical Symptoms of Calcific Tendinopathy

- Non symptomatic—incidental finding on radiological investigations
- Pain
  - Felt in the area of deposit
  - May present as:
    - Acute onset pain- sharp pain
    - Chronic pain

Pain may be due to:

- Chemical irritation of the tissue as the body attempts to break down and remove the calcium
- Increase in pressure within the tendon/ligament by the mass lesion effect of the calcific deposit

25.3 Clinical Signs of Calcific Tendinopathy

- Tenderness over the calcific deposit
- Swelling associated with the calcific deposit
- Effusion
- Reduced range of knee motion
  - Apparent—due to pain
  - True—due to associated stiffness

25.4 Investigations for Calcific Tendinopathy

- Plain radiographs to:
  - Confirm the presence of a calcific deposit
  - Determine the location of the calcific deposit in the anterior-posterior, proximal-distal and medial-lateral planes
- Ultrasound
- MRI scan
  - Look for other pathology

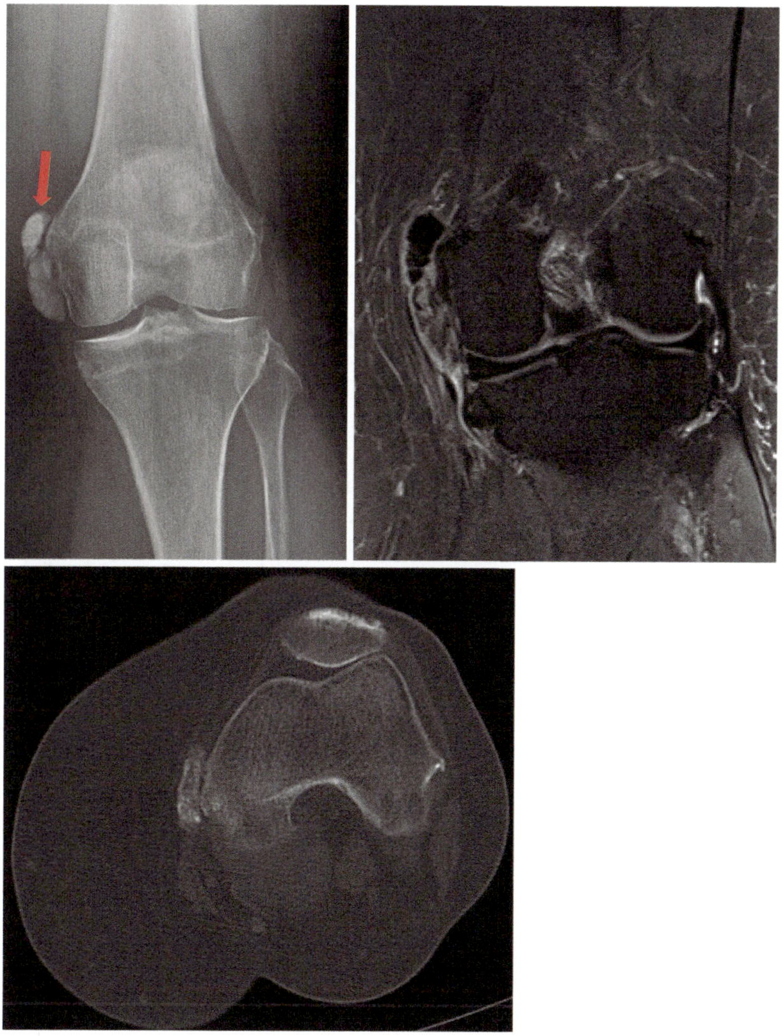

Calcification of the medial collateral ligament (red arrow (CT and MRI)

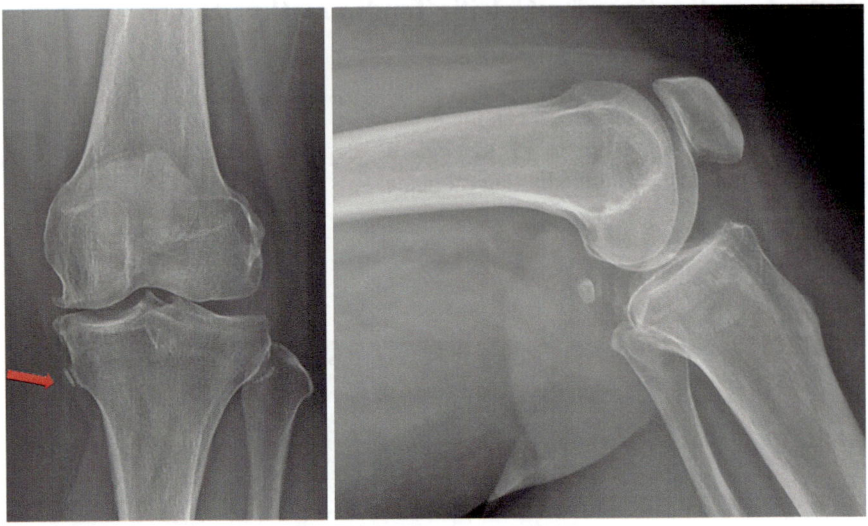

Cacific tendinopathy of the pes anserinus insertion

25.5 Management of Calcific Tendinopathy

25.5.1 Non-surgical [21–23]

- Observation and analgesia—spontaneous resolution of the calcific deposit may occur, or there may be improvement in symptoms even if the calcific deposit persists in the tissue
- Extracorporeal shock wave treatment (ECSW)
- Steroid injection around the involved tendon or ligament
- Calcific deposit barbotage +/− steroid injection

25.5.2 Surgical [24, 25]

- Open excision of the calcific deposit +/− repair of the residual defect in the tendon/ligament

At surgery an attempt is made to remove as much calcium as possible, and decompress the lesion. However, it is understandable that it may not be possible to remove all calcium as that could lead to substantial damage of the tendon/ligament.

25.6 Pellegrini-Stieda Disease

This is a condition whereby there is pain on the medial aspect of the knee associated with calcific deposition around the region of the femoral medial epicondyle and adductor tubercle. This may be associated with restriction of knee motion.

The exact soft tissue structures involved in calcification has been controversial—the proximal attachment of the superficial MCL, adductor magnus tendon, medial head of the the gastrocnemius, and medial patellofemoral ligament (MPFL) have been proposed as involved. Similarly, it is controversial as to whether this condition is encountered only after trauma, as cases occurring in the absence of trauma have been reported.

Management may be considered similar to that of calcific tendinopathy/ligamentopathy as described above. If surgical excision of the calcific deposits is performed, surgical repair or reconstruction of the superficial MCL may be necessary (if the ligament is found to be involved and be deficient following calcific deposit excision) [26–31].

Learning Pearls

- Patients need to be informed that pain from calcific deposits in tendons/ligaments may take a substantial time to improve post-surgery, or that it may not improve due to associated degeneration of the involved tendon/ligament.
- Calcification of the quadriceps insertion onto the patella (appearing as "whiskers" or "flecks") is common. These are considered traction enthesophytes, and are associated with underlying degenerative knee disease. They may also be more common in those who develop quadriceps tendon tear [32–34].
- Calcification may also be seen in bursae and management is similar to the above
- Tumoral calcinosis is a distinct entity characterised by massive extra-articular soft tissue deposits of calcium phosphate around large joints—it may be caused by renal failure, hyperparathyroidism, hypervitaminosis D, sarcoidosis, or be familial or idiopathic. Patients may present with pain, stiffness, or a mass. Treatment may involve control of calcium metabolism and excision of the deposits.

References

1. Oliva F, Via AG, Maffulli N. Physiopathology of intratendinous calcific deposition. BMC Med. 2012;10:95. https://doi.org/10.1186/1741-7015-10.
2. ElShewy MT. Calcific tendinitis of the rotator cuff. World J Orthop. 2016;7(1):55–60.

3. Hurt G, Baker CL Jr. Calcific tendinitis of the shoulder. Orthop Clin North Am. 2003;34(4):567–75.
4. Hamada J, Ono W, Tamai K, Saotome K, Hoshino T. Analysis of calcium deposits in calcific periarthritis. J Rheumatol. 2001;28(4):809–13.
5. Suzuki K, Potts A, Anakwenze O, Singh A. Calcific tendinitis of the rotator cuff: management options. J Am Acad Orthop Surg. 2014;22(11):707–17.
6. Grases F, Muntaner-Gimbernat L, Vilchez-Mira M, Costa-Bauzá A, Tur F, Prieto RM, Torrens-Mas M, Vega FG. Characterization of deposits in patients with calcific tendinopathy of the supraspinatus. Role of phytate and osteopontin. J Orthop Res. 2015;33(4):475–82.
7. Grases F, Sanchis P, Perello J, Isern B, Prieto RM, Fernandez-Palomeque C, Fiol M, Bonnin O, Torres JJ. Phytate (Myo-inositol hexakisphosphate) inhibits cardiovascular calcifications in rats. Front Biosci. 2006;11:136–42.
8. Hackett L, Millar NL, Lam P, Murrell GA. Are the symptoms of calcific tendinitis due to neoinnervation and/or neovascularization? J Bone Joint Surg Am. 2016;98(3):186–92.
9. Varghese B, Radcliffe GS, Groves C. Calcific tendonitis of the quadriceps. Br J Sports Med. 2006;40(7):652–4.
10. Peng X, Feng Y, Chen G, Yang L. Arthroscopic treatment of chronically painful calcific tendinitis of the rectus femoris. Eur J Med Res. 2013;18:49.
11. Webb SA, Hopper MA, Chitnavis J. Calcific tendonitis of the quadriceps tendon. J Surg Case Rep. 2018;2018(4):rjy053. https://doi.org/10.1093/jscr/rjy053.
12. Galletti L, Ricci V, Andreoli E, Galletti S. Treatment of a calcific bursitis of the medial collateral ligament: a rare cause of painful knee. J Ultrasound. 2019;22(4):471–6.
13. Doucet C, Gotra A, Reddy SMV, Boily M. Acute calcific tendinopathy of the popliteus tendon: a rare case diagnosed using a multimodality imaging approach and treated conservatively. Skeletal Radiol. 2017;46(7):1003–6.
14. Tennent TD, Goradia VK. Arthroscopic management of calcific tendinitis of the popliteus tendon. Arthroscopy. 2003;19(4):E35.
15. Tibrewal SB. Acute calcific tendinitis of the popliteus tendon—an unusual site and clinical syndrome. Ann R Coll Surg Engl. 2002;84(5):338–41.
16. Tsujii A, Tanaka Y, Yonetani Y, Iuchi R, Shiozaki Y, Horibe S. Symptomatic calcification of the anterior cruciate ligament: a case report. Knee. 2012;19(3):223–5.
17. Chan W, Chase HE, Cahir JG, Walton NP. Calcific tendinitis of biceps femoris: an unusual site and cause for lateral knee pain. BMJ Case Rep. 2016;2016:bcr2016215745. https://doi.org/10.1136/bcr-2016-215745.
18. Watura K, Greenish D, Williams M, Webb J. Acute calcific periarthiritis of the knee presenting with calcification within the lateral collateral ligament. BMJ Case Rep. 2015;2015:bcr2014209041. https://doi.org/10.1136/bcr-2014-209041.
19. White WJ, Sarraf KM, Schranz P. Acute calcific deposition in the lateral collateral ligament of the knee. J Knee Surg. 2013;26(Suppl 1):S116–9.
20. Schindler K, O'Keefe P, Bohn T, Sundaram M. Calcific tendonitis of the fibular collateral ligament. Orthopedics. 2006;29(4):282, 373–5.
21. De Zordo T, Ahmad N, Ødegaard F, Girtler MT, Jaschke W, Klauser AS, Chhem RK, Romagnoli C. US-guided therapy of calcific tendinopathy: clinical and radiological outcome assessment in shoulder and non-shoulder tendons. Ultraschall Med. 2011;32(Suppl 1):S117–23.
22. Del Castillo-González F, Ramos-Álvarez JJ, González-Pérez J, Jiménez-Herranz E, Rodríguez-Fabián G. Ultrasound-guided percutaneous lavage of calcific bursitis of the medial collateral ligament of the knee: a case report and review of the literature. Skeletal Radiol. 2016;45(10):1419–23.
23. Gatt DL, Charalambous CP. Ultrasound-guided barbotage for calcific tendonitis of the shoulder: a systematic review including 908 patients. Arthroscopy. 2014;30(9):1166–72.
24. Shenoy PM, Kim DH, Wang KH, Oh HK, Soo LC, Kim JH, Nha KW. Calcific tendinitis of popliteus tendon: arthroscopic excision and biopsy. Orthopedics. 2009;32(2):127.

25. Song K, Dong J, Zhang Y, Chen B, Wang F, Zhao J, Ji G. Arthroscopic management of calcific tendonitis of the medial collateral ligament. Knee. 2013;20(1):63–5.
26. Somford MP, Janssen RPA, Meijer D, Roeling TAP, Brown C Jr, Eygendaal D. The Pellegrini-Stieda lesion of the knee: an anatomical and radiological review. J Knee Surg. 2019;32(7):637–41.
27. Somford MP, Lorusso L, Porro A, Loon CV, Eygendaal D. The Pellegrini-Stieda lesion dissected historically. J Knee Surg. 2018;31(6):562–7.
28. Theivendran K, Lever CJ, Hart WJ. Good result after surgical treatment of Pellegrini-Stieda syndrome. Knee Surg Sports Traumatol Arthrosc. 2009;17(10):1231–3.
29. Wang JC, Shapiro MS. Pellegrini-Stieda syndrome. Am J Orthop (Belle Mead NJ). 1995;24(6):493–7.
30. Houston AN, Roy WA, Faust RA, Ewin DM, Espenan PA. Pellegrini-Stieda syndrome: report of 44 cases followed from original injury. South Med J. 1968;61(2):113–7.
31. Coltart WD. Pellegrini-Stieda lesion. Proc R Soc Med. 1938;31(3):180–1.
32. Trujeque L, Spohn P, Bankhurst A, Messner R, Searles R. Patellar whiskers and acute calcific quadriceps tendinitis in a general hospital population. Arthritis Rheum. 1977;20(7):1409–12.
33. Hardy JR, Chimutengwende-Gordon M, Bakar I. Rupture of the quadriceps tendon: an association with a patellar spur. J Bone Joint Surg Br. 2005;87(10):1361–3.
34. Ellanti P, Moriarity A, Wainberg N, Fhoghlu CN, McCarthy T. Association between patella spurs and quadriceps tendon ruptures. Muscles Ligaments Tendons J. 2015;5(2):88–91.

Chapter 26
Iliotibial Band Syndrome

Iliotibial band (ITB) syndrome is an overuse condition that is more common in activities that involve knee flexion and extension such as running, cycling or hiking. It may be seen following a recent change in activity (duration or level), inadequate warming for exercise, or in gait abnormalities such as foot overpronation, leg length discrepancy, or knee varus, which may put more strain on the ITB.

It has been traditionally thought that the ITB moves anterior to the lateral condyle of the femur with knee extension and slides posteriorly with 30° of knee flexion, rubbing over an underlying bursa. ITB syndrome was thus considered secondary to repetitive friction between the ITB and the underlying bursa and lateral femoral epicondyle. However, more recent anatomical studies have disputed the forth/back movement of the ITB. Instead, the apparent appearance has been attributed to alternate contraction of the anterior and posterior fibres of the ITB rather than translation. Furthermore, an underlying bursa has not been identified on anatomical studies but a fat pad has been located between the distal part of the ITB and bone. Hence, it is considered that repeated compression of this fat pad and its associated connective tissue may be involved in the pathogenesis of ITB syndrome. ITB irritation may also be caused by implants inserted close to the ITB, such as fixation devices (suture buttons) in anterior cruciate ligament reconstruction [1–13]. It may also be encountered post knee replacement arthroplasty (due to cement extrusion, prominent components-tibial insert, residual osteophytes). ITB syndrome has also been associated with a more prominent lateral epicondyle and varus thrust.

26.1 Clinical Symptoms of ITB Syndrome

- Pain on the outside of the knee with exercise
- Aggravated by activities that require knee flexion—running downhill, cycling, having the knee bent for prolonged periods of time
- Pain may be vague and dull, or sharp and substantial

C. Panayiotou Charalambous, *The Knee Made Easy*,
https://doi.org/10.1007/978-3-030-54506-2_26

26.2 Clinical Signs of ITB Syndrome

- Tenderness over the lateral femoral epicondyle
- Gait abnormalities—foot overpronation, leg length discrepancy, knee varus
- Tenderness over the distal part of the ITB aggravated by knee flexion/extension

26.3 Investigations for ITB Syndrome

- Plain radiographs
- MRI
- Ultrasound

26.4 Management of ITB Syndrome [1, 14–18]

26.4.1 Non-surgical

- Physiotherapy—stretching the ITB
- Local treatment, extracorporeal shock wave therapy (ECSW)
- Steroid injection between the ITB and femur

26.4.2 Surgical

- ITB lengthening
- ITB division
- ITB bursectomy/ debridement of connective tissue, fat pad
- Excision/removal of irritating factors

Learning Pearls

- A small amount of fluid under the ITB has been shown to be common in asymptomatic runners, hence its significance in symptomatic cases must be interpreted with caution.
- Fluid under the ITB may be of intra-articular origin (as connection between the two may occur), and hence clinical evaluation of the knee joint should be considered when indicated.

References

1. Strauss EJ, Kim S, Calcei JG, Park D. Iliotibial band syndrome: evaluation and management. J Am Acad Orthop Surg. 2011;19(12):728–36.
2. Fairclough J, Hayashi K, Toumi H, Lyons K, Bydder G, Phillips N, Best TM, Benjamin M. Is iliotibial band syndrome really a friction syndrome? J Sci Med Sport. 2007;10(2):74–6.
3. Jelsing EJ, Finnoff JT, Cheville AL, Levy BA, Smith J. Sonographic evaluation of the iliotibial band at the lateral femoral epicondyle: does the iliotibial band move? J Ultrasound Med. 2013;32(7):1199–206.
4. Takagi K, Inui H, Taketomi S, Yamagami R, Kono K, Nakazato K, Kawaguchi K, Kage T, Tanaka S. Iliotibial band friction syndrome after knee arthroplasty. Knee. 2020;27(1):263–73.
5. Everhart JS, Kirven JC, Higgins J, Hair A, Chaudhari AAMW, Flanigan DC. The relationship between lateral epicondyle morphology and iliotibial band friction syndrome: a matched case-control study. Knee. 2019;26(6):1198–203.
6. Flato R, Passanante GJ, Skalski MR, Patel DB, White EA, Matcuk GR Jr. The iliotibial tract: imaging, anatomy, injuries, and other pathology. Skeletal Radiol. 2017;46(5):605–22.
7. Aderem J, Louw QA. Biomechanical risk factors associated with iliotibial band syndrome in runners: a systematic review. BMC Musculoskelet Disord. 2015;16:356. https://doi.org/10.1186/s12891-015-0808-7.
8. Jelsing EJ, Maida E, Finnoff JT, Smith J. The source of fluid deep to the iliotibial band: documentation of a potential intra-articular source. PM R. 2014;6(2):134–8.
9. Stickley CD, Presuto MM, Radzak KN, Bourbeau CM, Hetzler RK. Dynamic varus and the development of iliotibial band syndrome. J Athl Train. 2018;53(2):128–34.
10. Hong JH, Kim JS. Diagnosis of iliotibial band friction syndrome and ultrasound guided steroid injection. Korean J Pain. 2013;26(4):387–91.
11. Taketomi S, Inui H, Hirota J, Nakamura K, Sanada T, Masuda H, Tanaka S, Nakagawa T. Iliotibial band irritation caused by the EndoButton after anatomic double-bundle anterior cruciate ligament reconstruction: report of two cases. Knee. 2013;20(4):291–4.
12. Cruz-López F, Mallen-Trejo A, Pascual-Vidriales C, Almazán-Díaz A, Ibarra-Ponce de León JC. [Iliotibial band friction syndrome due to bioabsorbable pins in ACL reconstruction]. Acta Ortop Mex. 2016;30(6):307–310.
13. Jelsing EJ, Finnoff J, Levy B, Smith J. The prevalence of fluid associated with the iliotibial band in asymptomatic recreational runners: an ultrasonographic study. PM R. 2013;5(7):563–7.
14. Fredericson M, Weir A. Practical management of iliotibial band friction syndrome in runners. Clin J Sport Med. 2006;16(3):261–8.
15. Hariri S, Savidge ET, Reinold MM, Zachazewski J, Gill TJ. Treatment of recalcitrant iliotibial band friction syndrome with open iliotibial band bursectomy: indications, technique, and clinical outcomes. Am J Sports Med. 2009;37(7):1417–24.
16. Barber FA, Boothby MH, Troop RL. Z-plasty lengthening for iliotibial band friction syndrome. J Knee Surg. 2007;20(4):281–4.
17. Pierce TP, Mease SJ, Issa K, Festa A, McInerney VK, Scillia AJ. Iliotibial band lengthening: an arthroscopic surgical technique. Arthrosc Tech. 2017;6(3):e785–9.
18. Walbron P, Jacquot A, Geoffroy JM, Sirveaux F, Molé D. Iliotibial band friction syndrome: an original technique of digastric release of the iliotibial band from Gerdy's tubercle. Orthop Traumatol Surg Res. 2018;104(8):1209–13.

Chapter 27
Quadriceps Tears

A condition whereby the quadriceps tendon tears. The quadriceps consists of rectus femoris, vastus medialis, vastus intermedius and vastus lateralis.

27.1 Causes of Quadriceps Tears [1–17]

Most often tears occur secondary to an acute trauma. However, weakness of the tendon due to intrinsic or extrinsic factors may predispose to tears occurring at a lower force than would be otherwise expected. Trauma is often the result of:

- Direct impact on the quadriceps tendon
- Forced hyperflexion (accompanied by substantial eccentric contraction of the quadriceps tendon to oppose such flexion)
- Traumatic lacerations of the tendon

27.1.1 Factors Predisposing to Quadriceps Tears

- Intrinsic factors
  These refer to changes originating within the tendon rather than due to an extrinsic cause. Such changes may be age related and include:
  - Degeneration
  - Hypovascularity
  - Reduced cellular component
  - Collagen fibre thinning and disorganisation
  - Increased concentrations of matrix metalloproteinase and reduced tissue inhibitors of matrix metalloproteinases causing a greater break down of collagen fibres

C. Panayiotou Charalambous, *The Knee Made Easy*,
https://doi.org/10.1007/978-3-030-54506-2_27

- Extrinsic factors
  These refer to external factors acting on the quadriceps tendon and include [9–11]:
  - Tensile overload (acute trauma or repetitive use)
  - Impingement/friction (by a distal femoral osteochondroma, femoral component of knee replacement arthroplasty, large loose body)
  - Iatrogenic disruption—in early post knee replacement arthroplasty, quadriceps tendon harvesting for ligamentous reconstruction
- Combination of intrinsic and extrinsic factors
  Several risk factors have been related to an increased risk of quadriceps tear (including bilateral or non-traumatic tear) including:
  - Chronic renal failure -dialysis
  - Fluoroquinolones antibiotic use (such as ciprofloxacin, levofloxacin)
  - Diabetes mellitus
  - Hyperparathyroidism
  - Gout
  - Systemic lupus erythromatosus(SLE)/rheumatoid arthritis
  - Systemic steroid use
  - Steroid injections into the tendon
  - Anabolic steroids
  - Obesity

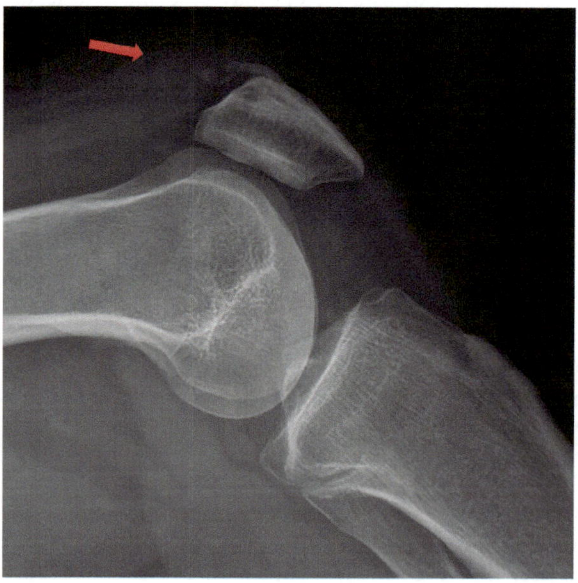

Gouty tophus distal quadriceps (red arrow)

27.2 Description of Quadriceps Tears

Quadriceps tears may be described in several ways and these are presented next.

According to the Precipitating Event

- Traumatic—the tendon tears suddenly (due to a substantial acute force)
- Spontaneous—(non-traumatic or with very minor trauma)—the tendon tears gradually over a long time (such as due to chronic repetitive loading or tendon degeneration). Tears occur without the application of substantial force
- Iatrogenic—as when surgically approaching the knee joint, harvesting the quadriceps tendon for ligament reconstruction (as in anterior cruciate ligament reconstruction)

According to the Site of the Tear

- Bony avulsions
- Mid-substance tears
- Musculotendinous junction tears

Quadriceps tears usually occur close to the tendon's insertion site (10–20 mm) or as avulsions from the patella rather than being much more proximal injuries of the tendon substance. The term "quadriceps tendon tear" is hence a misnomer. Quadriceps tears may occur at the mid-substance or at the musculotendinous junction rather than at the level of the bone tendon interface, but these are unusual.

According to the Length of the Tear

- Complete length tear (full)
- Incomplete length tear (partial)

The insertion of the quadriceps tendon on the patella is quite broad. It is thus possible to have a tear in the tendon which goes all the way transversely across its length (usually involving the medial and lateral retinacula) or one that involves only part of its length. If the whole of the tendon length is involved then this is described as a complete (or full) tear. If, however, only part of the quadriceps tendon length is involved then it is described as an incomplete length (or partial) tear.

According to the Tear Thickness

- Full thickness
- Partial thickness
  - Superficial site tear
  - Deep site tear

The insertion of the quadriceps tendon on the patella is thick. Hence, it is possible to have a tear in the tendon which goes all the way across the thickness (like a hole) described as a full thickness tear. Alternatively, it is possible for the deep surface or superficial surface of the tendon to pull off its attachment from the patella, giving rise to a partial thickness tear. In this situation there is no visible hole in the tendon.

Hence, in describing quadriceps tears, terminology is important. When describing tears as partial it is important to specify as to whether reference is made to tendon length or thickness.

According to the Degree of Tendon Retraction

Once a tendon avulses from the bone it retracts, that is the edge of the tendon moves away from its insertion site. This is due to:

- Muscle springing away from its insertion
- Muscle contracting
- Muscle shrinking
- Tendon substance lost

Following retraction of the quadriceps tendon stump, adhesions may form between the retracted tendon and the surrounding structures such as the femur. Such adhesions may limit a surgeon's ability to pull the tendon back to the patella. During attempted surgical reattachment of the tendon, release of such adhesions is essential in order to allow the tendon to be mobilised. However, despite release of adhesions it may still not be possible to return the tendon onto the patella due to changes in the muscle or tendon substance. Hence, alternative surgical techniques may be needed to bridge the gap.

According to Whether the Tear Can Be Surgically Repaired or Not

- Repairable
- Irreparable

Tendon tears may not be repairable due to several factors including:

- Excessive retraction—cannot reapproximate the tendon to bone
- Poor tendon quality—unable to hold sutures—sutures cutting through the tendon
- Poor bone quality—unable to hold suture anchors or sutures, such as in osteopenic bone (due to old age, immobility or other factors)

According to the Presence of Associated Muscle Atrophy or Fatty Infiltration
The muscle of a torn quadriceps tendon may atrophy (shrink) and undergo fatty infiltration (replaced by fat). Recognising the presence and extent of such atrophy is important as it may be associated with poorer clinical outcomes and may correlate with tear size [18–25].

Atrophy of quadriceps can be assessed quantitatively or qualitatively [13–15] by:

- Visual inspection
- Measurement of thigh girth
- Measurement of quadriceps volume and fatty infiltration on ultrasound, MRI or CT

Loss of muscle bulk and fatty infiltration may limit the success of surgical repair, even when a tendon can be physically reattached to bone.

According to the Timing of Presentation
Acute—presenting straight after the onset of the tear or shortly afterwards.
Chronic—presenting a substantial time after the onset of the tear due to factors including:

- Delayed presentation—by patient
- Missed diagnosis—by clinician
- Correct diagnosis made but surgery had to be delayed e.g. for medical reasons

27.3 Demographics of Quadriceps Tears

- Quadriceps tears have an incidence of about 1.37/100,000
- Most occur in men older than 40
- Spontaneous tears may occur in about 3.2% of cases

27.4 Clinical Symptoms of Quadriceps Tears

- History of trauma (major/minor)
- Sudden onset (even with no trauma)
- Pain—at rest or on exertion
- Weakness of leg (in one or multiple planes). Patient may complain that:
  - Cannot elevate the leg
  - Help the leg with the opposite one, after which leg elevation can be maintained e.g. getting in and out of bed
  - Can weightbear with leg straight but knee gives way when attempting to flex the knee
- Stiffness
- Difficulty in performing activities of daily life

27.5 Clinical Signs of Quadriceps Tears

These will depend on the severity and chronicity of the tear and include:

- Knee swelling, bruising—if acute tears
- Muscle wasting
- Tenderness over the distal quadriceps tendon
- Palpable gap at the distal insertion of the quadriceps on the patella
- Increased mobility of the patella medial/lateral and distal
- Quadriceps weakness
  - Reduced active motion—unable to straight leg raise
  - Resisted force
  - Extensor lag sign
- Stiffness—reduced passive motion
- Tendency to flick the knee into hyperextension during the stance phase of gait to achieve stability and stop the knee from giving way (seen in chronic tears whereby patients have found a way of compensating for the lost quadriceps activity) [26].
- Marked instability of the knee when flexing the knee such as upon tip-toe walking

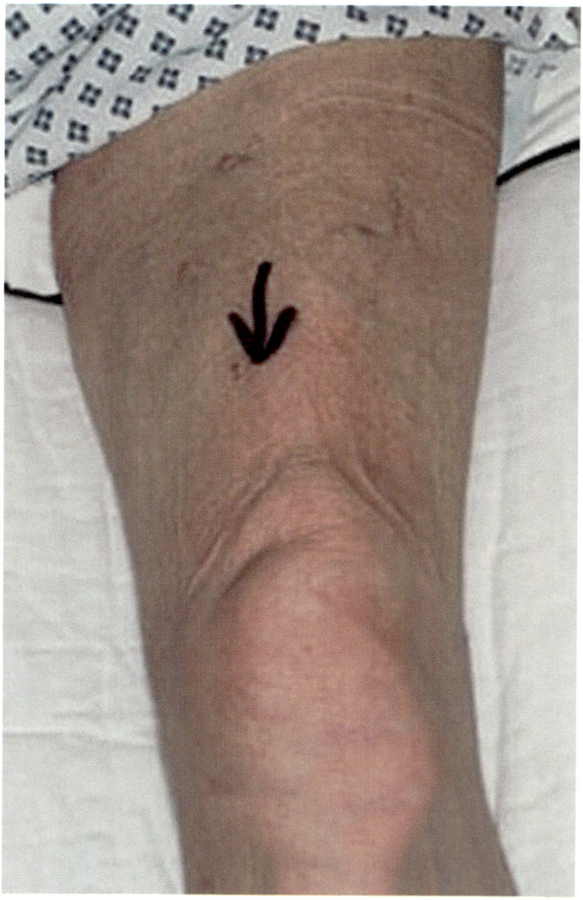

Visible dent just proximal to the patella, suggestive of quadriceps tendon tear

27.6 Investigations for Quadriceps Tears

- Plain radiograph to look for
  - Distal migration of the patella
- Ultrasound scan to assess
  - Extent of tear
  - Retraction of tendon stump

Dynamic US scan during knee flexion and extension may further help to identify the tear

- MRI to assess
  - Extent of tear
  - Retraction
  - Muscle atrophy
  - Fatty infiltration

  MRI is the investigation of choice.

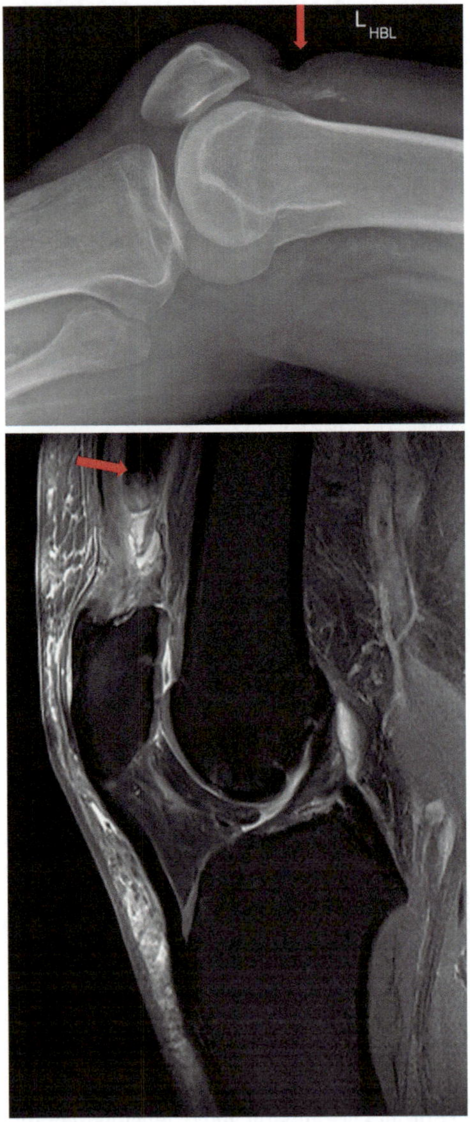

Quadriceps rupture, causing dent (red arrow) on anterior soft tissues. The patella displaces only slightly distally, by the intact patellar tendon. Quadriceps rupture and proximal retraction (red arrow)

Quadriceps rupture and proximal retraction (red arrow)

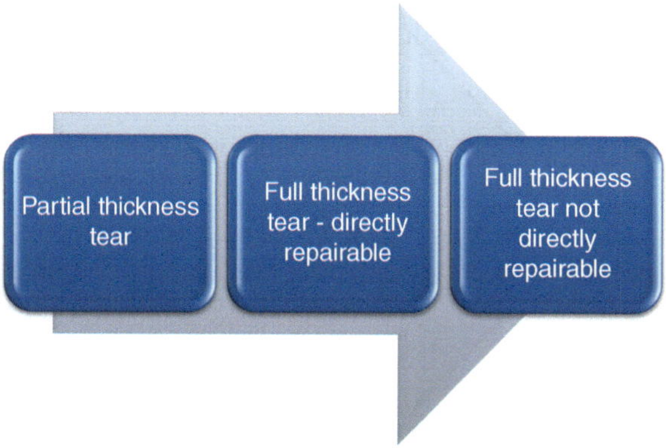

Quadriceps tears may be described according to the thickness of tendon involvement

27.7 Management of Quadriceps Tears [27–41]

Surgical management is the preferred treatment for a substantial quadriceps tear due to the functional disability it confers, but non-surgical management may be appropriate in partial length or partial thickness tears or in patients who have very limited mobility or are medically unfit to undergo surgery.

27.7.1 Non-surgical

- Analgesia
- Activity modification
- Bracing—in extension to:
  - Allow healing of partial tears
  - Support the knee in total tears in patients for whom surgery is not possible
- Physiotherapy
  - Local treatment—heat therapy, megapulse, ultrasound

27.7.2 Surgical

There are several surgical options [26–41] including:

If tendon tear is repairable:

- Quadriceps tear primary direct repair

If tendon tear is repairable but repair site under too much tension:

- Tendon lengthening

If tendon tear is repairable but distal stump is of very poor quality/degenerate:

- Augmentation with a local tendon or artificial graft

If the tendon tear is irreparable and cannot be approximated by tendon lengthening:

- Interposition grafts—autografts, synthetic, allografts
- Knee arthrodesis to maintain support of the knee for ambulation (in very rare cases)

27.7.2.1 Quadriceps Tendon Repair

In quadriceps tendon direct repair the aim is to reattach the tendon back to the patella from where it was avulsed. This may be achieved using:

- Suture anchors (screw like devices which are made either of metallic or non-metallic material and which have sutures attached to them). These anchors are inserted into the top end of the patella and the sutures are used to stitch the tendon down on to the bone.
- Sutures passed through bone tunnels in the patella—sutures are passed through the tendon. Tunnels are drilled through the knee. The sutures are passed through these tunnels and tied over a bone bridge.

The number and configuration of sutures, suture anchors and bone tunnels is determined by the exact technique used as well as the tendon and bone quality.

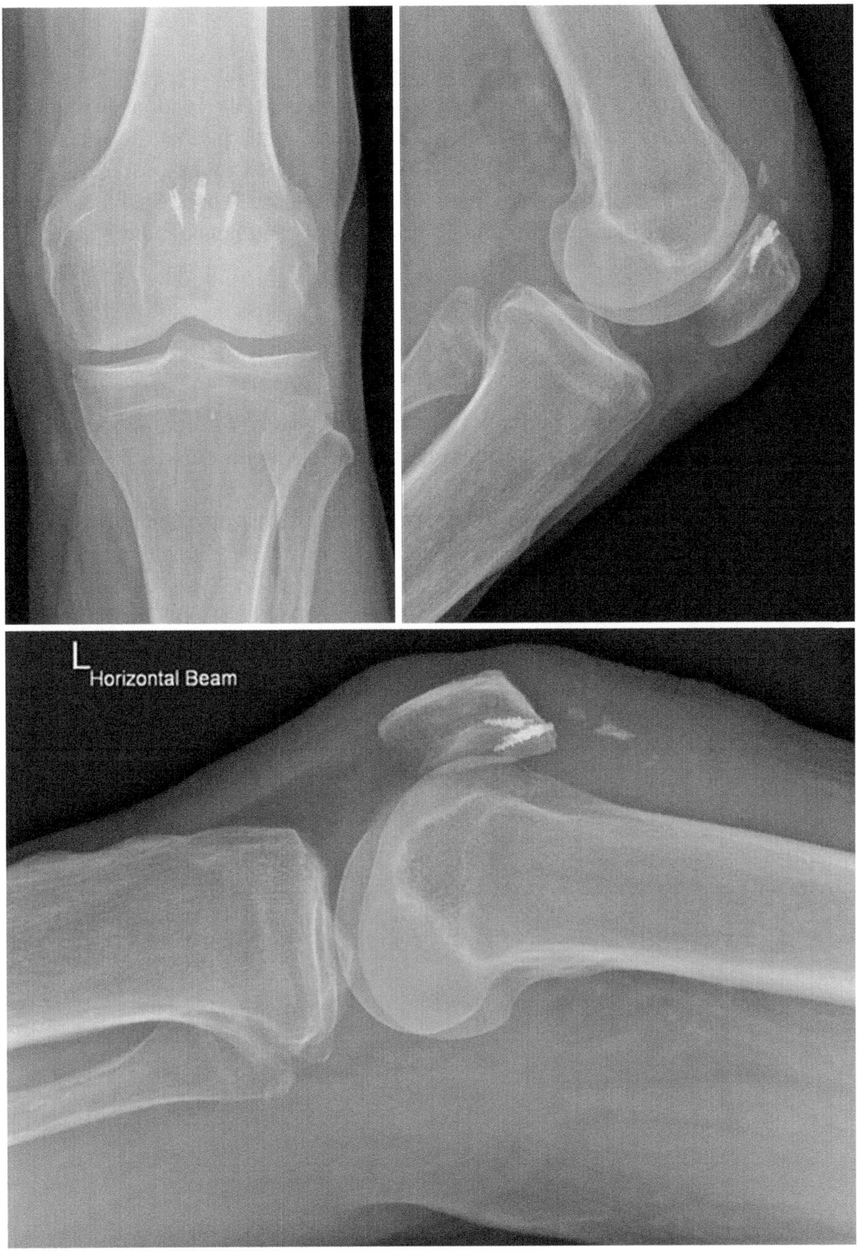

Bone suture anchors inserted into the patella and used to reattach a torn quadriceps tendon

27.7.2.2 Tendon Repair Augmentation

- There are cases where the free edge of the torn quadriceps tendon can be approximated to its bony origin to allow a repair, but the tendon substance is very degenerate and of poor quality. This raises concerns that the repair may fail due to the sutures cutting through the tendon. In such circumstances a synthetic ligament can be used to augment the site of the repair. Such a ligament provides a strong scaffold which can hold sutures and hence may increase the chance of a successful repair.

27.7.2.3 Tendon Lengthening

- V-Y plasty—a V superficial flap of the quadriceps tendon stump is constructed, which allows effective tendon lengthening, which is then sutured to the proximal tendon forming a Y configuration.
- Gradual tendon lengthening using an external fixator has also been described.

27.7.2.4 Tendon Bridging

In cases where the tendon is substantially retracted and cannot be reapproximated to its bony origin even with tendon lengthening several techniques may be utilised to bridge the gap:

- Local autograft (semitendinosus)
- Allograft
- Artificial ligament

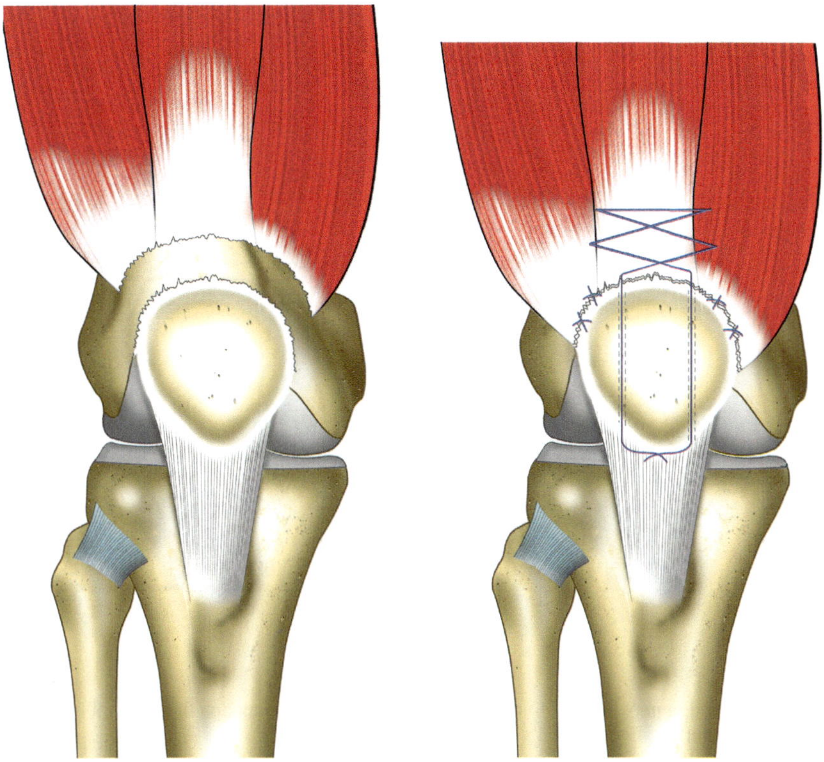

Quadriceps repair may be achieved via vertical drill holes in the patella

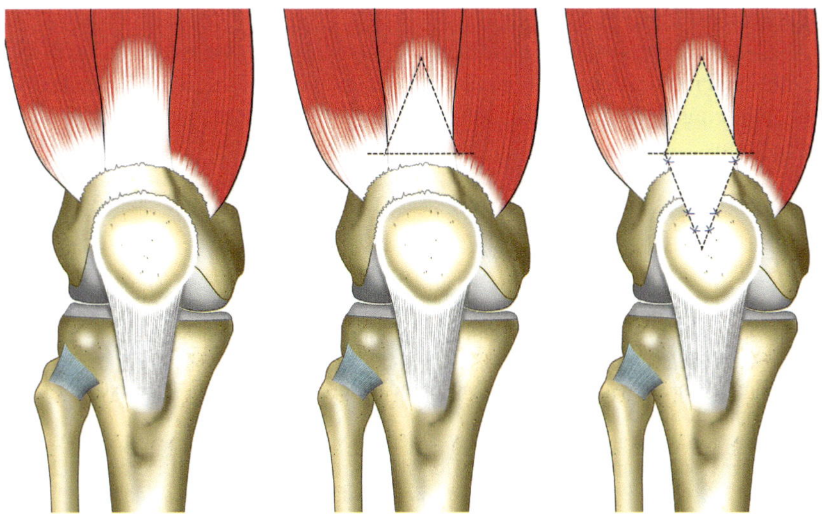

A V-Y advancement of the quadriceps may help approximate the quadriceps to the patella

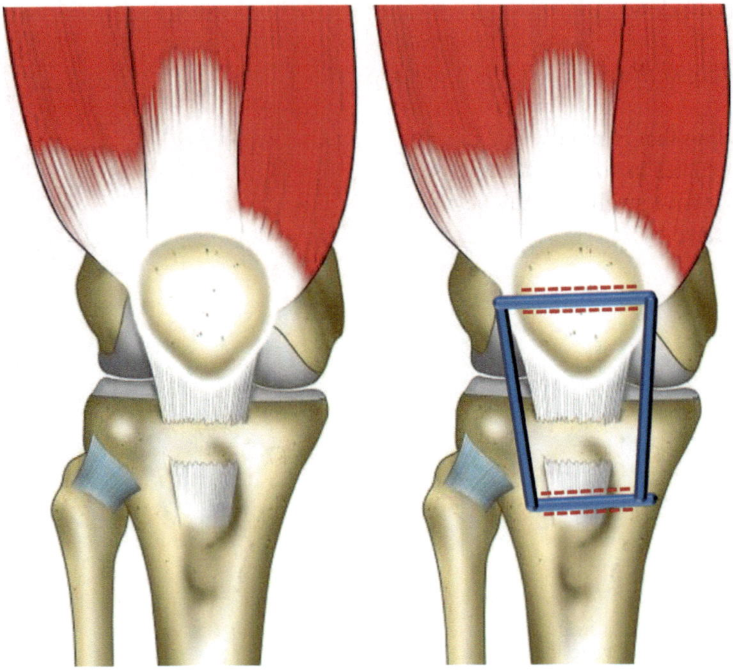

A hamstring tendon may be used to reconstruct a torn quadriceps tendon that can not be approximated to the patella

Learning Pearls
A substantial proportion of quadriceps tendon tears may be associated with an additional intra-articular injury, and this ought to be looked for either initially or following surgical repair if the patient were to continue with troublesome symptoms.

References

1. Pengas IP, Assiotis A, Khan W, Spalding T. Adult native knee extensor mechanism ruptures. Injury. 2016;47(10):2065–70.
2. Ibounig T, Simons TA. Etiology, diagnosis and treatment of tendinous knee extensor mechanism injuries. Scand J Surg. 2016;105(2):67–72.
3. Chhapan J, Sankineani SR, Chiranjeevi T, Reddy MV, Reddy D, Gurava Reddy AV. Early quadriceps tendon rupture after primary total knee arthroplasty. Knee. 2018;25(1):192–4.
4. Clayton RA, Court-Brown CM. The epidemiology of musculoskeletal tendinous and ligamentous injuries. Injury. 2008;39(12):1338–44.

5. Garner MR, Gausden E, Berkes MB, Nguyen JT, Lorich DG. Extensor mechanism injuries of the knee: demographic characteristics and comorbidities from a review of 726 patient records. J Bone Joint Surg Am. 2015;97(19):1592–6.
6. Varghese B, Radcliffe GS, Groves C. Calcific tendonitis of the quadriceps. Br J Sports Med. 2006;40(7):652–4.
7. Abram SG, Sharma AD, Arvind C. Atraumatic quadriceps tendon tear associated with calcific tendonitis. BMJ Case Rep. 2012;2012:bcr2012007031. https://doi.org/10.1136/bcr-012-007031.
8. Maffulli N, Del Buono A, Spiezia F, Longo UG, Denaro V. Light microscopic histology of quadriceps tendon ruptures. Int Orthop. 2012;36(11):2367–71.
9. Kannus P, Józsa L. Histopathological changes preceding spontaneous rupture of a tendon. A controlled study of 891 patients. J Bone Joint Surg Am. 1991;73(10):1507–25.
10. Arumilli B, Adeyemo F, Samarji R. Bilateral simultaneous complete quadriceps rupture following chronic symptomatic tendinopathy: a case report. J Med Case Rep. 2009;3:9031. https://doi.org/10.4076/1752-1947-3-9031.
11. Chua SY, Chang HC. Bilateral spontaneous rupture of the quadriceps tendon as an initial presentation of alkaptonuria—a case report. Knee. 2006;13(5):408–10.
12. Karistinos A, Paulos LE. “Ciprofloxacin-induced” bilateral rectus femoris tendon rupture. Clin J Sport Med. 2007;17(5):406–7.
13. Khaliq Y, Zhanel GG. Fluoroquinolone-associated tendinopathy: a critical review of the literature. Clin Infect Dis. 2003;36(11):1404–10.
14. Maddox PA, Garth WP Jr. Tendinitis of the patellar ligament and quadriceps (jumper’s knee) as an initial presentation of hyperparathyroidism. A case report. J Bone Joint Surg Am. 1986;68(2):288–92.
15. Ranger TA, Wong AM, Cook JL, Gaida JE. Is there an association between tendinopathy and diabetes mellitus? A systematic review with meta-analysis. Br J Sports Med. 2016;50(16):982–9.
16. Song Y, Wu J, Chen J. Spontaneous multiple tendon rupture in a hemodialysis patient. Intern Med. 2014;53(14):1583.
17. Muzi F, Gravante G, Tati E, Tati G. Fluoroquinolones-induced tendinitis and tendon rupture in kidney transplant recipients: 2 cases and a review of the literature. Transplant Proc. 2007;39(5):1673–5.
18. Maricar N, Callaghan MJ, Parkes MJ, Felson DT, O’Neill TW. Interobserver and Intraobserver reliability of clinical assessments in knee osteoarthritis. J Rheumatol. 2016;43(12):2171–8.
19. Marcon M, Ciritsis B, Laux C, Nanz D, Nguyen-Kim TD, Fischer MA, Andreisek G, Ulbrich EJ. Cross-sectional area measurements versus volumetric assessment of the quadriceps femoris muscle in patients with anterior cruciate ligament reconstructions. Eur Radiol. 2015;25(2):290–8.
20. Morse CI, Degens H, Jones DA. The validity of estimating quadriceps volume from single MRI cross-sections in young men. Eur J Appl Physiol. 2007;100(3):267–74.
21. Tracy BL, Ivey FM, Jeffrey Metter E, Fleg JL, Siegel EL, Hurley BF. A more efficient magnetic resonance imaging-based strategy for measuring quadriceps muscle volume. Med Sci Sports Exerc. 2003;35(3):425–33.
22. Inhuber S, Sollmann N, Schlaeger S, Dieckmeyer M, Burian E, Kohlmeyer C, Karampinos DC, Kirschke JS, Baum T, Kreuzpointner F, Schwirtz A. Associations of thigh muscle fat infiltration with isometric strength measurements based on chemical shift encoding-based water-fat magnetic resonance imaging. Eur Radiol Exp. 2019;3(1):45. https://doi.org/10.1186/s41747-019-0123-4.
23. Kulas AS, Schmitz RJ, Shultz SJ, Waxman JP, Wang HM, Kraft RA, Partington HS. Bilateral quadriceps and hamstrings muscle volume asymmetries in healthy individuals. J Orthop Res. 2018;36(3):963–70.
24. Davison MJ, Maly MR, Keir PJ, Hapuhennedige SM, Kron AT, Adachi JD, Beattie KA. Lean muscle volume of the thigh has a stronger relationship with muscle power than muscle strength in women with knee osteoarthritis. Clin Biomech (Bristol, Avon). 2017;41:92–7.

25. Kumar D, Karampinos DC, MacLeod TD, Lin W, Nardo L, Li X, Link TM, Majumdar S, Souza RB. Quadriceps intramuscular fat fraction rather than muscle size is associated with knee osteoarthritis. Osteoarthr Cartil. 2014;22(2):226–34.
26. Pocock CA, Trikha SP, Bell JS. Delayed reconstruction of a quadriceps tendon. Clin Orthop Relat Res. 2008;466(1):221–4.
27. Lee D, Stinner D, Mir H. Quadriceps and patellar tendon ruptures. J Knee Surg. 2013;26(5):301–8.
28. Mille F, Adam A, Aubry S, Leclerc G, Ghislandi X, Sergent P, Garbuio P. Prospective multicentre study of the clinical and functional outcomes following quadriceps tendon repair with suture anchors. Eur J Orthop Surg Traumatol. 2016;26(1):85–92.
29. Hart ND, Wallace MK, Scovell JF, Krupp RJ, Cook C, Wyland DJ. Quadriceps tendon rupture: a biomechanical comparison of transosseous equivalent double-row suture anchor versus transosseous tunnel repair. J Knee Surg. 2012;25(4):335–9.
30. Verdano MA, Zanelli M, Aliani D, Corsini T, Pellegrini A, Ceccarelli F. Quadriceps tendon tear rupture in healthy patients treated with patellar drilling holes: clinical and ultrasonographic analysis after 36 months of follow-up. Muscles Ligaments Tendons J. 2014;4(2):194–200.
31. Yilmaz C, Binnet MS, Narman S. Tendon lengthening repair and early mobilization in treatment of neglected bilateral simultaneous traumatic rupture of the quadriceps tendon. Knee Surg Sports Traumatol Arthrosc. 2001;9(3):163–6.
32. Shi SM, Shi GG, Laurent EM, Ninomiya JT. Modified V-Y turndown flap augmentation for quadriceps tendon rupture following total knee arthroplasty: a retrospective study. J Bone Joint Surg Am. 2019;101(11):1010–5.
33. Chekofsky KM, Spero CR, Scott WN. A method of repair of late quadriceps rupture. Clin Orthop Relat Res. 1980;(147):190–191.
34. Courtney PM, Edmiston TA, Pflederer CT, Levine BR, Gerlinger TL. Is there any role for direct repair of extensor mechanism disruption following total knee arthroplasty? J Arthroplast. 2018;33(7S):S244–8.
35. Maffulli N, Papalia R, Torre G, Denaro V. Surgical treatment for failure of repair of patellar and quadriceps tendon rupture with ipsilateral hamstring tendon graft. Sports Med Arthrosc Rev. 2017;25(1):51–5.
36. Unlu MC, Kaynak G, Caliskan G, Birsel O, Kesmezacar H. Late repair of quadriceps tendon ruptures with free hamstring autograft augmentation and tension relief in patients with predisposing systemic diseases. J Trauma. 2011;71(4):1048–53.
37. Chahla J, DePhillipo NN, Cinque ME, Kennedy NI, Lebus GF, Familiari F, Moatshe G, LaPrade RF. Open repair of quadriceps tendon with suture anchors and semitendinosus tendon allograft augmentation. Arthrosc Tech. 2017;6(6):e2071–7.
38. Morrey MC, Barlow JD, Abdel MP, Hanssen AD. Synthetic mesh augmentation of acute and subacute quadriceps tendon repair. Orthopedics. 2016;39(1):e9–e13.
39. Rust PA, Tanna N, Spicer DD. Repair of ruptured quadriceps tendon with Leeds-Keio ligament following revision knee surgery. Knee Surg Sports Traumatol Arthrosc. 2008;16(4):370–2.
40. Lamberti A, Loconte F, Spinarelli A, Baldini A. Bilateral extensor mechanism allograft reconstruction for chronic spontaneous rupture: a case report and review of the literature. JBJS Case Connect. 2019;9(2):e0058. https://doi.org/10.2106/JBJS.CC.18.00058.
41. Burnett RS, Berger RA, Paprosky WG, Della Valle CJ, Jacobs JJ, Rosenberg AG. Extensor mechanism allograft reconstruction after total knee arthroplasty. A comparison of two techniques. J Bone Joint Surg Am. 2004;86(12):2694–9.

Chapter 28
Patellar Tendon Tears

A condition whereby the patellar tendon tears.

28.1 Causes of Patellar Tendon Tears [1–13]

Most often tears occur secondary to an acute trauma. However, weakness of the tendon due to intrinsic or extrinsic factors may predispose to tears.

Trauma is often the result of:

- Direct impact on the patellar tendon
- Forced hyperflexion (accompanied by substantial eccentric contraction of the quadriceps to oppose such flexion)
- Traumatic lacerations of the tendon

28.1.1 Factors Predisposing to Patellar Tendon Tears

- Intrinsic factors

  These refer to changes originating within the tendon and include:

  - Degeneration
  - Hypovascularity
  - Reduced cellular component
  - Collagen fibre thinning and disorganisation

C. Panayiotou Charalambous, *The Knee Made Easy*,
https://doi.org/10.1007/978-3-030-54506-2_28

- Extrinsic factors
  These refer to external factors acting on the patellar tendon and include [9–11]:
  - Tensile overload (acute trauma or repetitive use)
  - Iatrogenic disruption—in early post knee replacement arthroplasty, patellar tendon harvesting for ligamentous reconstruction
- Combination of intrinsic and extrinsic factors
  Several risk factors have been related to an increased risk of patellar tendon tear (including bilateral or non-traumatic tears)
  - Chronic renal failure—dialysis
  - Fluoroquinolones antibiotic use (such as ciprofloxacin, levofloxacin)
  - Systemic lupus erythromatosus (SLE)
  - Statin use
  - PRP injections
  - Diabetes mellitus
  - Hyperparathyroidism
  - Rheumatoid arthritis
  - Systemic steroid use/steroid injections into the tendon
  - Anabolic steroids
  - Obesity

28.2 Description of Patellar Tendon Tears

Patellar tendon tears may be described in several ways and these are presented next.

According to the Precipitating Event

- Traumatic—the tendon tears suddenly (due to a substantial acute force)
- Spontaneous—(non-traumatic or with very minor trauma)—the tendon weakens or tears gradually over a long time (such as due to chronic repetitive loading or tendon degeneration). Tears occur without the application of substantial force
- Iatrogenic—as when surgically approaching the knee joint, harvesting the patellar tendon for ligament reconstruction (as in anterior cruciate ligament (ACL) reconstruction)

According to the Site of Tear

- Patellar avulsion
- Mid-substance tear
- Tibial tubercle avulsion

According to the Length of the Tear

- Complete length tear(full)
- Incomplete length tear(partial)

The patellar tendon is a broad tendon. It is thus possible to have a tear in the tendon which goes all the way transversely across its length or one that involves only part of its length.

According to Whether the Tear Can Be Surgically Repaired or Not

- Repairable
- Irreparable

Tendon tears may not be repairable due to several factors including:

- Poor tendon quality—unable to hold sutures—sutures cutting through the tendon
- Poor bone quality—unable to hold suture anchors or sutures, such as in osteopenic bone (due to old age, immobility or other factors)

According to the Timing of Presentation

Acute—presenting straight after the onset of the tear or shortly afterwards.

Chronic—presenting a substantial time after the onset of the tear due to factors including:

- Delayed presentation—by patient
- Missed diagnosis—by clinician
- Correct diagnosis made but surgery had to be delayed e.g. for medical reasons

28.3 Demographics of Patellar Tendon Tears [14]

- Patellar tendon tears have an incidence of about 0.68/100,000
- Mean age at tear is about 50 years for men and 70 for women
- Tears may be bilateral or may be associated with contralateral simultaneous quadriceps tendon tears (in underlying predisposing factors)

28.3.1 Clinical Symptoms of Patellar Tendon Tears

- History of trauma(major/minor)
- Sudden onset(even with no trauma)
- Pain—at rest or on exertion
- Weakness of leg (in one or multiple planes). Patient may complain that:
  - Cannot elevate the leg
  - Help the leg with the opposite one, after which leg elevation can be maintained e.g. getting in and out of bed
  - Can weightbear with leg straight but knee gives way when attempting to flex the knee
- Stiffness
- Difficulty in performing activities of daily life

28.3.2 Clinical Signs of Patellar Tendon Tears

These will depend on severity and chronicity of the tear and include:

- Knee swelling, bruising—if acute tears
- Muscle wasting
- Tenderness over the patellar tendon
- Palpable gap distal to the patella
- Proximal migration of the patella (due to pull of the quadriceps)
- Knee weakness
  - Reduced active motion—unable to straight leg raise
  - Resisted force
  - Extensor lag sign
- Stiffness—reduced passive motion
- Tendency to flick the knee into hyperextension during the stance phase of gait to achieve stability (encountered in chronic tears whereby patients try to compensate for the loss of the patellar tendon) [15].
- Marked knee instability

28.4 Investigations for Patellar Tendon Tears

- Plain radiograph to look for
  - Proximal migration of the patella
- Ultrasound scan

- MRI to assess:
  - Extent of tear
  - Site of tear

  MRI is the investigation of choice.

28.5 Management of Patellar Tendon Tears [15–27]

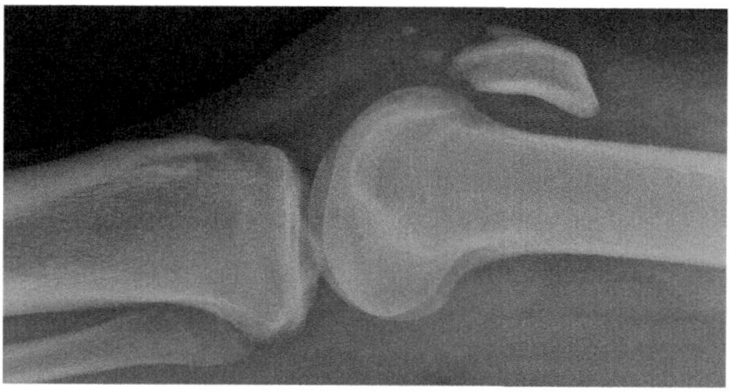

Proximal migration of the patella due to patellar tendon avulsion from its proximal tibial attachment

Surgical management is the preferred treatment for a complete patellar tendon tear due to the functional disability it confers, but non-surgical management may be appropriate in partial tears or in patients who have very limited mobility or are medically unfit to undergo surgery.

28.5.1 Non-surgical

- Analgesia
- Activity modification
- Bracing—in extension to:
  - Allow healing of partial tears
  - Support the knee in total tears in patients for whom surgery is not possible

28.5.2 Surgical

There are several surgical options including:

If tendon tear is repairable:

- Patellar avulsion—reattachment to the patella with suture anchors or vertical patellar tunnels
- Mid-substance tear—direct end to end repair +/reinforcement with sutures passing through patellar or tibial tunnels +/− temporary patellar box wire to protect repair
- Tibial tubercle avulsion—reattachment to the patella with suture anchors or transverse tibial tubercle tunnels

If the patellae tendon tear is repairable but repair site under too much tension:

- Augmentation with autograft tendon, allograft, artificial ligament

If the tendon tear is repairable but of very poor quality/degenerate:

- Augmentation with autograft tendon, allograft, artificial ligament

If the tendon tear is irreparable and cannot be approximated:

- Mobilisation of the patella to allow its distal migration (by extensive release of retinacula, quadriceps lengthening, external fixator distraction)
- Bridging with—autografts (quadriceps, hamstrings), synthetic, allografts
- Knee arthrodesis to maintain support of the knee for ambulation (in very rare cases)

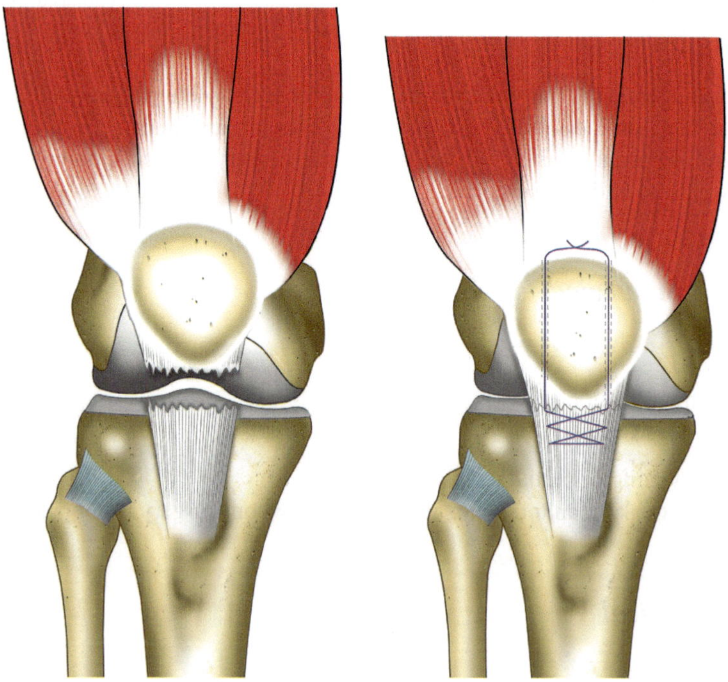

Patellar tendon avulsion from the inferior pole of the patella reattached via vertical drill holes in the patella

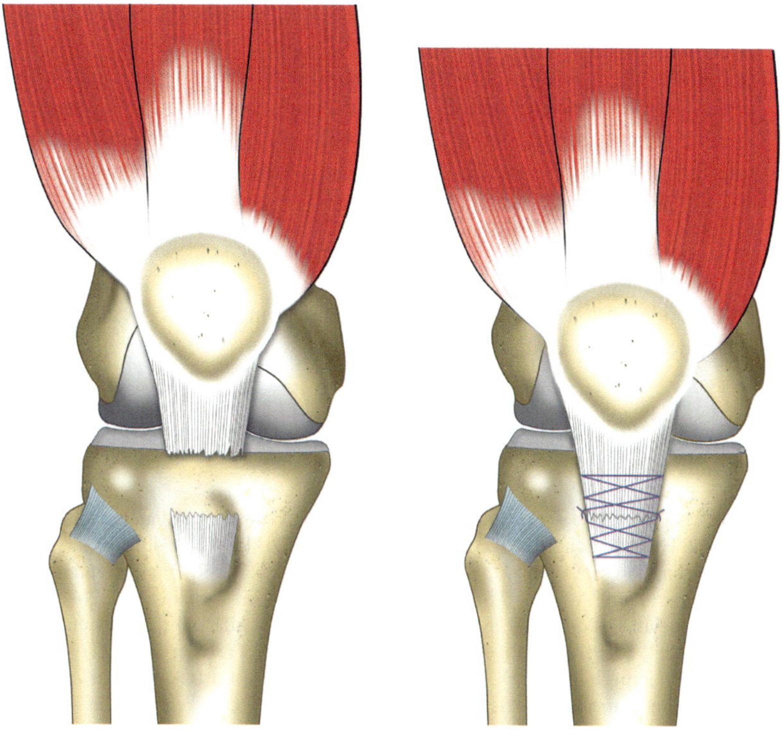

Direct side to side repair of a mid-substance patellar tendon tear

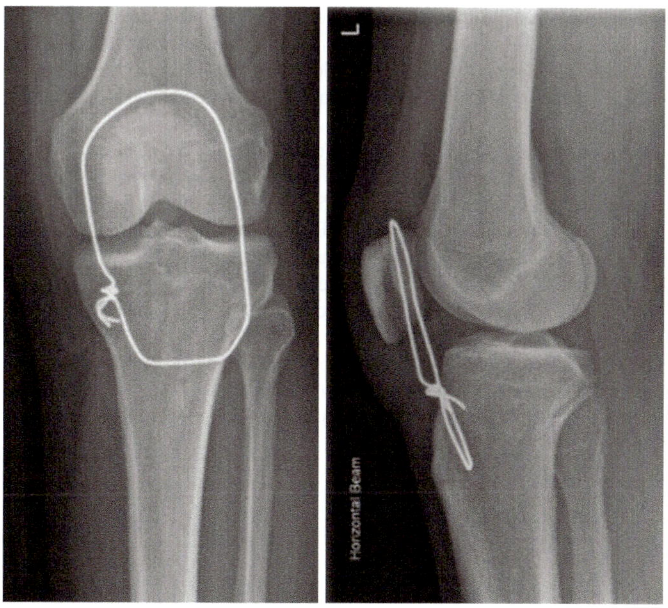

Following repair of a midsubstance patellar tendon tear a box wire may be used to temporarily protect the repair

Learning Pearls

- In the acutely injured knee a high index of suspicion and early radiological investigation may help identify patellar tendon tears at an early stage
- Patellar tendon ruptures may coexist with an ACL tear or other ligamentous knee injury (especially in traumatic injuries sustained in sports) [1, 11–13] and these should be:
  - Looked for in the acute stage clinically or with radiological investigations
  - Considered if a patient continues with on-going symptoms after patellar tendon surgery and rehabilitation

References

1. Boublik M, Schlegel T, Koonce R, Genuario J, Lind C, Hamming D. Patellar tendon ruptures in National Football League players. Am J Sports Med. 2011;39(11):2436–40.
2. Rosso F, Bonasia DE, Cottino U, Dettoni F, Bruzzone M, Rossi R. Patellar tendon: from tendinopathy to rupture. Asia Pac J Sports Med Arthrosc Rehabil Technol. 2015;2(4):99–107.
3. Foley J, Elhelali R, Moiloa D. Spontaneous simultaneous bilateral patellar tendon rupture. BMJ Case Rep. 2019;12(2). pii: e227931. https://doi.org/10.1136/bcr-2018-227931.
4. Redler A, Proietti L, Mazza D, Koverech G, Vadala A, De Carli A, Ferretti A. Rupture of the patellar tendon after platelet-rich plasma treatment: a case report. Clin J Sport Med. 2020;30(1):e20–2.
5. Albayrak İ, Küçük A, Arslan Ş, Özbek O. Spontaneous patellar tendon rupture in a case followed up for diagnosis of systemic lupus erythematosus. Eur J Rheumatol. 2014;1(4):159–60.
6. Kearns MC, Singh VK. Bilateral patellar tendon rupture associated with statin use. J Surg Case Rep. 2016;2016(5):rjw072. https://doi.org/10.1093/jscr/rjw072.
7. Chloros GD, Razavi A, Cheatham SA. Complete avulsion of the patellar tendon from the tibial tubercle in an adult without predisposing factors. J Orthop Sci. 2014;19(2):351–3.
8. Rosa B, Campos P, Barros A, Karmali S, Gonçalves R. Spontaneous bilateral patellar tendon rupture: case report and review of fluoroquinolone-induced tendinopathy. Clin Case Rep. 2016;4(7):678–81.
9. Jagow DM, Garcia BJ, Yacoubian SV, Yacoubian SV. Recurrent patellar tendon rupture in a patient after intramedullary nailing of the tibia: reconstruction using an Achilles tendon allograft. Am J Orthop (Belle Mead NJ). 2015;44(5):E153–5.
10. Rajani A, Dash KK, Mahajan NP, Kumar R. Bilateral spontaneous midsubstance patellar tendon rupture after bilateral total knee arthroplasty. J Orthop Case Rep. 2016;6(2):75–7.
11. Lobo JO, Cherian JJ, Sahu A. Case of acute concomitant rupture of anterior cruciate ligament and patellar tendon of knee: surgical decision making and outcome. J Orthop Case Rep. 2017;7(3):5–8.
12. Kim DH, Lee GC, Park SH. Acute simultaneous ruptures of the anterior cruciate ligament and patellar tendon. Knee Surg Relat Res. 2014;26(1):56–60.
13. Brunkhorst J, Johnson DL. Multiligamentous knee injury concomitant with a patellar tendon rupture. Orthopedics. 2015;38(1):45–8.

14. Clayton RA, Court-Brown CM. The epidemiology of musculoskeletal tendinous and ligamentous injuries. Injury. 2008;39(12):1338–44.
15. Palencia J, Alfayez SM, Alshammri AA, Serhan HS, Serro F, Alomar AZ. Late reconstruction of the patellar tendon in rheumatoid arthritis using bone-patellar tendon-bone allograft. Int J Surg Case Rep. 2016;27:66–9.
16. Benner RW, Shelbourne KD, Freeman H. Nonoperative management of a partial patellar tendon rupture after bone-patellar tendon-bone graft harvest for ACL reconstruction. J Knee Surg. 2013;26(Suppl 1):S123–7.
17. Regis D, Sandri A, Bizzotto N, Magnan B. Open patellar tendon avulsion from tibial tuberosity after ACL reconstruction successfully treated with suture anchors. Acta Biomed. 2019;90(12-S):196–201.
18. Gilmore JH, Clayton-Smith ZJ, Aguilar M, Pneumaticos SG, Giannoudis PV. Reconstruction techniques and clinical results of patellar tendon ruptures: evidence today. Knee. 2015;22(3):148–55.
19. Woodmass JM, Johnson JD, Wu IT, Krych AJ, Stuart MJ. Patellar tendon repair with ipsilateral semitendinosus autograft augmentation. Arthrosc Tech. 2017;6(6):e2177–81.
20. Core M, Anract P, Raffin J, Biau DJ. Traumatic patellar tendon rupture repair using synthetic ligament augmentation. J Knee Surg. 2019;33:804–9. https://doi.org/10.1055/s-0039-1688564.
21. Wiegand N, Naumov I, Vámhidy L, Warta V, Than P. Reconstruction of the patellar tendon using a Y-shaped flap folded back from the vastus lateralis fascia. Knee. 2013;20(2):139–43.
22. Lewis PB, Rue JP, Bach BR Jr. Chronic patellar tendon rupture: surgical reconstruction technique using 2 achilles tendon allografts. J Knee Surg. 2008;21(2):130–5.
23. Gomes JL, de Oliveira Alves JA, Zimmermann JM Jr. Reconstruction of neglected patellar tendon ruptures using the quadriceps graft. Orthopedics. 2014;37(8):527–9.
24. Kumar A, Rutherford-Davies J, Thorpe P, Newson A. Combined quadriceps lengthening (using an external ring fixator) and patellar tendon reconstruction (using a tendoachilles allograft) in a case of chronic patellar tendon rupture: a case report. Knee. 2020;27(2):598–606.
25. Haskoor JP, Busconi BD. Patellar tendon reconstruction using semitendinosus autograft with preserved distal insertion for treatment of patellar tendon rupture after bone-patellar tendon-bone ACL reconstruction: a case report. Orthop J Sports Med. 2019;7(10):2325967119877802. https://doi.org/10.1177/2325967119877802.
26. Valianatos P, Papadakou E, Erginoussakis D, Kampras D, Schizas N, Kouzoupis A. Treatment of chronic patellar tendon rupture with hamstrings tendon autograft. J Knee Surg. 2019;33:792–7. https://doi.org/10.1055/s-0039-1688499.
27. Beranger JS, Kajetanek C, Bayoud W, Pascal-Mousselard H, Khiami F. Return to sport after early surgical repair of acute patellar tendon ruptures. Orthop Traumatol Surg Res. 2020;106(3):503–7.

Chapter 29
Tibial Tubercle Apophysitis

The tibial tubercle develops at the anterior part of the proximal tibia as a secondary ossification centre which fuses with the tibia. This ossification centre is separated from the main tibia by a physis (apophysis) which is less resistant to tensile stresses than bone.

Tibial tubercle apophysitis (also known as Osgood Schlatter disease) is a disease of the tibial tubercle apophysis. Patellar tendon tensile forces (traction) brought about by powerful contractions of the quadriceps may lead to microtrauma and avulsion of apophyseal fragments, causing local inflammation and pain. This may also lead to failure of fusion of part of the apophysis and the development of an accessory ossicle which may persist into adulthood [1–6].

In a prospective radiographic study, Vergara-Amador et al. [7] showed that in girls the anterior tibial tubercle is ossified by 11 (50% at 10), fusion with the epiphysis starts at 12 and is complete by 17. In boys, this process is delayed by a year. A single centre of ossification is found in all.

29.1 Demographics of Tibial Tubercle Apophysitis

- More common in males as compared to females
- More common in those participating in sports involving running and jumping or repetitive knee flexion (football, volleyball, basketball, kneeling, squatting)
- Symptoms commoner in about 8–13 years in females and 10–15 years in males when growth spurt occurs (and quadriceps contractions are very strong)
- Bilateral in 30% of cases

C. Panayiotou Charalambous, *The Knee Made Easy*,
https://doi.org/10.1007/978-3-030-54506-2_29

29.2 Clinical Symptoms of Tibial Tubercle Apophysitis

- Asymptomatic—often discovered as an incidental finding on radiological imaging
- Pain:
  - Aggravated by running or jumping, improved by rest
  - Due to patellar tendon impingement caused by the mobile bony fragments
  - From the site of non-fusion due to inflammation caused by abnormal movement of the unfused fragments
- Clicking
- Swelling over the tibial tuberosity area

29.3 Clinical Signs of Tibial Tubercle Apophysitis

- Tibial tubercle or patellar tendon tenderness
- Prominent tibial tubercle

29.4 Investigations for Tibial Tubercle Apophysitis

- Plain radiographs:
  - Lateral view
    - Unfused ossicles, prominent tibial tubercle
- CT
  - Confirm the presence of tibial tubercle apophysitis
  - Further characterise the size and shape of the tibial tubercle apophysitis in planning surgery
- SPECT
  - Determine if the tibial tubercle area is the origin of the patient's symptoms
- MRI
  - Identify the relation of the patellar tendon to the unfused ossicles to determine whether reattachment of the tendon may be needed if the ossicles were to be excised

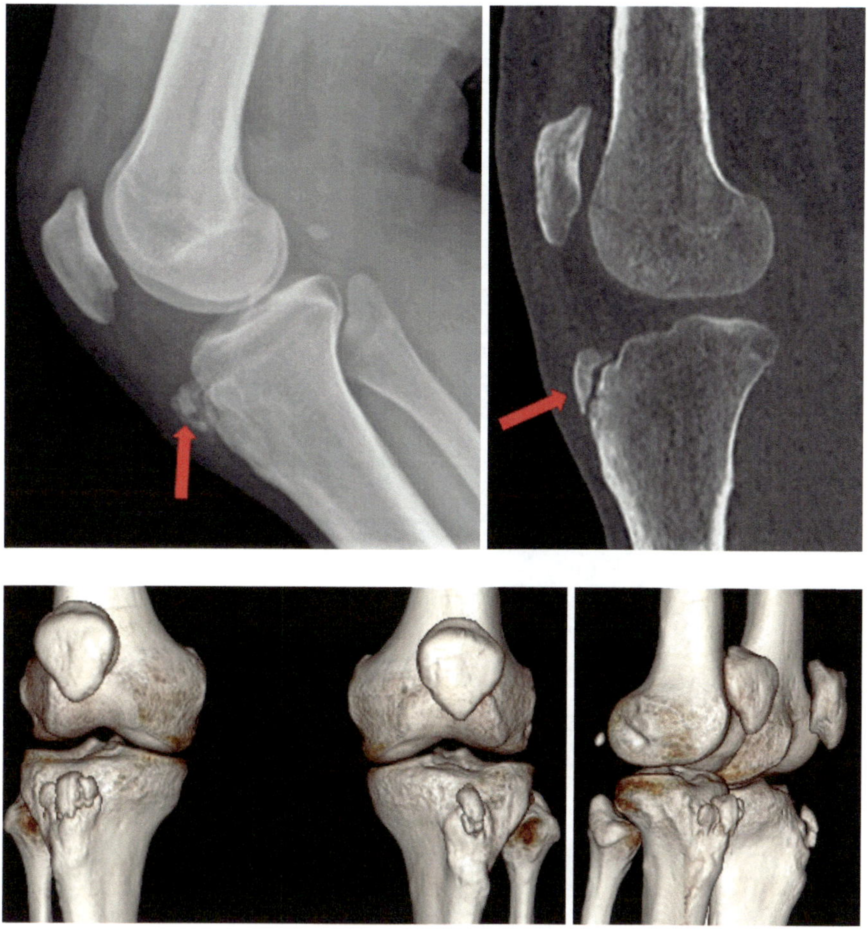

Tibial tubercle apophysitis with residual ossicles in adulthood

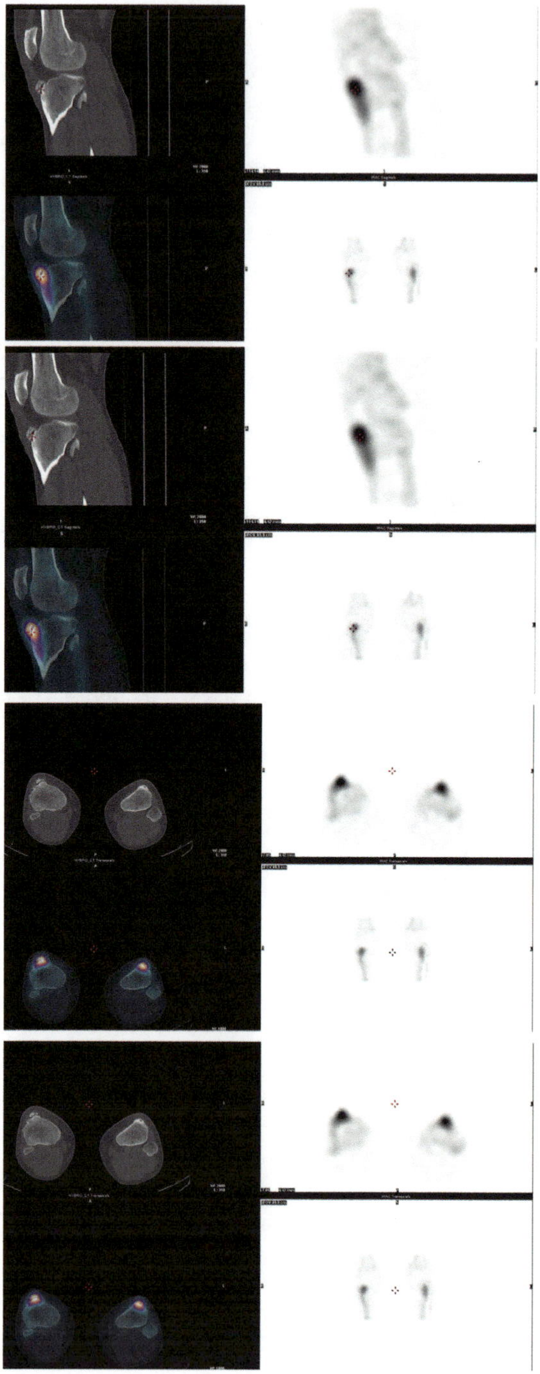

Tibial tubercle apophysitis with residual ossicles in adulthood (SPECT)

29.5 Management of Tibial Tubercle Apophysitis [8–16]

29.5.1 Non-surgical

- Leave alone
- Analgesia, anti-inflammatories, local treatment
- Rest, activity modification, load restriction(reduce exercise duration, intensity, frequency, minimise impact activities that require strong contraction of the quadriceps—running, jumping)
- Physiotherapy—improve quadriceps and hamstring flexibility, isometric, closed chain exercises, eccentric loading to address patellar tendinopathy
- Extracorporeal shockwave therapy (ECSW)
- Steroid injections:
  - Patellar tendon sheath
  - Non-fusion site

29.5.2 Surgical

- Arthroscopic or open tibial tubercle apophysitis mobile fragment excision
- Debridement and drilling of the tibial apophysis
- Osteotomy of the tibial tubercle—closing wedge to reduce the prominence of the tuberosity

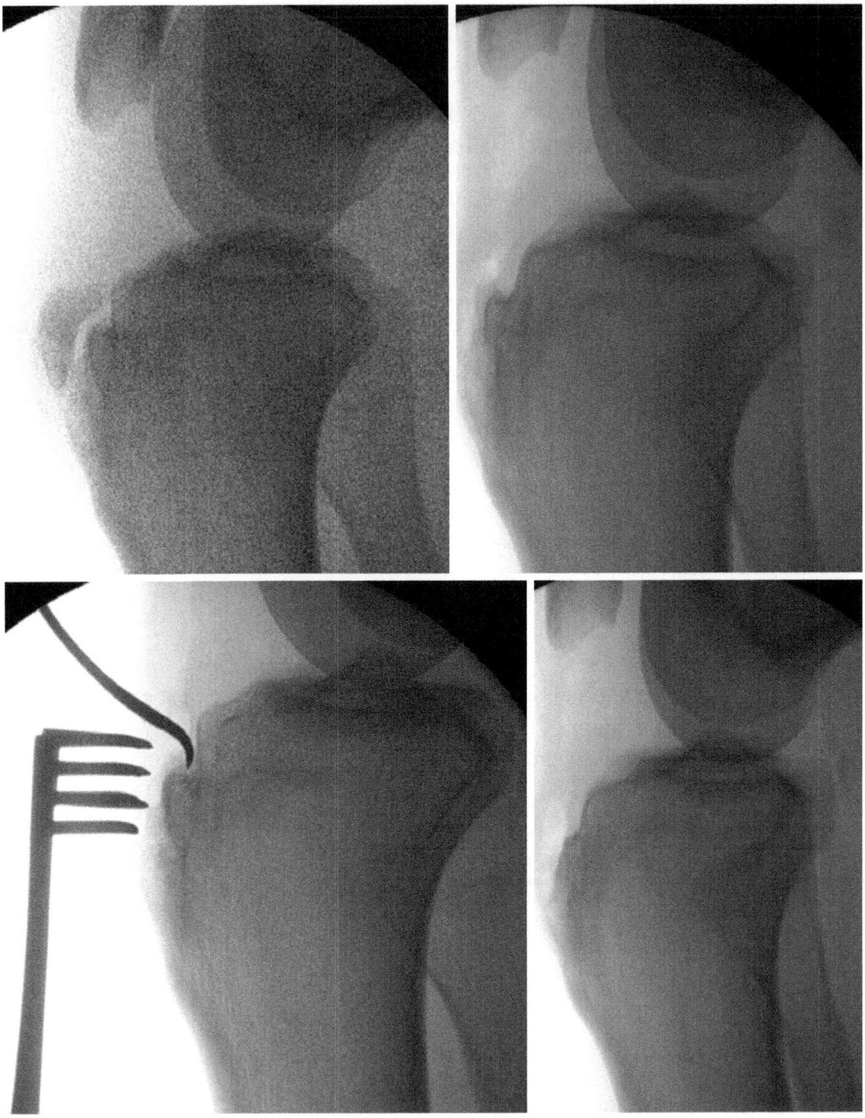

Removal of ossicles and debridement of tibial tubercle apophysitis in adulthood

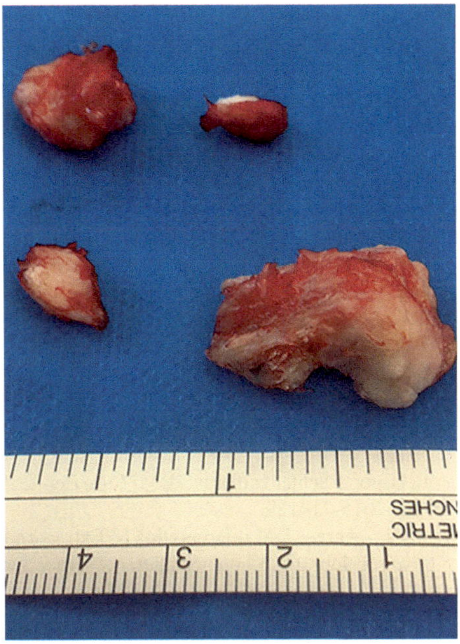

Excised residual unfused ossicles in tibial apophysitis

Learning Pearls

- In most cases symptoms settle with activity modification, or once growth spurt is completed, but in about 10% of individuals symptoms may continue into adulthood.
- The patellar tendon may show tendinopathy in association with tibial tubercle apophysitis, hence knee symptoms may persist despite debridement of the tibial tubercle.
- Following debridement or ossicle excision, reattachment of the patellar tendon may be necessary, if a substantial part of the tendon had to be lifted off the bone.
- Surgery for unresolved apophysitis in adults may be successful in most cases, but scar pain is a potential complication to be considered in those with frequent kneeling.

References

1. Nakase J, Goshima K, Numata H, Oshima T, Takata Y, Tsuchiya H. Precise risk factors for Osgood-Schlatter disease. Arch Orthop Trauma Surg. 2015;135(9):1277–81.
2. Watanabe H, Fujii M, Yoshimoto M, Abe H, Toda N, Higashiyama R, Takahira N. Pathogenic factors associated with Osgood-Schlatter disease in adolescent male soccer players: a prospective cohort study. Orthop J Sports Med. 2018;6(8):2325967118792192. https://doi.org/10.1177/2325967118792192.

3. Falciglia F, Giordano M, Aulisa AG, Poggiaroni A, Guzzanti V. Osgood Schlatter lesion: histologic features of slipped anterior tibial tubercle. Int J Immunopathol Pharmacol. 2011;24(1 Suppl 2):25–8.
4. Sailly M, Whiteley R, Johnson A. Doppler ultrasound and tibial tuberosity maturation status predicts pain in adolescent male athletes with Osgood-Schlatter's disease: a case series with comparison group and clinical interpretation. Br J Sports Med. 2013;47(2):93–7.
5. Arendt EA. Editorial commentary: tibial tubercle prominence after Osgood-Schlatter disease: what causes pain? Arthroscopy. 2017;33(8):1558–9.
6. Jamshidi K, Mirkazemi M, Izanloo A, Mirzaei A. Benign bone tumours of tibial tuberosity clinically mimicking Osgood-Schlatter disease: a case series. Int Orthop. 2019;43(11):2563–8.
7. Vergara-Amador E, Davalos Herrera D, Moreno LÁ. Radiographic features of the development of the anterior tibial tuberosity. Radiologia. 2016;58(4):294–300.
8. Circi E, Atalay Y, Beyzadeoglu T. Treatment of Osgood-Schlatter disease: review of the literature. Musculoskelet Surg. 2017;101(3):195–200.
9. Gerulis V, Kalesinskas R, Pranckevicius S, Birgeris P. Importance of conservative treatment and physical load restriction to the course of Osgood-Schlatter's disease. Medicina (Kaunas). 2004;40(4):363–9.
10. Morris E. Acupuncture in Osgood-Schlatter disease. BMJ Case Rep. 2016;2016:bcr2015214129. https://doi.org/10.1136/bcr-2015-214129.
11. Lohrer H, Nauck T, Schöll J, Zwerver J, Malliaropoulos N. Extracorporeal shock wave therapy for patients suffering from recalcitrant Osgood-Schlatter disease. Sportverletz Sportschaden. 2012;26(4):218–22.
12. Narayan N, Mitchell PD, Latimer MD. Complete resolution of the symptoms of refractory Osgood-Schlatter disease following percutaneous fixation of the tibial tuberosity. BMJ Case Rep. 2015;2015:bcr2014206734. https://doi.org/10.1136/bcr-2014-206734.
13. Nierenberg G, Falah M, Keren Y, Eidelman M. Surgical treatment of residual Osgood-Schlatter disease in young adults: role of the mobile osseous fragment. Orthopedics. 2011;34(3):176. https://doi.org/10.3928/01477447-20110124-07.
14. El-Husseini TF, Abdelgawad AA. Results of surgical treatment of unresolved Osgood-Schlatter disease in adults. J Knee Surg. 2010;23(2):103–7.
15. Circi E, Beyzadeoglu T. Results of arthroscopic treatment in unresolved Osgood-Schlatter disease in athletes. Int Orthop. 2017;41(2):351–6.
16. Pagenstert G, Wurm M, Gehmert S, Egloff C. Reduction osteotomy of the prominent Tibial tubercle after Osgood-Schlatter disease. Arthroscopy. 2017;33(8):1551–7.

Chapter 30
Fabella Pain Syndrome

This is a condition whereby the fabella causes posterolateral knee pain. There may be associated nerve symptoms due to compression of the common peroneal nerve [1–15]. This may be due to multiple underlying causes including:

- Arthritis of the fabello-fibular articulation
- Pressure effect of the fabella
- Fabellar injury—chronic overuse, acute trauma

30.1 Clinical Symptoms of Fabella Pain Syndrome

- Posterolateral knee pain
- Snapping
- Neurological dysfunction in the presence of nerve compression

30.2 Clinical Signs of Fabella Pain Syndrome

- Posterolateral knee tenderness
- Common peroneal nerve dysfunction

30.3 Investigations for Fabella Pain Syndrome [16–19]

- Plain radiographs
  - To evaluate the fabella

C. Panayiotou Charalambous, *The Knee Made Easy*,
https://doi.org/10.1007/978-3-030-54506-2_30

- Ultrasound
- MRI scan
  - Look for other pathology
- CT—to evaluate a fabellar fracture
- Nerve conduction studies/electromyography—if neurological symptoms or signs present

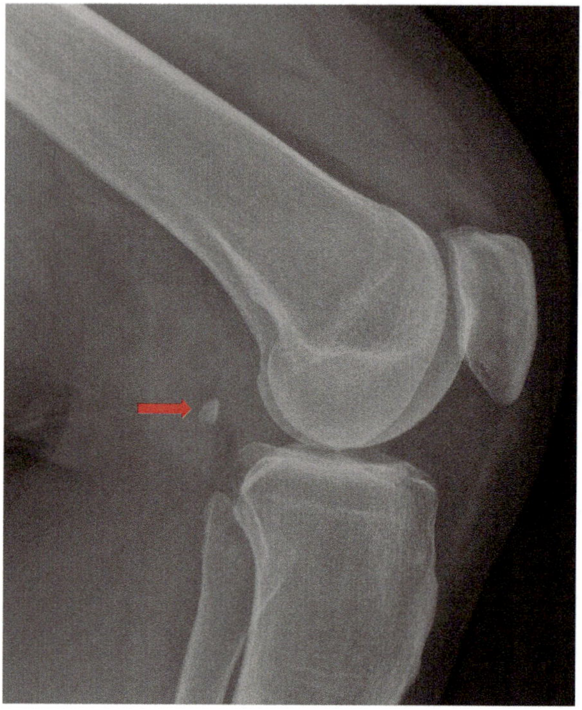

Fabella on Lateral view (red arrow)

30.4 Management of Fabella Pain Syndrome [20–25]

30.4.1 Non-surgical

- Physiotherapy—stretching of the lateral head of gastrocnemius
- Steroid injection around the fabella
- Extracorporeal shock wave therapy (ECSW)

30.4.2 Surgical

- Fabellectomy +/− decompression of common peroneal nerve

References

1. Berthaume MA, Bull AMJ. Human biological variation in sesamoid bone prevalence: the curious case of the fabella. J Anat. 2020;236(2):228–42.
2. Berthaume MA, Di Federico E, Bull AMJ. Fabella prevalence rate increases over 150 years, and rates of other sesamoid bones remain constant: a systematic review. J Anat. 2019;235(1):67–79.
3. Robertson A, Jones SC, Paes R, Chakrabarty G. The fabella: a forgotten source of knee pain? Knee. 2004;11(3):243–5.
4. Driessen A, Balke M, Offerhaus C, White WJ, Shafizadeh S, Becher C, Bouillon B, Höher J. The fabella syndrome—a rare cause of posterolateral knee pain: a review of the literature and two case reports. BMC Musculoskelet Disord. 2014;15:100. https://doi.org/10.1186/1471-2474-15-100.
5. Clarke AM, Matthews JG. Osteoarthritis of the fabella: a fourth knee compartment? J R Coll Surg Edinb. 1991;36(1):58.
6. Cherrad T, Louaste J, Bousbaä H, Amhajji L, Khaled R. Fracture of the fabella: an uncommon injury in knee. Case Rep Orthop. 2015;2015:396710.
7. Zhou F, Zhang F, Deng G, Bi C, Wang J, Wang Q, Wang Q. Fabella fracture with radiological imaging: a case report. Trauma Case Rep. 2017;12:19–23.
8. Hire JM, Oliver DL, Hubbard RC, Fontaine ML, Bojescul JA. Snapping knee caused by symptomatic fabella in a native knee. Am J Orthop (Belle Mead NJ). 2014;43(8):377–9.
9. Franceschi F, Longo UG, Ruzzini L, Leonardi F, Rojas M, Gualdi G, Denaro V. Dislocation of an enlarged fabella as uncommon cause of knee pain: a case report. Knee. 2007;14(4):330–2.
10. Agathangelidis F, Vampertzis T, Gkouliopoulou E, Papastergiou S. Symptomatic enlarged fabella. BMJ Case Rep. 2016;2016:bcr2016218085. https://doi.org/10.1136/bcr-2016-218085.
11. Patel A, Singh R, Johnson B, Smith A. Compression neuropathy of the common peroneal nerve by the fabella. BMJ Case Rep. 2013;2013:bcr2013202154. https://doi.org/10.1136/bcr-2013-202154.
12. Kim T, Chung H, Lee H, Choi Y, Son JH. A case report and literature review on fabella syndrome after high tibial osteotomy. Medicine (Baltimore). 2018;97(4):e9585. https://doi.org/10.1097/MD.0000000000009585.
13. Rankin I, Rehman H, Ashcroft GP. Fabella syndrome following de-rotation surgery to correct a femoral malunion. Open Orthop J. 2018;12:346–52.
14. Kimura T, Tanikawa H, Hasegawa T, Takeda K, Harato K, Kobayashi S, Niki Y, Okuma K. Late onset of the fabella syndrome after total knee arthroplasty. Case Rep Orthop. 2019;2019:3. https://doi.org/10.1155/2019/5219237.
15. Kwee TC, Heggelman B, Gaasbeek R, Nix M. Fabella fractures after total knee arthroplasty with correction of valgus malalignment. Case Rep Orthop. 2016;2016:5. https://doi.org/10.1155/2016/4749871.
16. Houghton-Allen BW. In the case of the fabella a comparison view of the other knee is unlikely to be helpful. Australas Radiol. 2001;45(3):318–9.
17. Dale KM, Boggess SB, Boggess B, Moorman CT 3rd. Ultrasound evaluation and surgical excision of a Fabella causing peroneal neuropathy in a track athlete. Case Rep Orthop. 2018;2018:5. https://doi.org/10.1155/2018/2371947.
18. Ehara S. Potentially symptomatic fabella: MR imaging review. Jpn J Radiol. 2014;32(1):1–5.

19. Heideman GM, Baynes KE, Mautz AP, DuBois MS, Roberts JW. Fabella fracture with CT imaging: a case report. Emerg Radiol. 2011;18(4):357–61.
20. Seol PH, Ha KW, Kim YH, Kwak HJ, Park SW, Ryu BJ. Effect of radial extracorporeal shock wave therapy in patients with fabella syndrome. Ann Rehabil Med. 2016;40(6):1124–8.
21. Zipple JT, Hammer RL, Loubert PV. Treatment of fabella syndrome with manual therapy: a case report. J Orthop Sports Phys Ther. 2003;33(1):33–9.
22. Ando Y, Miyamoto Y, Tokimura F, Nakazawa T, Hamaji H, Kanetaka M, Koshiishi A, Hirabayashi K, Anamizu Y, Miyazaki T. A case report on a very rare variant of popliteal artery entrapment syndrome due to an enlarged fabella associated with severe knee osteoarthritis. J Orthop Sci. 2017;22(1):164–8.
23. Dekker TJ, Crawford MD, DePhillipo NN, Kennedy MI, Grantham WJ, Schairer WW, LaPrade RF. Clinical presentation and outcomes associated with fabellectomy in the setting of fabella syndrome. Orthop J Sports Med. 2020;8(2):2325967120903722. https://doi.org/10.1177/2325967120903722.
24. Provencher MT, Sanchez G, Ferrari MB, Moatshe G, Chahla J, Akamefula R, LaPrade RF. Arthroscopy-assisted fabella excision: surgical technique. Arthrosc Tech. 2017;6(2):e369–74.
25. Dannawi Z, Khanduja V, Vemulapalli KK, Zammit J, El-Zebdeh M. Arthroscopic excision of the fabella. J Knee Surg. 2007;20(4):299–301.

Chapter 31
Knee Tendon Snapping Syndrome

Knee snapping is a condition whereby there is clicking or snapping during movement of a soft tissue structure across a bony or other prominence, with an associated resultant sound. This may be painful or painless [1–26].

Snapping may be:

- Intra-articular
- Extra-articular (tendon, ligament)

Snapping may be present for a long time before starting to cause troublesome symptoms. In some cases it may be bilateral but with only one side causing symptoms. Snapping may occur during knee flexion/extension or during internal/external rotation according to the structure involved and the underlying cause of the snapping.

Onset may be acute, related to a traumatic event, or come on gradually without a precipitating event.

31.1 Snapping of Knee Tendons

Tendons are commonly involved in snapping around the knee. A tendon crossing a joint may move back and forth with joint motion (snapping) catching on the intervening bone. This may be likened to the rope anchoring a boat to the dock cleat, and flipping upwards and downwards each time the boat is lifted by an incoming wave.

C. Panayiotou Charalambous, *The Knee Made Easy*,
https://doi.org/10.1007/978-3-030-54506-2_31

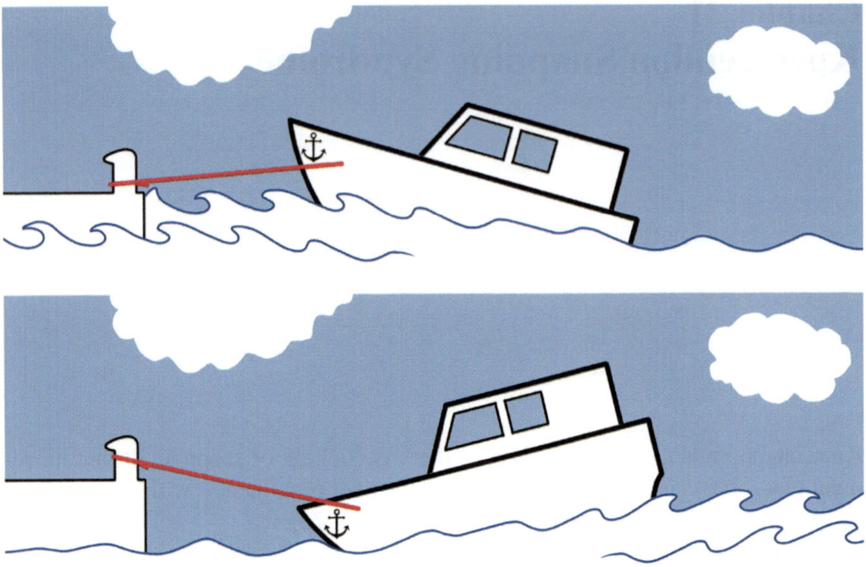

Tendon snapping is analogous to a boat rope flipping upwards and downwards with the incoming waves

Several tendons in the knee have been described as showing snapping, and these include:

- Sartorius
- Semitendinosus
- Gracilis
- Semimembranosus
- Biceps femoris
- Iliotibial band
- Popliteus

31.2 Causes of Snapping Tendons

Tendon snapping may be due to bony abnormalities, or due to changes in the soft tissues (muscles, bursae, ligaments) that are located close to the tendon path. These include:

- Bursal inflammation and fibrosis following acute trauma or chronic overuse
- Muscle fibrosis
- Abnormal bone morphology
- Prominence over which tendon snaps—exostosis, prominent anatomical ridge

- Fractures
  - Malunion
  - Excessive callus formation
- Mass lesions located in the pathway of the tendon:
  - Para-meniscal cyst, ganglion
  - Implant—such as knee replacement arthroplasty prosthesis, fracture fixation plate
- Anomalous insertion of the tendon—altering the normal relation between tendon and surrounding structures
- Soft tissue disruption—snapping in the presence of abnormal anatomy, due to disruption of the tissues surrounding and maintaining the normal position of the tendon (as due to trauma)

31.3 Clinical Symptoms of Knee Tendon Snapping Syndrome

- Pain (but snapping may also be painless)
- Visible snapping—reported by patient or others
- Audible and palpable crepitus with tendon movements

31.4 Clinical Signs of Knee Tendon Snapping Syndrome

- Palpable crepitus
- Audible snapping (friction sound, grating, snapping sound)
- Visible snapping—reported by patient or others
- Mass lesion—visible, palpable
- Tenderness over the tendon involved

31.5 Investigations for Knee Tendon Snapping Syndrome [21, 22]

- Radiological
  - Plain radiographs/CT scans to look for osseous causes of snapping
  - MRI, ultrasound to identify inflamed bursal tissue, soft tissue mass lesions, evaluate tendinopathy of involved tendon
  - Dynamic ultrasound to demonstrate tendon snapping during knee motion

31.6 Management of Knee Tendon Snapping Syndrome

31.6.1 Non-surgical: Successful in Most Cases

- Leave alone
- Analgesia
- Activity modification
- Physiotherapy—tendon stretching
- Extracorporeal shock wave therapy (ECSW)
- Steroid injections of inflamed bursae

31.6.2 Surgical (Open or Arthroscopic)

- Resection of prominence/mass lesion over which snapping occurs
- Division of the tendon insertion +/− stabilisation of the tendon in its anatomical location or reposition of the tendon to an alternative site
- Tendon lengthening

Learning Pearls

- The aim of non-surgical treatment is often to improve the troublesome symptoms of knee tendon snapping (such as pain) rather than abolish snapping per se. Non-troublesome snapping may then be left alone.

References

1. Reid L, Mofidi A. Bilateral snapping biceps femoris tendon: a case report and review of the literature. Eur J Orthop Surg Traumatol. 2019;29(5):1081–7.
2. Matar HE, Farrar NG. Snapping biceps femoris: clinical demonstration and operative technique. Ann R Coll Surg Engl. 2018;100(3):e59–61.
3. McNulty M, Carreau J, Hendrickson N, Bollier M. Case report: snapping biceps femoris tendon due to abnormal fibular morphology. Iowa Orthop J. 2017;37:81–4.
4. Fritsch BA, Mhaskar V. Anomalous biceps femoris tendon insertion leading to a snapping knee in a young male. Knee Surg Relat Res. 2017;29(2):144–9.
5. Karataglis D, Papadopoulos P, Fotiadou A, Christodoulou AG. Snapping knee syndrome in an athlete caused by the semitendinosus and gracilis tendons. A case report. Knee. 2008;15(2):151–4.
6. von Dercks N, Theopold JD, Marquass B, Josten C, Hepp P. Snapping knee syndrome caused by semitendinosus and semimembranosus tendons. A case report. Knee. 2016;23(6):1168–71.
7. de la Hera Cremades B, Escribano Rueda L, Lara Rubio A. Snapping knee caused by the thickening of the medial hamstrings. Rev Esp Cir Ortop Traumatol. 2017;61(3):200–2.

8. Protzman NM, Conkle SB, Busch MF. Snapping knee syndrome of the medial hamstrings. Orthopedics. 2015;38(10):e940–2.
9. Date H, Hayakawa K, Nakagawa K, Yamada H. Snapping knee due to the biceps femoris tendon treated with repositioning of the anomalous tibial insertion. Knee Surg Sports Traumatol Arthrosc. 2012;20(8):1581–3.
10. Vavalle G, Capozzi M. Symptomatic snapping knee from biceps femoris tendon subluxation: an unusual case of lateral pain in a marathon runner. J Orthop Traumatol. 2010;11(4):263–6.
11. Inui H, Taketomi S, Yamagami R, Tahara K, Tanaka S. Snapping pes syndrome after unicompartmental knee arthroplasty. Knee Surg Relat Res. 2016;28(2):172–5.
12. Yoong-Leong Oh J, Tan KK, Wong YS. 'Snapping' knee secondary to a tibial osteochondroma. Knee. 2008;15(1):58–60.
13. Crites BM, Lohnes J, Garrett WE Jr. Snapping popliteal tendon as a source of lateral knee pain. Scand J Med Sci Sports. 1998;8(4):243–4.
14. Fung DA, Frey S, Markbreiter L. Bilateral symptomatic snapping biceps femoris tendon due to fibular exostosis. J Knee Surg. 2008;21(1):55–7.
15. Geeslin AG, LaPrade RF. Surgical treatment of snapping medial hamstring tendons. Knee Surg Sports Traumatol Arthrosc. 2010;18(9):1294–6.
16. Bernhardson AS, LaPrade RF. Snapping biceps femoris tendon treated with an anatomic repair. Knee Surg Sports Traumatol Arthrosc. 2010;18(8):1110–2.
17. Gaine WJ, Mohammed A. Osteophyte impingement of the popliteus tendon as a cause of lateral knee joint pain. Knee. 2002;9(3):249–52.
18. Krause DA, Stuart MJ. Snapping popliteus tendon in a 21-year-old female. J Orthop Sports Phys Ther. 2008;38(4):191–5.
19. Bollen SR, Arvinite D. Snapping pes syndrome: a report of four cases. J Bone Joint Surg Br. 2008;90:334–5.
20. Song SJ, Bae DK, Park CH. Snapping knee due to a femoral osteochondroma after total knee arthroplasty. Knee Surg Relat Res. 2019;31(2):147–50.
21. Hung CY, Chang KV, Lam S. Dynamic sonography for snapping knee syndrome caused by the Gracilis tendon. J Ultrasound Med. 2018;37(3):803–4.
22. Guillin R, Marchand AJ, Roux A, Niederberger E, Duvauferrier R. Imaging of snapping phenomena. Br J Radiol. 2012;85(1018):1343–53.
23. Gali JC, Serafim BLC, Nassar SA, Gali Filho JC, LaPrade RF. Percutaneous lengthening of a regenerated semitendinosus tendon for medial hamstring snapping. Arthrosc Tech. 2019;8(3):e349–52.
24. Akagawa M, Kimura Y, Saito H, Kijima H, Saito K, Segawa T, Wakabayashi I, Kashiwagura T, Miyakoshi N, Shimada Y. Snapping pes syndrome caused by the Gracilis tendon: successful selective surgery with specific diagnosis by ultrasonography. Case Rep Orthop. 2020;2020:5. https://doi.org/10.1155/2020/1783813.
25. Hadeed MM, Post M, Werner BC. Partial fibular head resection technique for snapping biceps femoris. Arthrosc Tech. 2018;7(8):e859–62.
26. Saltzman BM, Collins MJ, Arns TA, Forsythe B. Unilateral snapping biceps femoris tendon with an anomalous insertion treated with anatomic repositioning and lengthening with a single suture anchor: a report of two cases. JBJS Case Connect. 2018;8(1):e13. https://doi.org/10.2106/JBJS.CC.16.00251.

Chapter 32
Knee Intra-articular Snapping Syndrome

This is a condition whereby there is movement of an intra-articular soft tissue structure across a bony, soft tissue prominence, or prosthetic hardware prominence, with an associated resultant sound [1–8]. This may be painful or painless. It may be troublesome or an incidental finding.

Causes of intra-articular snapping include:

- Mass lesion—ganglion, rheumatoid nodule
- Discoid meniscus
- Patellar clunk syndrome (cruciate sacrificing knee arthroplasty)

Patellar clunk syndrome—in this condition a soft tissue nodule forms at the superior pole of the patella. During knee flexion this moves distally to the intercondylar notch of the femoral prosthesis (usually of a cruciate substituting knee replacement arthroplasty). Upon knee extension (at about 30–45° flexion) this nodule catches on the proximal border of the notch, with snapping on this border upon further extension [9–15].

32.1 Clinical Symptoms of Knee Intra-articular Snapping Syndrome

- Pain (although snapping may be painless)
- Visible snapping—reported by patient or others
- Audible and palpable crepitus with knee motion

C. Panayiotou Charalambous, *The Knee Made Easy*,
https://doi.org/10.1007/978-3-030-54506-2_32

32.2 Clinical Signs of Knee Intra-articular Snapping Syndrome

- Palpable crepitus
- Audible snapping
- Visible snapping
- Mass lesion/swelling—visible, palpable
- Tenderness over the lesion

32.3 Investigations for Knee Intra-articular Snapping Syndrome

- Radiological
  - Plain radiographs/CT scans looking for osseous causes of snapping
  - MRI/ultrasound to identify intra-articular mass lesions, discoid meniscus
  - Dynamic ultrasound to demonstrate snapping during knee motion

32.4 Management of Knee Intra-articular Snapping Syndrome

32.4.1 Non-surgical

- Leave alone
- Analgesia
- Activity modification
- Steroid injections—intra-articular

32.4.2 Surgical (Open or Arthroscopic) [9–12]

- Resection of soft tissue structure causing snapping—open or arthroscopic
- Discoid meniscus:
  - Partial meniscectomy saucerization
  - Stabilisation—if unstable

Learning Pearls

- In cases presenting with knee snapping, if an extra-articular cause is not obvious the possibility of an intra-articular cause needs to be considered

References

1. Chen G, Zhang Z, Li J. Symptomatic discoid lateral meniscus: a clinical and arthroscopic study in a Chinese population. BMC Musculoskelet Disord. 2016;17:329. https://doi.org/10.1186/s12891-016-1188-3.
2. Harato K, Niki Y, Nagashima M, Masumoto K, Otani T, Toyama Y, Suda Y. Arthroscopic visualization of abnormal movement of discoid lateral meniscus with snapping phenomenon. Arthrosc Tech. 2015;4(3):e235–8.
3. Mine T, Ihara K, Kawamura H, Kuwabara Y. Intra-articular synovial cyst of the knee joint: a case report. J Orthop Surg (Hong Kong). 2010;18(2):248–50.
4. Liu PC, Chen CH, Huang HT, Chang JK, Chen JC, Tien YC, Hung SH. Snapping knee symptoms caused by an intra-articular ganglion cyst. Knee. 2007;14(2):167–8.
5. Yilmaz E, Karakurt L, Yildirim H, Ozercan R. Intra-articular lipoma causing snapping in the patellofemoral joint. Saudi Med J. 2007;28(6):955–8.
6. Mine T, Ihara K, Taguchi T, Tanaka H, Suzuki H, Hashimoto T, Kawai S. Snapping knee caused by intra-articular tumors. Arthroscopy. 2003;19(3):E21.
7. Torisu T, Yosida S, Takasita M. Painful snapping in rheumatoid knees. Int Orthop. 1997;21(6):361–3.
8. Yoo JH, Kim EH, Ryu HK. Arthroscopic removal of separated bipartite patella causing snapping knee syndrome. Orthopedics. 2008;31(7):717.
9. Frye BM, Floyd MW, Pham DC, Feldman JJ, Hamlin BR. Effect of femoral component design on patellofemoral crepitance and patella clunk syndrome after posterior-stabilized total knee arthroplasty. J Arthroplast. 2012;27(6):1166–70.
10. Dajani KA, Stuart MJ, Dahm DL, Levy BA. Arthroscopic treatment of patellar clunk and synovial hyperplasia after total knee arthroplasty. J Arthroplasty. 2010;25(1):97–103.
11. Schroer WC, Diesfeld PJ, Reedy ME, LeMarr A. Association of increased knee flexion and patella clunk syndrome after mini-subvastus total knee arthroplasty. J Arthroplasty. 2009;24(2):281–7.
12. Shoji H, Shimozaki E. Patellar clunk syndrome in total knee arthroplasty without patellar resurfacing. J Arthroplasty. 1996;11(2):198–201.
13. Geannette C, Miller T, Saboeiro G, Parks M. Sonographic evaluation of patellar clunk syndrome following total knee arthroplasty. J Clin Ultrasound. 2017;45(2):105–7.
14. Ip D, Ko PS, Lee OB, Wu WC, Lam JJ. Natural history and pathogenesis of the patella clunk syndrome. Arch Orthop Trauma Surg. 2004;124(9):597–602.
15. Costanzo JA, Aynardi MC, Peters JD, Kopolovich DM, Purtill JJ. Patellar clunk syndrome after total knee arthroplasty; risk factors and functional outcomes of arthroscopic treatment. J Arthroplasty. 2014;29(9 Suppl):201–4.

Chapter 33
Meniscal Tears

Tears of the meniscus disrupt the meniscal structure and are commonly encountered in the troublesome knee.

33.1 Causes of Meniscal Tears

- Acute trauma
  - Compressive forces
  - Shear forces
  - Torsional forces (such as internal rotation of the femur in relation to a fixed tibia)
- Chronic degeneration
  - Repetitive loading
  - Aging

33.2 Description of Meniscal Tears

Meniscal tears may be described in several ways and these are presented next.

According to the Precipitating Event

1. Acute traumatic—the meniscus tears suddenly (due to the application of substantial acute force)

C. Panayiotou Charalambous, *The Knee Made Easy*,
https://doi.org/10.1007/978-3-030-54506-2_33

2. Chronic—the meniscus tears gradually over a long time (such as due to chronic repetitive loading or meniscal degeneration). Tears occur with the application of no acute force or minimal force. The force required is much less than that expected to cause a tear in a healthy meniscus
3. Iatrogenic—as when performing arthroscopic or open surgery

According to the Site of the Tear

- Anterior Horn
- Body
- Posterior horn
- Meniscal root
- Combination

Meniscal tears most often involve the posterior horn.

According to the Meniscus Torn

1. Medial
2. Lateral
3. Both

Most degenerative tears affect the medial meniscus due to the amount of forces that normally pass through the medial tibiofemoral compartment.

Meniscal tears occurring at the same time as an anterior cruciate ligament (ACL) traumatic tear tend to involve the lateral meniscus. In contrast, those occurring at a subsequent stage, due to raised medial compartment pressures tend to involve the posterior horn of the medial meniscus [1–6].

According to Tear Thickness

1. Full thickness
2. Partial thickness
   (a) Superior surface
   (b) Inferior surface
   (c) Intrasubstance tear

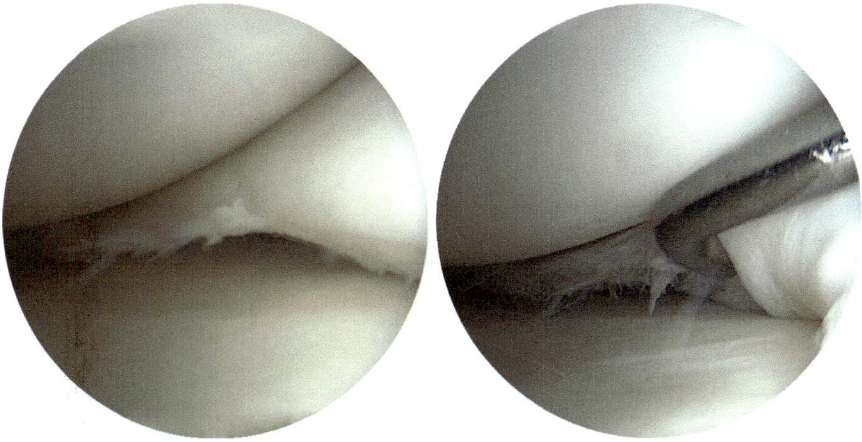

Degenerate meniscal tear

According to the Tear Shape

Tear shape is determined at surgery and may be:

- Longitudinal (including bucket handle tears)
- Radial
- Oblique
- Flap
- Horizontal
- Complex (no specific pattern, combinations of above)

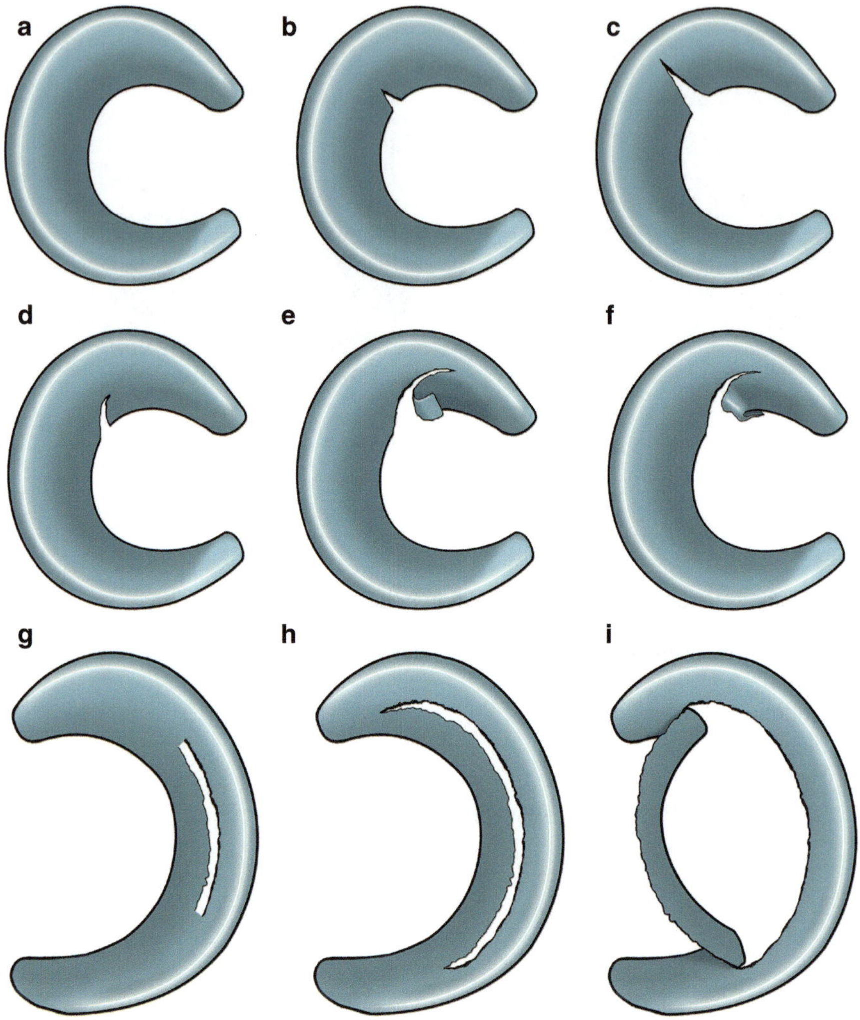

Meniscal tear patterns: (**a**) Intact meniscus. (**b**) Radial tear, inner margin. (**c**) Radial tear extending to outer part of meniscus. (**d**) Oblique tear, undisplaced. (**e**) Oblique tear, flap folded above the meniscus. (**f**) Oblique tear, flap folded under the meniscus. (**g**) Longitudinal tear, body of meniscus, undisplaced. (**h**) Longitudinal tear, across meniscal length, undisplaced. (**i**) Longitudinal tear displaced (bucket-handle tear)

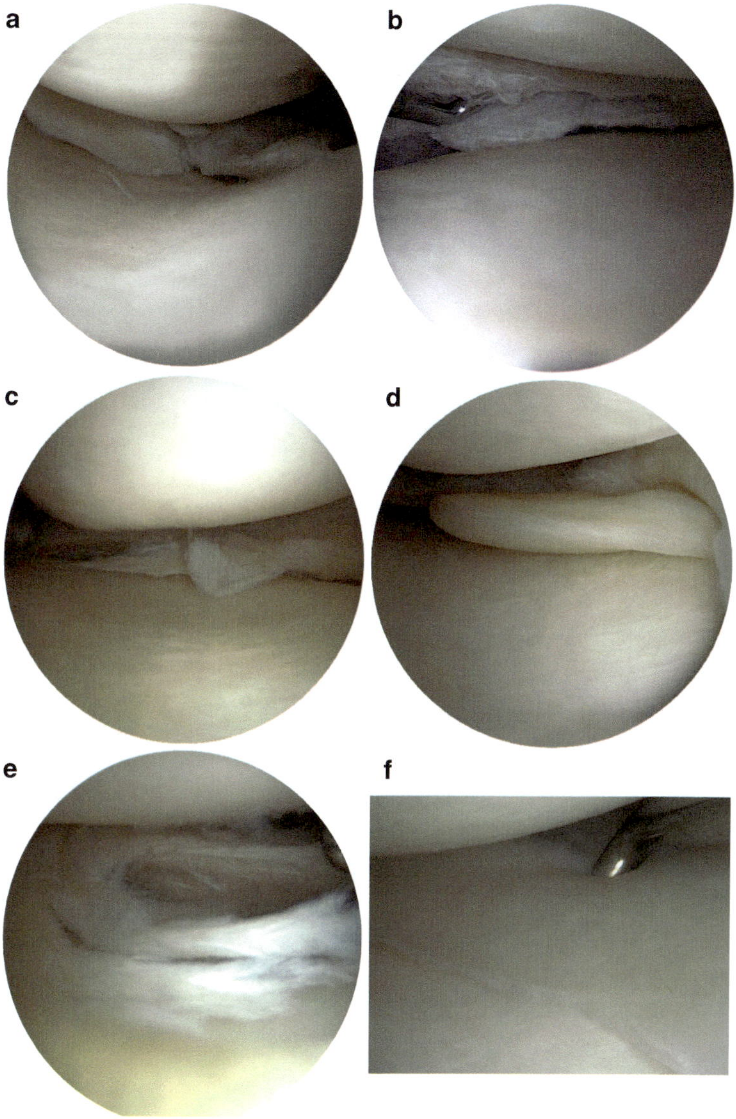

Meniscal tear patterns: (**a**) Posterior horn radial tear. (**b**) Horizontal degenerate tear. (**c**) Posterior horn degenerate complex tear. (**d**) Radial tear with a displaced flap. (**e**) Partial length longitudinal tear. (**f**) Peripheral menisco-capsular separation

According to Tear Size

Tear size is based on the anteroposterior length of the meniscus.

According to the Degree of Displacement

- Undisplaced
- Displaced

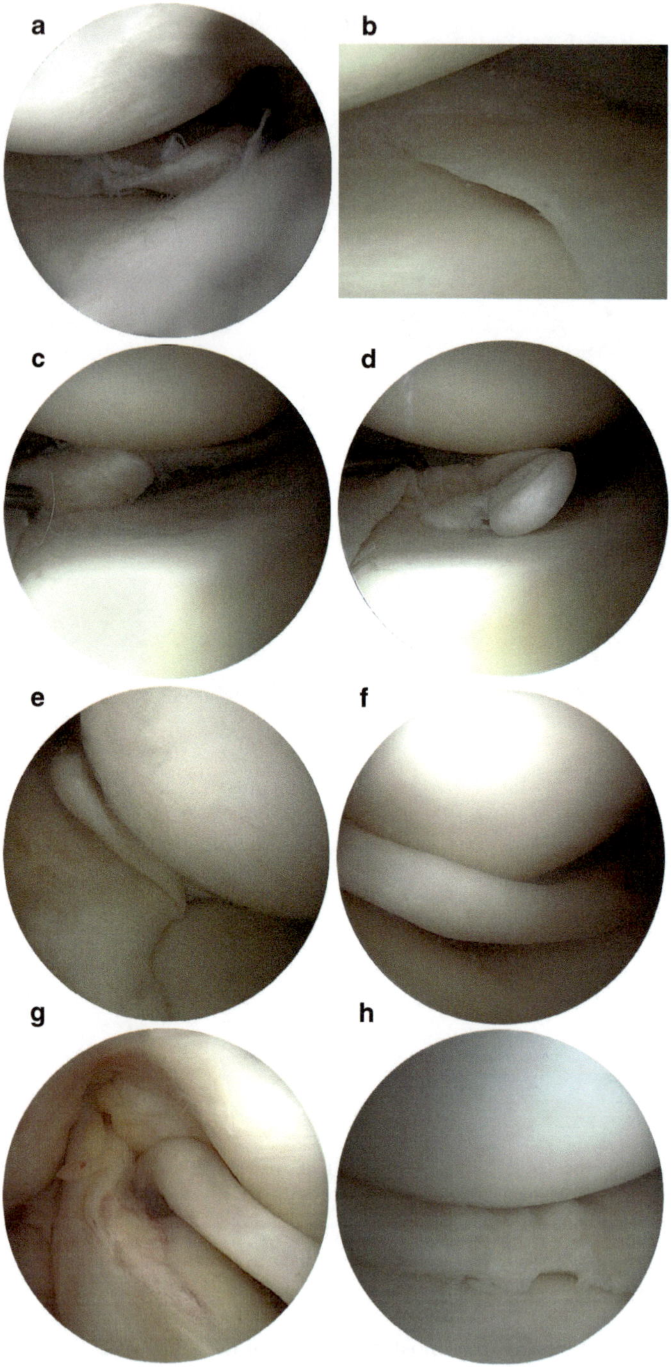

Displaced meniscal tear patterns: (**a**) Undisplaced radial tear extending to the outer periphery. (**b**) Undisplaced radial tear not extending to the outer periphery. (**c, d**) Displaced meniscal flap folded under the meniscus. (**e**) Displaced flap folded superior to the meniscal surface. (**f**) Displaced bucket handle tear. (**g**) Displaced bucket handle tear located in the femoral notch. (**h**) Displaced partial length longitudinal tear

According to the Degree of Displacement Reducibility

- Reducible
- Irreducible (may be stuck in a displaced position such as in the femoral notch area)

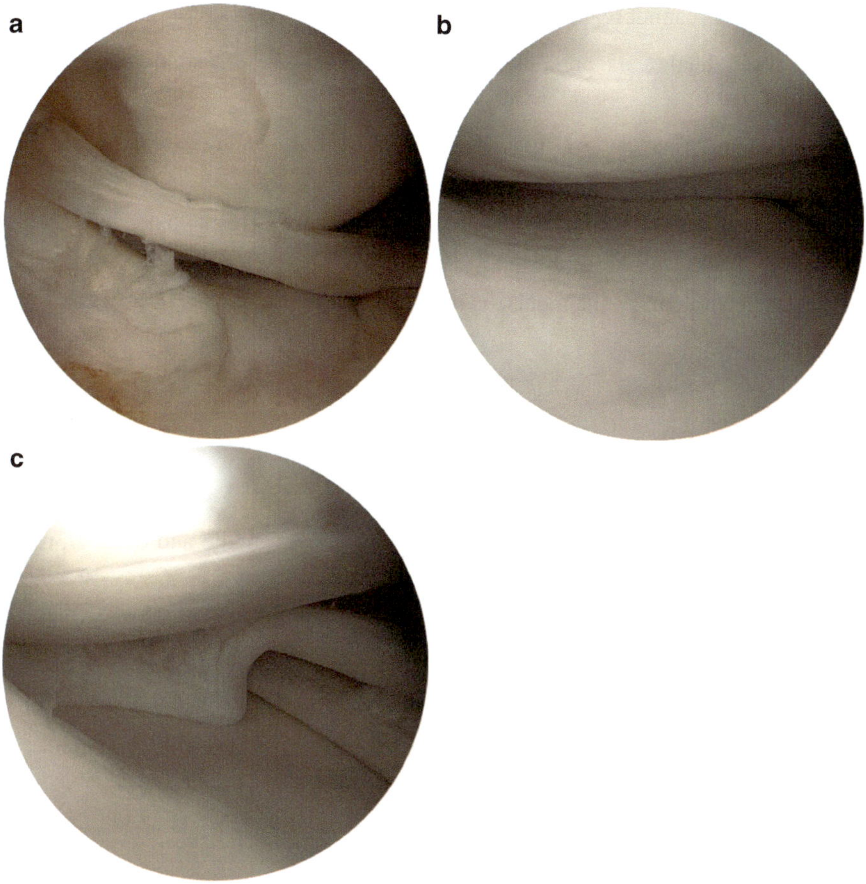

Bucket handle tear reducibility. (**a**) Bucket handle tear in femoral notch. (**b**) Reduced. (**c**) Re-displaced

According to the Presence of Associated Injuries

- Isolated
- Concomitant injuries
- Chondral
- Ligamentous
- Bony
- Combination of the above

According to whether the Tear Can Be Physically Repaired or Not

1. Repairable
2. Irreparable

Meniscal tears may not be repairable due to several factors including:

- Tear shape—cannot reapproximate the meniscal edges
  - Longitudinal tears are amenable to repair, repair of radial tears is also described
- Poor meniscal substance quality—unable to hold sutures—sutures cutting through the meniscus

The decision as to whether to repair a meniscal tear [7–15] also depends on the chances of such repair being successful. This may be influenced by:

- Vascularity of part of the meniscus involved by tear:
  - Outer 1/3rd
  - Middle 1/3rd
  - Inner 1/3rd
- May be described as:
  - Red on red (outer 1/3rd tears)
  - White on red (involving the junction between the middle and outer 1/3rd of the meniscus)
  - White on white (inner 1/3rd tears)
- Age of the patient
  - Children and young adults have a greater healing potential
- Chronicity of tear—the more chronic the tear the lower its healing potential
- Meniscal degeneration—increased degeneration impairs the biological ability of the meniscus to heal

33.3 Demographics of Meniscal Tears [16–20]

Prevalence:

- Haviv et al. [16] reported a low prevalence of isolated medial meniscal tears in young females with stable knees. Six females (of 111) and 87 males (of 480) younger than 30 years had isolated medial meniscus tears

- Culvenor et al. [17] performed a meta-analysis to estimate the prevalence of magnetic resonance imaging (MRI) features of osteoarthritis (OA) in asymptomatic uninjured knees. They included 63-studies (5397 knees in 4751 adults) and reported that the overall pooled prevalence of meniscal tears was 10% (7–13%), with significantly higher prevalence in older age:
  - <40 years old—meniscal tear prevalence—4% (2–7%)
  - ≥40 years old—meniscal tear prevalence—19% (13–26%)
- Cimino PM et al. [18] looked at the incidence of meniscal tears associated with acute ACL disruption in a series of 328 cases secondary to snow skiing accidents and reported:
  - 75 (23%) coexistent meniscal injuries:
    - 43 (13%) lateral meniscus
    - 32 (10%) medial meniscus
    - 32 (43%) of the 75 meniscal tears were peripheral detachments from the capsule (red-red tears)

33.4 Clinical Symptoms of Meniscal Tears

- Knee pain
  - Deep seated pain (constant or activity related)
  - Medial joint line pain
- Swelling (effusion, synovitis, parameniscal cyst)
- Clicking, catching, popping
- Locking
- Knee instability
- Neurological symptoms due to parameniscal cysts causing nerve compression

33.5 Clinical Signs of Meniscal Tears

- Joint line tenderness
- McMurray's test -pain/palpable clicking on loading and rotating the knee
- Thesally test
- Snapping
- Knee effusion, synovitis
- Visible or palpable parameniscal cyst
- Loss of motion (stiffness, loss of extension)

33.6 Investigations for Meniscal Tears [21–26]

- MRI
  - Medial meniscal tear—MRI sensitivity about 92%, specificity about 90% [15]
  - Lateral meniscal tear—MRI sensitivity about 80%, specificity about 95%

Sensitivity and specificity may however be influenced by the type and size of tear. They may be lower for peripheral meniscal detachments associated with ACL tears.

The post-partial meniscectomy meniscus and the repaired meniscus are more difficult to evaluate as compared to a meniscus which has not not had previous surgery. There may be overlap between the MRI expected post-surgical changes and a re-torn meniscus. A new meniscal tear is suggested by:

- High T2 signal reaching the articular surface
- Abnormal meniscal shape not explained by the previous surgery
- Displaced meniscal fragment
- Presence of contrast material within the meniscus substance (in MRI arthrogram examinations)

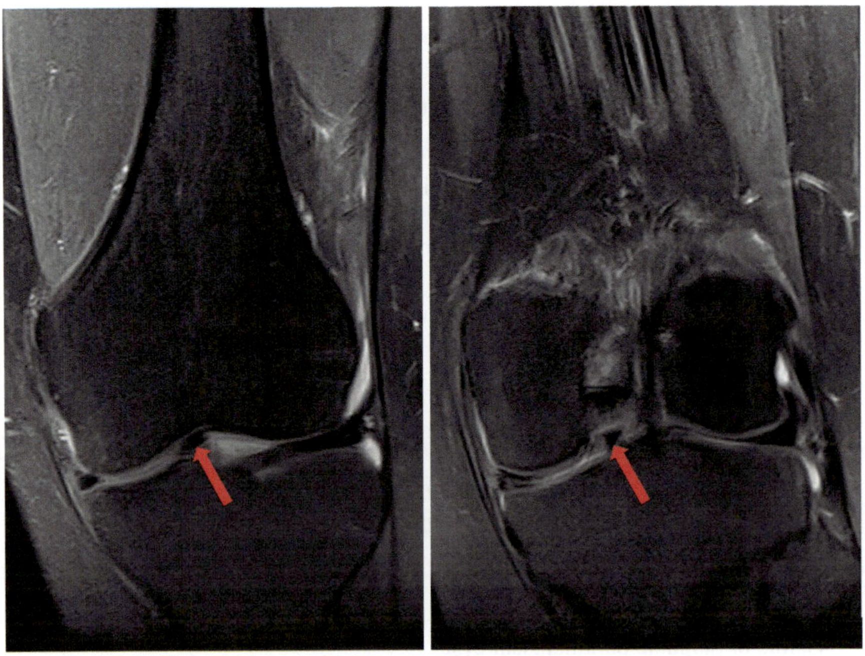

Bucket handle tear with fragment displaced in the femoral notch (red arrow)

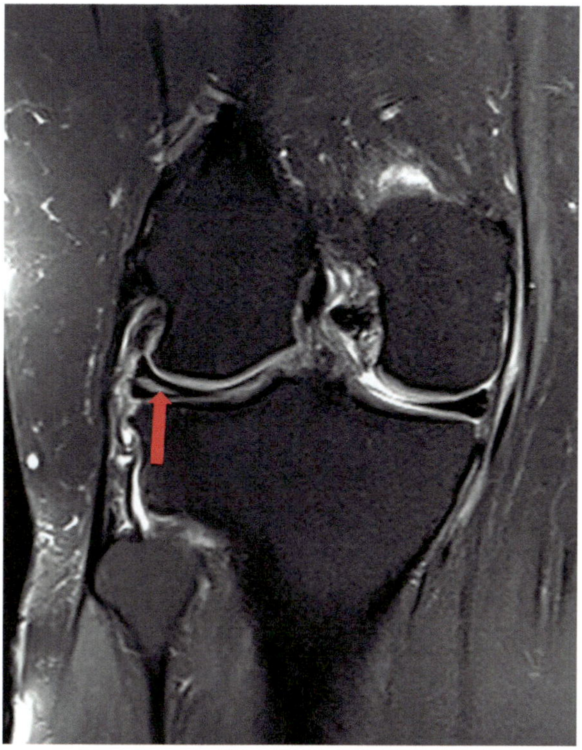

Lateral meniscal horizontal tear (red arrow)

33.7 Management of Meniscal Tears [27–35]

Treatment is directed towards the troubling symptoms:

33.7.1 Treatment for Pain

33.7.1.1 Non-surgical

- Leave alone
- Analgesia, activity modification
- Knee steroid injections
- Physiotherapy
  - Posterior capsular stretching to address contractures, to regain motion loss
  - Improve muscle strength and neuromuscular control
  - Increase lower extremity strengthening and core strengthening

33.7.1.2 Surgical

- Arthroscopic
  - Partial meniscectomy
  - Meniscal repair
  - Decompression of parameniscal cyst

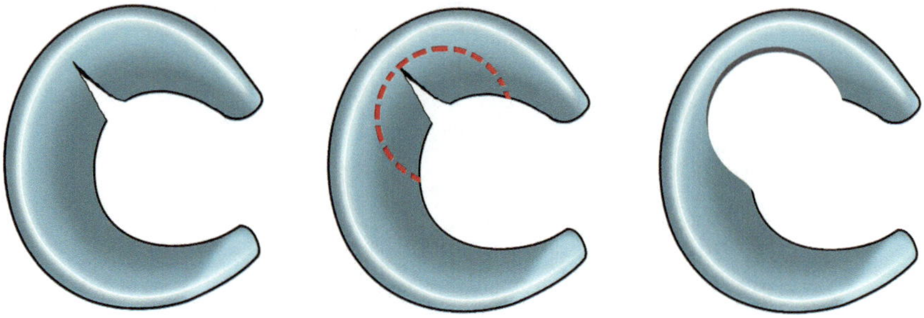

Partial meniscectomy of radial meniscal tear

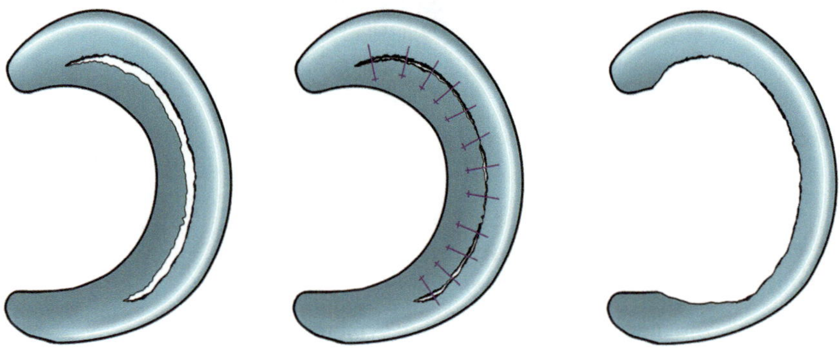

Meniscal repair or partial meniscectomy of a longitudinal meniscal tear

33.7.2 Treatment for Locking

33.7.2.1 Non-surgical

- Leave alone
- Physiotherapy
  - Improve knee muscle strength and neuromuscular control
  - Lower extremity strengthening and core strengthening

33.7.2.2 Surgical

- Arthroscopic surgery
  - Partial meniscectomy/debridement
  - Meniscal repair

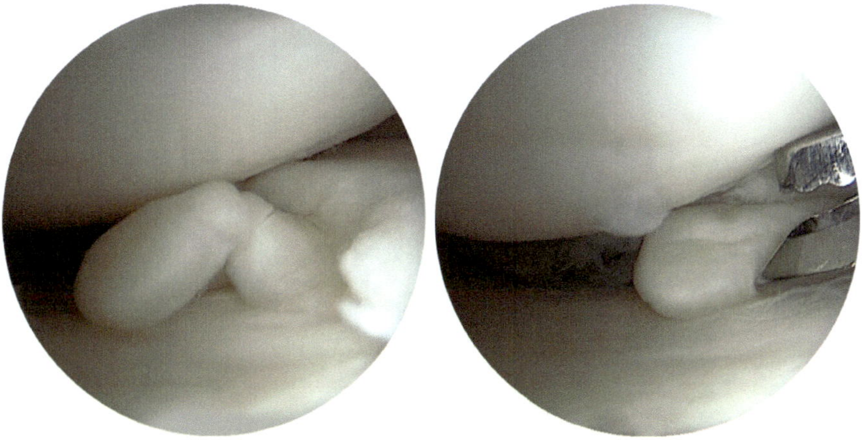

Arthroscopic partial meniscectomy of flap tear

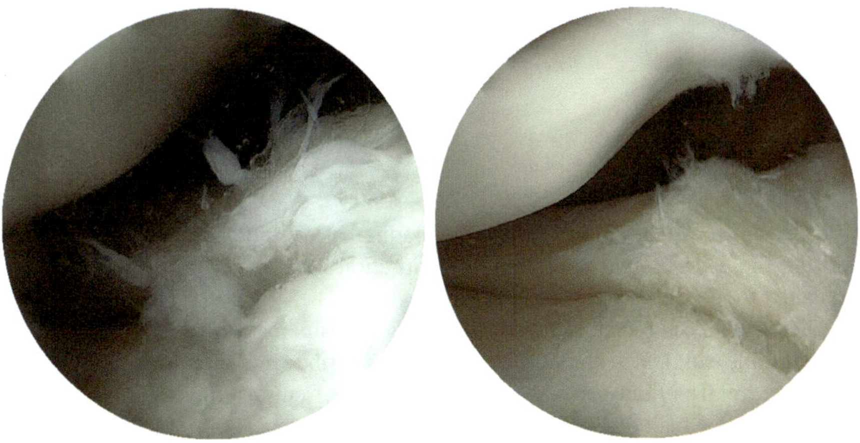

Arthroscopic debridement of complex meniscal tear

33.8 Meniscal Root Tear

Meniscal root tear refers to an avulsion of the posterior root of the meniscus, or a radial/oblique tear extending to the periphery of the meniscus close to its posterior root (within about 10 mm of its tibial insertion) [36–42]. This disrupts the tibial anchorage or continuity of the meniscus, which leads to meniscal extrusion, and defunctions the ability of the meniscus to resist hoop stresses.

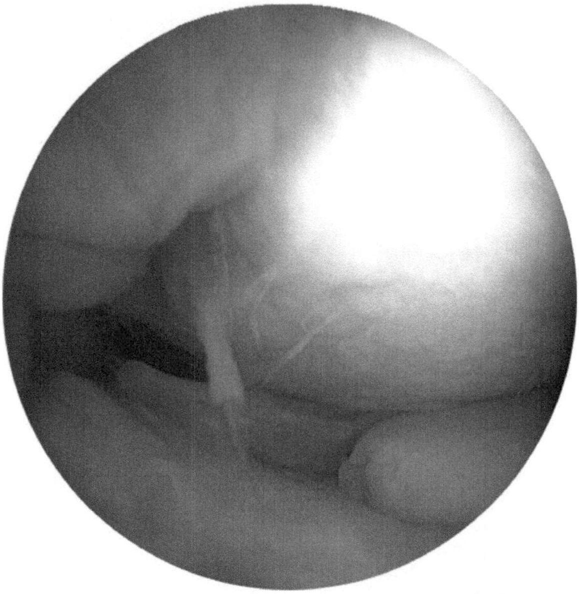

Meniscal root tear

Meniscal root tears may lead to overloading of the tibiofemoral compartment and the rapid development or rapid deterioration of articular cartilage degeneration and OA.

There have been recent suggestions that root repairs may halt such deterioration, and multiple surgical techniques have been described for meniscal root repairs, including tibial pullout sutures (involves passing of sutures through the meniscal root tear edge which are then brought through bony tunnels onto the outer surface of the proximal tibia, where the sutures are tied over a bone bridge or a surgical button).

It has been shown that lateral meniscal root tears tend to occur more often in younger male patients, are associated with less cartilage degeneration, and are more commonly associated with a ligament injury, as compared to medial posterior root tears. Lateral meniscal root repairs may confer better outcomes as compared to medial root repairs.

Although meniscal root repairs may be of benefit in acute tears in younger, high demand individuals, their role in older patients or in the presence of established degenerative changes is questioned, and should be viewed with high degree of caution.

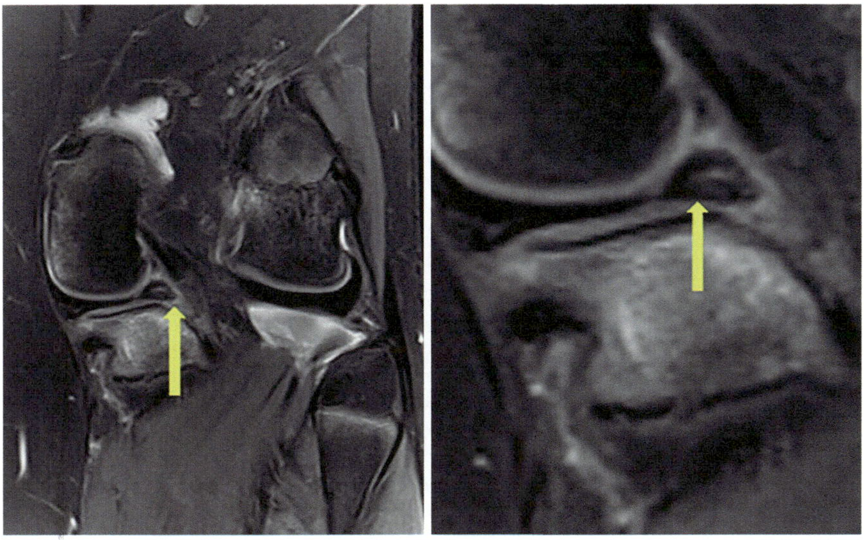

Posterior root lesion of the medial meniscus (yellow arrow)

33.9 Meniscal Extrusion

This refers to an external shift of the meniscus away from the knee joint, which leads to a reduction in the meniscal coverage of the tibial plateau.

It may signify defunction of the meniscus, either due to meniscal degeneration (with disruption of its matrix and circumferential collagen fibres) or due to a meniscal tear (body tear, or meniscal root/horn tear). This reduces the ability of the meniscus to take up hoop stresses when loaded. Meniscal damage has been shown to precede meniscal extrusion.

As the meniscal coverage of the tibial plateau decreases, the forces on the articular cartilage increase, which predisposes to development or progression of knee degeneration and OA. It has been shown that meniscal extrusion precedes the development of OA.

Meniscal extrusion is measured on MRI:

- As the distance by which the meniscus exceeds the margin of the tibial cartilage (osteochondral junction at the joint margin, excluding osteophytes)
- On a mid-coronal tibial slice (where the medial tibia spine appears the largest, or on the slice with the largest tibial width)

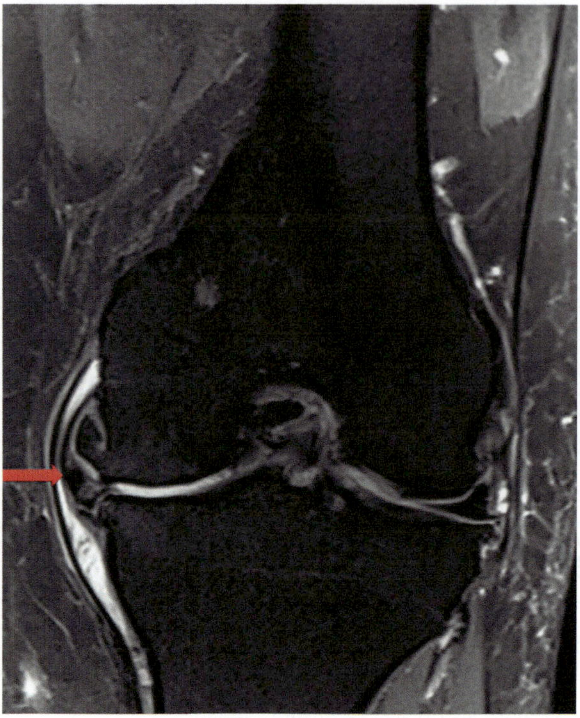

Knee osteoarthritis associated with large medial femoral osteophyte and extruded medial meniscus (red arrow)

Svensson et al. [43] studied 718 individuals free of radiographic tibiofemoral OA, aged 50–90 years, in the USA and reported that:

- Medial meniscal extrusion in middle-aged/older individuals without OA is around 3 mm
- Lateral meniscal extrusion in middle-aged/older individuals without OA is around 2 mm
- Meniscal damage is associated with medial meniscal extrusion >3 mm and less cartilage coverage

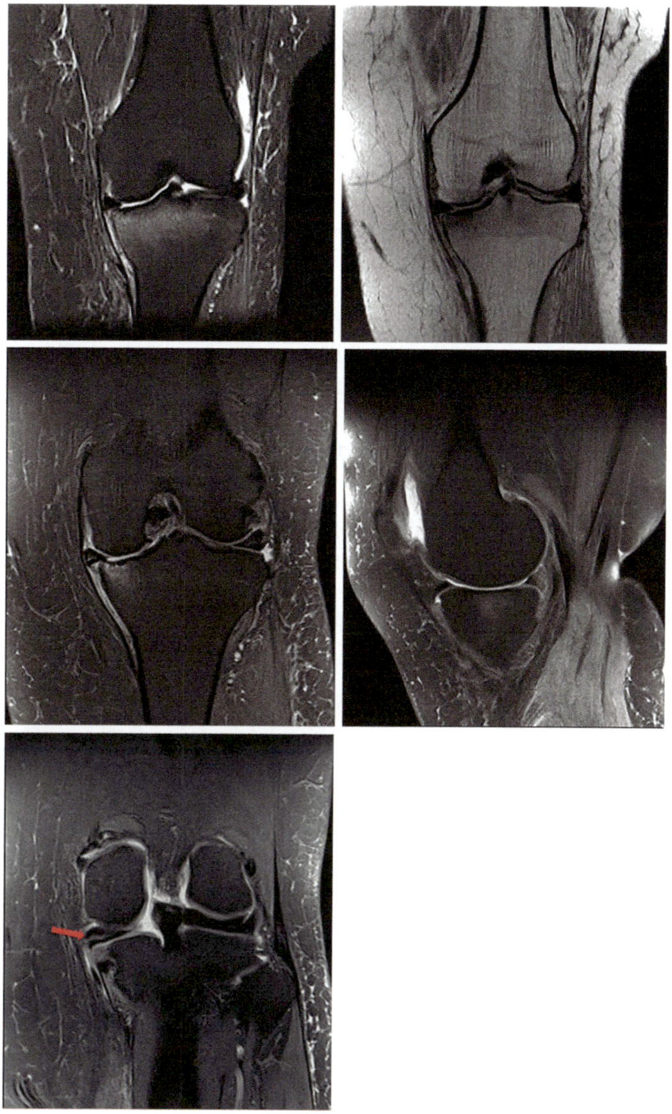

Posterior horn tear of the medial meniscus (red arrow) with meniscal extrusion and associated proximal medial tibia oedema. Oedema improved on follow up scan

Lerer et al. [44] reported a strong association between a medial meniscal extrusion that is greater than or equal to (≥) 3 mm and the presence of:

- Medial joint line osteophytes—77%
- Medial compartment articular cartilage loss—69%
- Medial meniscal root pathology—64%
- Meniscal radial tear—58%

A significant number of cases with no or minimal evidence of degeneration (20%) had ≥3 mm medial meniscal extrusion, suggesting that extrusion precedes, rather than follows, the development of OA.

Learning Pearls

- Not every meniscal tear needs to be dealt with. Many tears are incidental findings on radiological investigations or arthroscopic evaluation of the knee, and their presence needs to be correlated with clinical symptoms
- The overall beneficial effect of meniscal surgery has been questioned by multiple randomised trials that failed to show a difference in outcomes between those treated with meniscal surgery or sham surgery [43–47]
- In investigating and deciding how to manage meniscal tears (in particular whether surgery has any role to play) the following may be considered:
  - MRI may not fully characterise the type of tear
  - MRI is a static investigation hence may not demonstrate displacement in an intermittently displaced tear
  - It may be difficult to determine whether it is the mechanical symptoms or the pain which causes trouble to the patient, as these 2 symptoms may coexist
- Partial meniscectomy should be viewed with caution, especially in cases with coexistent arthritis
- Non-surgical methods should be tried prior to considering surgical intervention in most cases
- Early surgical intervention is considered for:
  - Displaced meniscal tear causing a locked knee
  - Traumatic meniscal tear in a young patient, for which surgical repair is warranted
- Long duration of symptoms (>1 year), radiological OA and resection of more than 50% of meniscus are associated with poorer outcomes following arthroscopic partial meniscectomy [29]. Total meniscectomy, removal of the peripheral meniscal rim, lateral meniscectomy, degenerative meniscal tears, associated chondral damage, arthritis and high BMI have also been related to a poor outcome following meniscectomy
- Rehabilitation of meniscal repairs varies amongst clinicians, but there is some evidence that early range of motion and weightbearing may not confer a detrimental effect on clinical outcomes

References

1. Arner JW, Irvine JN, Zheng L, Gale T, Thorhauer E, Hankins M, Abebe E, Tashman S, Zhang X, Harner CD. The effects of anterior cruciate ligament deficiency on the meniscus and articular cartilage: a novel dynamic in vitro pilot study. Orthop J Sports Med. 2016;4(4):2325967116639895. https://doi.org/10.1177/2325967116639895.
2. Nikolic DK. Lateral meniscal tears and their evolution in acute injuries of the anterior cruciate ligament of the knee. Arthroscopic analysis. Knee Surg Sports Traumatol Arthrosc. 1998;6:26–30.
3. Cipolla M, Scala A, Gianni E, Puddu G. Different patterns of meniscal tears in acute anterior cruciate ligament (ACL) ruptures and in chronic ACL-deficient knees. Classification, staging and timing of treatment. Knee Surg Sports Traumatol Arthrosc. 1995;3:130–4.
4. Hagino T, Ochiai S, Senga S, Yamashita T, Wako M, Ando T, Haro H. Meniscal tears associated with anterior cruciate ligament injury. Arch Orthop Trauma Surg. 2015;135(12):1701–6.
5. Yoo JC, Ahn JH, Lee SH, Yoon YC. Increasing incidence of medial meniscal tears in nonoperatively treated anterior cruciate ligament insufficiency patients documented by serial magnetic resonance imaging studies. Am J Sports Med. 2009;37(8):1478–83.
6. Feucht MJ, Bigdon S, Bode G, et al. Associated tears of the lateral meniscus in anterior cruciate ligament injuries: risk factors for different tear patterns. J Orthop Surg Res. 2015;10:34. Published 2015 Mar 18. https://doi.org/10.1186/s13018-015-0184-x.
7. Karia M, Ghaly Y, Al-Hadithy N, Mordecai S, Gupte C. Current concepts in the techniques, indications and outcomes of meniscal repairs. Eur J Orthop Surg Traumatol. 2019;29(3):509–20.
8. Moulton SG, Bhatia S, Civitarese DM, Frank RM, Dean CS, LaPrade RF. Surgical techniques and outcomes of repairing meniscal radial tears: a systematic review. Arthroscopy. 2016;32(9):1919–25.
9. Ferrari MB, Murphy CP, Gomes JLE. Meniscus repair in children and adolescents: a systematic review of treatment approaches, meniscal healing, and outcomes. J Knee Surg. 2019;32(6):490–8.
10. Eberbach H, Zwingmann J, Hohloch L, Bode G, Maier D, Niemeyer P, Südkamp NP. Feucht sport-specific outcomes after isolated meniscal repair: a systematic review. Knee Surg Sports Traumatol Arthrosc. 2018;26(3):762–71.
11. Mutsaerts EL, van Eck CF, van de Graaf VA, Doornberg JN, van den Bekerom MP. Surgical interventions for meniscal tears: a closer look at the evidence. Arch Orthop Trauma Surg. 2016;136(3):361–70.
12. Kurzweil PR, Lynch NM, Coleman S, Kearney B. Repair of horizontal meniscus tears: a systematic review. Arthroscopy. 2014;30(11):1513–9.
13. Espejo-Reina A, Serrano-Fernández JM, Martín-Castilla B, Estades-Rubio FJ, Briggs KK, Espejo-Baena A. Outcomes after repair of chronic bucket-handle tears of medial meniscus. Arthroscopy. 2014;30(4):492–6.
14. Turman KA, Diduch DR. Meniscal repair: indications and techniques. J Knee Surg. 2008;21(2):154–62.
15. Paxton ES, Stock MV, Brophy RH. Meniscal repair versus partial meniscectomy: a systematic review comparing reoperation rates and clinical outcomes. Arthroscopy. 2011;27(9):1275–88.
16. Haviv B, Bronak S, Thein R. Low prevalence of isolated medial meniscal tears in young females with stable knees. Orthopedics. 2015;38(3):e196–9.
17. Culvenor AG, Øiestad BE, Hart HF, Stefanik JJ, Guermazi A, Crossley KM. Prevalence of knee osteoarthritis features on magnetic resonance imaging in asymptomatic uninjured adults: a systematic review and meta-analysis. Br J Sports Med. 2019;53(20):1268–78.
18. Cimino PM. The incidence of meniscal tears associated with acute anterior cruciate ligament disruption secondary to snow skiing accidents. Arthroscopy. 1994;10(2):198–200.
19. Beals CT, Magnussen RA, Graham WC, Flanigan DC. The prevalence of meniscal pathology in asymptomatic athletes. Sports Med. 2016;46(10):1517–24.

20. Yeh PC, Starkey C, Lombardo S, Vitti G, Kharrazi FD. Epidemiology of isolated meniscal injury and its effect on performance in athletes from the National Basketball Association. Am J Sports Med. 2012;40(3):589–94.
21. Koo B, Lee SH, Yun SJ, Song JG. Diagnostic performance of magnetic resonance imaging for detecting meniscal ramp lesions in patients with anterior cruciate ligament tears: a systematic review and meta-analysis. Am J Sports Med. 2020;48:2051–9. https://doi.org/10.1177/0363546519880528.
22. Wang W, Li Z, Peng HM, Bian YY, Li Y, Qian WW, Weng XS, Jin J, Yang XY, Lin J. Accuracy of MRI diagnosis of meniscal tears of the knee: a meta-analysis and systematic review. J Knee Surg. 2019. https://doi.org/10.1055/s-0039-1694056.
23. Chapin R. Imaging of the postoperative meniscus. Radiol Clin North Am. 2018;56(6):953–64.
24. Vance K, Meredick R, Schweitzer ME, Lubowitz JH. Magnetic resonance imaging of the postoperative meniscus. Arthroscopy. 2009;25(5):522–30.
25. Cardello P, Gigli C, Ricci A, Chiatti L, Voglino N, Pofi E. Retears of postoperative knee meniscus: findings on magnetic resonance imaging (MRI) and magnetic resonance arthrography (MRA) by using low and high field magnets. Skeletal Radiol. 2009;38(2):149–56.
26. Pujol N, Panarella L, Selmi TA, Neyret P, Fithian D, Beaufils P. Meniscal healing after meniscal repair: a CT arthrography assessment. Am J Sports Med. 2008;36(8):1489–95.
27. van de Graaf VA, Wolterbeek N, Mutsaerts EL, Scholtes VA, Saris DB, de Gast A, Poolman RW. Arthroscopic partial meniscectomy or conservative treatment for nonobstructive meniscal tears: a systematic review and meta-analysis of randomized controlled trials. Arthroscopy. 2016;32(9):1855–65.
28. Rothermich MA, Cohen JA, Wright R. Stable meniscal tears left in situ at the time of arthroscopic anterior cruciate ligament reconstruction: a systematic review. J Knee Surg. 2016;29(3):228–34.
29. Eijgenraam SM, Reijman M, Bierma-Zeinstra SMA, van Yperen DT, Meuffels DE. Can we predict the clinical outcome of arthroscopic partial meniscectomy? A systematic review. Br J Sports Med. 2018;52(8):514–21.
30. Jeong HJ, Lee SH, Ko CS. Meniscectomy. Knee Surg Relat Res. 2012;24(3):129–36.
31. Salata MJ, Gibbs AE, Sekiya JK. A systematic review of clinical outcomes in patients undergoing meniscectomy. Am J Sports Med. 2010;38(9):1907–16.
32. Shanmugaraj A, Tejpal T, Ekhtiari S, Gohal C, Horner N, Hanson B, Khan M, Bhandari M. The repair of horizontal cleavage tears yields higher complication rates compared to meniscectomy: a systematic review. Knee Surg Sports Traumatol Arthrosc. 2020;28(3):915–25.
33. Fillingham YA, Riboh JC, Erickson BJ, Bach BR Jr, Yanke AB. Inside-out versus all-inside repair of isolated meniscal tears: an updated systematic review. Am J Sports Med. 2017;45(1):234–42.
34. Ayeni O, Peterson D, Chan K, Javidan A, Gandhi R. Suture repair versus arrow repair for symptomatic meniscus tears of the knee: a systematic review. J Knee Surg. 2012;25(5):397–402.
35. O'Donnell K, Freedman KB, Tjoumakaris FP. Rehabilitation protocols after isolated meniscal repair: a systematic review. Am J Sports Med. 2017;45(7):1687–97.
36. Chahla J, LaPrade RF. Meniscal root tears. Arthroscopy. 2019;35(5):1304–5.
37. Krych AJ, Hevesi M, Leland DP, Stuart MJ. Meniscal Root Injuries. J Am Acad Orthop Surg. 2019;28:491–9. https://doi.org/10.5435/JAAOS-D-19-00102.
38. Krych AJ, Bernard CD, Kennedy NI, Tagliero AJ, Camp CL, Levy BA, Stuart MJ. Medial vs. lateral meniscus root tears: is there a difference in injury presentation, treatment decisions, and surgical repair outcomes? Arthroscopy. 2020;36(4):1135–41. pii: S0749-8063(19)31087-4.
39. Sharif B, Ashraf T, Saifuddin A. Magnetic resonance imaging of the meniscal roots. Skeletal Radiol. 2020;49:661–76. https://doi.org/10.1007/s00256-020-03374-3.
40. Kwon OJ, Bin SI, Kim JM, Lee BS, Lee SM, Park JG, Yoon GW. There is no difference in radiographic outcomes after average 9 years after arthroscopic partial medial meniscectomy for both posterior horn tears and posterior horn root tears. Arthroscopy. 2020;36(2):524–32.

41. Lee BS, Bin SI, Kim JM, Park MH, Lee SM, Bae KH. Partial meniscectomy for degenerative medial meniscal root tears shows favorable outcomes in well-aligned, nonarthritic knees. Am J Sports Med. 2019;47(3):606–11.
42. Lansdown DA, Feeley BT. Editorial commentary: are we over-treating meniscal root tears? Arthroscopy. 2020;36(2):533–4.
43. Svensson F, Felson DT, Zhang F, Guermazi A, Roemer FW, Niu J, Aliabadi P, Neogi T, Englund M. Meniscal body extrusion and cartilage coverage in middle-aged and elderly without radiographic knee osteoarthritis. Eur Radiol. 2019;29(4):1848–54.
44. Lerer DB, Umans HR, Hu MX, Jones MH. The role of meniscal root pathology and radial meniscal tear in medial meniscal extrusion. Skeletal Radiol. 2004;33(10):569–74.
45. Sihvonen R, Paavola M, Malmivaara A, Itälä A, Joukainen A, Nurmi H, Kalske J, Järvinen TL, Finnish Degenerative Meniscal Lesion Study (FIDELITY) Group. Arthroscopic partial meniscectomy versus sham surgery for a degenerative meniscal tear. N Engl J Med. 2013;369(26):2515–24.
46. Hohmann E, Glatt V, Tetsworth K, Cote M. Arthroscopic partial meniscectomy versus physical therapy for degenerative meniscus lesions: how robust is the current evidence? A critical systematic review and qualitative synthesis. Arthroscopy. 2018;34(9):2699–708.
47. Lee SH, Lee OS, Kim ST, Lee YS. Revisiting arthroscopic partial meniscectomy for degenerative tears in knees with mild or no osteoarthritis: a systematic review and meta-analysis of randomized controlled trials. Clin J Sport Med. 2020;30(3):195–202. https://doi.org/10.1097/JSM.0000000000000585, Publish ahead of print.

Chapter 34
Discoid Meniscus Syndrome

This is a condition whereby the meniscus is of abnormal shape [1–5]. The meniscus is discoid in shape (like a plate). This may be due to failure of absorption of the central part of the meniscus during development or abnormal morphogenesis of the meniscus. The thickness of the discoid meniscus is also altered with the central part being thin, whereas the anterior and posterior parts are thickened. Its matrix may have reduced collagen content, and irregular orientation and disorganisation of collagen fibres, and hence altered biomechanical properties.

The lateral meniscus is most commonly affected, but cases of medial discoid meniscus have been described. Patients may present with pain or mechanical symptoms of snapping and instability. Discoid menisci may also be predisposed to degeneration and tears.

34.1 Demographics of Discoid Meniscus

Incidence [3, 6–8]:

- Lateral discoid meniscus—0.4 to 17%
- Medial discoid meniscus—0.1 to 0.3%
- Bilateral in about 20% of cases (80–95% in symptomatic discoid meniscus)
- Higher in Asian countries (Japan, Korea, India) as compared to western populations

C. Panayiotou Charalambous, *The Knee Made Easy*,
https://doi.org/10.1007/978-3-030-54506-2_34

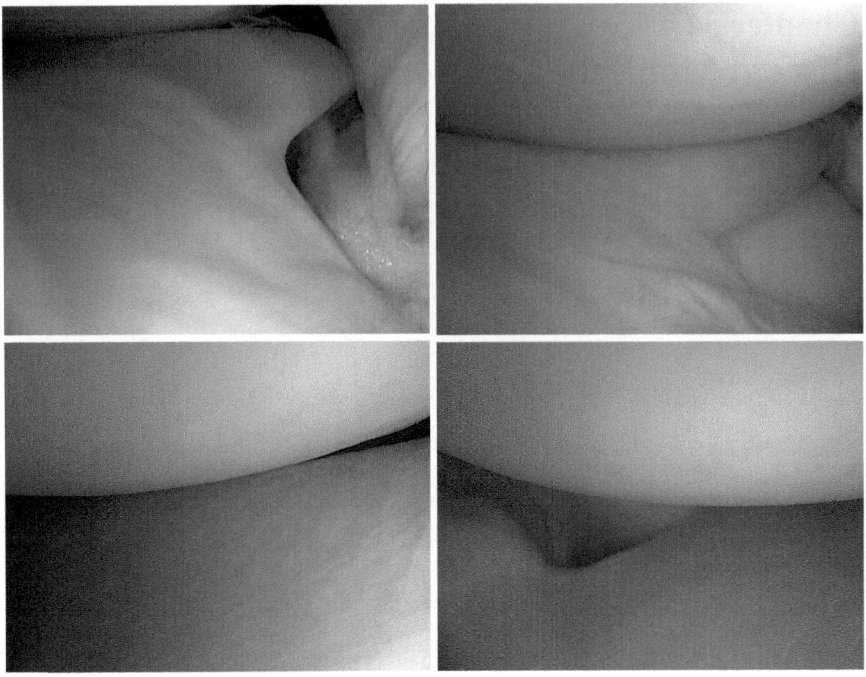

Discoid meniscus with intact periphery

34.2 Classification of Discoid Meniscus

Watanabe classification [9]

- Complete type—discoid shaped meniscus covers the whole of the tibial plateau and has normal posterior capsular attachment
- Incomplete type—covers less than 80% of the tibial plateau, with normal posterior capsular attachment
- Wrisberg type—more normally shaped than the complete or incomplete types but lacks the posterior meniscal attachments (coronary ligaments) with only the Wrisberg ligament (posterior meniscofemoral ligament) connecting the posterior horn.

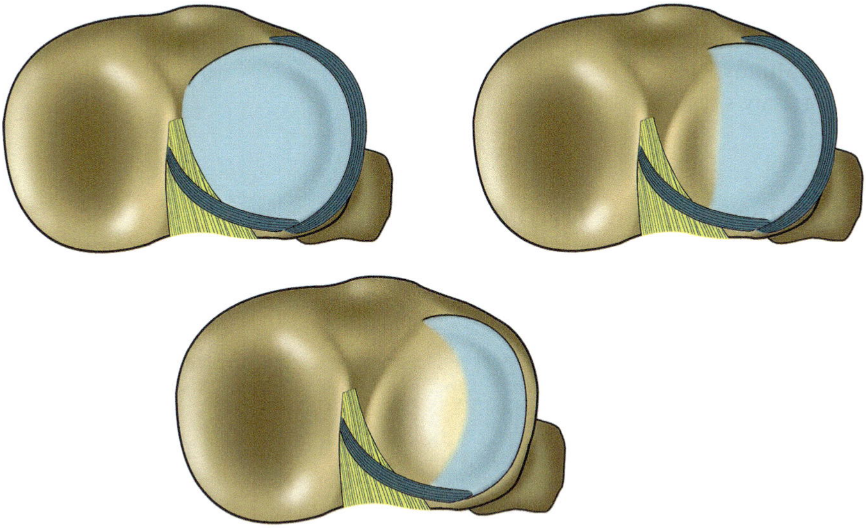

Watanabe discoid meniscus classification

34.3 Clinical Symptoms of Discoid Meniscus

- Pain
  - Deep seated pain (constant or activity related)
  - Lateral tibiofemoral joint line pain
- Clicking, catching, snapping, popping (arthroscopic evaluation of the discoid lateral meniscus has shown that on deep knee flexion from extension, the central part of the meniscus moves anteriorly with snapping. Upon extension from flexion, the central part returns to its previous posterior position, accompanied by snapping at 20–30° flexion [10]. Snapping may also be seen in peripheral rim instability, when the whole of the discoid lateral meniscus moves into the intercondylar notch and then reduces during knee flexion and extension [11]).
- Locking if there is an associated meniscal tear—these are often horizontal tears
- Swelling (synovitis, effusion)
- Neurological symptoms due to parameniscal cysts causing nerve compression

34.4 Clinical Signs of Discoid Meniscus

- Joint line tenderness
- Audible and palpable clicking/snapping on knee motion

- Knee effusion
- Limited knee motion
- McMurray's test
- Thessaly's test

34.5 Investigations for Discoid Meniscus

- MRI [12–14]

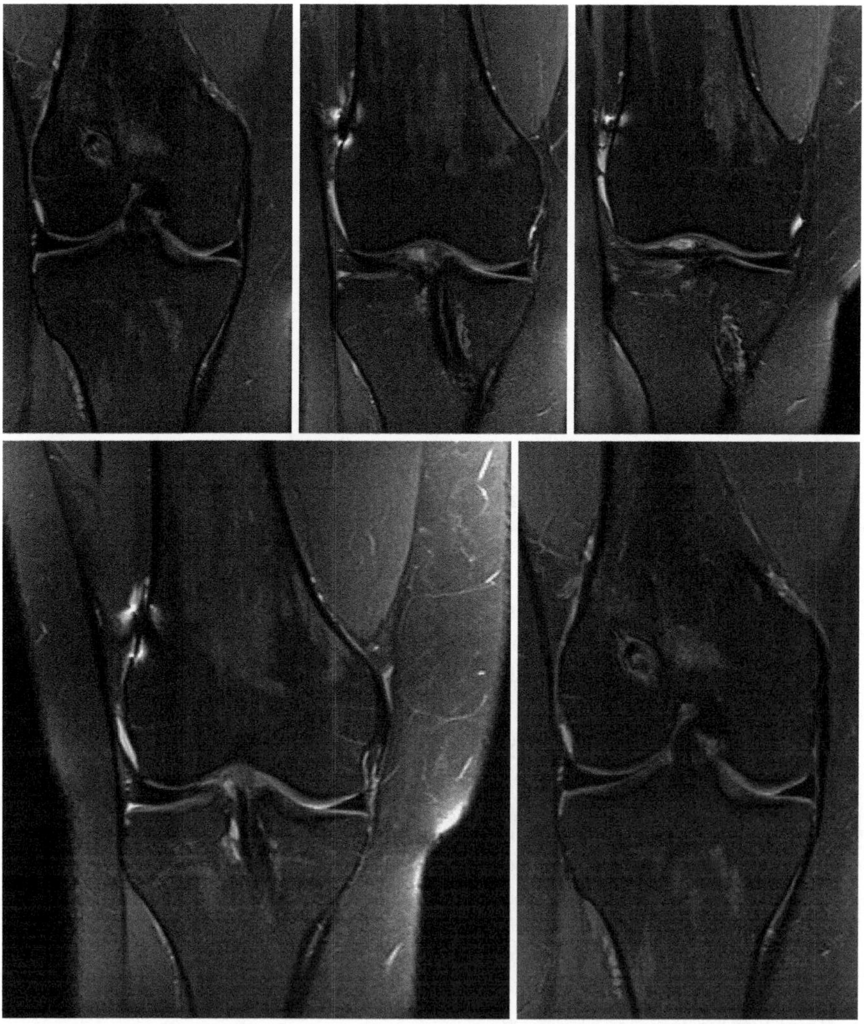

Previous ACL reconstruction with intact graft, discoid lateral meniscus

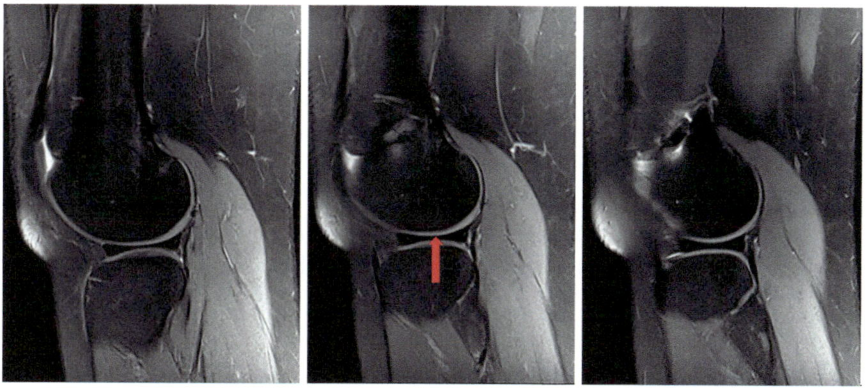

Discoid meniscus – bow tie appearance (red arrow) with continuity of the lateral meniscus in 3 consecutive sections

34.6 Management of Discoid Meniscus

Treatment is directed towards the troubling symptoms. If asymptomatic no intervention is needed as many do not become symptomatic.

34.6.1 Treatment for Pain

34.6.1.1 Non-surgical [15, 16]

- Leave alone
- Analgesia, activity modification
- Knee steroid injections
- Physiotherapy
  - Improve muscle strength and neuromuscular control
  - Increase lower extremity strengthening and core strengthening

34.6.1.2 Surgical [17–20]

- Arthroscopic
  - Partial meniscectomy (of the torn part)
  - Meniscal tear repair

34.6.2 *Treatment for Locking*

34.6.2.1 Non-surgical

- Leave alone
- Physiotherapy
  - Improve muscle strength and neuromuscular control
  - Lower extremity strengthening and core strengthening

34.6.2.2 Surgical

- Arthroscopic surgery
- Partial meniscectomy (+/– peripheral repair if peripheral instability is present)
- Saucerization—remove the central part of the meniscus to convert it from discoid to C-shaped meniscus (+/– peripheral repair) if peripheral instability is present
- Recently, successful repair of unstable peripheral longitudinal tears of a discoid meniscus without saucerization has also been reported (as saucerization may compromise the function of load transmission, predisposing to degenerative changes) [19]

34.7 Prognosis

- Lee et al. [17] reported unfavourable outcomes in >30% of patients following partial meniscectomy of discoid meniscus in 73 knee of patients younger than 40, at a mean follow up of 10 years. There was progression of arthritic changes in 70% and degeneration of the residual meniscus in 50%.
- Ohnishi et al. [18] reported that clinical outcomes following arthroscopic treatment of a symptomatic discoid meniscus was better in children aged <13 as compared to those aged >13.

References

1. Nicholson A, Petit L, Egger A, Saluan P, Carter CW. Current concepts: evaluation and treatment of discoid meniscus in the pediatric athlete. Am J Orthop (Belle Mead NJ). 2018;47(12). https://doi.org/10.12788/ajo.2018.0107.
2. Kushare I, Klingele K, Samora W. Discoid meniscus: diagnosis and management. Orthop Clin North Am. 2015;46(4):533–40.
3. Kim JG, Han SW, Lee DH. Diagnosis and treatment of discoid meniscus. Knee Surg Relat Res. 2016;28(4):255–62.

4. Papadopoulos A, Kirkos JM, Kapetanos GA. Histomorphologic study of discoid meniscus. Arthroscopy. 2009;25(3):262–8.
5. Song IS, Kim JB, Lee JK, Park BS. Discoid medial meniscus tear, with a literature review of treatments. Knee Surg Relat Res. 2017;29(3):237–42.
6. Papadopoulos A, Karathanasis A, Kirkos JM, Kapetanos GA. Epidemiologic, clinical and arthroscopic study of the discoid meniscus variant in Greek population. Knee Surg Sports Traumatol Arthrosc. 2009;17(6):600–6.
7. Bae JH, Lim HC, Hwang DH, Song JK, Byun JS, Nha KW. Incidence of bilateral discoid lateral meniscus in an Asian population: an arthroscopic assessment of contralateral knees. Arthroscopy. 2012;28(7):936–41.
8. Ahn JH, Lee SH, Yoo JC, Lee HJ, Lee JS. Bilateral discoid lateral meniscus in knees: evaluation of the contralateral knee in patients with symptomatic discoid lateral meniscus. Arthroscopy. 2010;26:1348–56.
9. Harato K, Niki Y, Nagashima M, Masumoto K, Otani T, Toyama Y, Suda Y, Watanabe M, Takeda S, Ikeuchi H. Atlas of arthroscopy. 3rd ed. Tokyo: Igaku-Shoin; 1979. p. 75–130.
10. Harato K, Niki Y, Nagashima M, Masumoto K, Otani T, Toyama Y, Suda Y. Arthroscopic visualization of abnormal movement of discoid lateral meniscus with snapping phenomenon. Arthrosc Tech. 2015;4(3):e235–8.
11. Yoo WJ, Choi IH, Chung CY. Discoid lateral meniscus in children: limited knee extension and meniscal instability in the posterior segment. J Pediatr Orthop. 2008;28:544–8.
12. Araki Y, Yamamoto H, Nakamura H, Tsukaguchi I. MR diagnosis of discoid lateral menisci of the knee. Eur J Radiol. 1994;18(2):92–5.
13. Samoto N, Kozuma M, Tokuhisa T, Kobayashi K. Diagnosis of discoid lateral meniscus of the knee on MR imaging. Magn Reson Imaging. 2002;20(1):59–64.
14. Sohn DW, Bin SI, Kim JM, Lee BS, Kim SJ. Discoid lateral meniscus can be overlooked by magnetic resonance imaging in patients with meniscal tears. Knee Surg Sports Traumatol Arthrosc. 2018;26(8):2317–23.
15. Liu WX, Zhao JZ, Huangfu XQ, He YH, Yang XG. Prevalence of bilateral discoid lateral menisci (DLM) in patients operated for symptomatic DLM with a follow-up study on their asymptomatic contralateral knees: a magnetic resonance imaging (MRI) assessment. BMC Musculoskelet Disord. 2015;16:172. https://doi.org/10.1186/s12891-015-0626-y.
16. Lee SH. Editorial commentary: why should the contralateral side be examined in patients with symptomatic discoid lateral meniscus? Arthroscopy. 2019;35(2):507–10.
17. Lee CR, Bin SI, Kim JM, Lee BS, Kim NK. Arthroscopic partial meniscectomy in young patients with symptomatic discoid lateral meniscus: an average 10-year follow-up study. Arch Orthop Trauma Surg. 2018;138(3):369–76.
18. Ohnishi Y, Nakashima H, Suzuki H, Nakamura E, Sakai A, Uchida S. Arthroscopic treatment for symptomatic lateral discoid meniscus: the effects of different ages, groups and procedures on surgical outcomes. Knee. 2018;25(6):1083–90.
19. Smuin DM, Swenson RD, Dhawan A. Saucerization versus complete resection of a symptomatic discoid lateral meniscus at short- and long-term follow-up: a systematic review. Arthroscopy. 2017;33(9):1733–42.
20. Kinugasa K, Hamada M, Yonetani Y, Matsuo T, Mae T, Nakata K, Horibe S. Discoid lateral meniscal repair without saucerization for adolescents with peripheral longitudinal tear. Knee. 2019;26(3):803–8.

Chapter 35
Parameniscal Cysts

This is a condition whereby a ganglion like cyst develops adjacent to the tibiofemoral joint line [1–4]. These are often the result of a horizontal meniscal tear extending to the periphery of the meniscus, which then acts as a one way valve allowing synovial fluid to get into the cyst but not escape back into the knee.

The cyst may vary in size (from tiny to very large) and may consist of one or multiple locules. Such cysts are located more frequently in relation to the lateral as compared to the medial meniscus. A large meniscal tear extending into the meniscocapsular junction is more likely to be associated with the occurrence of a parameniscal cyst. It has been suggested that a meniscal tear equal to or greater than 12 mm along its circumferential axis, as identified using MRI, is associated with parameniscal cyst formation. On occasion the cyst does not communicate with the knee joint, and is not associated with a meniscal tear.

C. Panayiotou Charalambous, *The Knee Made Easy*,
https://doi.org/10.1007/978-3-030-54506-2_35

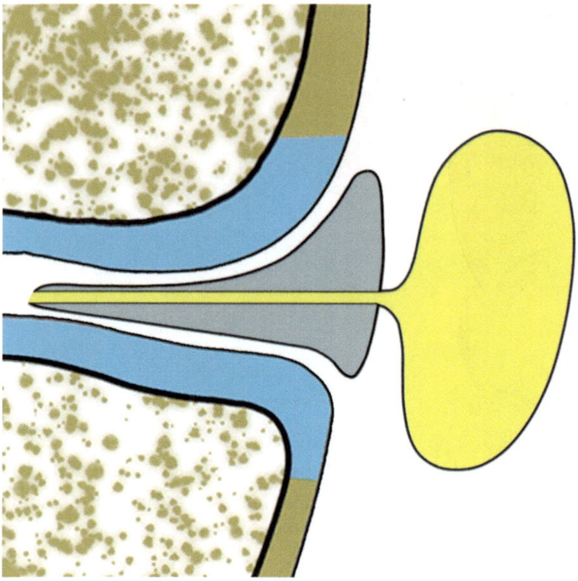

Parameniscal cyst secondary to a horizontal meniscal tear

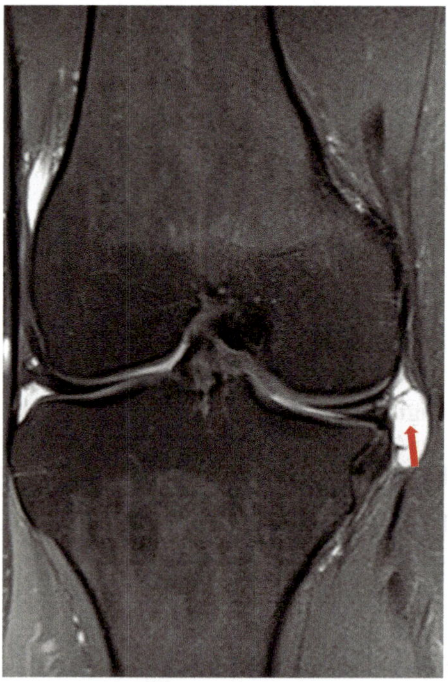

Medial parameniscal cyst (red arrow)

35.1 Clinical Symptoms of Parameniscal Cysts

- None—incidental findings on clinical or radiological evaluation of the knee
- Pain—dull
- Neurological symptoms (neurogenic pain, weakness, loss of muscle bulk) due to nerve compression (of the peroneal nerve, saphenous nerve) [5]
- Symptoms arising from an associated meniscal tear—clicking, knee pain, locking
- Mass lesion, if very large—snapping tendons, popliteal artery compression [6]

35.2 Clinical Signs of Parameniscal Cysts

- Cystic swelling related to the tibiofemoral joint line
- May feel very tense due to the pressure of its contents, to the extent that it may be mistaken as being of bony origin (such as osteoma)
- Size and tension may vary with joint position
  - Less prominent/disappears in flexion whilst larger and more tense in extension [7, 8]
  - Lateral parameniscal cysts may be more prominent with external rotation of the lower leg with the knee in 45° flexion, and show reduced prominence/disappearance with internal rotation of the lower leg [6]
- Neurological dysfunction—altered sensation, muscle weakness, muscle wasting
- Tendon snapping
- Signs of arterial compromise
- Lateral parameniscal cysts are often more easily apparent due to lack of much soft tissue coverage on the lateral side of the knee. Hence, they may be identifiable at an earlier, stage, when they are smaller.

35.3 Investigations for Parameniscal Cysts

- MRI
- Ultrasound

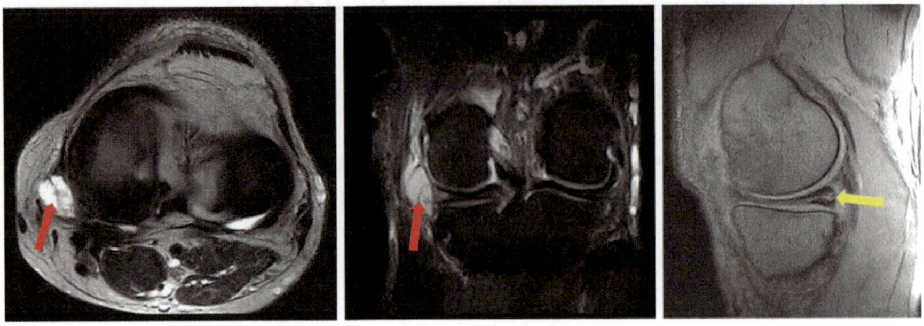

Medial parameniscal cyst (red arrow), associated with a horizontal tear of the medial meniscus (yellow arrow) (MRI)

35.4 Management of Parameniscal Cysts

In dealing with parameniscal cysts it is important to determine if they are contributing to any of the patient's symptoms or whether they are non-symptomatic. If non-symptomatic they are left alone. If symptomatic then options for treatment are as below:

35.4.1 Non-surgical

- Leave alone if symptoms not troublesome enough to warrant intervention
- Knee steroid injection—to reduce inflammation related to underlying knee degeneration or meniscal tear
- Aspiration of the cyst under ultrasound guidance and cyst steroid injection

35.4.2 Surgical [9–11]

- Arthroscopic partial meniscectomy +/− arthroscopic decompression of the cyst through the meniscal tear
- Arthroscopic partial meniscectomy+/− percutaneous needle decompression of the cyst
- Arthroscopic partial meniscectomy +/− open cyst excision
- Arthroscopic cyst decompression through a capsular window (if no associated meniscal tear)

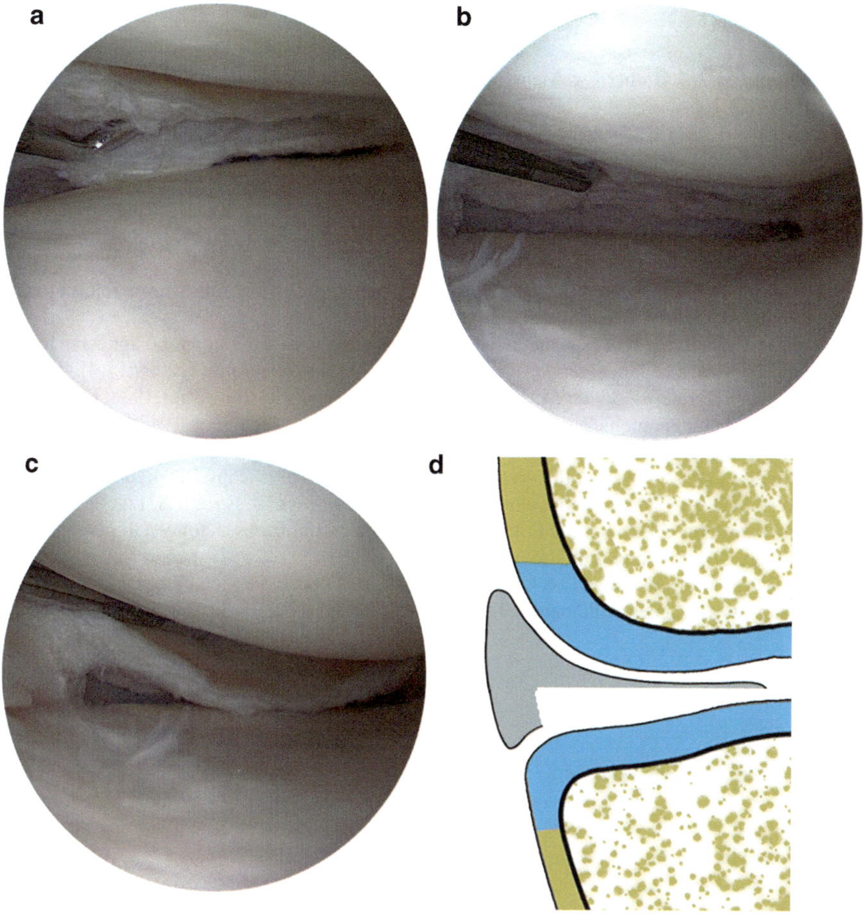

Partial meniscectomy with removal of the inferior lip of a horizontal tear to treat a parameniscal cyst

Learning Pearls

- Many of the parameniscal cysts detected radiologically are incidental findings, and may coexist with other knee disorders. Hence, the presence of a parameniscal cyst should be correlated with the patient's symptoms prior to planning any intervention.
- Open cyst excision is not commonly utilised
- Arthroscopic partial meniscectomy without cyst decompression has been shown to be equally effective to concomitant cyst decompression.
- Excellent short and medium-term outcomes have been described following partial meniscectomy without cyst decompression for patients with meniscal cysts and associated meniscal tears [11]

References

1. Cowden CH 3rd, Barber FA. Meniscal cysts: treatment options and algorithm. J Knee Surg. 2014;27(2):105–11.
2. De Smet AA, Graf BK, del Rio AM. Association of parameniscal cysts with underlying meniscal tears as identified on MRI and arthroscopy. AJR Am J Roentgenol. 2011;196(2):W180–6.
3. Wu CC, Hsu YC, Chiu YC, Chang YC, Lee CH, Shen HC, Huang GS. Parameniscal cyst formation in the knee is associated with meniscal tear size: an MRI study. Knee. 2013;20(6):556–61.
4. Anderson JJ, Connor GF, Helms CA. New observations on meniscal cysts. Skeletal Radiol. 2010;39(12):1187–91.
5. Thompson AT, Gallacher PD, Rees R. Lateral meniscal cyst causing irreversible peroneal nerve palsy. J Foot Ankle Surg. 2013;52(4):505–7.
6. Pinar H, Boya H, Satoglu IS, Oztekin HH. A contribution to Pisani's sign for diagnosing lateral meniscal cysts: a technical report. Knee Surg Sports Traumatol Arthrosc. 2009;17(4):402.
7. McMurray TP. Internal derangements of the knee joint. Ann R Coll Surg Engl. 1948;3(4):210–9.
8. Pisani AJ. Pathognomonic sign for cyst of the knee cartilage. Arch Surg. 1947;54(2):188–90.
9. Hulet C, Souquet D, Alexandre P, Locker B, Beguin J, Vielpeau C. Arthroscopic treatment of 105 lateral meniscal cysts with 5-year average follow-up. Arthroscopy. 2004;20(8):831–6.
10. Iorio R, Mazza D, Drogo P, Massafra C, Viglietta E, Conteduca J, Ferretti A. Lateral meniscal cysts: long-term clinical and radiological results of a partial meniscectomy and percutaneous decompressive needling. Int Orthop. 2020;44(3):487–93.
11. Kumar NS, Jakoi AM, Swanson CE, Tom JA. Is formal decompression necessary for parameniscal cysts associated with meniscal tears? Knee. 2014;21(2):501–3.

Chapter 36
Meniscal Deficiency Knee Syndrome

This is a condition whereby there is troublesome pain in the medial or lateral tibiofemoral compartment, following substantial meniscal resection [1, 2]. This may be due to loss of the cushion effect of the meniscus, leading to abnormal loading of the subchondral bone (compartment overloading). In the presence of meniscal deficiency, the contact area decreases and hence contact pressures increase. This may occur in the absence or in the presence of articular degenerative changes.

36.1 Clinical Symptoms of Meniscal Deficiency Knee Syndrome

- Deep seated knee pain in affected compartment—localised/diffuse
- Loss of motion
- Joint line pain—of the compartment of which meniscus was excised
- Pain upon impact activities or normal weightbearing
- Intermittent swelling (effusion/synovitis)
- Abnormal knee noise (clicking/clunking)
- Apparent instability

36.2 Clinical Signs of Meniscal Deficiency Knee Syndrome

- Muscle atrophy—related to disuse or tendon tear
- Diffuse knee swelling—effusion
- Painful knee motion—pain is worse on loading the tibiofemoral joint
- Knee weakness if associated quadriceps or other periarticular muscle atrophy and weakness

C. Panayiotou Charalambous, *The Knee Made Easy*,
https://doi.org/10.1007/978-3-030-54506-2_36

- Associated malalignment—varus/valgus deformity, flexion deformity
- Loss of knee motion
  - Apparent stiffness, due to pain
  - True stiffness

36.3 Investigations for Meniscal Deficiency Knee Syndrome

- Plain radiographs:
  - AP, lateral, skyline, notch view
  - Long leg film to assess alignment
- MRI:
  - To define the location, size and shape of any residual meniscus and determine any associated chondral disruption
  - Determine ligamentous disruption

36.4 Management of Meniscal Deficiency Knee Syndrome

36.4.1 Non-surgical

- Leave alone
- Activity modification
- Simple analgesia
- Physiotherapy to:
  - Strengthen the periarticular muscles of the knee
  - Maintain active motion
  - Stretch contracted soft tissues to regain motion
- Knee injections—steroid, viscosupplementation, PRP

36.4.2 Surgical [3–12]

- Arthroscopic debridement of residual meniscal tears or chondral lesions
- Realignment procedures (osteotomy) to offload the overloaded compartment if associated malalignment:
  - Distal femoral
  - Proximal tibial

- Stabilisation procedures, if associated ligamentous instability
- Meniscal transplantation +/− chondral restoration, if associated chondral disruption amenable to restoration procedures +/− realignment procedures +/− stabilisation procedures
  - Meniscal allograft
  - Meniscal artificial scaffold
- Knee arthroplasty
  - Unicompartmental
    - Medial
    - Lateral
  - Total arthroplasty (with or without patellar resurfacing)

Survival of meniscal allograft transplantation has been reported as 96.7% at 1 year, 87% at 5 years and 82.2% at 7 years. Knees without significant chondral damage had better survivorship (95% at 5 years) than knees with full thickness chondral wear (77% survivorship at 5 years). It was also shown that 77% of athletes may return to sporting activity.

References

1. Rao AJ, Erickson BJ, Cvetanovich GL, Yanke AB, Bach BR Jr, Cole BJ. The meniscus-deficient knee: biomechanics, evaluation, and treatment options. Orthop J Sports Med. 2015;3(10):2325967115611386. https://doi.org/10.1177/2325967115611386.
2. Hannon MG, Ryan MK, Strauss EJ. Meniscal allograft transplantation a comprehensive historical and current review. Bull Hosp Jt Dis (2013). 2015;73(2):100–8.
3. Liu JN, Agarwalla A, Gomoll AH. High tibial osteotomy and medial meniscus transplant. Clin Sports Med. 2019;38(3):401–16.
4. Leong NL, Southworth TM, Cole BJ. Distal femoral osteotomy and lateral meniscus allograft transplant. Clin Sports Med. 2019;38(3):387–99.
5. Bloch B, Asplin L, Smith N, Thompson P, Spalding T. Higher survivorship following meniscal allograft transplantation in less worn knees justifies earlier referral for symptomatic patients: experience from 240 patients. Knee Surg Sports Traumatol Arthrosc. 2019;27(6):1891–9.
6. Gitelis ME, Frank RM, Meyer MA, Cvetanovich G, Cole BJ. 5 points on meniscal allograft transplantation. Am J Orthop (Belle Mead NJ). 2018;47(9). https://doi.org/10.12788/ajo.2018.0069.
7. Cotter EJ, Frank RM, Waterman BR, Wang KC, Redondo ML, Cole BJ. Meniscal allograft transplantation with concomitant osteochondral allograft transplantation. Arthrosc Tech. 2017;6(5):e1573–80.
8. Saltzman BM, Meyer MA, Leroux TS, Gilelis ME, Debot M, Yanke AB, Cole BJ. The influence of full-thickness chondral defects on outcomes following meniscal allograft transplantation: a comparative study. Arthroscopy. 2018;34(2):519–29.
9. Jauregui JJ, Wu ZD, Meredith S, Griffith C, Packer JD, Henn RF 3rd. How should we secure our transplanted meniscus? A meta-analysis. Am J Sports Med. 2018;46(9):2285–90.

10. Saltzman BM, Griffin JW, Wetters N, Meyer MA, Cole BJ, Yanke AB. Concomitant arthroscopic meniscal allograft transplantation and anterior cruciate ligament reconstruction. Arthrosc Tech. 2016;5(5):e1161–71.
11. Schüttler KF, Pöttgen S, Getgood A, Rominger MB, Fuchs-Winkelmann S, Roessler PP, Ziring E, Efe T. Improvement in outcomes after implantation of a novel polyurethane meniscal scaffold for the treatment of medial meniscus deficiency. Knee Surg Sports Traumatol Arthrosc. 2015;23(7):1929–35.
12. Chalmers PN, Karas V, Sherman SL, Cole BJ. Return to high-level sport after meniscal allograft transplantation. Arthroscopy. 2013;29(3):539–44.

Chapter 37
Medial Plica Syndrome

A condition whereby a medial plica causes pain due to inflammation or thickening. Onset of symptoms may be post-traumatic or occur in the absence of an injury [1–6].

There are two entities of medial plica syndrome:

1. Seen in the absence of underlying arthritis
2. Seen in the presence of underlying arthritis or medial femoral condyle cartilage degeneration, whereby the plica may contribute to chondral damage due to a repetitive impingement and friction effect. The contact pressure on the medial femoral condyle has been shown to be related to the Young's modulus (stiffness) of the plica [6].

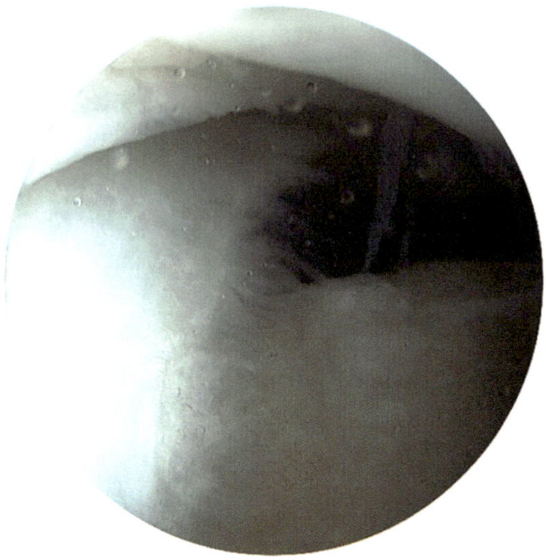

Thickened medial plica

C. Panayiotou Charalambous, *The Knee Made Easy*,
https://doi.org/10.1007/978-3-030-54506-2_37

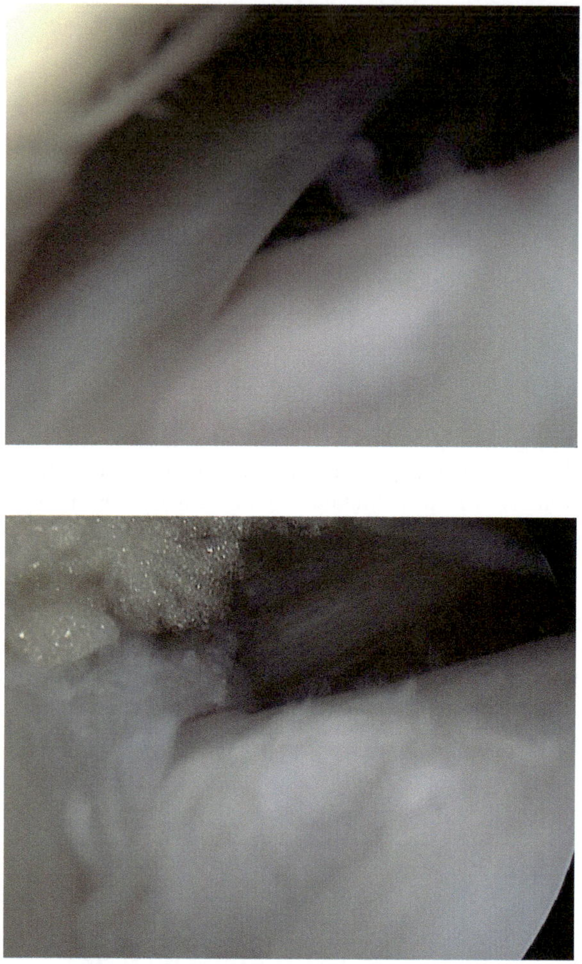

Medial plica with underlying chondral disruption

37.1 Clinical Symptoms of Medial Plica Syndrome

- Anteromedial pain:
  - Worse on going up stairs
  - Worse on knee flexion
- Clicking, snapping
- Pseudolocking

37.2 Clinical Signs of Medial Plica Syndrome

- Tenderness medial to the patella
- Tender medial femoral condyle
- Palpable thickened medial cord (can be rolled under the examiner's fingers, reproducing the patient's symptoms)
- MPP test [7]

37.3 Investigations for Medial Plica Syndrome [8, 9]

- Ultrasound—dynamic
- MRI

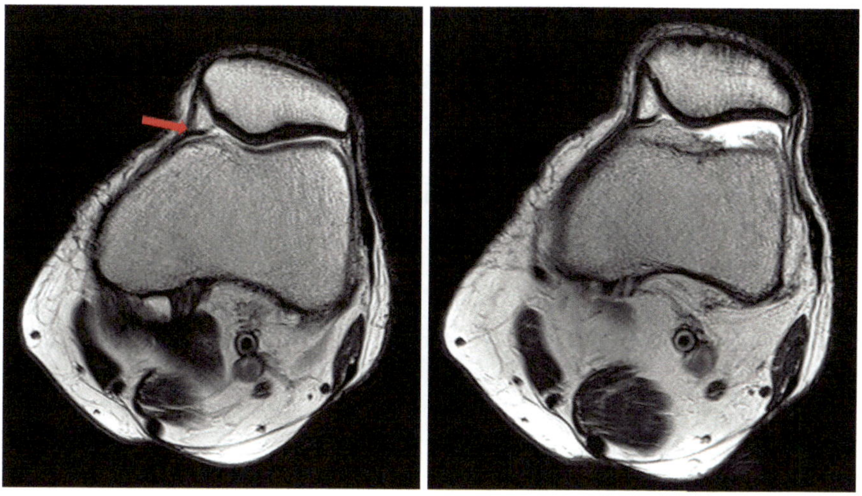

Medial plica projecting over the medial femoral condyle

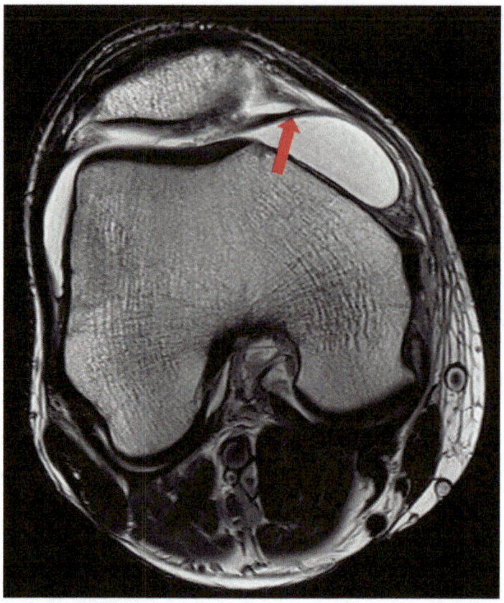

Thickened medial plica (red arrow)

37.4 Management of Medial Plica Syndrome

37.4.1 Non-surgical [10, 11]

- Analgesia/anti-inflammatories
- Physiotherapy:
  - Local massage
  - Quadriceps stretching
- Intra-articular steroid injections

37.4.2 Surgical Management [12, 13]

- Arthroscopic resection (along with resection of the medial retinaculum in cases of underlying arthritis of the medial compartment or the medial patellar facet)

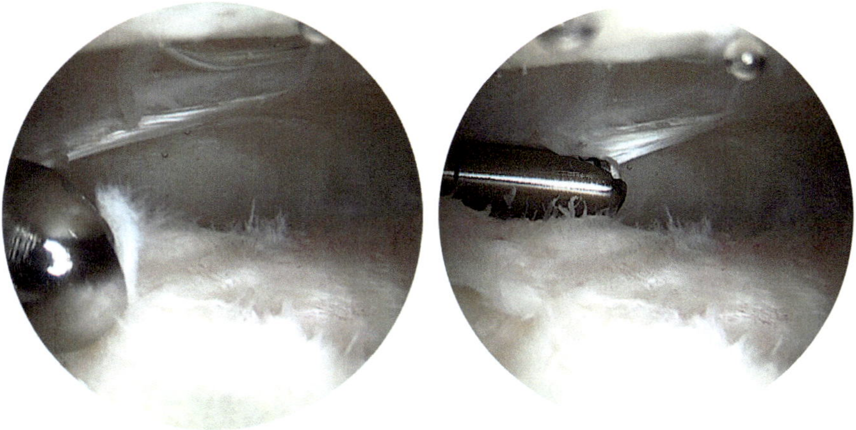

Arthroscopic resection of thickened medial plica

References

1. Hufeland M, Treder L, Kubo HK, Verde PE, Krauspe R, Patzer T. Symptomatic medial synovial plica of the knee joint: an underestimated pathology in young patients. Arch Orthop Trauma Surg. 2019;139(11):1625–31.
2. Lyu SR, Lee CC, Hsu CC. Medial abrasion syndrome: a neglected cause of knee pain in middle and old age. Medicine (Baltimore). 2015;94(16):e736. https://doi.org/10.1097/MD.0000000000000736.
3. Bellary SS, Lynch G, Housman B, Esmaeili E, Gielecki J, Tubbs RS, Loukas M. Medial plica syndrome: a review of the literature. Clin Anat. 2012;25(4):423–8.
4. Kan H, Arai Y, Nakagawa S, Inoue H, Hara K, Minami G, Inoue A, Kanamura H, Ikoma K, Fujiwara H, Kubo T. Characteristics of medial plica syndrome complicated with cartilage damage. Int Orthop. 2015;39(12):2489–94.
5. Yang CC, Lin CY, Wang HS, Lyu SR. Matrix metalloproteases and tissue inhibitors of metalloproteinases in medial plica and pannus-like tissue contribute to knee osteoarthritis progression. PLoS One. 2013;8(11):e79662. https://doi.org/10.1371/journal.pone.0079662.
6. Liu DS, Zhuang ZW, Lyu SR. Relationship between medial plica and medial femoral condyle—a three-dimensional dynamic finite element model. Clin Biomech (Bristol, Avon). 2013;28(9–10):1000–5.
7. Kim SJ, Jeong JH, Cheon YM, Ryu SW. MPP test in the diagnosis of medial patellar plica syndrome. Arthroscopy. 2004;20(10):1101–3.

8. Stubbings N, Smith T. Diagnostic test accuracy of clinical and radiological assessments for medial patella plica syndrome: a systematic review and meta-analysis. Knee. 2014;21(2):486–90.
9. Paczesny L, Kruczynski J. Medial plica syndrome of the knee: diagnosis with dynamic sonography. Radiology. 2009;251(2):439–46.
10. Amatuzzi MM, Fazzi A, Varella MH. Pathologic synovial plica of the knee: results of conservative treatment. Am J Sports Med. 1990;18:466–9.
11. Camanho GL. Treatment of pathological synovial plicae of the knee. Clinics (Sao Paulo). 2010;65(3):247–50.
12. Gerrard AD, Charalambous CP. Arthroscopic excision of medial knee plica: a meta-analysis of outcomes. Knee Surg Relat Res. 2018;30(4):356–63.
13. Paczesny L, Zabrzynski J, Kentzer R, Gryckiewicz S, Lewandowski B, Szwedowski D, Kruczynski J. A 10-year follow-up on arthroscopic medial plica syndrome treatments with special reference to related cartilage injuries. Cartilage. 2019;6:1947603519892310. https://doi.org/10.1177/1947603519892310.

Chapter 38
Suprapatellar Plica Syndrome

This is a condition whereby a suprapatellar plica causes pain due to inflammation or thickening. A complete plica that hinders communication between the main knee joint and suprapatellar bursa may lead to bursitis and swelling. Onset of symptoms may be post-traumatic or occur in the absence of an injury [1–14].

38.1 Clinical Symptoms of Suprapatellar Plica Syndrome

- Suprapatellar—anterior knee pain worse on going up stairs, prolonged knee flexion (sitting, squatting)
- Clicking
- Giving way
- Recurrent or progressive knee swelling, soft tissue mass
- Pseudolocking
- Audible/felt snapping
- Swelling

C. Panayiotou Charalambous, *The Knee Made Easy*,
https://doi.org/10.1007/978-3-030-54506-2_38

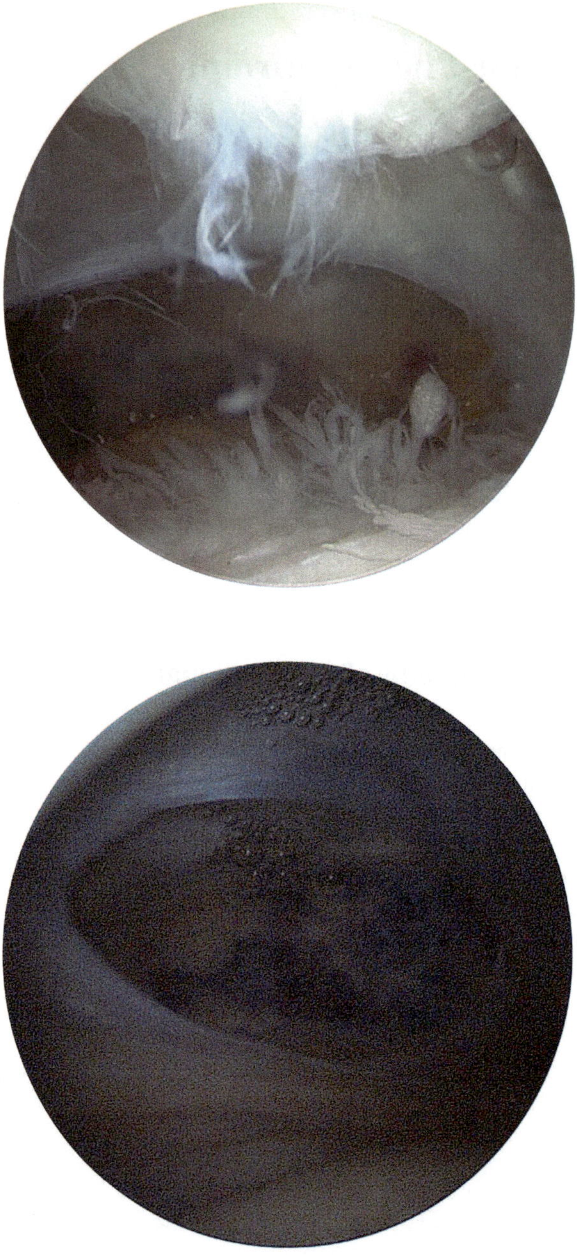

Suprapatellar plica

38.2 Clinical Signs of Suprapatellar Plica Syndrome

- Tenderness just proximal to the patella
- Effusion, soft tissue swelling
- Palpable suprapatellar cord
- Swelling/mass
- Reduced patellar mobility (due to tethering of the patella by the plica)

38.3 Investigations for Suprapatellar Plica Syndrome

- Ultrasound
- MRI

38.4 Management of Suprapatellar Plica Syndrome

38.4.1 Non-surgical Management

- Analgesia/anti-inflammatories
- Physiotherapy:
  - Local massage
  - Quadriceps stretching
- Intra-articular or suprapatellar bursa aspiration of synovial fluid
- Intra-articular or suprapatellar bursa steroid injection

38.4.2 Surgical Management

- Arthroscopic resection

References

1. Zmerly H, Moscato M, Akkawi I. Management of suprapatellar synovial plica, a common cause of anterior knee pain: a clinical review. Acta Biomed. 2019;90(12-S):33–8.
2. Akao M, Ikemoto T, Takata T, Kitamoto K, Deie M. Suprapatellar plica classification and suprapatellar plica syndrome. Asia Pac J Sports Med Arthrosc Rehabil Technol. 2019;17:10–5.
3. Kim SJ, Shin SJ, Koo TY. Arch type pathologic suprapatellar plica. Arthroscopy. 2001;17(5):536–8.
4. Bae DK, Nam GU, Sun SD, Kim YH. The clinical significance of the complete type of suprapatellar membrane. Arthroscopy. 1998;14(8):830–5.
5. Blatz DJ, Fleming R, McCarroll J. Suprapatellar plica: a study of their occurrence and role in internal derangement of the knee in active duty personnel. Orthopedics. 1981;4(2):181–5.
6. Pipkin G. Lesions of the suprapatellar plica. J Bone Joint Surg Am. 1950;32A(2):363–9.
7. Gülman B, Kopuz C, Yazici M, Karaismailoglu N. Morphological variants of the suprapatellar septum. An anatomical study in neonatal cadavers. Surg Radiol Anat. 1994;16(4):363–6.
8. Strover AE, Rouholamin E, Guirguis N, Behdad H. An arthroscopic technique of demonstrating the pathomechanics of the suprapatellar plica. Arthroscopy. 1991;7(3):308–10.
9. Adachi N, Ochi M, Uchio Y, Kawasaki K, Yamasaki K. The complete type of suprapatellar plica in a professional baseball pitcher: consideration of a cause of anterior knee pain. Arthroscopy. 2004;20(9):987–91.
10. Ehlinger M, Moser T, Adam P, Simon P, Bonnomet F. Complete suprapatellar plica presenting like a tumor. Orthop Traumatol Surg Res. 2009 Oct;95(6):447–50.
11. De Mot P, Brys P, Samson I. Non perforated septum supra-patellaris mimicking a soft tissue tumour. JBR-BTR. 2003;86(5):262–4.
12. Ziswiler M, Radü EW, Romero J. Chondrocalcinosis in an isolated suprapatellar pouch with recurrent effusion. Arthroscopy. 2002;18(3):E14.
13. Pekmezci M, Atay OA, Kerimoğlu U, Aydingöz U, Tetik O, Doral MN. A complete supra-patellar plica with an unusual presentation. Knee Surg Sports Traumatol Arthrosc. 2006;14(9):872–4.
14. Bojinca V, Malitchi R, Micu M. Refractory knee synovitis due to suprapatellar plica persistence—the role of ultrasonography in diagnosis and management. Med Ultrason. 2016;18(1):134–5.

Chapter 39
Infrapatellar Plica Syndrome

The infrapatellar plica extends from the anterior part of the intercondylar notch to the infrapatellar fat pad at the tip of the patella. Infrapatellar plica syndrome is a condition whereby an infrapatellar plica causes pain due to inflammation or thickening. Onset of symptoms may be post traumatic or occur in the absence of an injury [1–11].

39.1 Clinical Symptoms of Infrapatellar Plica Syndrome

- Infrapatellar pain worse on going up stairs
  - Worse on knee extension
- Limited knee extension, flexion deformity

39.2 Clinical Signs of Infrapatellar Plica Syndrome

- Tenderness over the proximal part of the patellar tendon with the knee in extension
- Reduced knee extension due to plica thickening

39.3 Investigations for Infrapatellar Plica Syndrome

- MRI may show abnormalities in the fat pad along the line of the plica [12, 13]

C. Panayiotou Charalambous, *The Knee Made Easy*,
https://doi.org/10.1007/978-3-030-54506-2_39

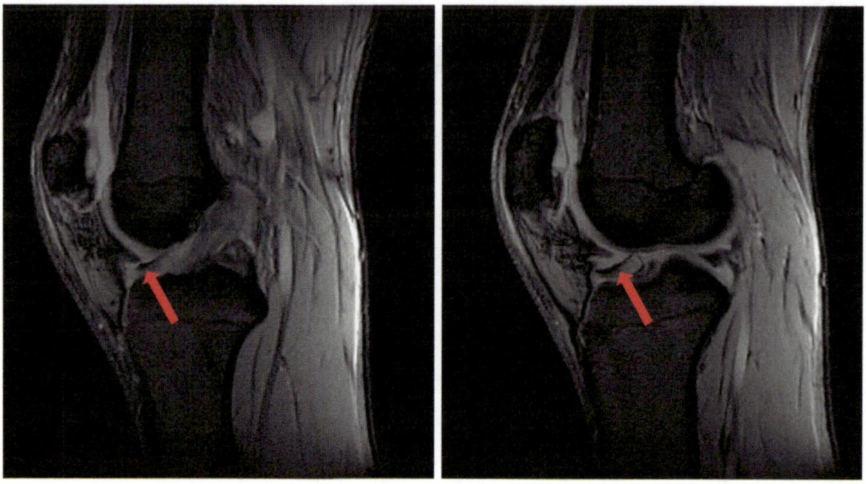

Thickened infrapatellar plica (red arrow)

39.4 Management of Infrapatellar Plica Syndrome

39.4.1 Non-surgical

- Analgesia/anti-inflammatories
- Physiotherapy:
  - Local massage
- Intra-articular steroid injections

39.4.2 Surgical

- Arthroscopic resection

Learning Pearls

- A thickened infrapatellar plica may impinge on the intercondylar notch and trochlea leading to chondral damage and dysfunction as well as anterior knee pain. Such chondral damage may also limit knee extension

References

1. Norris M, Corbo G, Banga K, Johnson M, Sandig M, Smallman T, Getgood A, Burkhart TA. The biomechanical and morphological characteristics of the ligamentum mucosum and its potential role in anterior knee pain. Knee. 2018;25(6):1134–41.
2. Demirag B, Ozturk C, Karakayali M. Symptomatic infrapatellar plica. Knee Surg Sports Traumatol Arthrosc. 2006;14(2):156–60.
3. Boyd CR, Eakin C, Matheson GO. Infrapatellar plica as a cause of anterior knee pain. Clin J Sport Med. 2005;15(2):98–103.
4. Kim SJ, Kim JY, Lee JW. Pathologic infrapatellar plica. Arthroscopy. 2002;18(5):E25.
5. Kim SJ, Min BH, Kim HK. Arthroscopic anatomy of the infrapatellar plica. Arthroscopy. 1996;12(5):561–4.
6. Kim SJ, Choe WS. Pathological infrapatellar plica: a report of two cases and literature review. Arthroscopy. 1996;12(2):236–9.
7. Smallman TV, Portner OT, Race A, Shekitka K, Mann K. Arthroscopic untethering of the fat pad of the knee: release or resection of the infrapatellar plica (Ligamentum Mucosum) and related structures for anterior knee pain. Arthrosc Tech. 2018;7(5):e575–88.
8. Radu A, Discepola F, Volesky M, Munk PL, Le H. Posterior Hoffa's fat pad impingement secondary to a thickened infrapatellar plica: a case report and review of the literature. J Radiol Case Rep. 2015;9(3):20–6.
9. Apostolopoulos AP, McConnell B, Manta A, Zafiropoulos G. The incidence of infrapatellar plicae in the elderly Welsh population. Folia Morphol (Warsz). 2012;71(3):194–7.
10. Lee YH, Song HT, Kim S, Kim SJ, Suh JS. Infrapatellar plica of the knee: revisited with MR arthrographies undertaken in the knee flexion position mimicking operative arthroscopic posture. Eur J Radiol. 2012;81(10):2783–7.
11. Ozcan M, Copuroğlu C, Ciftdemir M, Turan FN, Calpur OU. Does an abnormal infrapatellar plica increase the risk of chondral damage in the knee. Knee Surg Sports Traumatol Arthrosc. 2011;19(2):218–21.
12. Kosarek FJ, Helms CA. The MR appearance of the infrapatellar plica. AJR Am J Roentgenol. 1999;172(2):481–4.
13. Cothran RL, McGuire PM, Helms CA, Major NM, Attarian DE. MR imaging of infrapatellar plica injury. AJR Am J Roentgenol. 2003;180(5):1443–7.

Chapter 40
Patellofemoral Pain Syndrome

This is a condition whereby the patient experiences pain in the patellofemoral (PF) joint in the absence of a localised chondral defect or PF arthritis [1–15]. There may be associated PF cartilage softening.

PF pain is a common condition. Smith et al. [15] assessed the incidence of PF pain through a systematic review and meta-analysis. They included 23 studies. Annual prevalence for PF pain in the general population was reported as 22.7%, and amongst adolescents as 28.9%.

The pooled estimate for point prevalence was:

- In adolescents overall—7.2% (95% CI: 6.3–8.3%)
- In female adolescent athletes—22.7% (95% CI: 17.4–28.0%)

A number of factors contributing to this pain have been proposed although not consistently shown across individuals. In the biomechanics section it has been described how hip, knee and foot factors may contribute to the forces acting on the PF joint, and these factors must be considered when dealing with this condition. These may be divided into external or internal factors as below:

External factors

- Overuse—frequency, duration, intensity—overzealous, recent change
- PF compression activities—worse on prolonged knee flexion—going to movie, sitting in car, deep squats, ascending/descending stairs
  - Ascending requires concentric contraction of the quadriceps—may not cause symptoms
  - Descending—requires eccentric contraction- increased compression—pain

Internal factors

- Core muscles weakness/imbalance

C. Panayiotou Charalambous, *The Knee Made Easy*,
https://doi.org/10.1007/978-3-030-54506-2_40

- Hip—weak muscles
  - Abductors
  - External rotators
  - Extensors
- Knee:
  - Weak quadriceps, imbalanced quadriceps
  - Tight quadriceps, iliotibial band, patellar retinacula, gastrocnemius—increases PF compression upon knee flexion
  - Tight hamstrings—increased PF forces upon knee extension, may be associated with increased hamstring-quadriceps coactivation
  - Imbalanced hamstrings—biceps femoris showing more activity in PF pain—imbalance between lateral and medial hamstrings, with the lateral contracting earlier than the medial hamstrings.
- Foot—Hyperpronation and reduced ankle dorsiflexion lead to higher PF compression
- Patellar malalignment, maltracking, high riding patella due to:

  Soft tissue imbalance (over laxity/over tightness) including:

  - Tight lateral retinaculum or iliotibial tract leading to lateral maltracking
  - Medial retinaculum hyperlaxity leading to lateral maltracking
  - Quadriceps imbalance between vastus medialis and vastus lateralis leading to maltracking and abnormal loading

  Bony

  - Femoral intorsion
  - Tibial external rotation/internal rotation
  - Lateralization of the tibial tubercle (cadaveric studies have shown that lateralisation of the tibial tubercle increases the lateral PF contact pressures which are reduced by tubercle medialization)
  - High riding patella (patella alta), low lying patella (patella baja)
  - Knee valgus

Different subgroups have been described with regards to what is considered to be the main soft tissue driver behind their PF pain, including: hip abductor weakness, quadriceps weakness, patella hypermobility, patella hypomobility with pronated foot posture, lower limb biarticular muscle tightness [4].

Hence, the underlying pathogenesis of PF pain is not uniform amongst cases. Thus symptoms may not be consistent, and treatment needs to be individualised. In many cases various non-surgical modalities may need to be tried, as it is difficult to predict at an individual level who will be benefit from an individual intervention and who will not.

40.1 Clinical Symptoms of Patellofemoral Pain Syndrome

- Pain
  - Anterior knee
    - Central—behind the patella
    - Anterolateral—due to compression of the lateral patellar facet on the lateral femoral condyle
    - Anteromedial—lateral retinaculum tightness causes tension on the medial retinaculum
  - Worse on activities that include hyperflexion or prolonged flexion (squatting, sitting for prolonged time)
  - Worse going up and down stairs
- Clicking
- Instability, knee gives way

40.2 Clinical Signs of Patellofemoral Pain Syndrome

- Tender patellar articular surface
- Tenderness of the patellar edges
- PF crepitus
- Pain on patellar compression test
- Quadriceps weakness
- Hamstring or quadriceps tightness
- Hip abductors/external rotators weakness
- Lateral retinacula tightness—lateral tilting of patella, reduced medial mobility
- Iliotibial band tightness—lateral titling patella, lateral facet compression, lower leg external rotation
- Patellar maltracking—J sign, subluxation, dislocation
- Knee valgus
- Knee recurvatum
- Internal femoral torsion
- External tibial torsion
- Foot planovalgus deformity
- Flexion contracture—(post-surgery, trauma, tight hamstrings) leads to quadriceps overactivity
- Increased clinical Q angle (but this is controversial—a systematic review has shown that Q angle is not related to risk of PF pain)
- Leg length inequality (as measured from the anterior superior iliac spine to the medial malleolus—greater than 15 mm is considered finally significant)
  - Long leg—pronation of the foot and subtalar joint
  - Short leg—supination of foot to equalise leg length

40.3 Investigations for Patellofemoral Pain Syndrome

- Plain radiographs
  - AP—knee alignment
  - Lateral—evaluate patellar height, look for bipartite patella
  - Skyline—evaluate patellar tilting, degenerative changes
  - Long leg film—to further evaluate clinically detected coronal alignment deformities
- MRI to assess:
  - PF articular cartilage
  - Exclude other intra-articular lesions
  - Assess tibial tubercle lateralization
  - Determine patellar/trochlear articular cartilage overlap, assess patellar height
- CT to assess:
  - Rotational alignment—femur/tibia

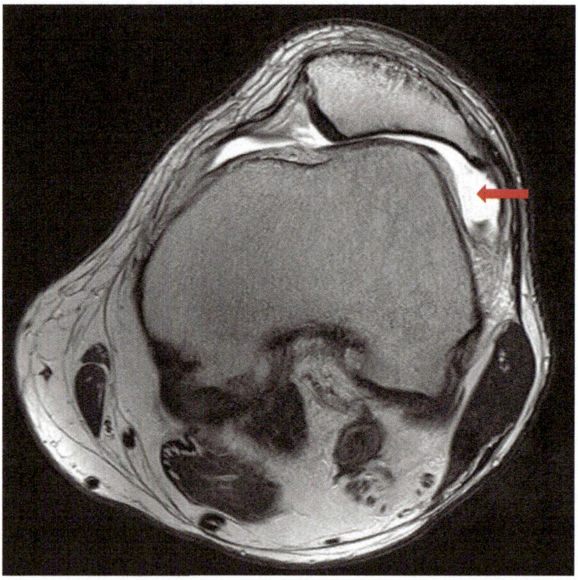

Effusion associated with patellofemoral degeneration and lateral patellar subluxation

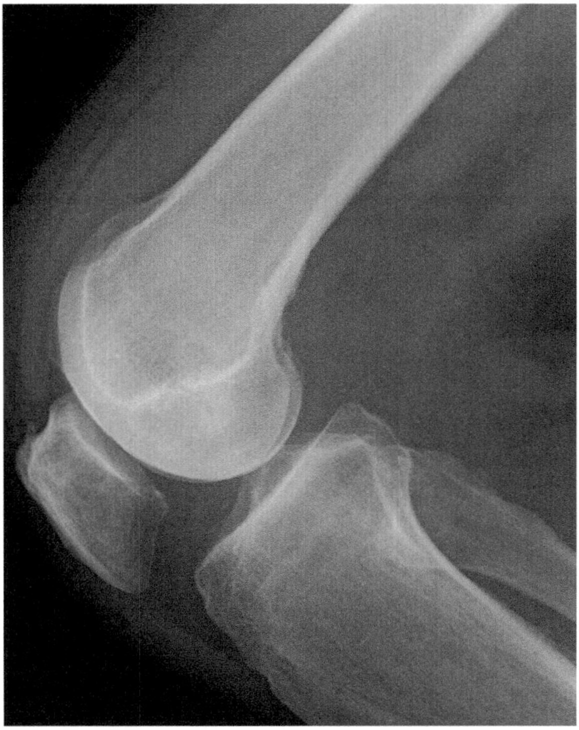

Low lying patella—Patellar baja

40.4 Management of Patellofemoral Pain Syndrome [16–49]

In considering the management of PF pain syndrome, an ala carte approach may be utilised whereby deficiencies that could affect PF biomechanics are identified and addressed, initially using non-surgical means. Such deficiencies may involve the:

- Core
- Hip
- Femur
- Knee
- Tibia
- Ankle
- Foot

40.4.1 Non-surgical

The overall aim is to improve flexibility, alignment, muscular control, and strength. At the same time, pain control measures aiming to address peripherally generated pain and centrally processed pain are applied. Such measures include:

- Restoration of knee motion, stretching and strengthening of hip and knee periarticular muscles
  - Quadriceps stretching and strengthening
  - Hamstring stretching
  - Hip abductors and external rotators strengthening
  - Iliotibial band and lateral retinaculum stretching
- Improvement in core stability
- Proprioception training
- Knee external devices—patellar bracing to improve proprioception and postural control, medial patellar taping, medial directed realignment brace
- Foot orthoses
  - Medial arch support if planovalgus deformity
  - Heel raise to address leg length inequality
- Pain control:
  - Analgesia, TENS, heat therapy, acupuncture
  - Psychological support
- Steroid/hyaluronic acid/PRP intra-articular injections

40.4.2 Surgical

Although several surgical procedures have been described their effectiveness is controversial and their results are highly unpredictable. Hence, they need to be approached with high caution.

These aim to improve the biomechanics of the PF joint, by addressing patellar alignment and tracking, with the aim of reducing PF compression pressures. Such procedures are used according to the deficit present and include:

- Tibial tubercle translation:
  - Anterior translation—to reduce PF compression, and PF forces
  - Distal translation—to reduce patella alta
  - Medial translation—to reduce lateral patellar tracking
- Femoral/tibial osteotomies—to address coronal and rotational malalignment

- Lateral retinacula release (arthroscopic or open)—to reduce lateral patellar tilting and tracking. This may have a role in lateral patellar compression syndrome, a condition whereby the patient experiences pain in the PF joint due to compression between the lateral articular facet of the patella and the lateral part of the femoral trochlea. This may occur in the absence of a localised chondral defect or PF arthritis.

40.5 Natural History of PF Pain

PF pain is self-resolving in many cases but in a substantial group of patients it may become chronic with previous studies reporting [50, 51]:

- Up to 90% having symptoms at 4 years post diagnosis
- 25% having significant symptoms at 20 year follow-up post presentation

Nimon et al. [51] described a consecutive series of females with adolescent idiopathic anterior knee pain treated non-surgically. At a mean follow-up of 16 years, 22% reported no pain, 71% felt that their symptoms were better than at presentation, and most (88%) used analgesia rarely or not at all, whilst 90% participated regularly in sports. However, about 1 in 4 continued to have significant symptoms for up to 20 years following presentation. No features could be identified to predict those patients in whom symptoms would persist.

The authors concluded that routine surgical treatment of idiopathic anterior knee pain in adolescents is not justified as the vast majority of patients will spontaneously improve and a reliable way that will identify those cases that will not improve spontaneously is not available.

Learning Pearls

- It is difficult to predict at an individual level the effects of a particular intervention
- PF overloading may affect both patellar facets similarly or one more than the other (usually lateral facet more than the medial facet).
- Saltychev et al. [25] in a systematic review and metanalysis showed that there is no evidence that a single treatment modality works for all patients with PF pain. Instead, there is some evidence that some modalities may be helpful for some subgroups.

References

1. Fulkerson JP. A practical guide to understanding and treating patellofemoral pain. Am J Orthop (Belle Mead NJ). 2017;46(2):101–3.
2. Gaitonde DY, Ericksen A, Robbins RC. Patellofemoral pain syndrome. Am Fam Physician. 2019;99(2):88–94.
3. Petersen W, Ellermann A, Gösele-Koppenburg A, Best R, Rembitzki IV, Brüggemann GP, Liebau C. Patellofemoral pain syndrome. Knee Surg Sports Traumatol Arthrosc. 2014;22(10):2264–74.
4. Selfe J, Callaghan M, Witvrouw E, Richards J, Dey MP, Sutton C, Dixon J, Martin D, Stokes M, Janssen J, Ritchie E, Turner D. Targeted interventions for patellofemoral pain syndrome (TIPPS): classification of clinical subgroups. BMJ Open. 2013;3(9):e003795. https://doi.org/10.1136/bmjopen-2013-003795.
5. Halabchi F, Mazaheri R, Seif-Barghi T. Patellofemoral pain syndrome and modifiable intrinsic risk factors; how to assess and address? Asian J Sports Med. 2013;4(2):85–100.
6. Lankhorst NE, Bierma-Zeinstra SM, van Middelkoop M. Factors associated with patellofemoral pain syndrome: a systematic review. Br J Sports Med. 2013;47(4):193–206.
7. Motealleh A, Kordi Yoosefinejad A, Ghoddosi M, Azhdari N, Pirouzi S. Trunk postural control during unstable sitting differs between patients with patellofemoral pain syndrome and healthy people: a cross-sectional study. Knee. 2019;26(1):26–32.
8. Tahmasebi MN, Aghaghazvini L, Mirkarimi SS, Zehtab MJ, Sheidaie Z, Sharafatvaziri A. The influence of Tibial tuberosity-trochlear groove distance on development of patellofemoral pain syndrome. Arch Bone Jt Surg. 2019;7(1):46–51.
9. Meira EP, Brumitt J. Influence of the hip on patients with patellofemoral pain syndrome: a systematic review. Sports Health. 2011;3(5):455–65.
10. Willson JD, Kernozek TW, Arndt RL, Reznichek DA, Scott Straker J. Gluteal muscle activation during running in females with and without patellofemoral pain syndrome. Clin Biomech (Bristol, Avon). 2011;26(7):735–40.
11. Kaya D, Citaker S, Kerimoglu U, Atay OA, Nyland J, Callaghan M, Yakut Y, Yüksel I, Doral MN. Women with patellofemoral pain syndrome have quadriceps femoris volume and strength deficiency. Knee Surg Sports Traumatol Arthrosc. 2011;19(2):242–7.
12. Felicio LR, de Carvalho CAM, Dias CLCA, Vigário PDS. Electromyographic activity of the quadriceps and gluteus medius muscles during/different straight leg raise and squat exercises in women with patellofemoral pain syndrome. J Electromyogr Kinesiol. 2019;48:17–23.
13. Lindberg U, Lysholm J, Gillquist J. The correlation between arthroscopic findings and the patellofemoral pain syndrome. Arthroscopy. 1986;2(2):103–7.
14. Witvrouw E, Werner S, Mikkelsen C, Van Tiggelen D, Vanden Berghe L, Cerulli G. Clinical classification of patellofemoral pain syndrome: guidelines for non-operative treatment. Knee Surg Sports Traumatol Arthrosc. 2005;13(2):122–30.
15. Smith BE, Selfe J, Thacker D, Hendrick P, Bateman M, Moffatt F, Rathleff MS, Smith TO, Logan P. Incidence and prevalence of patellofemoral pain: a systematic review and meta-analysis. PLoS One. 2018;13(1):e0190892. https://doi.org/10.1371/journal.pone.0190892.
16. Emamvirdi M, Letafatkar A, Khaleghi Tazji M. The effect of valgus control instruction exercises on pain, strength, and functionality in active females with patellofemoral pain syndrome. Sports Health. 2019;11(3):223–37.
17. Motealleh A, Mohamadi M, Moghadam MB, Nejati N, Arjang N, Ebrahimi N. Effects of Core neuromuscular training on pain, balance, and functional performance in women with patellofemoral pain syndrome: a clinical trial. J Chiropr Med. 2019;18(1):9–18.
18. Foroughi F, Sobhani S, Yoosefinejad AK, Motealleh A. Added value of isolated Core postural control training on knee pain and function in women with patellofemoral pain syndrome: a randomized controlled trial. Arch Phys Med Rehabil. 2019;100(2):220–9.

19. Scali K, Roberts J, McFarland M, Marino K, Murray L. Is multi-joint or single joint strengthening more effective in reducing pain and improving function in women with patellofemoral pain syndrome? A systematic review and meta-analysis. Int J Sports Phys Ther. 2018;13(3):321–34.
20. Kölle T, Alt W, Wagner D. Immediate effects of an elastic patellar brace on pain, neuromuscular activity and knee kinematics in subjects with patellofemoral pain. Arch Orthop Trauma Surg. 2020;140:905–12. https://doi.org/10.1007/s00402-020-03378-7.
21. Logan CA, Bhashyam AR, Tisosky AJ, Haber DB, Jorgensen A, Roy A, Provencher MT. Systematic review of the effect of taping techniques on patellofemoral pain syndrome. Sports Health. 2017;9(5):456–61.
22. Peters JS, Tyson NL. Proximal exercises are effective in treating patellofemoral pain syndrome: a systematic review. Int J Sports Phys Ther. 2013;8(5):689–700.
23. Park SK, Stefanyshyn DJ. Greater Q angle may not be a risk factor of patellofemoral pain syndrome. Clin Biomech (Bristol, Avon). 2011;26(4):392–6.
24. Chen S, Chang WD, Wu JY, Fong YC. Electromyographic analysis of hip and knee muscles during specific exercise movements in females with patellofemoral pain syndrome: an observational study. Medicine (Baltimore). 2018;97(28):e11424. https://doi.org/10.1097/MD.0000000000011424.
25. Saltychev M, Dutton RA, Laimi K, Beaupré GS, Virolainen P, Fredericson M. Effectiveness of conservative treatment for patellofemoral pain syndrome: a systematic review and meta-analysis. J Rehabil Med. 2018;50(5):393–401.
26. Earl JE, Hoch AZ. A proximal strengthening program improves pain, function, and biomechanics in women with patellofemoral pain syndrome. Am J Sports Med. 2011;39(1):154–63.
27. Moyano FR, Valenza MC, Martin LM, Caballero YC, Gonzalez-Jimenez E, Demet GV. Effectiveness of different exercises and stretching physiotherapy on pain and movement in patellofemoral pain syndrome: a randomized controlled trial. Clin Rehabil. 2013;27(5):409–17.
28. Chevidikunnan MF, Al Saif A, Gaowgzeh RA, Mamdouh KA. Effectiveness of core muscle strengthening for improving pain and dynamic balance among female patients with patellofemoral pain syndrome. J Phys Ther Sci. 2016;28(5):1518–23.
29. Plastaras C, McCormick Z, Nguyen C, Rho M, Nack SH, Roth D, Casey E, Carneiro K, Cucchiara A, Press J, McLean J, Caldera F. Is hip abduction strength asymmetry present in female runners in the early stages of patellofemoral pain syndrome? Am J Sports Med. 2016;44(1):105–12.
30. Alba-Martín P, Gallego-Izquierdo T, Plaza-Manzano G, Romero-Franco N, Núñez-Nagy S, Pecos-Martín D. Effectiveness of therapeutic physical exercise in the treatment of patellofemoral pain syndrome: a systematic review. J Phys Ther Sci. 2015;27(7):2387–90.
31. Clijsen R, Fuchs J, Taeymans J. Effectiveness of exercise therapy in treatment of patients with patellofemoral pain syndrome: systematic review and meta-analysis. Phys Ther. 2014;94(12):1697–708.
32. Santos TR, Oliveira BA, Ocarino JM, Holt KG, Fonseca ST. Effectiveness of hip muscle strengthening in patellofemoral pain syndrome patients: a systematic review. Braz J Phys Ther. 2015;19(3):167–76.
33. Esculier JF, Roy JS, Bouyer LJ. Lower limb control and strength in runners with and without patellofemoral pain syndrome. Gait Posture. 2015;41(3):813–9.
34. Felicio LR, Masullo Cde L, Saad MC, Bevilaqua-Grossi D. The effect of a patellar bandage on the postural control of individuals with patellofemoral pain syndrome. J Phys Ther Sci. 2014;26(3):461–4.
35. Petersen W, Ellermann A, Rembitzki IV, Scheffler S, Herbort M, Brüggemann GP, Best R, Zantop T, Liebau C. Evaluating the potential synergistic benefit of a realignment brace on patients receiving exercise therapy for patellofemoral pain syndrome: a randomized clinical trial. Arch Orthop Trauma Surg. 2016;136(7):975–82.
36. Swart NM, van Linschoten R, Bierma-Zeinstra SM, van Middelkoop M. The additional effect of orthotic devices on exercise therapy for patients with patellofemoral pain syndrome: a systematic review. Br J Sports Med. 2012;46(8):570–7.

37. Barton CJ, Menz HB, Crossley KM. The immediate effects of foot orthoses on functional performance in individuals with patellofemoral pain syndrome. Br J Sports Med. 2011;45(3):193–7.
38. Barton CJ, Munteanu SE, Menz HB, Crossley KM. The efficacy of foot orthoses in the treatment of individuals with patellofemoral pain syndrome: a systematic review. Sports Med. 2010;40(5):377–95.
39. Barton CJ, Menz HB, Levinger P, Webster KE, Crossley KM. Greater peak rearfoot eversion predicts foot orthoses efficacy in individuals with patellofemoral pain syndrome. Br J Sports Med. 2011;45(9):697–701.
40. Barton CJ, Menz HB, Crossley KM. Effects of prefabricated foot orthoses on pain and function in individuals with patellofemoral pain syndrome: a cohort study. Phys Ther Sport. 2011;12(2):70–5.
41. Kettunen JA, Harilainen A, Sandelin J, Schlenzka D, Hietaniemi K, Seitsalo S, Malmivaara A, Kujala UM. Knee arthroscopy and exercise versus exercise only for chronic patellofemoral pain syndrome: 5-year follow-up. Br J Sports Med. 2012;46(4):243–6.
42. Fulkerson JP, Schutzer SF. After failure of conservative treatment for painful patellofemoral malalignment: lateral release or realignment? Orthop Clin North Am. 1986;17(2):283–8.
43. Jenny JY, Sader Z, Henry A, Jenny G, Jaeger JH. Elevation of the tibial tubercle for patellofemoral pain syndrome. An 8- to 15-year follow-up. Knee Surg Sports Traumatol Arthrosc. 1996;4(2):92–6.
44. Chen JB, Chen D, Xiao YP, Chang JZ, Li T. Efficacy and experience of arthroscopic lateral patella retinaculum releasing through/outside synovial membrane for the treatment of lateral patellar compression syndrome. BMC Musculoskelet Disord. 2020;21(1):108. https://doi.org/10.1186/s12891-020-3130-y.
45. Krompinger WJ, Fulkerson JP. Lateral retinacular release for intractable lateral retinacular pain. Clin Orthop Relat Res. 1983;(179):191–193.
46. Karlsson J, Lansinger O, Swärd L. Anterior advancement of the tibial tuberosity in the treatment of the patellofemoral pain syndrome. Arch Orthop Trauma Surg. 1985;103(6):392–5.
47. Klinge SA, Fulkerson JP. Fifteen-year minimum follow-up of anteromedial tibial tubercle transfer for lateral and/or distal patellofemoral arthrosis. Arthroscopy. 2019;35(7):2146–51.
48. Middleton KK, Gruber S, Shubin Stein BE. Why and where to move the tibial tubercle: indications and techniques for tibial tubercle osteotomy. Sports Med Arthrosc Rev. 2019;27(4):154–60.
49. Fulkerson JP. Anteromedialization of the tibial tuberosity for patellofemoral malalignment. Clin Orthop Relat Res. 1983;(177):176–81.0.
50. Pappas E, Wong-Tom WM. Prospective predictors of patellofemoral pain syndrome: a systematic review with meta-analysis. Sports Health. 2012;4(2):115–20.
51. Nimon G, Murray D, Sandow M, Goodfellow J. Natural history of anterior knee pain: a 14- to 20-year follow-up of nonoperative management. J Pediatr Orthop. 1998;18(1):118–22.

Chapter 41
Infrapatellar Fat Pad Dysfunction

This refers to dysfunction of the infrapatellar (Hoffa's) fat pad (located behind the patellar tendon) [1–10]. Dysfunction may be due to fat pad:

- Inflammation
- Fibrosis
- Chondrogenesis
- Osteogenesis

Dysfunction may be due to fat pad:

- Acute trauma
  - Blunt injury on the front of the knee, intra-articular knee fracture, patellar dislocation
- Degenerative/chronic microtrauma
  - Main body of fat pad—impingement between femur and tibia
  - Superior part of fat pad—impingement between femur and patellar tendon
- Neoplastic—fat pad contains pluripotent stem cells which may differentiate to chondrocytes or osteoblasts, giving rise to chondromas, or osteochondromas
- Post-surgery—open/arthroscopic

Dysfunction may be primary, originating within the fat pad, or secondary to another condition of the knee joint.

41.1 Clinical Symptoms of Infrapatellar Fat Pad Dysfunction

- Pain in the front of the knee, behind patella

C. Panayiotou Charalambous, *The Knee Made Easy*,
https://doi.org/10.1007/978-3-030-54506-2_41

- Worse on knee extension/hyperextension
- Worse going up and down stairs
- Knee clicking
- Swelling at the infrapatellar area

41.2 Clinical Signs of Infrapatellar Fat Pad Dysfunction

- Tender patellar tendon and peri-tendon area
- Infrapatellar crepitus
- Quadriceps weakness
- Hoffa's test positive—pain on palpation of the medial and lateral edge of the patellar tendon whilst extending the knee from 90° flexion
- Hyperextension test positive—passive hyperextension of the knee reproduces pain in the infrapatellar area
- Patellar malalignment
  - Patella alta
  - Lateral malalignment/maltracking

41.3 Investigations for Infrapatellar Fat Pad Dysfunction [11–13]

- Plain radiographs—assess patella height, calcification in fat pad
  - AP, lateral, skyline
- MRI to assess:
  - Fat pad—oedema, fibrosis, synovitis, mass lesions
  - Femoral articular cartilage—evidence of impingement
  - Determine patellar/trochlear articular cartilage overlap, patellar height
  - Other causes of anterior knee pain
    - PF articular cartilage
    - Patellar tendon
    - Infrapatellar plica
    - Exclude other intra-articular lesions
  - Assess tibial tubercle lateralization

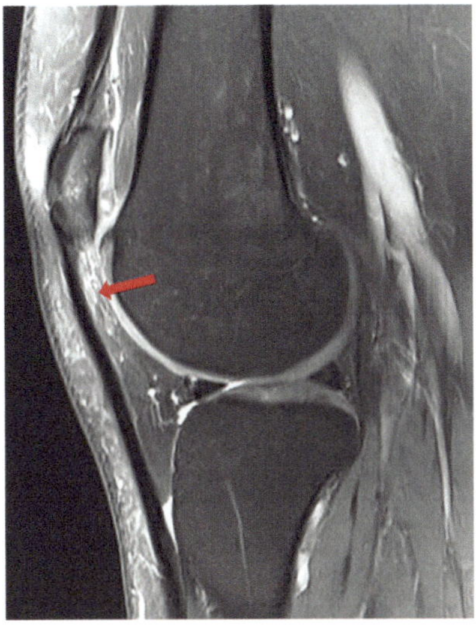

Infrapatellar fat pad oedema (red arrow) associated with high riding patella

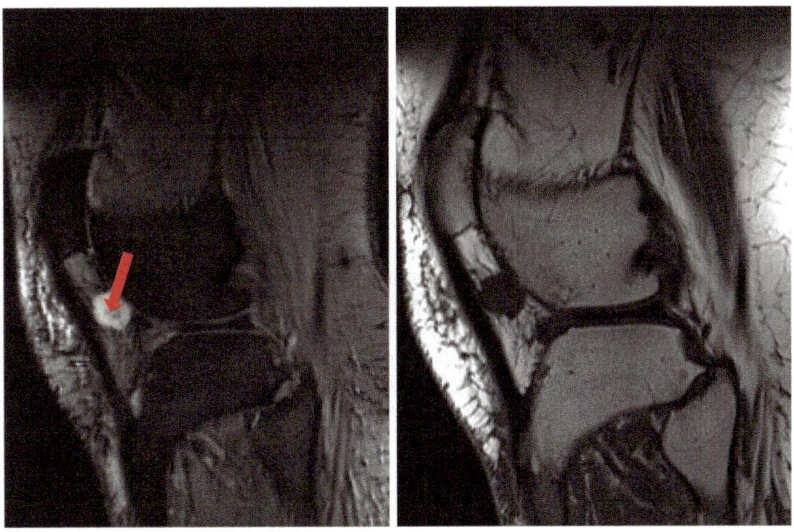

Patellofemoral osteoarthritis with associated necrosis of the infrapatellar fat pad (red arrow)

41.4 Management of Infrapatellar Fat Pad Dysfunction [13–15]

41.4.1 Non-surgical

- Restore knee motion, strengthen periarticular muscles, reduce forces on patellar tendon
- Quadriceps stretching and strengthening
- Patellar tendon taping, bracing
- Steroid injections into fat pad

41.4.2 Surgical

- Fat pad excision—open or arthroscopic

References

1. Leese J, Davies DC. An investigation of the anatomy of the infrapatellar fat pad and its possible involvement in anterior pain syndrome: a cadaveric study. J Anat. 2020;237:20–8. https://doi.org/10.1111/joa.13177.
2. Okita Y, Oba H, Miura R, Morimoto M, Gamada K. Movement and volume of infrapatellar fat pad and knee kinematics during quasi-static knee extension at 30 and 0° flexion in young healthy individuals. Knee. 2020;27(1):71–80.
3. Stephen JM, Sopher R, Tullie S, Amis AA, Ball S, Williams A. The infrapatellar fat pad is a dynamic and mobile structure, which deforms during knee motion, and has proximal extensions which wrap around the patella. Knee Surg Sports Traumatol Arthrosc. 2018;26(11):3515–24.
4. Singh VK, Shah G, Singh PK, Saran D. Extraskeletal ossifying chondroma in Hoffa's fat pad: an unusual cause of anterior knee pain. Singap Med J. 2009;50(5):e189–92.
5. Goyal R, Chopra R, Singh S, Kamra P. Ganglion cyst of Hoffa's fat pad of knee-a rare cause of knee pain and swelling—a case report and literature review. J Clin Orthop Trauma. 2019;10(Suppl 1):S215–7.
6. Trompeter A, Servant C. Case report. An unusual cause of a patient presenting with an acutely locked knee: multiple benign fat pad cysts. Arch Orthop Trauma Surg. 2009;129(8):1123–5.
7. Aynaci O, Kerimoglu S, Ozturk C, Saracoglu M, Yildiz K. Intraarticular fibroma of the tendon sheath arising from the infrapatellar fat pad in the knee joint. Arch Orthop Trauma Surg. 2009;129(3):291–4.
8. Yilmaz E, Karakurt L, Ozercan I, Ozdemir H. A ganglion cyst that developed from the infrapatellar fat pad of the knee. Arthroscopy. 2004;20(7):e65–8.
9. Bennell K, Hodges P, Mellor R, Bexander C, Souvlis T. The nature of anterior knee pain following injection of hypertonic saline into the infrapatellar fat pad. J Orthop Res. 2004;22(1):116–21.

10. Delcogliano A, Galli M, Menghi A, Belli P. Localized pigmented villonodular synovitis of the knee: report of two cases of fat pad involvement. Arthroscopy. 1998;14(5):527–31.
11. Draghi F, Ferrozzi G, Urciuoli L, Bortolotto C, Bianchi S. Hoffa's fat pad abnormalities, knee pain and magnetic resonance imaging in daily practice. Insights Imaging. 2016;7(3):373–83.
12. Mezian K, Chang KV, Zámečník D, Mezian H, Özçakar L. Herniation of Hoffa's fat pad through the lateral retinaculum: usefulness of dynamic ultrasonography to diagnose a lateral knee mass. Am J Phys Med Rehabil. 2018;97(11):e113. https://doi.org/10.1097/PHM.0000000000000934.
13. Dragoo JL, Johnson C, McConnell J. Evaluation and treatment of disorders of the infrapatellar fat pad. Sports Med. 2012;42(1):51–67.
14. Rooney A, Wahba AJ, Smith TO, Donell ST. The surgical treatment of anterior knee pain due to infrapatellar fat pad pathology: a systematic review. Orthop Traumatol Surg Res. 2015;101(4):469–75.
15. Smallman TV, Portner OT, Race A, Shekitka K, Mann K. Arthroscopic untethering of the fat pad of the knee: release or resection of the infrapatellar plica (Ligamentum Mucosum) and related structures for anterior knee pain. Arthrosc Tech. 2018;7(5):e575–88.

Chapter 42
Suprapatellar Fat Pad Dysfunction

This refers to dysfunction of the superficial suprapatellar (quadriceps) fat pad (located behind the distal quadriceps, anterior to the suprapatellar recess). This may have multiple causes [1–4].

Dysfunction may be due to fat pad:

- Acute trauma:
  - Blunt injury on front of the knee, intra-articular fracture
- Degenerative/chronic micro-trauma
  - Repeated hyperflexion with compression between he proximal pole of the patella and femur and fat pad and trochlea
  - Impingement by:
    - Spur
    - Femoral component post knee arthroplasty
- Neoplastic
- Post-surgery—fibrosis

42.1 Clinical Symptoms of Suprapatellar Fat Pad Dysfunction

- Pain in the front of the knee, suprapatellar area, related to the distal quadriceps tendon
- Worse on knee flexion
- Worse going up and down stairs
- Clicking
- Swelling suprapatellar area/diffuse

C. Panayiotou Charalambous, *The Knee Made Easy*,
https://doi.org/10.1007/978-3-030-54506-2_42

42.2 Clinical Signs of Suprapatellar Fat Pad Dysfunction

- Tender distal quadriceps area
- Quadriceps weakness
- Patellar malalignment
  - Patella alta
  - Lateral tracking

42.3 Investigations for Suprapatellar Fat Pad Dysfunction [5–8]

- Plain radiographs—assess patellar height, anterior femoral spurs, prominent anterior femoral component flange
  - AP, lateral, skyline
- MRI to assess:
  - Fat pad—oedema, fibrosis, synovitis, mass lesions
  - Mass effect (deep border of fat pad appears convex)
  - Distal quadriceps tendon enthesopathy
  - Other intra-articular lesions and causes of anterior knee pain

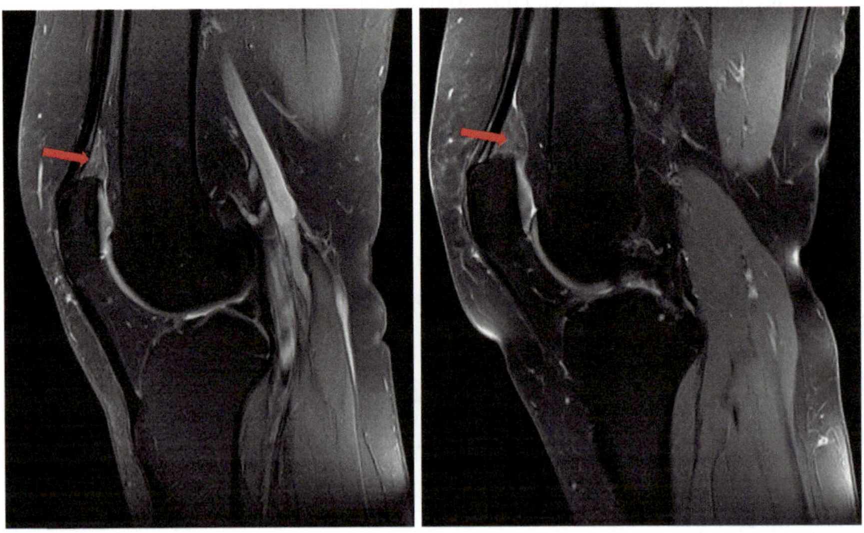

Bilateral Suprapatellar fat pad oedema and mass effect (convexity of its deep surface) due to impingement (red arrow)

42.4 Management of Suprapatellar Fat Pad Dysfunction

42.4.1 Non-surgical [9]

- Restore knee motion, strengthen periarticular muscles, reduce forces on quadriceps tendon
- Quadriceps stretching and strengthening
- Steroid injections into fat pad (ultrasound guided)

42.4.2 Surgical

- Fat pad excision—open or arthroscopic

References

1. Koyama S, Tensho K, Shimodaira H, Iwaasa T, Horiuchi H, Kato H, Saito N. A case of prefemoral fat pad impingement syndrome caused by hyperplastic fat pad. Case Rep Orthop. 2018;2018:3583049. https://doi.org/10.1155/2018/3583049.
2. Wang J, Han W, Wang X, Pan F, Liu Z, Halliday A, Jin X, Antony B, Cicuttini F, Jones G, Ding C. Mass effect and signal intensity alteration in the suprapatellar fat pad: associations with knee symptoms and structure. Osteoarthr Cartil. 2014;22(10):1619–26.
3. Jarraya M, Diaz LE, Roemer FW, Arndt WF, Goud AR, Guermazi A. MRI findings consistent with peripatellar fat pad impingement: how much related to patellofemoral maltracking? Magn Reson Med Sci. 2018;17(3):195–202.
4. Matcuk GR Jr, Cen SY, Keyfes V, Patel DB, Gottsegen CJ, White EA. Superolateral hoffa fat-pad edema and patellofemoral maltracking: predictive modeling. AJR Am J Roentgenol. 2014;203(2):W207–12.
5. Tsavalas N, Karantanas AH. Suprapatellar fat-pad mass effect: MRI findings and correlation with anterior knee pain. AJR Am J Roentgenol. 2013;200(3):W291–6.
6. Can TS, Yilmaz BK, Özdemir S. Magnetic resonance imaging of the quadriceps fat pad oedema pattern in relation to patellofemoral joint pathologies. Pol J Radiol. 2019;84:e375–80.
7. Shabshin N, Schweitzer ME, Morrison WB. Quadriceps fat pad edema: significance on magnetic resonance images of the knee. Skeletal Radiol. 2006;35(5):269–74.
8. Fontanella CG, Belluzzi E, Rossato M, Olivotto E, Trisolino G, Ruggieri P, Rubini A, Porzionato A, Natali A, De Caro R, Vettor R, Ramonda R, Macchi V, Favero M. Quantitative MRI analysis of infrapatellar and suprapatellar fat pads in normal controls, moderate and end-stage osteoarthritis. Ann Anat. 2019;221:108–14.
9. Ozdemir ZM, Aydingoz U, Korkmaz MF, Tunay VB, Ergen FB, Atay O, Baysal O. Ultrasonography-guided injection for quadriceps fat pad edema: preliminary report of a six-month clinical and radiological follow-up. J Belg Soc Radiol. 2016;100(1):78. https://doi.org/10.5334/jbr-btr.1148.

Chapter 43
Prefemoral Fat Pad Dysfunction

This refers to dysfunction of the prefemoral fat pad (located on the anterior aspect of the distal femur, behind the suprapatellar recess), which may have multiple causes [1–6].

Dysfunction may be due to fat pad:

- Inflammation
- Fibrosis

Dysfunction may be due to:

- Acute trauma:
  - Blunt injury on front of the knee, intra-articular fracture
- Degenerative/chronic micro-trauma
  - Impingement by a superior patellar osteophyte (involving the superior central part)
  - Patellofemoral (PF) friction syndrome—involving the lateral part of the fat pad
- Neoplastic
- Post-surgery—fibrosis

43.1 Clinical Symptoms of Prefemoral Fat Pad Dysfunction

- Pain in the front of the knee, suprapatellar area
- Clicking/catching

C. Panayiotou Charalambous, *The Knee Made Easy*,
https://doi.org/10.1007/978-3-030-54506-2_43

43.2 Clinical Signs of Prefemoral Fat Pad Dysfunction

- Tender suprapatellar area
- Patellar malalignment
  - Patella alta
  - Lateral tracking

43.3 Investigations for Prefemoral Fat Pad Dysfunction

- Plain radiographs—assess patellar height, superior patellar osteophyte
  - AP, lateral, skyline
- MRI to assess:
  - Fat pad—oedema, fibrosis, synovitis, mass lesions
  - Other intra-articular lesions and causes of anterior knee pain

43.4 Management of Prefemoral Fat Pad Dysfunction

43.4.1 Non-surgical

- Restore knee motion, strengthen periarticular muscles
- Quadriceps stretching and strengthening to reduce PF compression
- Steroid injections into fat pad (ultrasound guided)

43.4.2 Surgical

- Fat pad excision—open or arthroscopic

References

1. Shibata K, Okada K, Wakasa M, Saito I, Saito A, Takahashi Y, Sato H, Takahashi H, Kashiwagura T, Kimura Y. Ultrasonographic morphological changes in the prefemoral fat pad associated with knee osteoarthritis. J Med Ultrasound. 2018;26(2):94–9.
2. Borja MJ, Jose J, Vecchione D, Clifford PD, Lesniak BP. Prefemoral fat pad impingement syndrome: identification and diagnosis. Am J Orthop (Belle Mead NJ). 2013;42(1):E9–11.
3. Soder RB, Mizerkowski MD, Petkowicz R, Baldisserotto M. MRI of the knee in asymptomatic adolescent swimmers: a controlled study. Br J Sports Med. 2012;46(4):268–72.
4. van Middelkoop M, Macri EM, Eijkenboom JF, van der Heijden RA, Crossley KM, Bierma-Zeinstra SMA, de Kanter JL, Oei EH, Collins NJ. Are patellofemoral joint alignment and shape associated with structural magnetic resonance imaging abnormalities and symptoms among people with patellofemoral pain? Am J Sports Med. 2018;46(13):3217–26.
5. Koyama S, Tensho K, Shimodaira H, Iwaasa T, Horiuchi H, Kato H, Saito N. A case of prefemoral fat pad impingement syndrome caused by hyperplastic fat pad. Case Rep Orthop. 2018;2018:3583049.
6. Cilengir AH, Cetinoglu YK, Kazimoglu C, Gelal MF, Mete BD, Elmali F, Tosun O. The relationship between patellar tilt and quadriceps patellar tendon angle with anatomical variations and pathologies of the knee joint. Eur J Radiol. 2021;139:109719.

Chapter 44
Patellar Tendon Lateral Femoral Condyle Friction Syndrome

This is a condition where the patient experiences chronic pain in the anterior and lateral part of the knee, due to repetitive close contact between the proximal part of the patellar tendon and the lateral femoral condyle. This causes impingement of the underlying fat pad in extension, as well as patellar tendon microtrauma.

The fat pad is squeezed between the superior posterior and lateral part of the patellar tendon and femoral condyle. This is associated with patella alta and leads to oedema of the superolateral part of the infrapatellar fat pad [1–4].

Li et al. [3] described two types of shape of the anteroinferior part of the lateral femoral condyle—a sharp and a blunt morphology as assessed by MRI. They reported that a sharp lateral femoral condyle was correlated with lateral femoral condyle friction syndrome in patients with patella alta.

44.1 Clinical Symptoms of Patellar Tendon Lateral Femoral Condyle Friction Syndrome

- Pain
  - Anterolateral part of the knee
- Worse on activities that include hyperextension—such as sports (basketball, volleyball)
- Worse going up and down stairs
- Instability, knee gives way

C. Panayiotou Charalambous, *The Knee Made Easy*,
https://doi.org/10.1007/978-3-030-54506-2_44

44.2 Clinical Signs of Patellar Tendon Lateral Femoral Condyle Friction Syndrome

- Tenderness:
  - Proximal part of the infrapatellar fat pad
  - Proximal part of the patellar tendon
  - Anterior part of the lateral femoral condyle
- Patella alta
- Patellar malalignment/maltracking (lateral)

44.3 Investigations for Patellar Tendon Lateral Femoral Condyle Friction Syndrome

- Plain radiographs
  - AP, lateral, skyline to look for:
    - Patella alta
    - Lateral patellar subluxation/tilting
- MRI—may demonstrate:
  - Oedema like signal involving the:
    - Inferolateral part of the patellofemoral (PF) articulation
    - Superolateral part of the body of the infrapatellar fat pad
    - Soft tissues between lateral patellar retinaculum and lateral femoral condyle
  - Partial patellar tendon tears
  - Patellar cartilage defects

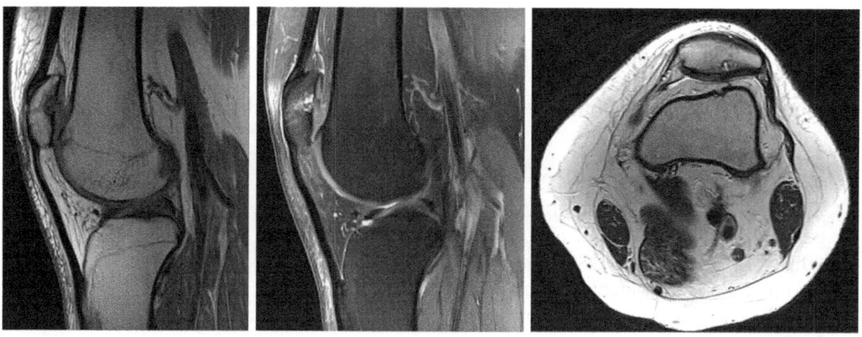

Patellar chondral lesion with underlying subchondral cyst, along with oedema of the upper part of the fat pad

44.4 Management of Patellar Tendon Lateral Femoral Condyle Friction Syndrome

44.4.1 *Non-surgical*

- Restoration of knee motion, strengthening of periarticular muscles
- Quadriceps stretching and strengthening
- Lateral patellar retinaculum stretching
- Proprioception training
- Improvement of core stability
- Patellar taping, bracing
- Steroid intra-articular fat pad injections

44.4.2 *Surgical*

Although several surgical procedures have been described their effectiveness is questionable and are better avoided.

These aim to address:

- Patella alta—tibial tubercle distalization
- Lateral patellar maltracking—tibial tubercle medialization, correction of knee valgus alignment
- Inflamed fat pad—excision

References

1. Touraine S, Lagadec M, Petrover D, Genah I, Parlier-Cuau C, Bousson V, Laredo JD. A ganglion of the patellar tendon in patellar tendon-lateral femoral condyle friction syndrome. Skeletal Radiol. 2013;42(9):1323–7.
2. Li J, Sheng B, Yu F, Guo C, Lv F, Lv F, Yang H. Quantitative magnetic resonance imaging in patellar tendon-lateral femoral condyle friction syndrome: relationship with subtle patellofemoral instability. Skeletal Radiol. 2019;48(8):1251–9.
3. Li J, Sheng B, Liu X, Yu F, Lv F, Lv F, Yang H. Sharp margin of antero-inferior lateral femoral condyle as a risk factor for patellar tendon-lateral femoral condyle friction syndrome. Eur Radiol. 2020;30(4):2261–9.
4. Chung CB, Skaf A, Roger B, Campos J, Stump X, Resnick D. Patellar tendon-lateral femoral condyle friction syndrome: MR imaging in 42 patients. Skeletal Radiol. 2001;30(12):694–7.

Chapter 45
Bipartite/Tripartite Patella Pain Syndrome

This is a condition where the patella may consist of 2 or 3 separate fragments, with pain arising from the junction between these fragments. It is considered to be a developmental abnormality with failure of the ossification centres of the patella to unite in early life. The tissue interposed between the fragments may consist of fibrous, fibrocartilage and hyaline cartilage components [1–4]. There may be variable mobility between the fragments.

45.1 Demographics of Bipartite Patella

- Rates of 0.8–6% in the general population have been described
- About 3 times more common in males compared to females
- Only about 1–2% of bipartite patella cases may be symptomatic

The junction between fragments may cause pain, related to fragment mobility. The onset of such pain may be:

- Acute—following trauma to the patella which stresses the junction between fragments
- Chronic—due to tensile forces by the:
  - Quadriceps (vastus lateralis) contractions
  - Pull of the lateral retinaculum during knee flexion

C. Panayiotou Charalambous, *The Knee Made Easy*,
https://doi.org/10.1007/978-3-030-54506-2_45

45.2 Classification

Oohashi [3] reported different types of bipartite/tripartite patella along with their relative frequencies:

1. Superolateral bipartite—83%
2. Lateral bipartite—12%
3. Superolateral and lateral tripartite—4%
4. Superolateral tripartite—1%

45.3 Clinical Symptoms of Bipartite Patella

- Most cases are not symptomatic but represent an incidental finding on radiological investigations of the knee
- Anterior knee pain
  - Exacerbated by movements of the knee
  - Worse during or after strenuous activity
  - Onset may be related to trauma of the patella

45.4 Clinical Signs of Bipartite Patella

- Localised tenderness—over the fragment site
- Patellofemoral (PF) crepitus
- Quadriceps wasting

45.5 Investigations for Bipartite Patella

- Plain radiographs—anteroposterior, skyline
- CT—to define the shape and size of the fragment

- MRI [5–7]:
  - Asymptomatic bipartite patella shows:
    - Intact but thinned cartilage along the border between the main patellar body and bipartite fragment
    - Fluid within the cleft
    - The synchondrosis may show cartilage, fibrous union, or fluid between the fragments
    - Lack of bone marrow oedema or high signal within the patellar body or the separate fragments
  - Symptomatic bipartite patella:
    - Bone marrow oedema within the bipartite fragment
- SPECT—to confirm that the synchondrosis is the source of pain

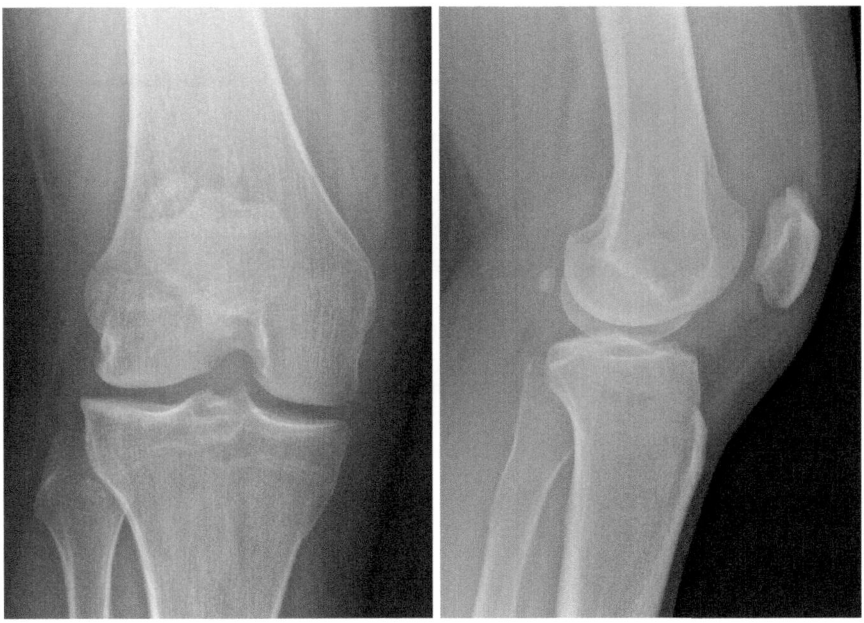

Bipartite patella, more evident on the AP view

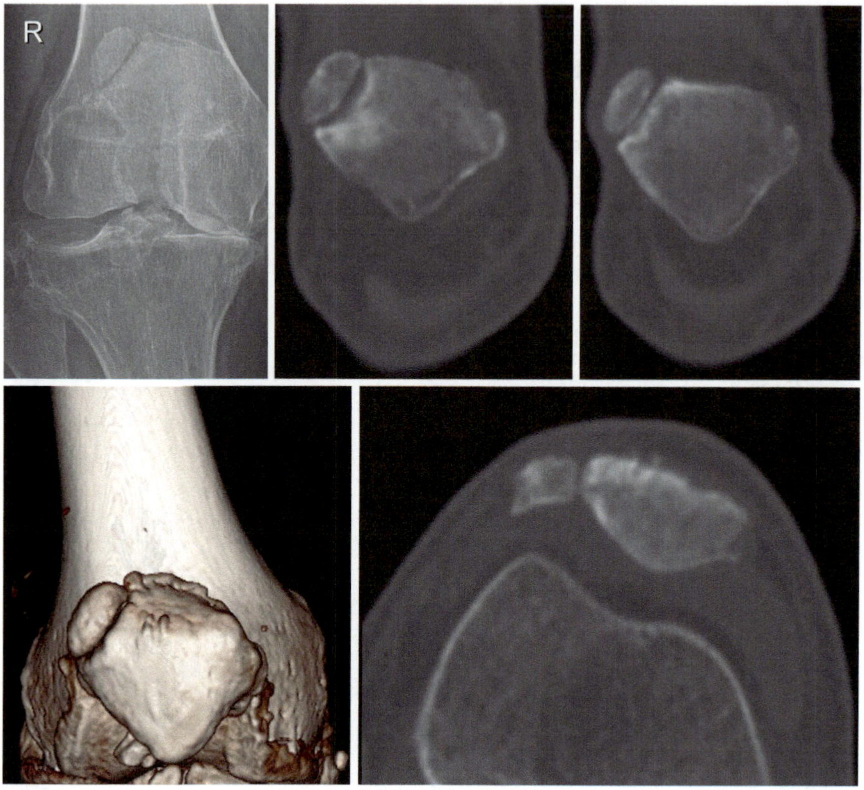

Bipartite patella associated with tibiofemoral arthritis– plain radiograph and CT

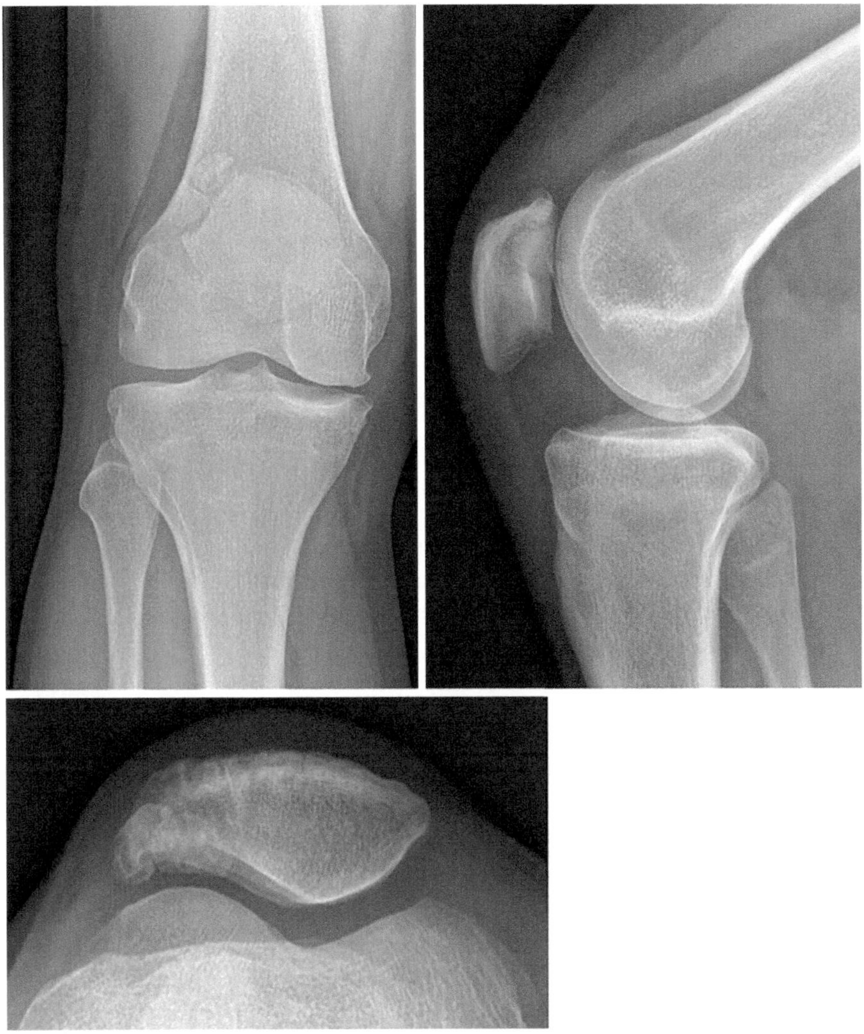

Tripartite patella

45.6 Management of Bipartite Patella

45.6.1 Non-surgical [8, 9]

- Leave alone
- Activity modification, rest, avoid strenuous activities

- NSAIDs (topical, systemic)
- Physiotherapy:
  - Stretching of the lateral retinaculum/vastus lateralis
  - Extraxcorporeal shock wave therapy (ECSW)
- External devices—bracing
- Low-intensity pulsed ultrasound—to stimulate bone union of the fragments
- Injection of the junction between fragments
  - Viscosupplementation
  - Steroid

45.6.2 *Surgical* [10–15]

- Fragment fixation
- Fragment excision (open or arthroscopic)
- Soft tissue release from the fragment (lateral retinaculum/vastus lateralis)
- Arthroscopic lateral retinaculum release without fragment excision

45.7 Prognosis of Treatment of Bipartite Patella

Matic et al [16] carried out a systematic review to determine the most effective intervention in allowing athletes with symptomatic bipartite patella to return to their prior activity levels. They included 20 articles with a total of 125 patients (130 knees) and reported:

- Overall treatment results—84% made a full return to sports
- Of those having surgical treatment—86% returned fully to their sport without symptoms
- Excision of the painful fragment—91% returned to sports with no symptoms and 9% returned but with residual symptoms

McMahon [12] in a similar systematic review reported relief of pain in 84% of cases, with 98% being able to return to their preoperative activity levels following surgery.

Learning Pearls

- Bipartite patella may be mistaken for a fracture following an acute injury to the knee. Its location, and cortication of the junction between the fragments may help distinguish it from an acute injury
- The articular cartilage is often intact across the junction between fragments, hence arthroscopic identification of the junction may be difficult

- Six months of non-surgical intervention is usually utilised prior to considering surgery

References

1. Ogden JA, McCarthy SM, Jokl P. The painful bipartite patella. J Pediatr Orthop. 1982;2(3):263–9.
2. Oohashi Y, Noriki S, Koshino T, Fukuda M. Histopathological abnormalities in painful bipartite patellae in adolescents. Knee. 2006;13(3):189–93.
3. Oohashi Y, Koshino T, Oohashi Y. Clinical features and classification of bipartite or tripartite patella. Knee Surg Sports Traumatol Arthrosc. 2010;18(11):1465–9.
4. Oohashi Y. Developmental anomaly of ossification type patella partita. Knee Surg Sports Traumatol Arthrosc. 2015;23(4):1071–6.
5. O'Brien J, Murphy C, Halpenny D, McNeill G, Torreggiani WC. Magnetic resonance imaging features of asymptomatic bipartite patella. Eur J Radiol. 2011;78(3):425–9.
6. Kavanagh EC, Zoga A, Omar I, Ford S, Schweitzer M, Eustace S. MRI findings in bipartite patella. Skeletal Radiol. 2007;36(3):209–14.
7. Akdag T, Guldogan ES, Coskun H, Turan A, Hekimoglu B. Magnetic resonance imaging for diagnosis of bipartite patella: usefulness and relationship with symptoms. Pol J Radiol. 2019;84:e491–7.
8. Atesok K, Doral MN, Lowe J, Finsterbush A. Symptomatic bipartite patella: treatment alternatives. J Am Acad Orthop Surg. 2008;16(8):455–61.
9. Kumahashi N, Uchio Y, Iwasa J, Kawasaki K, Adachi N, Ochi M. Bone union of painful bipartite patella after treatment with low-intensity pulsed ultrasound: report of two cases. Knee. 2008;15(1):50–3.
10. Felli L, Formica M, Lovisolo S, Capello AG, Alessio-Mazzola M. Clinical outcome of arthroscopic lateral retinacular release for symptomatic bipartite patella in athletes. Arthroscopy. 2018;34(5):1550–8.
11. Ferrari MB, Sanchez A, Sanchez G, Schantz K, Ellera Gomes JL, Provencher MT. Arthroscopic bony resection for treatment of symptomatic bipartite patella. Arthrosc Tech. 2017;6(4):e1003–7. https://doi.org/10.1016/j.eats.2017.03.013.
12. McMahon SE, LeRoux JA, Smith TO, Hing CB. The management of the painful bipartite patella: a systematic review. Knee Surg Sports Traumatol Arthrosc. 2016;24(9):2798–805.
13. Matic GT, Flanigan DC. Efficacy of surgical interventions for a bipartite patella. Orthopedics. 2014;37(9):623–8.
14. Vieira TD, Thaunat M, Saithna A, Carnesecchi O, Choudja E, Cavalier M, Vendrame JRB, Ockuly AC, Sonnery-Cottet B. Surgical technique for arthroscopic resection of painful bipartite patella. Arthrosc Tech. 2017;6(3):e751–5. https://doi.org/10.1016/j.eats.2017.02.007.
15. Radha S, Shenouda M, Konan S, Lavelle J, Church S. Successful treatment of painful synchondrosis of bipartite patella after direct trauma by operative fixation: a series of six cases. Open Orthop J. 2017;11:390–6. https://doi.org/10.2174/1874325001711010390.
16. Matic GT, Flanigan DC. Return to activity among athletes with a symptomatic bipartite patella: a systematic review. Knee. 2015;22(4):280–5. https://doi.org/10.1016/j.knee.2015.01.005.

Chapter 46
Knee Bursal Dysfunction

This is a condition where there is disease of one or more bursae around the knee [1–40]. The bursae are lined by synovium, hence may be affected by any disorder that can affect synovium. These include:

- Inflammation—overuse, trauma, crystal arthropathy (gout)
- Infection
- Neoplasia
  - Benign
  - Malignant

  Haemorrhagic—bleeding into bursa

46.1 Clinical Symptoms of Bursal Dysfunction

- Pain
  - Acute
  - Chronic
- Swelling at bursa site
- Leg swelling—if bursa tears—mimicking deep venous thrombosis
- Mass pressure effect—vascular obstruction, neurological symptoms, tendon snapping, bone erosion
- Limitation of motion—popliteal bursa limiting knee flexion

C. Panayiotou Charalambous, *The Knee Made Easy*,
https://doi.org/10.1007/978-3-030-54506-2_46

46.2 Clinical Signs of Bursal Dysfunction

- Visible swelling in area of anatomical bursa
- Palpable swelling
  - Cystic
  - Not pulsatile
  - Compressible
  - Reducible—popliteal bursa may be emptied by the application of pressure when the knee is in flexion, but not in extension
  - Hot, red, tender—if acute inflammation/infection
- Signs due to mass pressure effects—weak/diminished pulses, venous congestion, neurological signs
- Diffuse leg swelling—if bursa tear

46.3 Investigations for Bursal Dysfunction [41–45]

- Plain radiographs to look for bony abnormalities that may have led to bursal dysfunction or may be secondary to bursal dysfunction, calcification of a bursa
- MRI—to determine nature, dimensions and relations of swelling
- Ultrasound scan—allows more localised evaluation of a swelling as well as its vascular supply

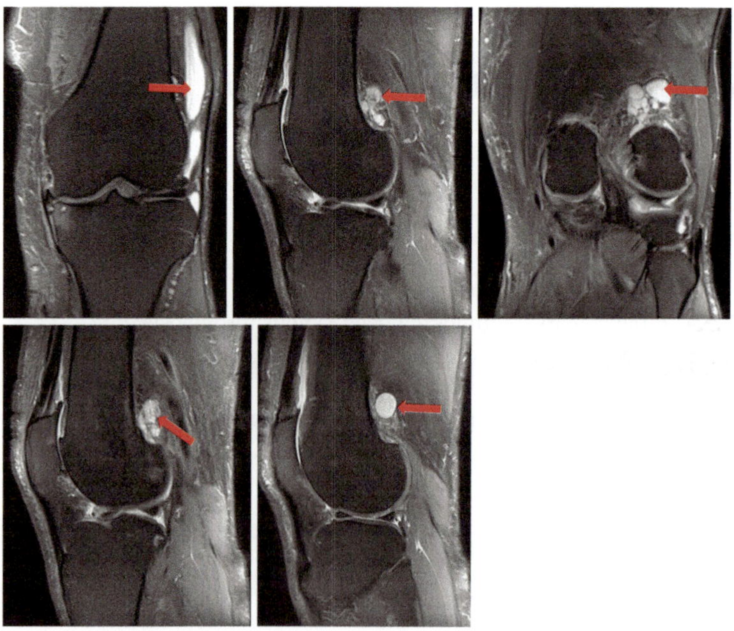

Bursal collection (red arrow) related to the lateral head of the gastrocnemius muscle in a knee with substantial osteoarthritis (MRI)

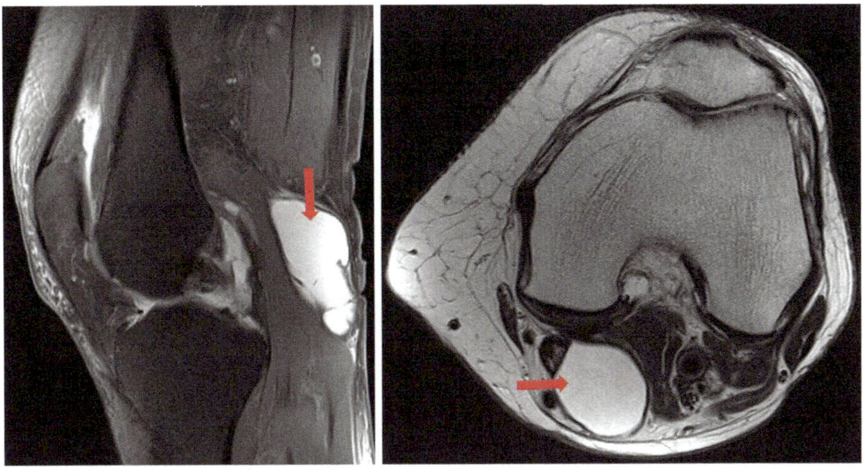

Large popliteal bursa

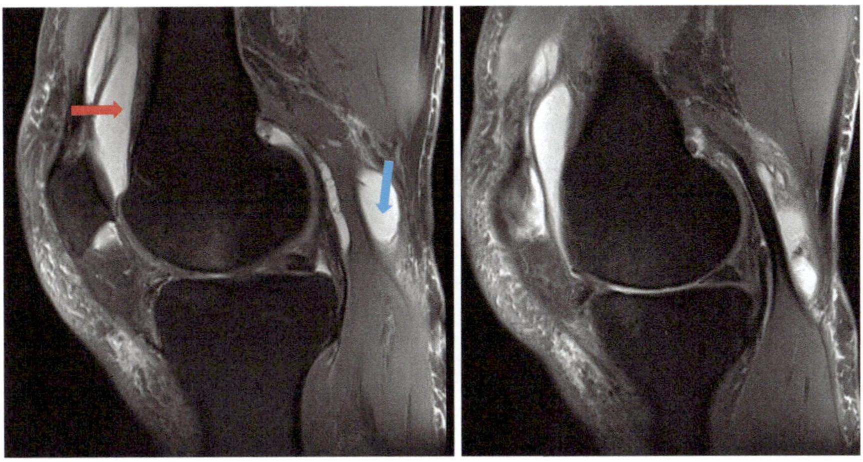

Large patellar effusion (red arrow) and associated popliteal bursa (blue arrow)

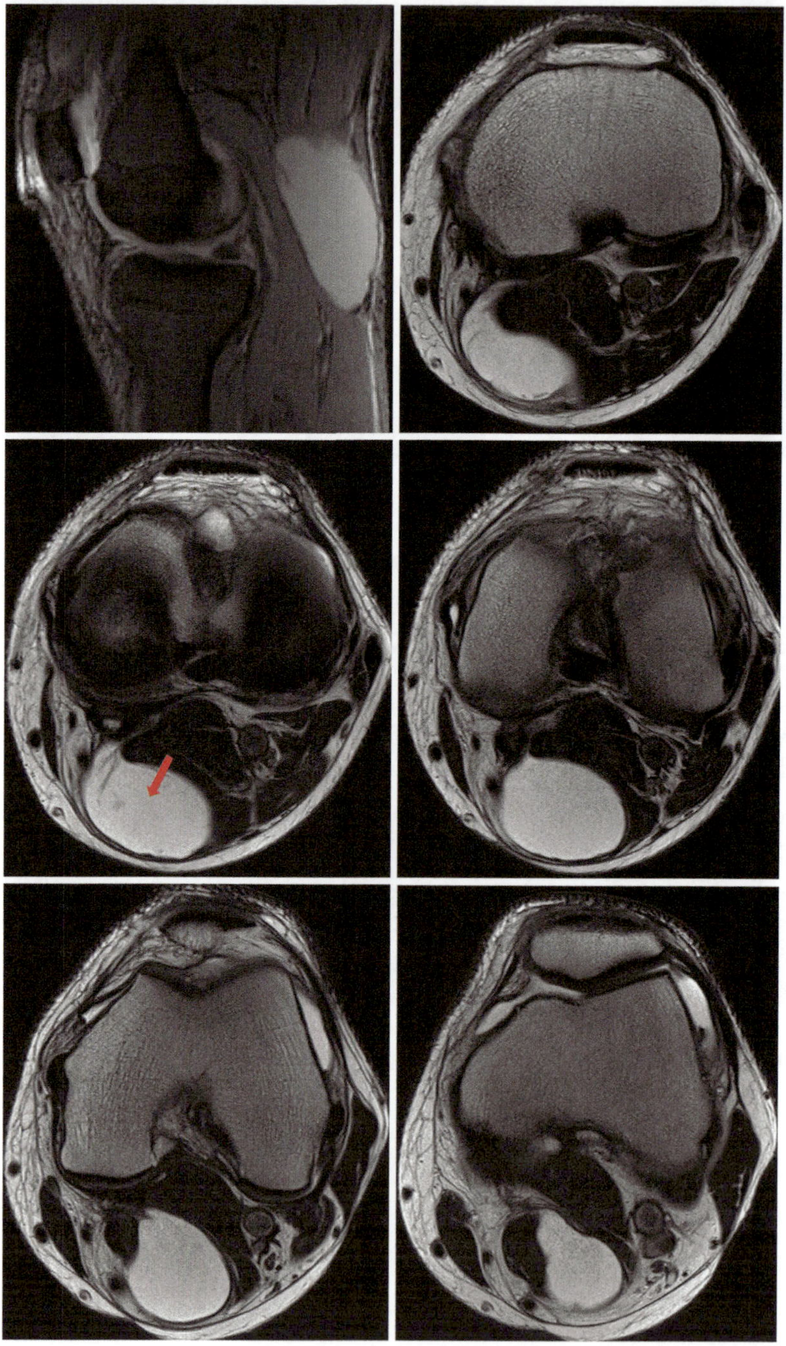

Large popliteal cyst associated with a degenerative medial meniscal tear and minor osteoarthritis. Axial MRI images show its deep origin and location (red arrow)

46.4 Management of Bursal Dysfunction [46–57]

Inflammatory bursitis may be treated with non-surgical or surgical means as below:

46.4.1 Non-surgical

- Expectant
- Anti-inflammatories
- Manage underlying disorder (such as gout)
- Aspiration +/− steroid injection

46.4.2 Surgical

- Incision and drainage +/− bursa excision

Infective bursitis may be treated with:

- Antibiotic treatment
- Surgical—incision and drainage +/− bursa excision

Neoplastic bursitis—management is as per neoplastic lesions

Haemmorhagic bursitis—address underlying haematological condition, drain bursa if very painful or pressure effect

Some of the specific bursae involved in inflammatory bursitis around the knee are described below:

Popliteal bursitis: this bursa is also known as the gastrocnemius-semimembranosus bursa/Baker's cyst. It is located between the posterior aspect of the medial femoral condyle, the medial head of gastrocnemius and semimembranosus. It usually communicates with the knee joint through an opening in the posterior part of the capsule [9–11].

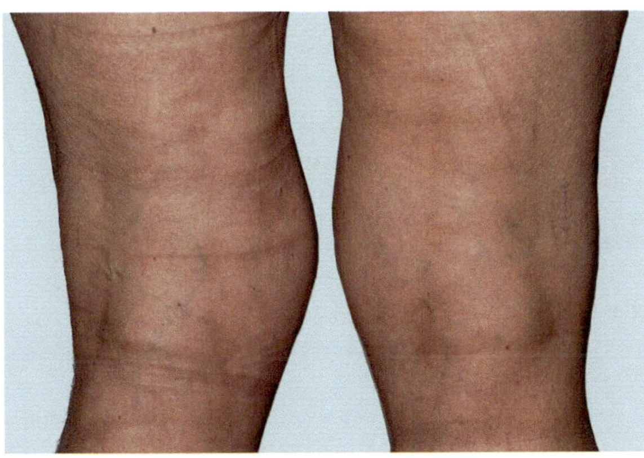

Posterior knee swelling due to enlarged popliteal bursa

It may extend proximally along the distal semimbranosous tendon or tear and extend distally into the calf (mimicking deep venous thrombosis). Patients often present with a working diagnosis of lower leg deep venous thrombosis, only to find out that they have a ruptured popliteal cyst. Most of these are treated with observation, but in cases with severely troublesome symptoms intervention may be necessary. This may be:

Non-surgical: aspiration and steroid injection.

Surgical: arthroscopic decompression, or, very rarely, open excision.

Prepatellar bursitis—housemaid's knee—presents as a swelling in front of the patella. Seen in individuals who spend time kneeling (such as housemaids!!). It is also reported in wrestlers, carpet and floor layers.

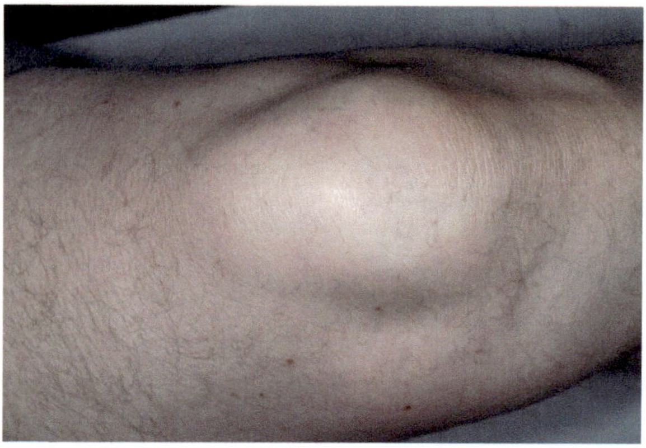

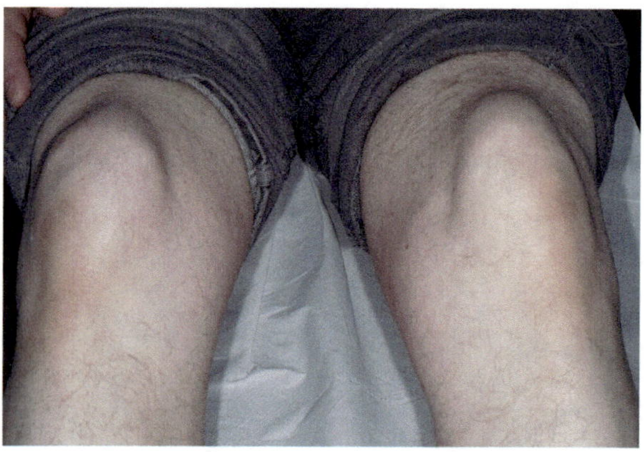

Enlarged Prepatellar bursa

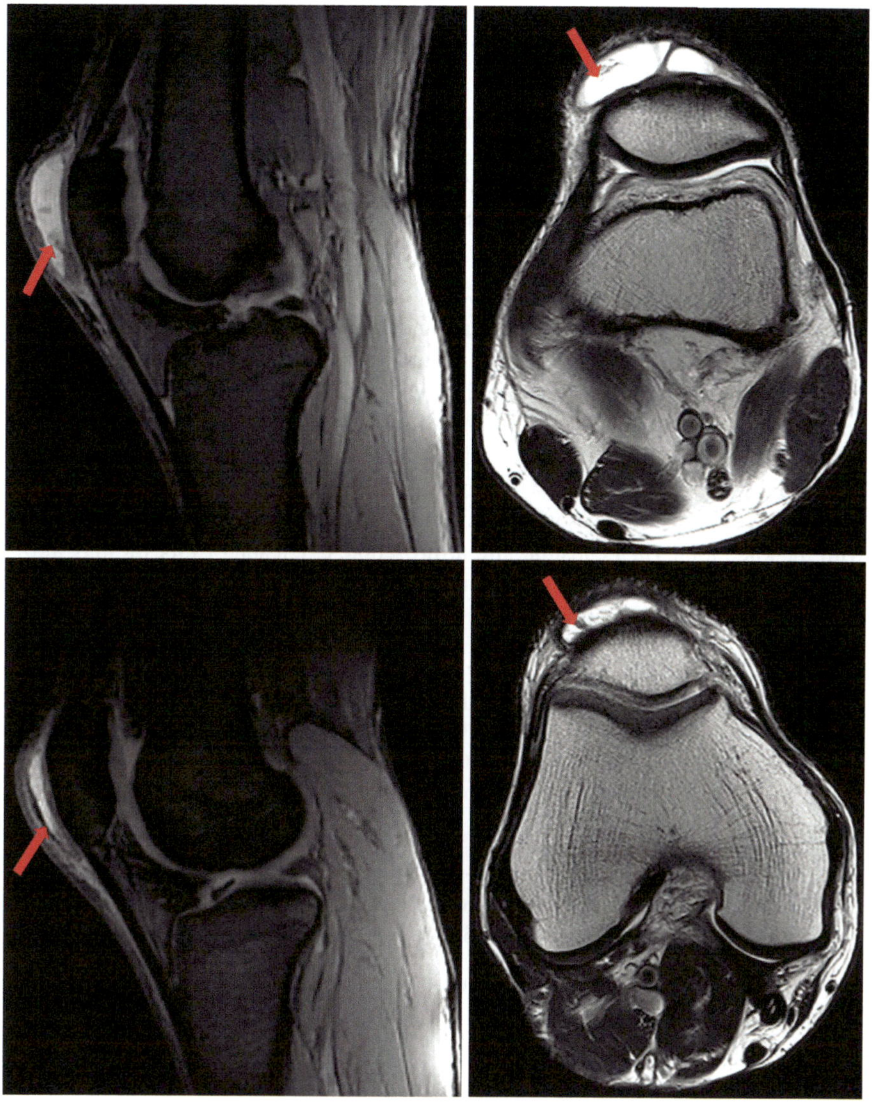

Bilateral prepatellar bursitis (red arrow) (MRI)

Superficial infrapatellar bursitis—clergyman's bursitis—this bursa is located between the patellar tendon and skin. It presents as a swelling in front of the patellar tendon (hence inferior to the location of the prepatellar bursa). Seen in individuals who spend time in deep flexion kneeling (such as clergymen!!), carpet and floor layers.

Suprapatellar bursitis—this bursa is located between the distal quadriceps and femoral shaft. A transverse septum separating the suprapatellar bursa from the main knee joint may persist into adulthood, limiting fluid flow between the two. It can thus present as painful swelling proximal to the patella. Spontaneous tear mimicking deep venous thrombosis has also been reported. Arthroscopic excision of the septum may help improve symptoms.

Deep infrapatellar bursitis—this bursa is located between the posterior aspect of the patellar tendon and proximal tibia, hence pain may be felt more deeply and swelling may not be very obvious. It may mimic patellar tendinopathy. It may contain ossicles in tibial tubercle apophysitis, and it has also been reported in enthesopathy of ankylosing spondylitis.

Medial collateral ligament bursitis—this bursa is located between the superficial and deep layers of the medial collateral ligament (MCL). It may cause pain at the medial aspect of the knee, aggravated by valgus stressing. It may also present as a medial knee swelling located next to the femur, the tibia or at the level of the tibiofemoral joint line. A MCL enlarged bursa may communicate with the knee joint through a capsular slit. MRI demonstrates fluid in the bursa between the deep and superficial layers of the MCL. Ultrasound guided aspiration +/− steroid injection may help symptoms. In cases where the bursa is not resolving and is communicating with the knee joint via a capsular slit, arthroscopic extension of this slit may allow decompression of the bursa. Differential diagnosis includes parameniscal cyst due to meniscocapsular separation or meniscal-capsular tear.

Lateral collateral ligament—biceps femoris bursitis—this bursa extends around the lateral, anterior, and anteromedial part of the distal quarter of the lateral collateral ligament (LCL), close to its insertion on the fibular head, deep to the anterior arm of the long head of the biceps femoris. The bursa can aid in the identification of the LCL during surgical stabilisation of the lateral part of the knee.

Pes anserinus bursitis—the pes anserinus describes the conjoined insertion of three tendons on the proximal tibia—sartorius, gracilis and semitendinosus. This bursa is located between the pes anserinus tendons, MCL and proximal tibia. Pes anserinus bursitis is seen more commonly in:

- Medial compartment osteoarthritis or knee inflammatory arthritis
- Females
- Obesity
- Hamstring overuse
- Impact activities including running, basketball, racquet sports
- Diabetes mellitus
- Total knee replacement arthroplasty
- Proximal medial tibial osteochondromas

Clinical Symptoms of Pes Anserinus Bursitis

- Pain on the medial aspect of knee
  - Aggravated by:
    - Standing from sitting

  - Crossing legs (as sartorius, gracilis and semitendinosus work together to cross legs)

Clinical Signs of Pes Anserinus Bursitis

- Tenderness over the pes anserinus area and along the distal part of the pes anserinus tendons
- Swelling at the pes anserinus area

Investigations for Pes Anserinus Bursitis

- Plain radiographs—looking for associated bony lesion (medial tibial osteochondroma)
- Ultrasound
- MRI

Management of Pes Anserinus Bursitis

Non-surgical

- Rest, ice, elevation
- Anti-inflammatories
- Manage underlying condition—gout in crystal arthropathy
- Ultrasound guided aspiration and steroid injection

Surgical

Very rare—debridement and bursal excision

References

1. Jensen LK, Mikkelsen S, Loft IP, Eenberg W. Work-related knee disorders in floor layers and carpenters. J Occup Environ Med. 2000;42(8):835–42.
2. Mysnyk MC, Wroble RR, Foster DT, Albright JP. Prepatellar bursitis in wrestlers. Am J Sports Med. 1986;14(1):46–54.
3. Sharrard WJ. Pressure effects on the knee in kneeling miners. Ann R Coll Surg Engl. 1965;36:309–24.
4. LaPrade RF. The anatomy of the deep infrapatellar bursa of the knee. Am J Sports Med. 1998;26(1):129–32.
5. Taylor PW. Inflammation of the deep infrapatellar bursa of the knee. Arthritis Rheum. 1989;32(10):1312–4.
6. Le Manac'h AP, Ha C, Descatha A, Imbernon E, Roquelaure Y. Prevalence of knee bursitis in the workforce. Occup Med (Lond). 2012;62(8):658–60.
7. Lieber SB, Fowler ML, Zhu C, Moore A, Shmerling RH, Paz Z. Clinical characteristics and outcomes of septic bursitis. Infection. 2017;45(6):781–6.
8. Zeng X, Xie L, Qiu Z, Sun K. Compression neuropathy of common peroneal nerve caused by a popliteal cyst: a case report. Medicine (Baltimore). 2018;97(16):e9922. https://doi.org/10.1097/MD.0000000000009922.
9. Kim JS, Lim SH, Hong BY, Park SY. Ruptured popliteal cyst diagnosed by ultrasound before evaluation for deep vein thrombosis. Ann Rehabil Med. 2014;38(6):843–6.
10. Kim KI, Lee SH, Ahn JH, Kim JS. Arthroscopic anatomic study of posteromedial joint capsule in knee joint associated with popliteal cyst. Arch Orthop Trauma Surg. 2014;134(7):979–84.

11. Marimuthu C, Rangarajan N, Abraham VT, Subbiah R. Tubercular popliteal cyst as a primary presentation in an adult: a case report and review of the literature. JBJS Case Connect. 2013;3(4 Suppl 6):e128–35. https://doi.org/10.2106/JBJS.CC.M.00163.
12. Chang CY, Shih YC, Wang HJ, Hsieh MS. Popliteal cyst rupture in a haemophiliac presenting as refractory recurrent right lower leg haemorrhage. Haemophilia. 2011;17(2):320–2.
13. Froelich JM, Hillard-Sembell D. Symptomatic loose bodies of the knee located in a popliteal cyst. Orthopedics. 2009;32(12):918. https://doi.org/10.3928/01477447-20091020-26.
14. Moretti B, Patella V, Mouhsine E, Pesce V, Spinarelli A, Garofalo R. Multilobulated popliteal cyst after a failed total knee arthroplasty. Knee Surg Sports Traumatol Arthrosc. 2007;15(2):212–6.
15. Sansone V, Sosio C, da Gama Malchér M, De Ponti A. An unusual cause of popliteal cyst. Arthroscopy. 2004;20(4):432–4.
16. Tashjian RZ, Nickisch F, Dennison D. Ruptured septic popliteal cyst associated with psoriatic arthritis. Orthopedics. 2004;27(2):231–3.
17. Robertson CM, Robertson RF, Strazerri JC. Proximal dissection of a popliteal cyst with sciatic nerve compression. Orthopedics. 2003;26(12):1231–2.
18. Rodriguez V, Shaughnessy WJ, Schmidt KA, Slaby JA, Gilchrist GS, Pruthi RK. Haemorrhage into a popliteal cyst: an unusual complication of haemophilia A. Haemophilia. 2002;8(5):725–8.
19. Ikeda M, Fujimori Y, Tankawa H, Iwata H. Compression syndrome of the popliteal vein and artery caused by popliteal cyst. Angiology. 1984;35(4):245–51.
20. Krag DN, Stansel HC Jr. Popliteal cyst producing complete arterial occlusion. A case report. J Bone Joint Surg Am. 1982;64(9):1369–70.
21. Schmitt BP, Kraag GR, Kelton JG. Acute calf pain and swelling in the arthritic patient: rupture of a popliteal cyst or deep venous thrombosis? Can Med Assoc J. 1981;125(1):54–6.
22. Akagi R, Saisu T, Segawa Y, Sasho T, Moriya H, Takahashi K, Kamegaya M. Natural history of popliteal cysts in the pediatric population. J Pediatr Orthop. 2013;33(3):262–8.
23. Hammoudeh M, Siam AR, Khanjar I. Anterior dissection of popliteal cyst causing anterior compartment syndrome. J Rheumatol. 1995;22(7):1377–9.
24. Hamabuchi M, Takeda Z. Isolated tuberculosis of the popliteal cyst. Nihon Geka Hokan. 1990;59(4):337–43.
25. Colak C, Ilaslan H, Sundaram M. Bony changes of the tibia secondary to pes anserine bursitis mimicking neoplasm. Skeletal Radiol. 2019;48(11):1795–801.
26. El-Khoury GY, Corbett AJ, Summers TB. A complete plica synovialis suprapatellaris, with diffuse pigmented villonodular synovitis limited to an isolated non-communicating suprapatellar bursa. Skeletal Radiol. 1985;13(2):164–8.
27. Yamamoto T, Akisue T, Marui T, Hitora T, Nagira K, Mihune Y, Matsui N, Yoshiya S, Kurosaka M. Isolated suprapatellar bursitis: computed tomographic and arthroscopic findings. Arthroscopy. 2003;19(2):E10.
28. Alvarez-Nemegyei J. Risk factors for pes anserinus tendinitis/bursitis syndrome: a case control study. J Clin Rheumatol. 2007;13(2):63–5.
29. Nur H, Aytekin A, Gilgil E. Medial collateral ligament bursitis in a patient with knee osteoarthritis. J Back Musculoskelet Rehabil. 2018;31(4):589–91.
30. Aydingoz U, Oguz B, Aydingoz O, Comert RB, Akgun I. The deep infrapatellar bursa: prevalence and morphology on routine magnetic resonance imaging of the knee. J Comput Assist Tomogr. 2004;28(4):557–61.
31. Andersen-Ranberg F, Hejgaard N. Ruptured semimembranosus bursa—an unusual complication following sports injury of the knee. Br J Sports Med. 1986;20(1):23–4.
32. Lindgren PG. Gastrocnemio-semimembranosus bursa and its relation to the knee joint. IV. Clinical considerations. Acta Radiol Diagn (Stockh). 1978;19(4):609–22.
33. Schickendantz MS, Watson JT. Mycobacterial prepatellar bursitis. Clin Orthop Relat Res. 1990;258:209–12.
34. Waters P, Kasser J. Infection of the infrapatellar bursa. A report of two cases. J Bone Joint Surg Am. 1990;72(7):1095–6.

35. Minami S, Miyake Y, Kinoshita H. Lipoma arborescens arising in the extra-articular bursa of the knee joint. SICOT J. 2016;2:28. https://doi.org/10.1051/sicotj/2016019.
36. Uysal F, Akbal A, Gökmen F, Adam G, Reşorlu M. Prevalence of pes anserine bursitis in symptomatic osteoarthritis patients: an ultrasonographic prospective study. Clin Rheumatol. 2015;34(3):529–33.
37. Cao Y, Jones G, Han W, Antony B, Wang X, Cicuttini F, Ding C. Popliteal cysts and subgastrocnemius bursitis are associated with knee symptoms and structural abnormalities in older adults: a cross-sectional study. Arthritis Res Ther. 2014;16(2):R59. https://doi.org/10.1186/ar4496.
38. Manning BT, Lewis N, Tzeng TH, Saleh JK, Potty AG, Dennis DA, Mihalko WM, Goodman SB, Saleh KJ. Diagnosis and management of extra-articular causes of pain after total knee arthroplasty. Instr Course Lect. 2015;64:381–8.
39. Huang TW, Wang CJ, Huang SC. Polyethylene-induced pes anserinus bursitis mimicking an infected total knee arthroplasty: a case report and review of the literature. J Arthroplasty. 2003;18(3):383–6.
40. Pavlov H, Steinbach L, Fried SH. A posterior ascending popliteal cyst mimicking thrombophlebitis following total knee arthroplasty (TKA). Clin Orthop Relat Res. 1983;179:204–8.
41. Tiwari V, Sampath Kumar V, Poudel RR, Kumar A, Khan SA. Pes Anserinus bursitis due to tibial spurs in children. Cureus. 2017;9(7):e1427. https://doi.org/10.7759/cureus.1427.
42. Stahnke M, Mangham DC, Davies AM. Calcific haemorrhagic bursitis anterior to the knee mimicking a soft tissue sarcoma: report of two cases. Skeletal Radiol. 2004;33(6):363–6.
43. Demeyere N, De Maeseneer M, Van Roy P, Osteaux M, Shahabpour M. Imaging of semimembranosus bursitis: MR findings in three patients and anatomical study. JBR-BTR. 2003;86(6):332–4.
44. Draghi F, Corti R, Urciuoli L, Alessandrino F, Rotondo A. Knee bursitis: a sonographic evaluation. J Ultrasound. 2015;18(3):251–7.
45. Zeiss J, Booth RL Jr, Woldenberg LS, Saddemi SR. Post-traumatic synovitis presenting as a mass in the suprapatellar bursa of the knee. MRI appearance. Clin Imaging. 1993;17(1):81–5.
46. Homayouni K, Foruzi S, Kalhori F. Effects of kinesiotaping versus non-steroidal anti-inflammatory drugs and physical therapy for treatment of pes anserinus tendino-bursitis: a randomized comparative clinical trial. Phys Sportsmed. 2016;44(3):252–6.
47. Khosrawi S, Taheri P, Ketabi M. Investigating the effect of extracorporeal shock wave therapy on reducing chronic pain in patients with pes anserine bursitis: a randomized, clinical- controlled trial. Adv Biomed Res. 2017;6:70. https://doi.org/10.4103/2277-9175.190999.
48. Dinham JM. Popliteal cysts in children. The case against surgery. J Bone Joint Surg Br. 1975;57(1):69–71.
49. Malinowski K, Synder M, Sibiński M. Selected cases of arthroscopic treatment of popliteal cyst with associated intra-articular knee disorders primary report. Ortop Traumatol Rehabil. 2011;13(6):573–82.
50. Meric G, Sargin S, Atik A, Budeyri A, Ulusal AE. Endoscopic versus open bursectomy for prepatellar and olecranon bursitis. Cureus. 2018;10(3):e2374. https://doi.org/10.7759/cureus.2374.
51. Jiang J, Ni L. Arthroscopic internal drainage and cystectomy of popliteal cyst in knee osteoarthritis. J Orthop Surg Res. 2017;12(1):182. https://doi.org/10.1186/s13018-017-0670-4.
52. Yang B, Wang F, Lou Y, Li J, Sun L, Gao L, Liu F. A comparison of clinical efficacy between different surgical approaches for popliteal cyst. J Orthop Surg Res. 2017;12(1):158. https://doi.org/10.1186/s13018-017-0659-z.
53. Roland GC, Beagley MJ, Cawley PW. Conservative treatment of inflamed knee bursae. Phys Sportsmed. 1992;20(2):66–77.
54. Sarifakioglu B, Afsar SI, Yalbuzdag SA, Ustaömer K, Bayramoğlu M. Comparison of the efficacy of physical therapy and corticosteroid injection in the treatment of pes anserine tendino-bursitis. J Phys Ther Sci. 2016;28(7):1993–7.
55. Zhou XN, Li B, Wang JS, Bai LH. Surgical treatment of popliteal cyst: a systematic review and meta-analysis. J Orthop Surg Res. 2016;11:22. https://doi.org/10.1186/s13018-016-0356-3.

56. Gu H, Bi Q, Chen J. Arthroscopic treatment of popliteal cyst using a figure-of-four position and double posteromedial portals. Int Orthop. 2019;43(6):1503–8.
57. Dillon JP, Freedman I, Tan JS, Mitchell D, English S. Endoscopic bursectomy for the treatment of septic pre-patellar bursitis: a case series. Arch Orthop Trauma Surg. 2012;132(7):921–5.

Chapter 47
Osteonecrosis of the Knee

This is a condition where there is interruption of the blood supply to the distal femur, proximal tibia or patella. As a result, the bone undergoes necrosis [1–6]. Osteonecrosis of the knee is much rarer as compared to osteonecrosis of the femoral or humeral head.

Three different entities of osteonecrosis of the knee have been described

- Spontaneous osteonecrosis of the knee (SPONK)
- Secondary osteonecrosis
- Post-surgical (including arthroscopic osteonecrosis)

These three entities are considered to have specific underlying pathogenesis, clinical and radiological features but with some overlap in these parameters. Hence, common features are initially presented followed by their distinct characteristics.

47.1 Causes of Osteonecrosis of the Knee [7–42]

- Idiopathic (spontaneous osteonecrosis of the knee—SPONK)
- Secondary
  - Trauma
  - Surgery
    - Post-arthroscopy
    - Post-open surgical approaches disrupting blood supply—as in patellar necrosis
  - Steroid use—including intra-articular injections
  - Alcohol abuse
  - Metabolic—Gaucher's disease
  - Haematological—Haemoglobinopathies—sickle cell disease

C. Panayiotou Charalambous, *The Knee Made Easy*,
https://doi.org/10.1007/978-3-030-54506-2_47

- Connective tissue disorders—lupus
- Inflammatory arthritis—rheumatoid arthritis
- Infective—bacterial or non-bacterial
- Dysbaric—Caisson disease

47.2 Demographics [8, 9]

- SPONK—more common in women in their sixth decade of life
- Secondary osteonecrosis—more common in younger patients

47.3 Distribution of Osteonecrosis

- SPONK most commonly affects the subchondral bone of the weightbearing part of the medial femoral condyle, although other parts of the knee may be involved. Usually unilateral
- Secondary osteonecrosis may affect any part of the femur or tibia including metaphysis or diaphysis. Secondary osteonecrosis may affect both knees and multiple joints
- Post-surgical (arthroscopic) osteonecrosis also seems to affect most commonly the medial femoral condyle but the lateral compartment and patella may also be involved

47.4 Pathogenesis

Disruption of the blood supply may involve the arterial inflow or venous outflow. It may be due to external mechanical factors causing compression or disruption of blood vessels, or due to internal occlusion of the vessel lumen. Necrosis may also be due to a traumatic event that damages the bone primarily.

It is considered that the pathogenesis of the 3 entities may differ [10–12]:

- SPONK may be due to subchondral insufficiency fracture
  This would be in line with:
  - Their most common location: weightbearing part of medial femoral condyle that is associated with high loading forces
  - Association with meniscal injuries or partial meniscectomy
  - Association with osteoarthritis and osteopenia
- Secondary osteonecrosis is considered to be due to vascular occlusion secondary to one of multiple factors
- Post-surgical osteonecrosis may be:

- Related to altered biomechanics as a result of the procedure
- Due to trauma as a result of the arthroscopic instrumentation
- Due to disruption of the blood supply to the bone (as in fat pad excision associated with patellar osteonecrosis)

47.5 Clinical Symptoms of Osteonecrosis of the Knee

- Knee pain
  - At rest and on activity, pain on weightbearing
  - Night pain, disturbing sleep
  - Onset:
    - Acute in SPONK—may be so severe that patient presents acutely to the emergency room
    - Gradual, slow onset in secondary osteonecrosis
    - Temporal relation to arthroscopy or other surgery (6–8 weeks post arthroscopy)
- Stiffness
- Apparent weakness
- Clicking/clucking, if collapsed or arthritic knee
- Locking or popping, if loose chondral or osteochondral fragments

47.6 Clinical Signs of Osteonecrosis of the Knee

- Painful knee motion
- Loss of knee motion
  - Apparent due to pain
  - True stiffness
- Localised tenderness
- Effusion/synovitis

47.7 Investigations for Osteonecrosis of the Knee

- Radiological [13–15]
  - Plain radiographs (may be normal in early stages of the disease)
  - MRI scan

- SPONK
- Secondary Osteonecrosis
- Post-surgical osteonecrosis

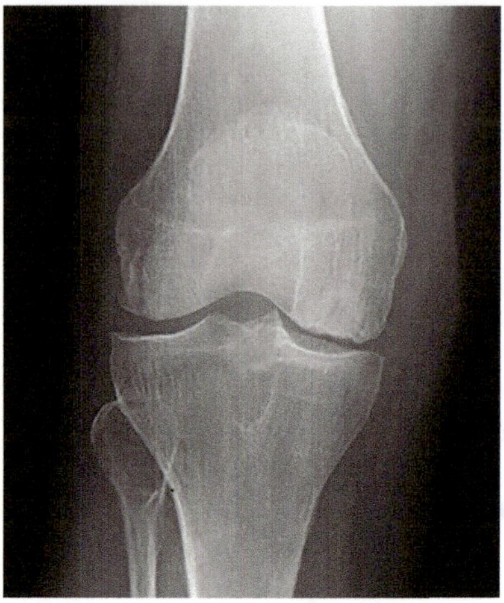

Medial femoral condyle spontaneous osteonecrosis

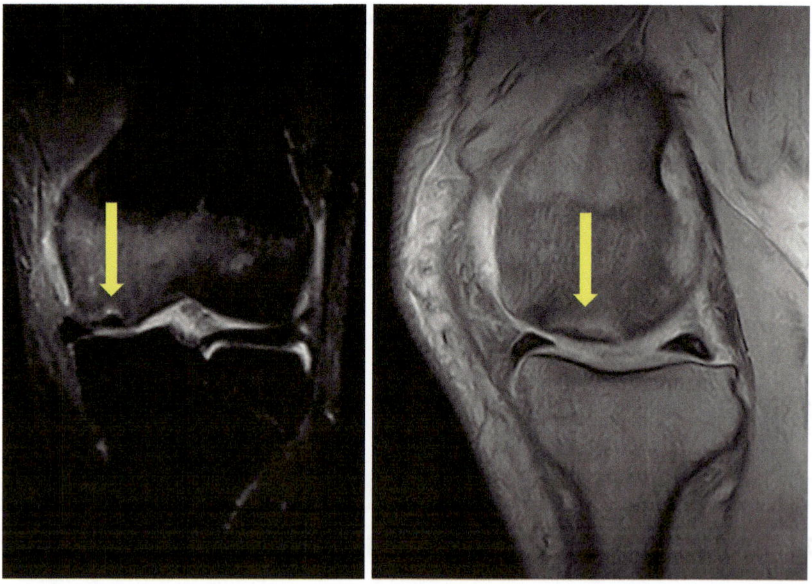

SPONK of the medial femoral condyle associated with medial meniscal extrusion (MRI)

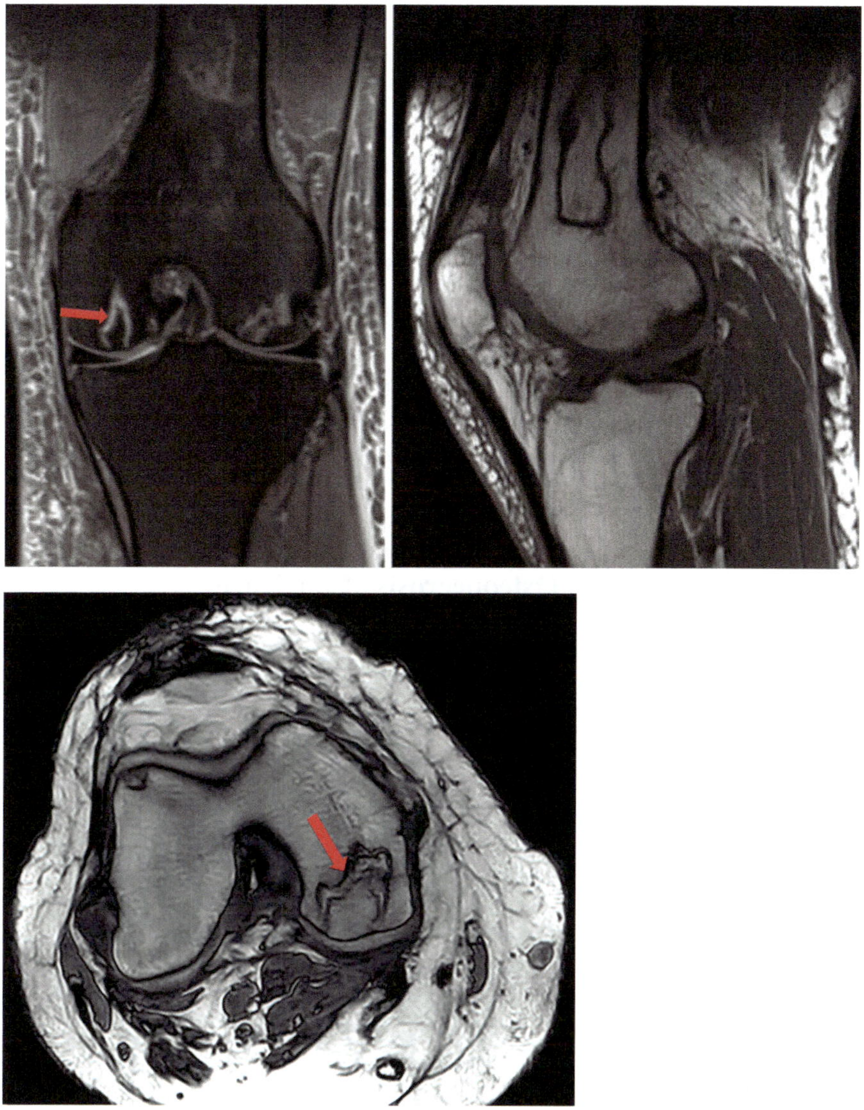

Secondary necrosis of the distal femur—geographic appearence (red arrow) (MRI)

47.8 Classification of SPONK

Koshino [40, 41]

- Stage I—No abnormal radiograph findings, but marrow signal changes on MRI
- Stage II—Flattening of the convexity (weightbearing part) of the femoral condyle or subchondral radiolucency surrounded by sclerosis or both
- Stage III—Sclerotic halo around radiolucent area and subchondral collapse
- Stage IV—Degenerative changes involving the tibiofemoral articulation

  Agglietti Modification [42]

- Stage I—Normal radiographs
- Stage II—Flattening of the affected condyle
- Stage III—Subchondral radiolucent lesion surrounded by limited sclerosis
- Stage IV—Substantial sclerosis and subchondral bone collapse
- Stage V—Degenerative changes

47.9 Management of Osteonecrosis of the Knee

This will depend on clinical symptoms and disease stage and is described below.

47.9.1 Non-surgical [43–49]

- Leave alone
- Analgesia
- Eliminate risk factors
- Activity modification to minimise loading of the involved part of the knee (6–12 weeks of non-weightbearing in cases of involvement of the tibiofemoral joint)
- Physiotherapy to maintain joint mobility and avoid stiffness
- External devices:
  - Bracing to reduce loading of the involved compartment
  - Foot orthotics to reduce loading of the involved compartment
- Bisphosphonates (their use has been described but no strong evidence for their electiveness. They are believed to reduce bone resorption and hence limit collapse and disease progression)

47.9.2 Surgical [46, 50–61]

- Joint preserving (in the absence of degenerative changes)

  - Knee debridement with removal of chondral flaps and loose bodies/drilling/decompression of affected area
  - Core decompression ± grafting
  - Resurfacing of osteochondral lesion—microfracture/transplant techniques/synthetic button
  - Osteotomy (high tibial/distal femoral)—to unload the lesion

- Joint arthroplasty (for degenerative changes)

  - Partial replacement
  - Total knee replacement

47.10 Natural History of Osteonecrosis of the Knee [62–68]

47.10.1 SPONK

- Prognosis is inversely related to the extent of disease (size, depth, presence of collapse)
- Spontaneous resolution in those with MRI changes but normal radiographs is possible
- Varus deformity and deeper lesions >20 mm are associated with a worse prognosis
- Smaller lesions and lesions in earlier stages of the disease may be more likely to resolve spontaneously. It has been suggested that lesions:

  - <3.5 cm are likely to resolve
  - 3.5-5 cm are unpredictable
  - >5 cm are likely to progress

- Medial tibial plateau SPONK may be associated with a poor prognosis with most lesions progressing to degenerative changes or collapse

47.10.2 Secondary Osteonecrosis

It has been reported that in asymptomatic secondary necrosis due to steroid use in systemic lupus erythromatosus, with no collapse, spontaneous repair may occur in about 50% of joints, with complete disappearance in some. About 15% of lesions may enlarge, usually related to an increase in steroid use, and 22% may progress to collapse. Larger lesions confer poorer prognosis [65].

Learning Pearls

- In early stages, no specific signs may be apparent and plain radiographs may be normal, hence diagnosis may be overlooked

- Late presentation is common, as symptoms may not be apparent until the disease has substantially progressed and degenerative changes set in.
- AVN should be considered when encountering:
  - Pain in the knee of no obvious origin
  - A patient at high risk of AVN (female in sixth decade of life with acute onset non-traumatic pain, post-arthroscopy ongoing pain, steroid use or alcohol abuse)
- Secondary osteonecrosis may occur very early following high steroid treatment (within 1–5 months, mean 3.1 months in SLE) [68]
- Classification of osteonecrosis: Classifying osteonecrosis into:
  - Pre-collapse
  - Post-collapse

  is more appropriate as may guide treatment:
  - In the pre-collapse state, collapse preventing interventions (limited weightbearing, bisphosphonates, drilling, and decompression) may be utilised
  - In the post-collapse state resurfacing techniques, unloading osteotomy, or replacement arthroplasty are more appropriate

References

1. Zywiel MG, McGrath MS, Seyler TM, Marker DR, Bonutti PM, Mont MA. Osteonecrosis of the knee: a review of three disorders. Orthop Clin North Am. 2009;40(2):193–211.
2. Low K, Mont MA, Hungerford DS. Steroid-associated osteonecrosis of the knee: a comprehensive review. Instr Course Lect. 2001;50:489–93.
3. Mont MA, Baumgarten KM, Rifai A, Bluemke DA, Jones LC, Hungerford DS. Atraumatic osteonecrosis of the knee. J Bone Joint Surg Am. 2000;82(9):1279–90.
4. Narváez J, Narváez JA, Rodriguez-Moreno J, Roig-Escofet D. Osteonecrosis of the knee: differences among idiopathic and secondary types. Rheumatology (Oxford). 2000;39(9):982–9.
5. Mont MA, Marker DR, Zywiel MG, Carrino JA. Osteonecrosis of the knee and related conditions. J Am Acad Orthop Surg. 2011;19(8):482–94.
6. Karim AR, Cherian JJ, Jauregui JJ, Pierce T, Mont MA. Osteonecrosis of the knee: review. Ann Transl Med. 2015;3(1):6. https://doi.org/10.3978/j.issn.2305-5839.2014.11.13.
7. Pape D, Seil R, Anagnostakos K, Kohn D. Postarthroscopic osteonecrosis of the knee. Arthroscopy. 2007;23(4):428–38.
8. Di Caprio F, Meringolo R, Navarra MA, Mosca M, Ponziani L. Postarthroscopy Osteonecrosis of the Knee: Current Concepts. Joints. 2017;5(4):229–36.
9. Zywiel MG, Armocida FM, McGrath MS, Bonutti PM, Mont MA. Bicondylar spontaneous osteonecrosis of the knee: a case report. Knee. 2010;17(2):167–71.
10. Ohdera T, Miyagi S, Tokunaga M, Yoshimoto E, Matsuda S, Ikari H. Spontaneous osteonecrosis of the lateral femoral condyle of the knee: a report of 11 cases. Arch Orthop Trauma Surg. 2008;128(8):825–31.

11. Marx A, Beier A, Taheri P, Röpke M, Kalinski T, Halder AM. Post-arthroscopic osteonecrosis of the medial tibial plateau: a case series. J Med Case Rep. 2016;10(1):291.
12. Lansdown DA, Shaw J, Allen CR, Ma CB. Osteonecrosis of the Knee After Anterior Cruciate Ligament Reconstruction: A Report of 5 Cases. Orthop J Sports Med. 2015;3(3):2325967115576120. https://doi.org/10.1177/2325967115576120.
13. Son IJ, Kim MK, Kim JY, Kim JG. Osteonecrosis of the knee after arthroscopic partial meniscectomy. Knee Surg Relat Res. 2013;25(3):150–4.
14. Chambers C, Craig JG, Zvirbulis R, Nelson F. Spontaneous osteonecrosis of knee after arthroscopy is not necessarily related to the procedure. Am J Orthop (Belle Mead NJ). 2015;44(6):E184–9.
15. Jeong HJ, Kim D, Cho SK, Kim Y, Bae SC, Sung YK. Clinical characteristics of multifocal osteonecrosis in Korean patients with rheumatic disease. Int J Rheum Dis. 2018;21(6):1301–8.
16. Flouzat-Lachaniete CH, Roussignol X, Poignard A, Mukasa MM, Manicom O, Hernigou P. Multifocal joint osteonecrosis in sickle cell disease. Open Orthop J. 2009;3:32–5.
17. Shigemura T, Nakamura J, Kishida S, Harada Y, Takeshita M, Takazawa M, Takahashi K. The incidence of alcohol-associated osteonecrosis of the knee is lower than the incidence of steroid-associated osteonecrosis of the knee: an MRI study. Rheumatology (Oxford). 2012;51(4):701–6.
18. Haque W, Kadikoy H, Pacha O, Maliakkal J, Hoang V, Abdellatif A. Osteonecrosis secondary to antiphospholipid syndrome: a case report, review of the literature, and treatment strategy. Rheumatol Int. 2010;30(6):719–23.
19. Hauzeur JP, Malaise M, Gangji V. Osteonecrosis in inflammatory bowel diseases: a review of the literature. Acta Gastroenterol Belg. 2009;72(3):327–34.
20. Yang WM, Zhao CQ, Lu ZY, Yang WY, Lin DK, Cao XW. Clinical Characteristics and Treatment of Spontaneous Osteonecrosis of Medial Tibial Plateau: A Retrospective Case Study. Chin Med J (Engl). 2018;131(21):2544–50.
21. Lee JH, Wang SI, Noh SJ, Ham DH, Kim KB. Osteonecrosis of the medial tibial plateau after intra-articular corticosteroid injection: a case report. Medicine (Baltimore). 2019;98(44):e17248. https://doi.org/10.1097/MD.0000000000017248.
22. McCurdie DFK, Roi DD, Sahu DA, Sandhu DGS. Severe bilateral knee osteonecrosis in a young man with human immunodeficiency virus. Radiol Case Rep. 2018;14(2):208–12.
23. Barbosa M, Cotter J. Osteonecrosis of both knees in a woman with Crohn's disease. World J Gastrointest Pharmacol Ther. 2016;7(4):579–83.
24. Daltro G, Franco BA, Faleiro TB, Rosário DAV, Daltro PB, Meyer R, Fortuna V. Use of autologous bone marrow stem cell implantation for osteonecrosis of the knee in sickle cell disease: a preliminary report. BMC Musculoskelet Disord. 2018;19(1):158. https://doi.org/10.1186/s12891-018-2067-x.
25. Roach R, Miller D, Griffiths D. Multifocal osteonecrosis predominantly affecting the knees secondary to chronic alcohol ingestion: a case report and review. Acta Orthop Belg. 2006;72(2):234–6.
26. Carstensen SE, Domson GF. Patellar Osteonecrosis Following Knee Arthroscopy. Orthopedics. 2019;42(6):e552–4.
27. Noh JH, Roh YH. Osteonecrosis of bipartite patella following total knee arthroplasty without lateral release. Acta Orthop Traumatol Turc. 2019;53(1):74–6.
28. Boretto JG, Altube G, Gallucci GL, Narvaez HR, De Carli P. Femoral Osteonecrosis after Medial Femoral Condyle Bone Graft Harvest. Plast Reconstr Surg Glob Open. 2018;6(6):e1792. https://doi.org/10.1097/GOX.0000000000001792.
29. Takeda M, Higuchi H, Kimura M, Kobayashi Y, Terauchi M, Takagishi K. Spontaneous osteonecrosis of the knee: histopathological differences between early and progressive cases. J Bone Joint Surg Br. 2008;90(3):324–9.
30. Akamatsu Y, Mitsugi N, Hayashi T, Kobayashi H, Saito T. Low bone mineral density is associated with the onset of spontaneous osteonecrosis of the knee. Acta Orthop. 2012;83(3):249–55.

31. Nelson FR, Craig J, Francois H, Azuh O, Oyetakin-White P, King B. Subchondral insufficiency fractures and spontaneous osteonecrosis of the knee may not be related to osteoporosis. Arch Osteoporos. 2014;9:194.
32. Oda S, Fujita A, Moriuchi H, Okamoto Y, Otsuki S, Neo M. Medial meniscal extrusion and spontaneous osteonecrosis of the knee. J Orthop Sci. 2019;24(5):867–72.
33. Muscolo DL, Costa-Paz M, Ayerza M, Makino A. Medial meniscal tears and spontaneous osteonecrosis of the knee. Arthroscopy. 2006;22(4):457–60.
34. Robertson DD, Armfield DR, Towers JD, Irrgang JJ, Maloney WJ, Harner CD. Meniscal root injury and spontaneous osteonecrosis of the knee: an observation. J Bone Joint Surg Br. 2009;91(2):190–5.
35. Hussain ZB, Chahla J, Mandelbaum BR, Gomoll AH, LaPrade RF. The role of meniscal tears in spontaneous osteonecrosis of the knee: a systematic review of suspected etiology and a call to revisit nomenclature. Am J Sports Med. 2019;47(2):501–7.
36. Yasuda T, Ota S, Fujita S, Onishi E, Iwaki K, Yamamoto H. Association between medial meniscus extrusion and spontaneous osteonecrosis of the knee. Int J Rheum Dis. 2018;21(12):2104–11.
37. Sung JH, Ha JK, Lee DW, Seo WY, Kim JG. Meniscal extrusion and spontaneous osteonecrosis with root tear of medial meniscus: comparison with horizontal tear. Arthroscopy. 2013;29(4):726–32.
38. Yamagami R, Taketomi S, Inui H, Tahara K, Tanaka S. The role of medial meniscus posterior root tear and proximal tibial morphology in the development of spontaneous osteonecrosis and osteoarthritis of the knee. Knee. 2017;24(2):390–5.
39. Kidwai AS, Hemphill SD, Griffiths HJ. Radiologic case study. Spontaneous osteonecrosis of the knee reclassified as insufficiency fracture. Orthopedics. 2005;28(3):236, 333–6.
40. Koshino T, Okamoto R, Takamura K, Tsuchiya K. Arthroscopy in spontaneous osteonecrosis of the knee. Orthop Clin North Am. 1979;10(3):609–18.
41. Koshino T. Calcified plate and flattening of the femoral condyle with spontaneous osteonecrosis. Bull Hosp Jt Dis. 1993 Summer;53(3):29–33.
42. Aglietti P, Insall JN, Buzzi R, Deschamps G. Idiopathic osteonecrosis of the knee. Aetiology, prognosis and treatment. J Bone Joint Surg Br. 1983;65(5):588–97.
43. Yates PJ, Calder JD, Stranks GJ, Conn KS, Peppercorn D, Thomas NP. Early MRI diagnosis and non-surgical management of spontaneous osteonecrosis of the knee. Knee. 2007;14(2):112–6.
44. Osmani F, Thakkar S, Vigdorchik J. The Utility of Conservative Treatment Modalities in the Management of Osteonecrosis. Bull Hosp Jt Dis. 2017;75(3):186–92.
45. Uchio Y, Ochi M, Adachi N, Shu N. Effectiveness of an insole with a lateral wedge for idiopathic osteonecrosis of the knee. J Bone Joint Surg Br. 2000;82(5):724–7.
46. Marti CB, Rodriguez M, Zanetti M, Romero J. Spontaneous osteonecrosis of the medial compartment of the knee: a MRI follow-up after conservative and operative treatment, preliminary results. Knee Surg Sports Traumatol Arthrosc. 2000;8(2):83–8.
47. Jureus J, Lindstrand A, Geijer M, Roberts D, Tägil M. Treatment of spontaneous osteonecrosis of the knee (SPONK) by a bisphosphonate. Acta Orthop. 2012;83(5):511–4.
48. Breer S, Oheim R, Krause M, Marshall RP, Amling M, Barvencik F. Spontaneous osteonecrosis of the knee (SONK). Knee Surg Sports Traumatol Arthrosc. 2013;21(2):340–5.
49. Meier C, Kraenzlin C, Friederich NF, Wischer T, Grize L, Meier CR, Kraenzlin ME. Effect of ibandronate on spontaneous osteonecrosis of the knee: a randomized, double-blind, placebo-controlled trial. Osteoporos Int. 2014;25(1):359–66.
50. Lieberman JR, Varthi AG, Polkowski GG 2nd. Osteonecrosis of the knee - which joint preservation procedures work? J Arthroplast. 2014;29(1):52–6.
51. Marulanda G, Seyler TM, Sheikh NH, Mont MA. Percutaneous drilling for the treatment of secondary osteonecrosis of the knee. J Bone Joint Surg Br. 2006;88(6):740–6.
52. von Keudell A, Gomoll AH, Bryant T, Minas T. Spontaneous osteonecrosis of the knee treated with autologous chondrocyte implantation, autologous bone-grafting, and osteotomy: a report

of two cases with follow-up of seven and nine years. J Bone Joint Surg Am. 2011;93(24):e149. https://doi.org/10.2106/JBJS.K.00242.
53. Akgun I, Kesmezacar H, Ogut T, Kebudi A, Kanberoglu K. Arthroscopic microfracture treatment for osteonecrosis of the knee. Arthroscopy. 2005;21(7):834–43.
54. Yoon C, Chang MJ, Chang CB, Choi JH, Lee SA, Kang SB. Does unicompartmental knee arthroplasty have worse outcomes in spontaneous osteonecrosis of the knee than in medial compartment osteoarthritis? A systematic review and meta-analysis. Arch Orthop Trauma Surg. 2019;139(3):393–403.
55. Kamenaga T, Hiranaka T, Hida Y, Fujishiro T, Okamoto K. Unicompartmental knee arthroplasty for spontaneous osteonecrosis of the medial tibial plateau. Knee. 2018;25(4):715–21.
56. Fukuoka S, Fukunaga K, Taniura K, Sasaki T, Takaoka K. Medium-term clinical results of unicompartmental knee arthroplasty for the treatment for spontaneous osteonecrosis of the knee with four to 15 years of follow-up. Knee. 2019;26(5):1111–6.
57. Greco NJ, Lombardi AV Jr, Hurst JM, Morris MJ, Berend KR. Medial Unicompartmental Knee Arthroplasty for the Treatment of Focal Femoral Osteonecrosis. J Bone Joint Surg Am. 2019;101(12):1077–84.
58. Tarumi E, Nakagawa Y, Mukai S, Yabumoto H, Nakamura T. The clinical outcomes and the ability to sit straight in the Japanese style following high tibial osteotomy combined with osteochondral autologous transfer for osteonecrosis of the medial femoral condyle. J Orthop Sci. 2019;24(1):136–41.
59. Chalmers BP, Mehrotra KG, Sierra RJ, Pagnano MW, Taunton MJ, Abdel MP. Reliable outcomes and survivorship of primary total knee arthroplasty for osteonecrosis of the knee. Bone Joint J. 2019;101-B(11):1356–61.
60. Early S, Tírico LEP, Pulido PA, McCauley JC, Bugbee WD. Long-Term Retrospective Follow-Up of Fresh Osteochondral Allograft Transplantation for Steroid-Associated Osteonecrosis of the Femoral Condyles artilage. 2018;31:1947603518809399. https://doi.org/10.1177/1947603518809399.
61. Mont MA, Rifai A, Baumgarten KM, Sheldon M, Hungerford DS. Total knee arthroplasty for osteonecrosis. J Bone Joint Surg Am. 2002;84(4):599–603.
62. Akamatsu Y, Kobayashi H, Kusayama Y, Aratake M, Kumagai K, Saito T. Predictive factors for the progression of spontaneous osteonecrosis of the knee. Knee Surg Sports Traumatol Arthrosc. 2017;25(2):477–84.
63. Nakayama H, Iseki T, Kanto R, Daimon T, Kashiwa K, Yoshiya S. Analysis of risk factors for poor prognosis in conservatively managed early-stage spontaneous osteonecrosis of the knee. Knee. 2016;23(1):25–8.
64. Juréus J, Lindstrand A, Geijer M, Robertsson O, Tägil M. The natural course of spontaneous osteonecrosis of the knee (SPONK): a 1- to 27-year follow-up of 40 patients. Acta Orthop. 2013;84(4):410–4.
65. Nakamura J, Harada Y, Oinuma K, Iida S, Kishida S, Takahashi K. Spontaneous repair of asymptomatic osteonecrosis associated with corticosteroid therapy systemic lupus erythematosus: 10-year minimum follow-up with MRI. Lupus. 2010;19(11):1307–14.
66. Takao M, Sugano N, Nishii T, Miki H, Yoshikawa H. Spontaneous regression of steroid-related osteonecrosis of the knee. Clin Orthop Relat Res. 2006;452:210–5.
67. Satku K, Kumar VP, Chong SM, Thambyah A. The natural history of spontaneous osteonecrosis of the medial tibial plateau. J Bone Joint Surg Br. 2003;85(7):983–8.
68. Oinuma K, Harada Y, Nawata Y, Takabayashi K, Abe I, Kamikawa K, Moriya H. Osteonecrosis in patients with systemic lupus erythematosus develops very early after starting high dose corticosteroid treatment. Ann Rheum Dis. 2001;60(12):1145–8.

Chapter 48
Chondral Disruption of the Knee

A condition whereby there is disruption of the articular cartilage of the knee. This may be described in various ways as below:

According to the Extent of Articular Cartilage Involvement

- Localised
- Diffuse

According to the Anatomical Location of Such Disruption

- Femoral condyle
- Femoral trochlea
- Tibial plateau
- Patellar
- Combined
- Weightbearing vs. non-weightbearing area

According to the Thickness of Articular Cartilage Disruption

- Partial thickness
- Full thickness—not involving bone
- Full thickness—involving subchondral bone

According to the Stability of the Disrupted Cartilage

- Stable
- Unstable
- Loose body

According to the Appearance of the Articular Cartilage Damage

- Fibrillations/crevices/cracks
- Flaps
- Cartilage loss with bone exposed

C. Panayiotou Charalambous, *The Knee Made Easy*,
https://doi.org/10.1007/978-3-030-54506-2_48

According to the Shape of the Articular Cartilage Damage

- Circular
- Rectangular
- Oval
- Other

According to the Walls of the Articular Cartilage Defect

- Fully contained
- Partially contained
- Non-contained (open)

48.1 Causes of Cartilage Loss

- Acute trauma—shear forces, compressive forces through cartilage/subchondral bone
- Chronic, repeated minor trauma
- Infection
- Joint immobilisation
- Instability—leading to abnormal cartilage loading, with some areas overloaded at the expense of others
- Malalignment—leading to abnormal cartilage loading, with some areas overloaded at the expense of others

Damage may be initially microscopic to the cartilage cells and extracellular matrix, but as it progresses it can lead to a chondral fracture short of the subchondral bone or a chondral fracture reaching the subchondral bone.

48.2 Classification of Chondral Disruption

48.2.1 Outerbridge Classification of Chondral Dysfunction

The Outerbridge classification [1, 2] (initially described for chondral defects of the patella) is frequently utilised:

- Grade 0—normal
- Grade I—cartilage with softening and swelling
- Grade II—a partial-thickness defect with fissures on the surface that do not reach the subchondral bone or exceed 1.5 cm in diameter
- Grade III—fissuring to the level of the subchondral bone in an area with a diameter more than 1.5 cm
- Grade IV—exposed subchondral bone

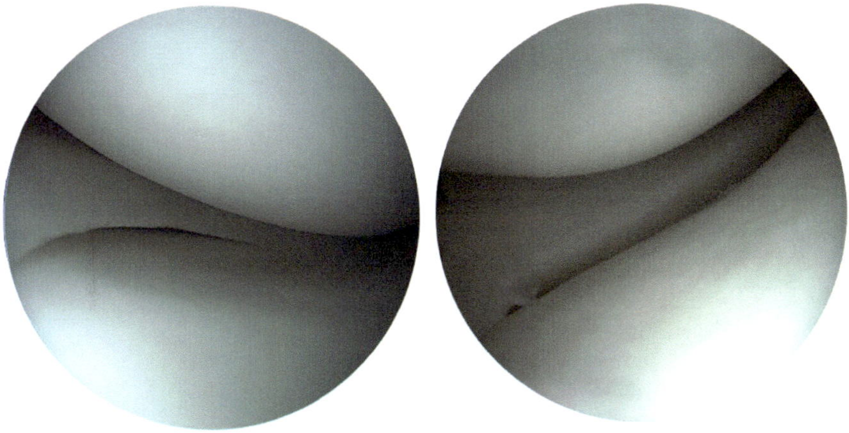

Intact articular cartilage

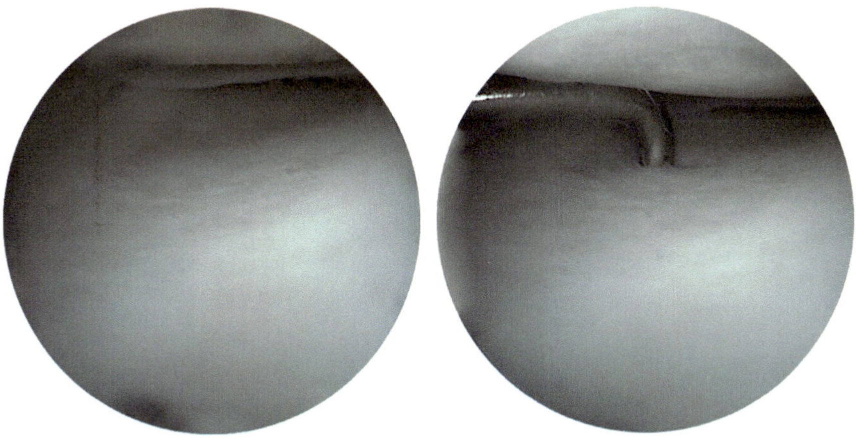

Grade I

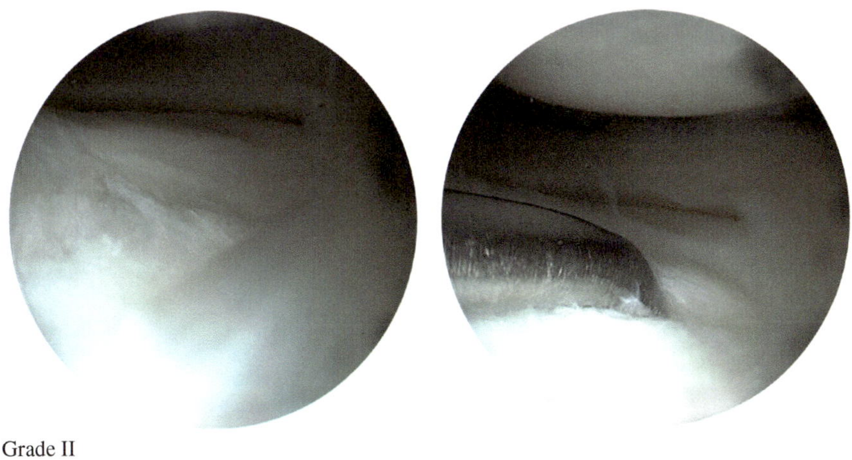

Grade II

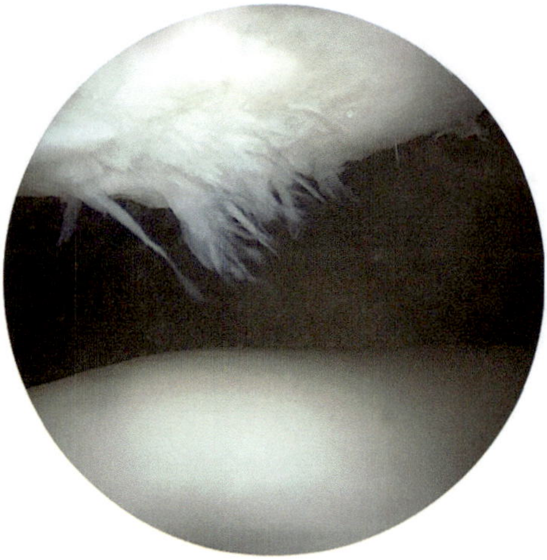

Grade III

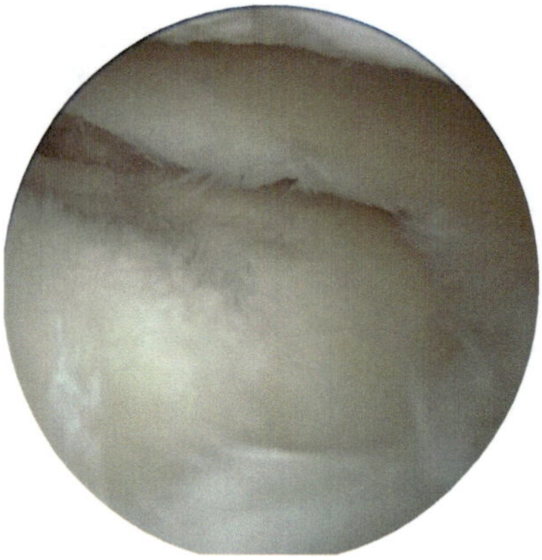

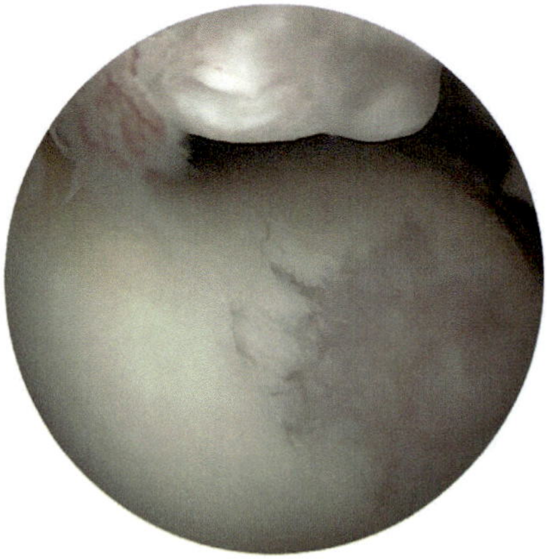

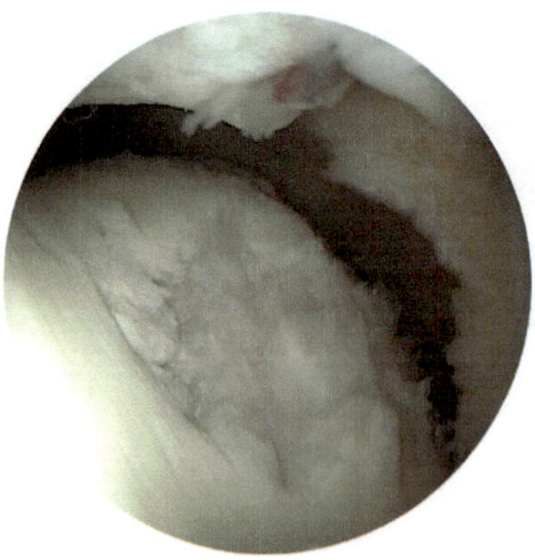

Grade IV

48.3 Demographics of Articular Cartilage Disruption [2–6]

In a study of 25,124 knee arthroscopies performed from 1989 to 2004 the following were reported [3]:

- Chondral lesions—in 60% of cases
- Type of chondral lesion
  - Localized focal osteochondral or chondral lesion—67%
  - Osteoarthritis—29%
  - Osteochondritis dissecans—2%
  - Other—1%
- Of the lesions—isolated lesion—30%
- Location of the cartilage lesion
  - Patellar articular surface—36%
  - Medial femoral condyle –34%
- Severity of cartilage lesion
  - Grade 2 (Outerbridge classification) most frequent—42%
- Associated articular lesions
  - Medial meniscus tear—37%
  - Anterior cruciate ligament (ACL) tear—36%
- Cases with 1 to 3 localized grade III and IV cartilage lesions in individuals under 40 years old—in 7%

Amongst 508 primary ACL tear cases, the following rates of severe chondral lesions (Outerbridge grades 3 or 4) were observed at the time of reconstruction [4]:

- Medial femoral condyle—10%
- Lateral femoral condyle—5%
- Medial tibial plateau—1%
- Lateral tibial plateau—3%
- Patellar—7%
- Trochlear—3%

A systematic review of studies investigating the incidence of articular cartilage injury in association with acute ACL tears [5] reported this to be between 16% and 46%.

48.4 Clinical Symptoms of Articular Cartilage Disruption

- Deep seated knee pain—localised/diffuse
- Painful knee motion

- Pain is worse on loading the patella in flexion such as in squatting, prolonged sitting, kneeling, going up and down stairs
- Loss of motion
- Intermittent swelling (effusion/synovitis)
- Abnormal knee noise (clicking/clunking)
- Locking (apparent/true if loose bodies)

48.5 Clinical Signs of Articular Cartilage disruption [6, 7]

- Muscle atrophy—related to disuse
- Diffuse knee swelling/effusion
- Femoral/tibial condyle or patellar tenderness
- Associated malalignment—varus/valgus deformity, flexion deformity
- Loss of knee motion
  - Apparent due to pain
  - True stiffness
- Knee muscle weakness

48.6 Investigations for Articular Cartilage Disruption

- Plain radiographs:
  - AP, lateral, skyline, notch view
  - Long leg film to assess alignment
- MRI
  - Define the location, size and shape of chondral disruption
  - Determine the presence of associated subchondral fluid
  - Evaluate the presence of loose, detached fragments

48.7 Management of Localised Chondral Disruption

48.7.1 Non-surgical [8–10]

- Leave alone
- Activity modification

- Simple analgesia
- Physiotherapy to:
  - Strengthen the periarticular muscles of the knee
  - Maintain active motion
  - Stretch contracted soft tissues to regain lost motion
- Knee injections—steroid, viscosupplementation, PRP

48.7.2 Surgical [11–22]

- Arthroscopic debridement of partial or full thickness lesions
- Removal of loose bodies
- Surgical fixation of acute osteochondral lesions
- Resurfacing procedures for chronic full thickness lesions:
  - Microfracture
  - Microfracture with artificial scaffold coverage
  - Autologous chondrocyte implantation (ACI)
  - Matrix autologous chondrocyte implantation (MACI)
  - Osteochondral grafting (autograft/allograft)
  - Metal button replacement (contoured focal articular femoral condyle resurfacing)
- Realignment procedures (osteotomy) to offload the area of chondral disruption:
  - Distal femoral
  - Proximal tibial
- Knee replacement arthroplasty
  - Unicompartmental
    - Medial
    - Lateral
    - Patellofemoral (PF)
  - Bicompartmental
  - Total (with or without patellar resurfacing)

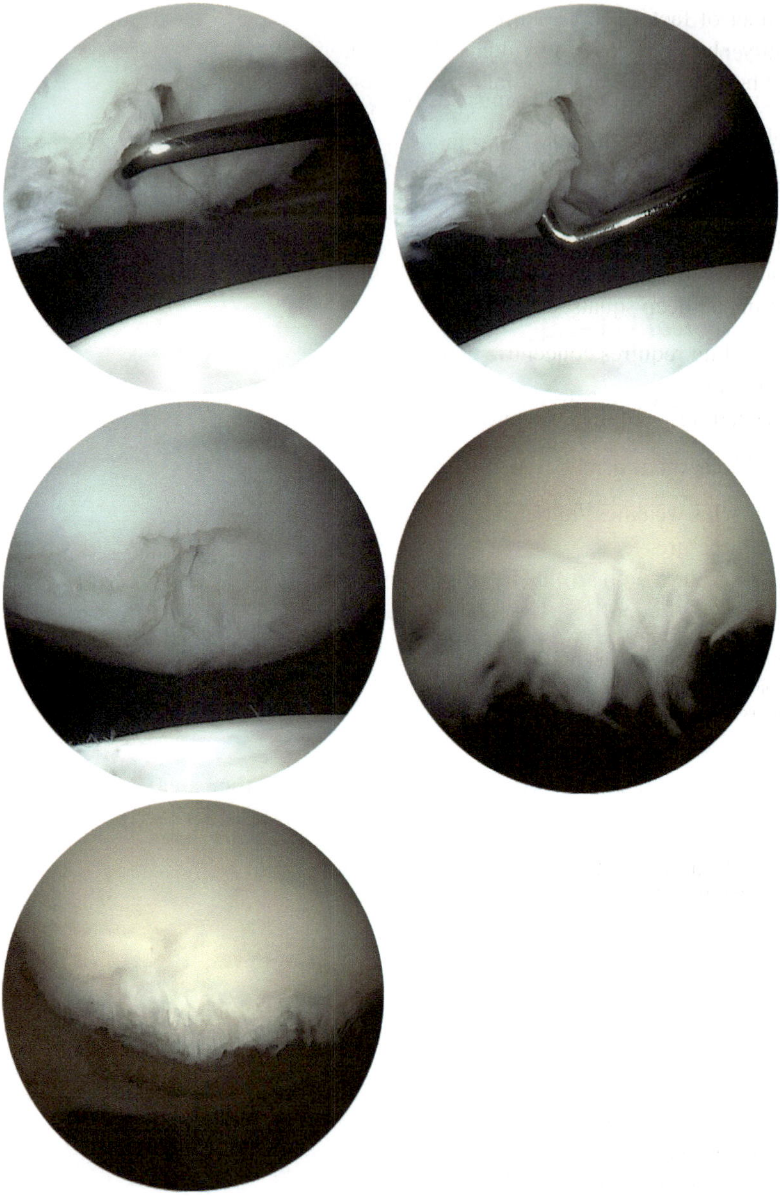

Patellar chondral disruption, debribed to stable margins

Learning Pearls

- The size of the lesion may guide as to the resurfacing procedure to be used [12–14]:

  - <2.5 cm^2 microfracture—larger defects may increase subchondral contact and pressures predisposing to failure
  - <4 cm^2—ACI
  - >4cm^2—osteochondral grafting

- Randomised trials have shown similar outcomes following microfracture versus chondrocyte transplantation [15–17]
- Cartilage restoration techniques are avoided in:
  - Inflammatory arthropathy
  - Instability
  - Joint malalignment
  - Kissing lesions (this refers to a similar lesion present on opposing articular surfaces)
  - Infection
- Presence of joint space narrowing, osteophytes, subchondral cyst formation or subchondral sclerosis are indicative of joint degeneration, and hence they are relative contraindications for the isolated treatment of chondral disruption
- The results of microfracture may be:
  - Better in those younger than 14
  - Deteriorate after 18 months
- Ligament instability or malalignment may need to be addressed along with cartilage resurfacing using an unloading or a stabilisation procedure
- In dealing with PF defects, osteochondral grafting has poor results due to the differential thickness between the donor and recipient site and also due to the shape of the patellar facets

References

1. Outerbridge RE. Further studies on the etiology of chondromalacia patellae. J Bone Joint Surg Br. 1964;46:179–90.
2. Outerbridge RE. The etiology of chondromalacia patellae. J Bone Joint Surg Br. 1961;43-B:752–7.
3. Widuchowski W, Widuchowski J, Trzaska T. Articular cartilage defects: study of 25,124 knee arthroscopies. Knee. 2007;14(3):177–82.
4. Borchers JR, Kaeding CC, Pedroza AD, Huston LJ, Spindler KP, Wright RW, MOON Consortium and the MARS study group. Intra-articular findings in primary and revision anterior cruciate ligament reconstruction surgery: a comparison of the MOON and MARS study groups. Am J Sports Med. 2011;39(9):1889–93.
5. Brophy RH, Zeltser D, Wright RW, Flanigan D. Anterior cruciate ligament reconstruction and concomitant articular cartilage injury: incidence and treatment. Arthroscopy. 2010;26(1):112–20.

6. Logerstedt DS, Scalzitti DA, Bennell KL, Hinman RS, Silvers-Granelli H, Ebert J, Hambly K, Carey JL, Snyder-Mackler L, Axe MJ, McDonough CM. Knee pain and mobility impairments: meniscal and articular cartilage lesions revision 2018. J Orthop Sports Phys Ther. 2018;48(2):A1–A50.
7. Wang HJ, Ao YF, Jiang D, Gong X, Wang YJ, Wang J, Yu JK. Relationship between quadriceps strength and patellofemoral joint chondral lesions after anterior cruciate ligament reconstruction. Am J Sports Med. 2015;43(9):2286–92.
8. Wilk KE, Briem K, Reinold MM, Devine KM, Dugas J, Andrews JR. Rehabilitation of articular lesions in the athlete's knee. J Orthop Sports Phys Ther. 2006;36(10):815–27.
9. Gobbi A, Karnatzikos G, Kumar A. Long-term results after microfracture treatment for full-thickness knee chondral lesions in athletes. Knee Surg Sports Traumatol Arthrosc. 2014;22(9):1986–96.
10. Benthien JP, Behrens P. Autologous matrix-induced Chondrogenesis (AMIC): combining microfracturing and a collagen I/III matrix for articular cartilage resurfacing. Cartilage. 2010;1(1):65–8.
11. Steinwachs MR, Gille J, Volz M, Anders S, Jakob R, De Girolamo L, Volpi P, Schiavone-Panni A, Scheffler S, Reiss E, Wittmann U. Systematic review and meta-analysis of the clinical evidence on the use of autologous matrix-induced Chondrogenesis in the knee. Cartilage. 2019;11:1947603519870846. https://doi.org/10.1177/1947603519870846.
12. Gao L, Orth P, Cucchiarini M, Madry H. Autologous matrix-induced Chondrogenesis: a systematic review of the clinical evidence. Am J Sports Med. 2019;47(1):222–31.
13. Karataglis D, Green MA, Learmonth DJ. Autologous osteochondral transplantation for the treatment of chondral defects of the knee. Knee. 2006;13(1):32–5.
14. Solheim E, Hegna J, Øyen J, Harlem T, Strand T. Results at 10 to 14 years after osteochondral autografting (mosaicplasty) in articular cartilage defects in the knee. Knee. 2013;20(4):287–90.
15. Familiari F, Cinque ME, Chahla J, Godin JA, Olesen ML, Moatshe G, LaPrade RF. Clinical outcomes and failure rates of osteochondral allograft transplantation in the knee: a systematic review. Am J Sports Med. 2018;46(14):3541–9.
16. Richardson JB, Caterson B, Evans EH, Ashton BA, Roberts S. Repair of human articular cartilage after implantation of autologous chondrocytes. J Bone Joint Surg Br. 1999;81(6):1064–8.
17. Biant LC, Bentley G, Vijayan S, Skinner JA, Carrington RW. Long-term results of autologous chondrocyte implantation in the knee for chronic chondral and osteochondral defects. Am J Sports Med. 2014;42(9):2178–83.
18. Nawaz SZ, Bentley G, Briggs TW, Carrington RW, Skinner JA, Gallagher KR, Dhinsa BS. Autologous chondrocyte implantation in the knee: mid-term to long-term results. J Bone Joint Surg Am. 2014;96(10):824–30.
19. Bartlett W, Skinner JA, Gooding CR, Carrington RW, Flanagan AM, Briggs TW, Bentley G. Autologous chondrocyte implantation versus matrix-induced autologous chondrocyte implantation for osteochondral defects of the knee: a prospective, randomised study. J Bone Joint Surg Br. 2005;87(5):640–5.
20. Ebert JR, Schneider A, Fallon M, Wood DJ. Es GC. A comparison of 2-year outcomes in patients undergoing tibiofemoral or patellofemoral matrix-induced autologous chondrocyte implantation. Am J Sports Med. 2017;45(14):3243–53.
21. Schlechter JA, Nguyen SV, Fletcher KL. Utility of Bioabsorbable Fixation of Osteochondral Lesions in the Adolescent Knee: Outcomes Analysis With Minimum 2-Year Follow-up. Orthop J Sports Med. 2019;7(10):2325967119876896. https://doi.org/10.1177/2325967119876896.
22. Zamborsky R, Danisovic L. Surgical techniques for knee cartilage repair: an updated large-scale systematic review and network meta-analysis of randomized controlled trials. Arthroscopy. 2020;36(3):845–58.

Chapter 49
Osteochondritis Dissecans of the Knee

Osteochondritis dissecans (OCD) is a condition whereby there is localised dysfunction of the subchondral bone leading to detachment of part of the subchondral bone along with its overlying cartilage. It may be viewed as a fracture with an osteochondral fragment (subchondral bone plus cartilage) [1–7].

49.1 Demographics of Osteochondritis Dissecans [8, 9]

- More common in adolescence, but may occur at any age
- More common in males as compared to females
- Can involve any area of the knee (femur, tibia, patella) but the lateral (weightbearing) part of the medial femoral condyle is most commonly involved (about 85% of cases)
- 20 to 30% bilateral

49.2 Pathogenesis of Osteochondritis Dissecans

Several theories have been proposed including [10–12]:

- Compromise of the vascular supply of the subchondral bone
- Micro-splits in the articular cartilage (due to acute trauma or chronic overload) which allow the escape of synovial fluid into the subchondral bone
- Ischemia (vascular spasm, fat emboli, infection or thrombosis) leading to bone necrosis
- Trauma leading to subchondral fracture and resultant necrosis of the adjacent subchondral bone
  - Acute trauma
  - Repetitive trauma

C. Panayiotou Charalambous, *The Knee Made Easy*,
https://doi.org/10.1007/978-3-030-54506-2_49

    - Repetitive contact/impingement between the tibial spine and medial femoral condyle with internal rotation of the tibia—more likely in narrow femoral notch
- Abnormal ossification of the growing bones—physeal irregularities
  - Impaired cartilage blood supply, chondronecrosis and impaired ossification
- Underlying genetic predisposition

49.3 Clinical Symptoms of Osteochondritis Dissecans

- Deep seated knee pain
- Painful knee motion
- Loss of motion
- Intermittent swelling
- Abnormal knee noise (clicking/clunking)
- Locking (apparent/true if loose bodies)

49.4 Clinical Signs of Osteochondritis Dissecans

- Muscle atrophy—related to disuse
- Localised tenderness of involved area (medial femoral condyle easier to palpate in flexion)
- Knee effusion/synovitis
- Associated malalignment—varus/valgus deformity, flexion deformity
- Loss of knee motion
  - Apparent due to pain
  - True stiffness
- Walking with leg in external rotation to minimise impingement (and hence resultant pain) between the medial tibial spine and lateral part of the medial femoral condyle where lesion is often located
- Internal rotation of the tibia during knee extension from 90° to 30° of flexion, reproduces pain. The pain is relieved by externally rotating the tibia (Wilson's test). Although absent in most patients with medial femoral condyle OCD, if present it may signify resolution of the lesion when the test becomes negative [12, 13]
- Knee weakness if associated quadriceps or other periarticular muscle atrophy

49.5 Investigations for Osteochondritis Dissecans

- Plain radiographs:
  - AP and lateral radiographs
  - Notch view—allows better evaluation of the medial femoral condyle
  - Long leg film to assess alignment

- MRI
  - To define the location, size and stability of the lesion
  - Determine the presence of associated subchondral fluid
  - Evaluate the presence of loose, detached fragments
- Arthroscopic evaluation of fragment stability

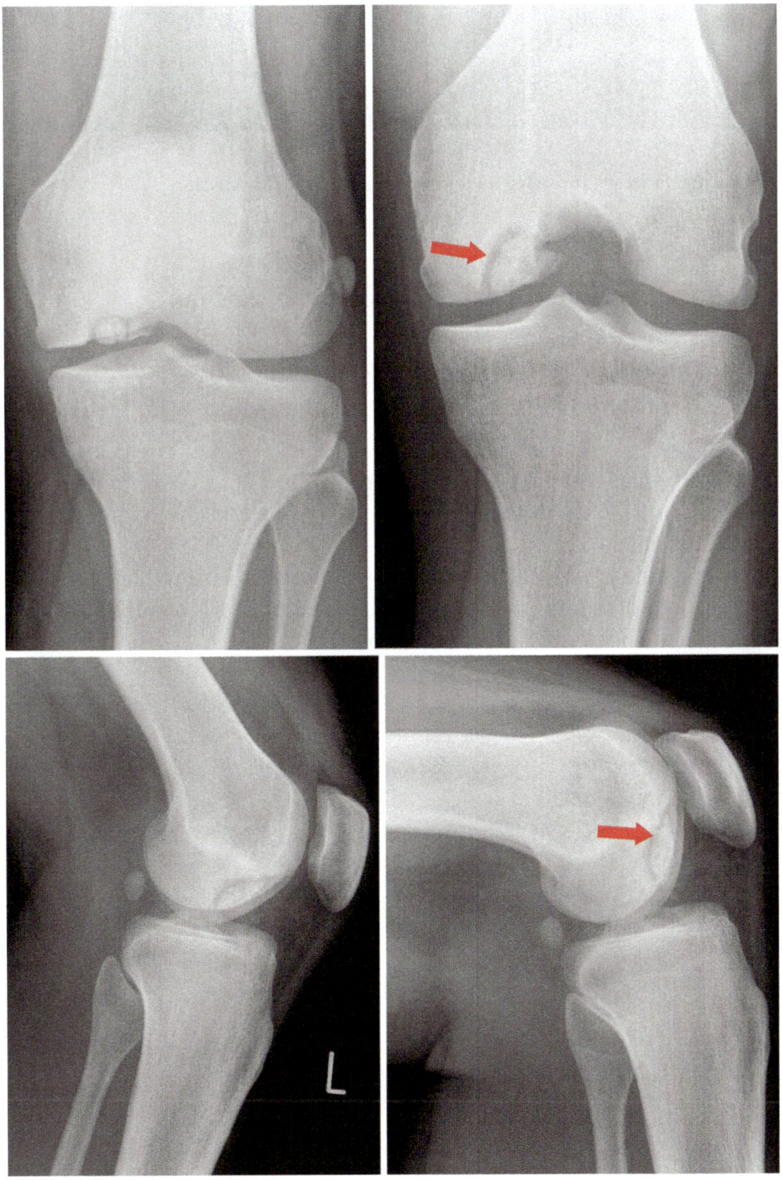

Osteochondritis dissecans of the medial femoral condyle (red arrow), more evident in the notch view

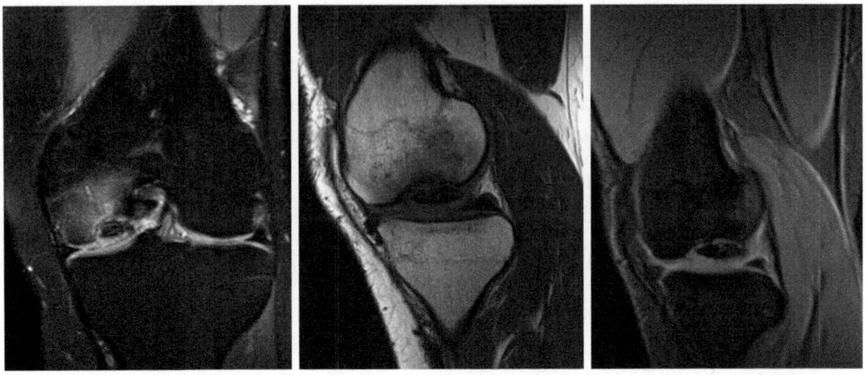

Osteochondritis dissecans involving the medial femoral condyle (MRI)

49.6 Classification of Osteochondritis Dissecans

49.6.1 Dipaola MRI Classification of Osteochondritis Dissecans [14]

- I Articular cartilage is thickened but intact
- II Articular cartilage is breached; low signal rim behind the fragment indicates fibrous attachment
- III Articular cartilage is breached; high signal (equal to that of fluid) behind the fragment indicates loss of attachment and presence of synovial fluid between fragment and underlying subchondral bone
- IV Formation of loose bodies

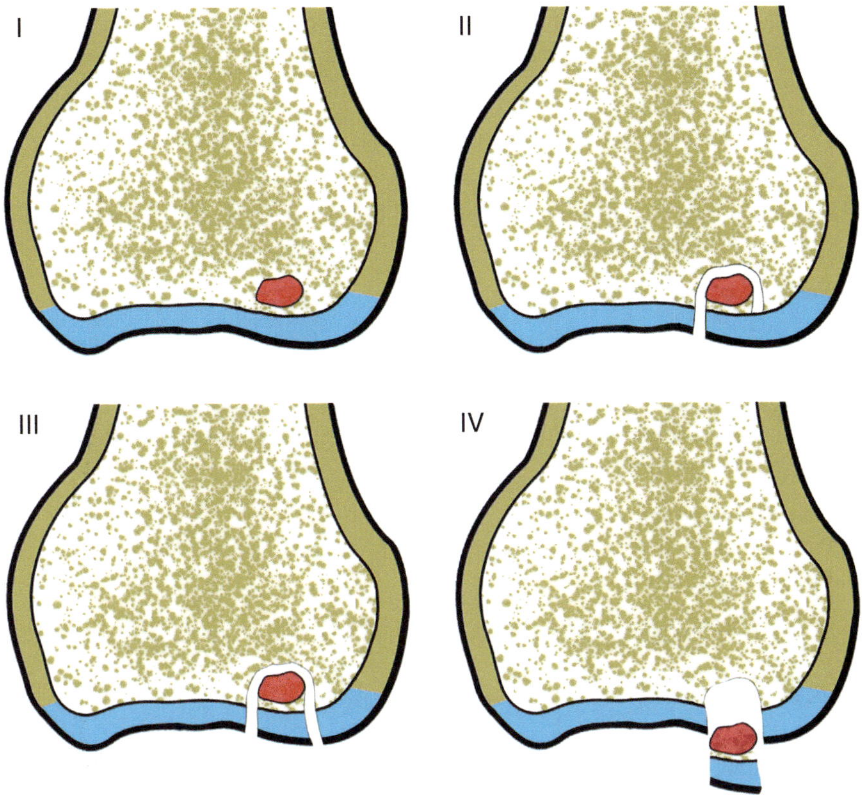

Dipaola classification of OCD

These findings may guide as to the stability of the lesion [14–17].

- Stable lesions—Stages I and II
- Unstable lesions—there is fluid between the surrounding subchondral bone and detached fragment

49.6.2 Macroscopic (Arthroscopic) ICRS Classification [18]

1. Cartilage intact but softened
2. Partial discontinuity of cartilage and stable on probing
3. Complete discontinuity, unstable on probing, but in situ—"dead in situ"

4. Displaced fragment (loose within bed or loose body)

49.7 Management of Osteochondritis Dissecans

Management may be non-surgical or surgical [17, 19–34].

Some of the factors to consider in choosing management are:

- Presence of open/closed physes
  - OCD lesions in the presence of open physes have a high rate of successful management and healing with non-surgical treatment.
  - OCD lesions in the presence of closed physes have a low rate of successful management with non-surgical treatment and in these surgery may be considered at an earlier stage.
- Clinical symptoms
- Patient compliance
- Fragment stability

49.7.1 Non-surgical

- Leave alone
- Simple analgesia
- Activity modification—guided by pain, avoid impact activities but maintain range of motion and muscle bulk
- Physiotherapy to:
  - Strengthen the periarticular muscles of the knee
  - Maintain motion-active
  - Stretch contracted soft tissues to regain motion

49.7.2 Surgical

- If lesion in situ:
  - Subchondral drilling (antegrade/retrograde)
  - Fix in situ—smooth pins
- If lesion is loose/detached—reposition and fix (if technically feasible)
- If lesion is loose-detached and cannot be repositioned and fixed then:
  - Removal of loose fragment, defect debridement and management as for chondral disruption:
  - Resurfacing ± re-alignment procedure ± stabilisation procedure

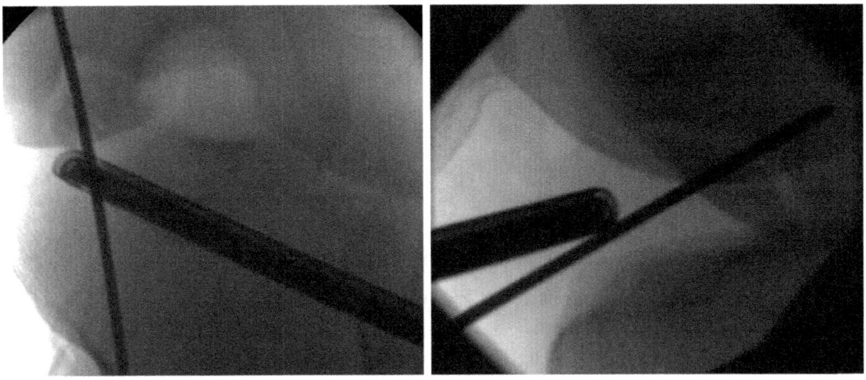

Drilling of an osteochondritis dissecans lesion involving the medial femoral condyle (intra-operative screening)

49.8 Natural History of Osteochondritis Dissecans [35–37]

Poor prognosis is associated with:

- Closed physes
- Older than 20 age
- Unstable lesion

Hevesi M et al. [35] looked at the outcomes of OCD in 95 skeletally immature patients (70 male, 25 female, mean age 12.5 ± 2.0 years) followed for a mean of 14 years (range, 2–40 years). Of these, 53 were managed surgically and 42 non-surgically. At final follow-up, 13(14%) reported persistent knee pain (8 treated surgically vs. 5 treated non-surgically). Risk factors for ongoing knee pain were female sex, patellar lesions, and unstable lesions.

- 4 cases (8%) treated surgically and 2 cases (5%) treated non-surgically developed symptomatic osteoarthritis at a mean of 28.6 years
- OCD cases had a total knee replacement arthroplasty (TKR) at a mean age of 52 years, younger than the rest of their institution's population.

Sanders TL et al. [37] looked at 86 patients (mean age 21.4 years) with OCD lesions treated non-surgically. At a mean ± SD follow-up of 12.6 ± 9.8 years from diagnosis, 13 patients (15%) were diagnosed with arthritis. This corresponded to a cumulative incidence of 5% at 5 years, 10% at 10 years, 20% at 25 years, and 30% at 35 years. The cumulative incidence of replacement arthroplasty was 1% at 5 years, 3% at 10 years, 8% at 25 years, and 8% at 35 years. BMI greater than 25 kg/m^2, patellar lesions, and diagnosis as an adult, were associated with an increased risk of arthritis.

Learning Pearls

- Management of OCD may be considered similar to that of a fracture, and hence similar principles may be applied in their management (non-surgical or surgical).
- Non-surgical management may vary from casting and non-weightbearing to free mobilisation of the knee with full weightbearing but limiting high impact and high demand activities. There is no convincing evidence as to which approach is more superior. The pain level and potential patient's compliance may guide as to which approach to use.
- Some OCD cases seen with closed physes may have arisen prior to physeal closure, but some may arise following physeal closure

References

1. Shea KG, Richmond CG, Ganley TJ. Osteochondritis Dissecans in the Skeletally Immature Knee. Instr Course Lect. 2018;67:403–12.
2. Masquijo J, Kothari A. Juvenile osteochondritis dissecans (JOCD) of the knee: current concepts review. EFORT Open Rev. 2019;4(5):201–12.
3. Andriolo L, Crawford DC, Reale D, Zaffagnini S, Candrian C, Cavicchioli A, Filardo G. Osteochondritis dissecans of the knee: etiology and pathogenetic mechanisms. A Systematic Review Cartilage. 2018;1:1947603518786557–290. https://doi.org/10.1177/1947603518786557.
4. Price MJ, Tuca M, Nguyen J, Silberman J, Luderowski E, Uppstrom TJ, Green DW. Juvenile osteochondritis Dissecans of the trochlea: a cohort study of 34 trochlear lesions associated with sporting activities that load the patellofemoral joint. J Pediatr Orthop. 2018;16:103–9. https://doi.org/10.1097/BPO.0000000000001174.
5. Bruns J, Werner M, Habermann C. Osteochondritis Dissecans: etiology, pathology, and imaging with a special focus on the knee joint. Cartilage. 2018;9(4):346–62.
6. Heyworth BE, Kocher MS. Dissecans of the Knee. JBJS Rev. 2015;3(7) https://doi.org/10.2106/JBJS.RVW.N.00095Osteochondritis.
7. Årøen A. OCD: an unsolved puzzle in articular cartilage problems. Osteoarthr Cartil. 2018;26(12):1573–4.
8. Weiss JM, Shea KG, Jacobs JC Jr, Cannamela PC, Becker I, Portman M, Kessler JI. Incidence of osteochondritis Dissecans in adults. Am J Sports Med. 2018;46(7):1592–5.
9. Pareek A, Sanders TL, Wu IT, Larson DR, Saris DBF, Krych AJ. Incidence of symptomatic osteochondritis dissecans lesions of the knee: a population-based study in Olmsted County. Osteoarthr Cartil. 2017;25(10):1663–71.
10. Markolf KL, Du PZ, McAllister DR. Contact force between the tibial spine and medial femoral condyle: A biomechanical study. Clin Biomech. 2018;60:9–12.
11. Olstad K, Shea KG, Cannamela PC, Polousky JD, Ekman S, Ytrehus B, Carlson CS. Juvenile osteochondritis dissecans of the knee is a result of failure of the blood supply to growth cartilage and osteochondrosis. Osteoarthr Cartil. 2018;26(12):1691–8.
12. Chow RM, Guzman MS, Dao Q. Intercondylar notch width as a risk factor for medial femoral condyle osteochondritis Dissecans in skeletally immature patients. J Pediatr Orthop. 2016;36(6):640–4.
13. Wilson JN. A diagnostic sign in osteochondritis dissecans of the knee. J Bone Joint Surg Am. 1967;49(3):477–80.

14. Conrad JM, Stanitski CL. Osteochondritis dissecans: Wilson's sign revisited. Am J Sports Med. 2003;31(5):777–8.
15. Dipaola JD, Nelson DW, Colville MR. Characterizing osteo-chondral lesions by magnetic resonance imaging. Arthroscopy. 1991;7:101–4.
16. Quatman CE, Quatman-Yates CC, Schmitt LC, Paterno MV. The clinical utility and diagnostic performance of MRI for identification and classification of knee osteochondritis dissecans. J Bone Joint Surg Am. 2012;94(11):1036–44.
17. De Smet AA, Ilahi OA, Graf BK. Untreated osteochondritis dissecans of the femoral condyles: prediction of patient outcome using radiographic and MR findings. Skelet Radiol. 1997;26(8):463–7.
18. Dwyer T, Tin CR, Kendra R, Sermer C, Chahal J, Ogilvie-Harris D, Whelan D, Murnaghan L, Nauth A, Theodoropoulos J. Reliability and validity of the arthroscopic international cartilage repair society classification system: correlation with histological assessment of depth. Arthroscopy. 2017;33(6):1219–24.
19. Jones MH, Williams AM. Osteochondritis dissecans of the knee: a practical guide for surgeons. Bone Joint J. 2016;98-B(6):723–9.
20. Andriolo L, Candrian C, Papio T, Cavicchioli A, Perdisa F, Filardo G. Osteochondritis Dissecans of the knee - conservative treatment strategies: a systematic review. Cartilage. 2019;10(3):267–77.
21. Cahill BR, Ahten SM. The three critical components in the conservative treatment of juvenile osteochondritis dissecans (JOCD). Physician, parent, and child. Clin Sports Med. 2001;20(2):287–98.
22. Aglietti P, Buzzi R, Bassi PB, Fioriti M. Arthroscopic drilling in juvenile osteochondritis dissecans of the medial femoral condyle. Arthroscopy. 1994;10(3):286–91.
23. Anderson AF, Richards DB, Pagnani MJ. Hovis WD Antegrade drilling for osteochondritis dissecans of the knee. Arthroscopy. 1997;13(3):319–24.
24. Nuelle CW, Farr J. Internal fixation of osteochondritis Dissecans lesions in the patellofemoral joint. J Knee Surg. 2018;31(3):206–11.
25. Kouzelis A, Plessas S, Papadopoulos AX, Gliatis I, Lambiris E. Herbert screw fixation and reverse guided drillings, for treatment of types III and IV osteochondritis dissecans. Knee Surg Sports Traumatol Arthrosc. 2006;14(1):70–5.
26. Herring MJ, Knudsen ML, Macalena JA. Open Reduction, Bone Grafting, and Internal Fixation of Osteochondritis Dissecans Lesion of the Knee. JBJS Essent Surg Tech. 2019;9(3):e23. https://doi.org/10.2106/JBJS.ST.18.00035.
27. Randsborg PH, Kjennvold S, Røtterud JH. Arthroscopic Fixation of Osteochondritis Dissecans of the Knee Using a Motorized Pick and Headless Compression Screws. Arthrosc Tech. 2019;8(10):e1115–20. https://doi.org/10.1016/j.eats.2019.05.031.
28. Schlechter JA, Nguyen SV, Fletcher KL. Utility of Bioabsorbable Fixation of Osteochondral Lesions in the Adolescent Knee: Outcomes Analysis With Minimum 2-Year Follow-up. Orthop J Sports Med. 2019;7(10):2325967119876896. https://doi.org/10.1177/2325967119876896.
29. Wang K, Waterman B, Dean R, Redondo M, Cotter E, Manning B, Yanke A, Cole B. The Influence of Physeal Status on Rate of Reoperation After Arthroscopic Screw Fixation for Symptomatic Osteochondritis Dissecans of the Knee. Arthroscopy. 2019. pii: S0749–8063(19)30797–2
30. Leland DP, Bernard CD, Camp CL, Nakamura N, Saris DBF, Krych AJ. Does internal fixation for unstable osteochondritis dissecans of the skeletally mature knee work? A Systematic Review Arthroscopy. 2019;35(8):2512–22.
31. Sacolick DA, Kirven JC, Abouljoud MM, Everhart JS, Flanigan DC. The treatment of adult osteochondritis Dissecans with autologous cartilage implantation: a systematic review. J Knee Surg. 2019;32(11):1102–10.
32. Roffi A, Andriolo L, Ditino A, Balboni F, Papio T, Zaffagnini S, Filardo G. Long-term results of matrix-assisted autologous chondrocyte transplantation combined with autologous bone grafting for the treatment of juvenile osteochondritis Dissecans. J Pediatr Orthop. 2020;40(2):e115–21. https://doi.org/10.1097/BPO.0000000000001404.

33. Jones KJ, Cash BM, Arshi A, Williams RJ 3rd. Fresh Osteochondral Allograft Transplantation for Uncontained, Elongated Osteochondritis Dissecans Lesions of the Medial Femoral Condyle. Arthrosc Tech. 2019;8(3):e267–73.
34. Filardo G, Andriolo L, Soler F, Berruto M, Ferrua P, Verdonk P, Rongieras F, Crawford DC. Treatment of unstable knee osteochondritis dissecans in the young adult: results and limitations of surgical strategies-the advantages of allografts to address an osteochondral challenge. Knee Surg Sports Traumatol Arthrosc. 2019;27(6):1726–38.
35. Hevesi M, Sanders TL, Pareek A, Milbrandt TA, Levy BA, Stuart MJ, Saris DBF, Krych AJ. Osteochondritis Dissecans in the knee of skeletally immature patients: rates of persistent pain, osteoarthritis, and arthroplasty at mean 14-Years' follow-up. Cartilage. 2018;1:1947603518786545–299. https://doi.org/10.1177/1947603518786545.
36. Ananthaharan A, Randsborg PH. Epidemiology and patient-reported outcome after juvenile osteochondritis dissecans in the knee. Knee. 2018;25(4):595–601.
37. Sanders TL, Pareek A, Johnson NR, Carey JL, Maak TG, Stuart MJ, Krych AJ. Nonoperative Management of Osteochondritis Dissecans of the Knee: Progression to Osteoarthritis and Arthroplasty at Mean 13-Year Follow-up. Orthop J Sports Med. 2017;5(7):2325967117704644. https://doi.org/10.1177/2325967117704644.

Chapter 50
Knee Arthritis

Several types of arthritis may affect the knee joint [1–23]. These include:

- *Osteoarthritis (OA)*—condition whereby there is degeneration of the articular cartilage of the knee joint
- *Inflammatory arthritis*—condition whereby there is destruction of the articular cartilage of the knee joint due to an inflammatory process. Causes include:
  - Sero-positive arthritis—rheumatoid arthritis
  - Sero-negative arthritis (e.g. psoriatic)
  - Crystal arthropathy (gout, pseudogout)
  - Infective arthritis
  - Reactive arthritis
- *Neurogenic arthropathy*—condition whereby there is degeneration of the articular cartilage of the knee joint associated with a loss of sensory innervation of the affected limb

  OA is considered next.

50.1 Osteoarthritis Compartment Involvement

This may be limited to one compartments or involve multiple compartments. The medial compartment is most frequently affected, with lower rates of involvement of the lateral and patellofemoral (PF) compartments.

Felson et al. [8] looked at knees with radiographic OA in individuals from the USA and China and reported:

C. Panayiotou Charalambous, *The Knee Made Easy*,
https://doi.org/10.1007/978-3-030-54506-2_50

- Isolated medial compartment involvement rates:
  - USA—85%
  - Chinese—60%

Wise et al. [9] looked at knee OA in White and African Americans and reported:

- Isolated medial compartment OA rates:
  - White Americans—79%
  - African American—64%

Wang WJ et al. [10] in a study of Chinese patients awaiting total knee replacement arthropathy (TKR) for end-stage primary OA, reported involvement rates of:

- Medial compartment—92%
- Lateral compartment −32%
- PF compartment—34%
- Isolated lateral compartment −7%

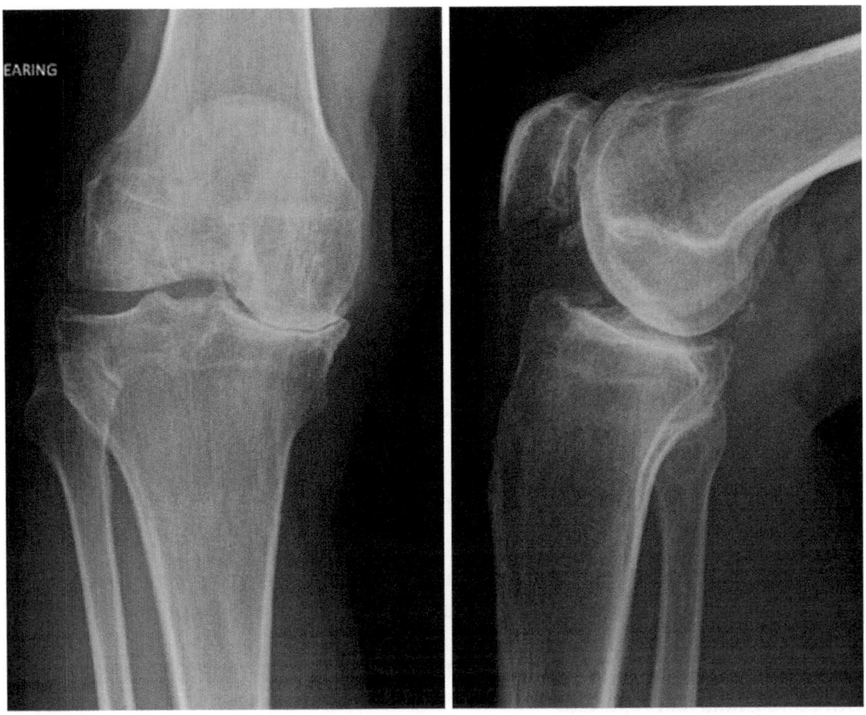

Medial compartment osteoarthritis (loss of joint space, subchondral sclerosis, osteophyte formation)

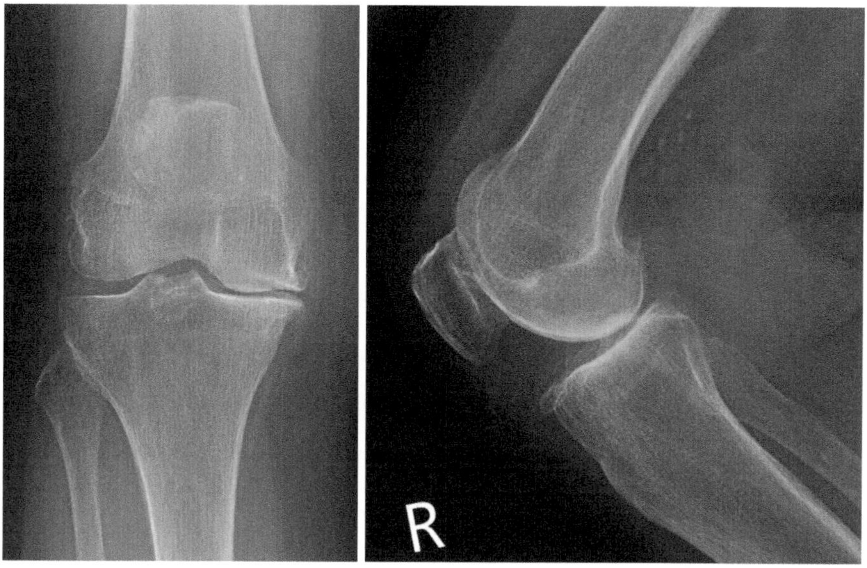

Medial compartment osteoarthritis (loss of joint space, subchondral sclerosis, osteophyte formation)

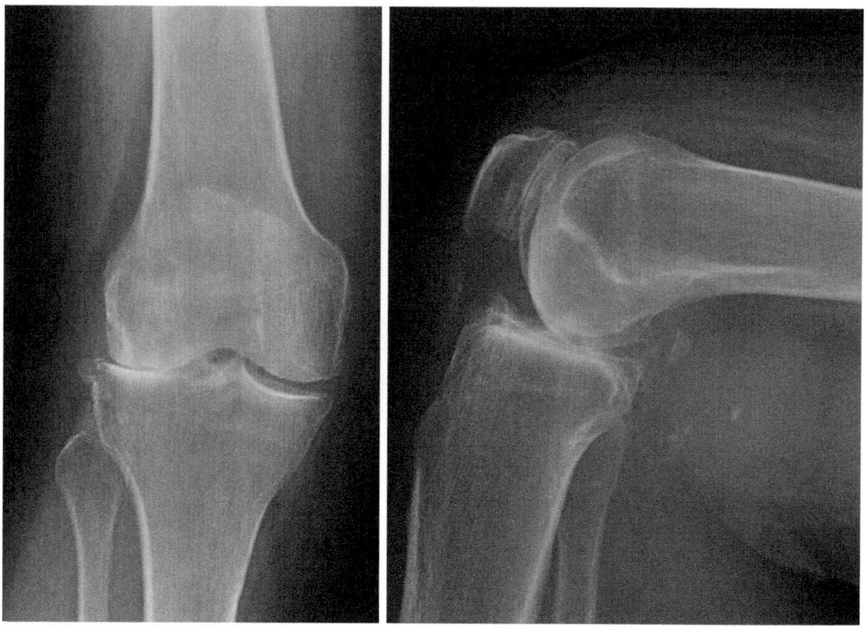

Lateral compartment osteoarthritis

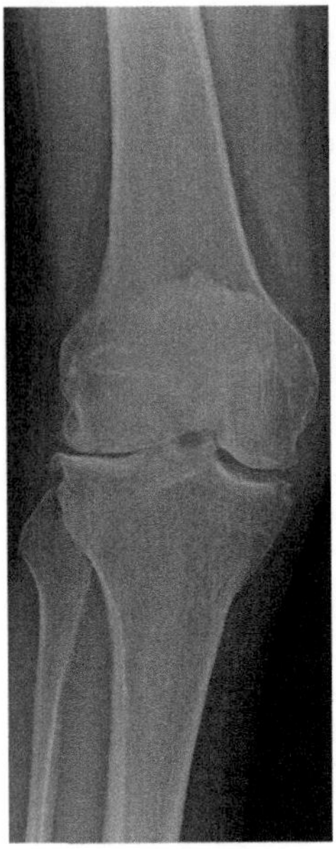

Lateral compartment osteoarthritis, with valgus alignment

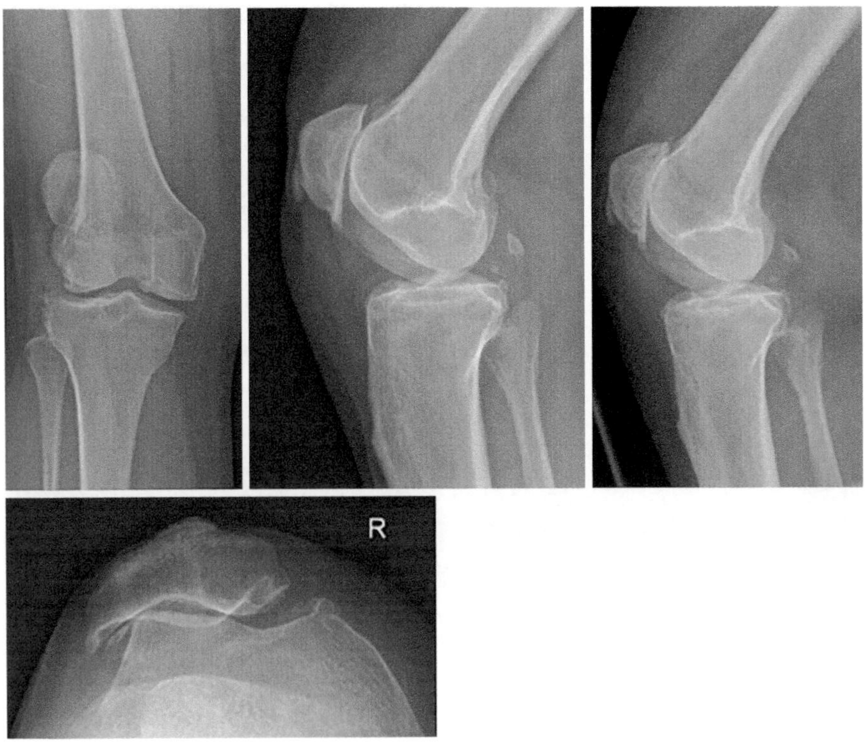

Patellofemoral osteoarthritis with lateral patellar subluxation. The tibiofemoral joint is preserved

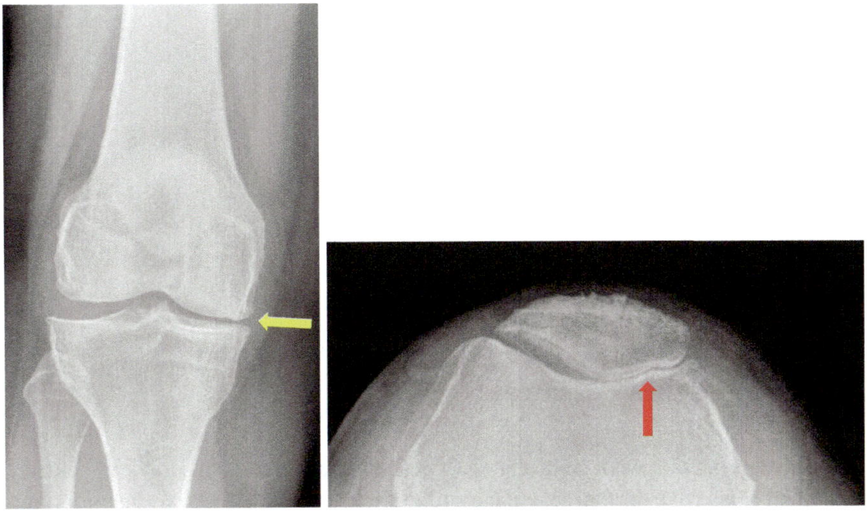

Medial (yellow arrow) and patellofemoral (red arrow) compartment osteoarthritis

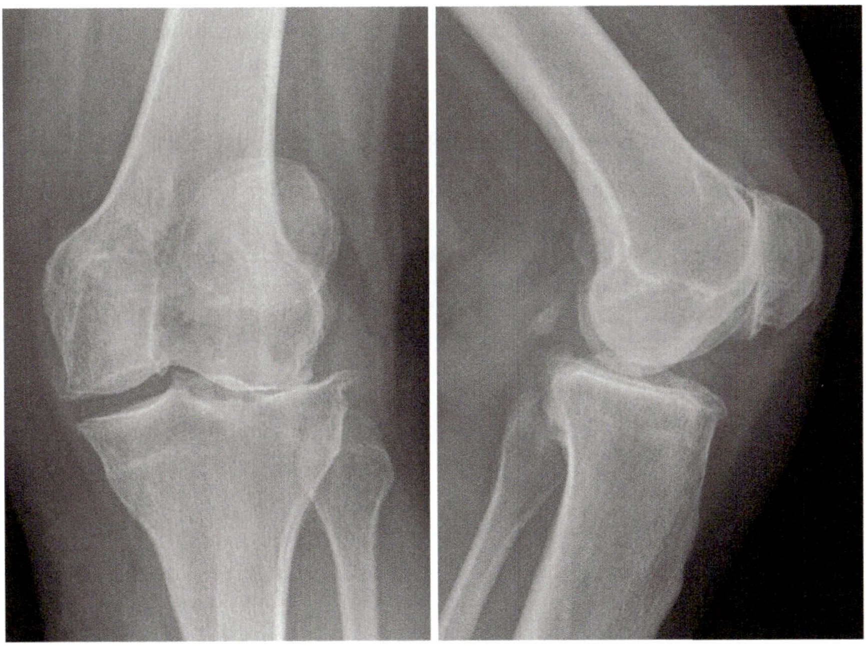

Lateral and patellofemoral compartment osteoarthritis

50.2 Causes of OA

These include:

- Primary
- Secondary
  - Post-traumatic
  - Osteonecrosis
  - Instability

50.3 Pathogenesis of OA

- Passive process—wear and tear as a result of chronic use. However, elderly patients may have normal articular cartilage hence other factors may be important.
- Overloading due to abnormal biomechanics (due to malalignment, instability, loss of meniscal protection, articular cartilage collapse due to osteonecrosis)
- Active process—an inflammatory component has been demonstrated, which when initiated may propagate the destruction of articular cartilage. Atukorala I et al. [11] showed that effusion-synovitis and infrapatellar fat pad synovitis strongly predicted the development of radiographic OA.

  Several conditions may increase the risk of osteoarthritis:

- Varus alignment and obesity are related to an increased risk of developing medial compartment osteoarthritis
- Female sex and valgus malalignment are associated with a higher risk of lateral compartment osteoarthritis
- PF arthritis—associated with patellar instability, patellar malalignment, posterior cruciate ligament (PCL) injury

a

b

c

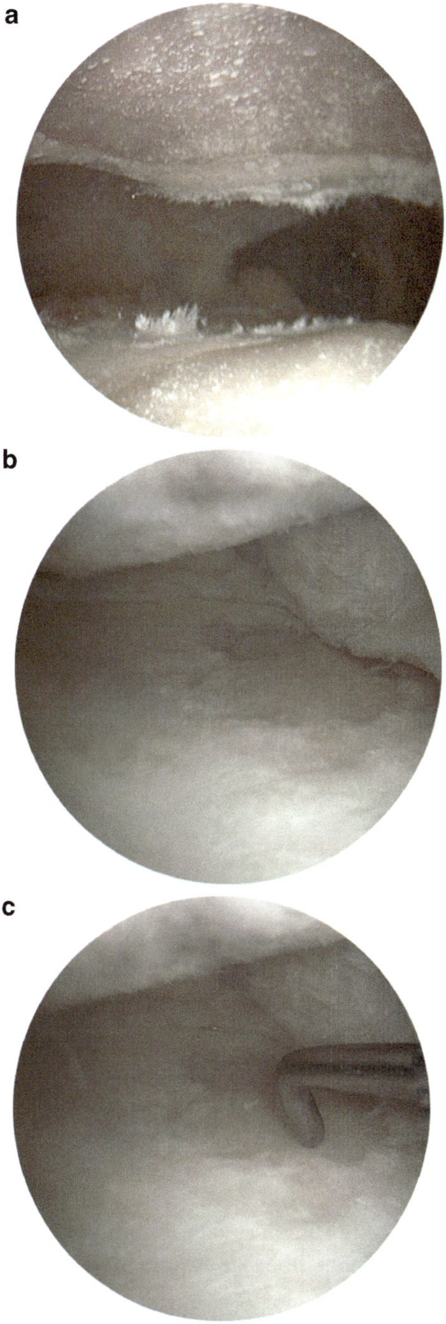

Knee arthritis. (**a**) Patellofemoral joint. (**b**, **c**) Medial compartment

50.4 Clinical Symptoms of Knee OA

- Deep seated knee pain
- Loss of motion
- Painful knee motion
- Leg weakness
- Instability
- Swelling:
  - Diffuse
  - Localised
- Locking/catching
- Crepitus, clunking

50.5 Clinical Signs of Knee OA

- Muscle atrophy—related to disuse
- Diffuse knee swelling—may vary from small to large
  - Effusion
  - Synovitis
- Localised knee swelling due to associated bursitis—popliteal, pes anserinus
- Malalignment—coronal-varus/valgus, sagittal-flexion deformity, rotational
- Tenderness
- Crepitus
- Loss of knee motion
  - Apparent stiffness—due to pain
  - True stiffness
- Knee weakness, if associated quadriceps or other periarticular muscle atrophy and weakness

50.6 Investigations for Osteoarthritis

These aim to confirm the presence of OA, differentiate it from other causes of arthritis, determine its extent, as well as provide information to guide non-surgical or surgical intervention (alignment, bone stock, integrity of soft tissues).

- Plain radiographs—anteroposterior, Rosenberg view, lateral, skyline

  - OA—loss of joint space, subchondral sclerosis, subchondral cysts, osteophyte formation. This contrasts with rheumatoid arthritis below:
  - RA—joint space narrowing, marginal erosions (that occur in the outer part of the joint), periarticular osteopenia, soft tissue swelling, minimal reactive bone formation
  - Long leg film to assess alignment
- CT—to define in detail:
  - Coronal/sagittal/rotational alignment
  - Bone loss and cystic areas in planning surgical intervention
- MRI—to identify early articular cartilage loss (not visible on plain radiographs), associated lesions that may be amenable to less invasive interventions (synovitis, meniscal tears)
- White cell bone scan—to detect inflammatory component

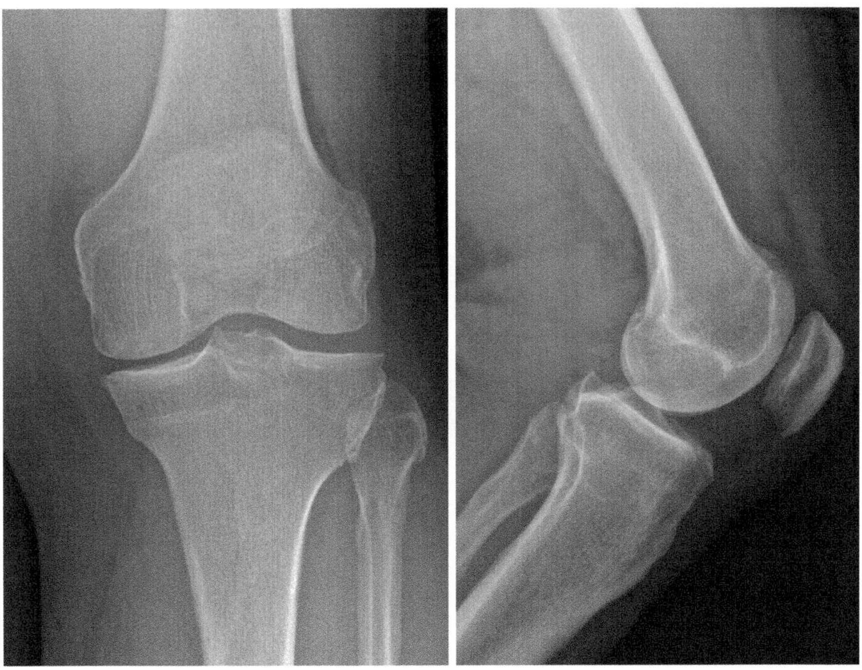

Early medial compartment osteoarthritis with joint space loss (compared to lateral compartment)

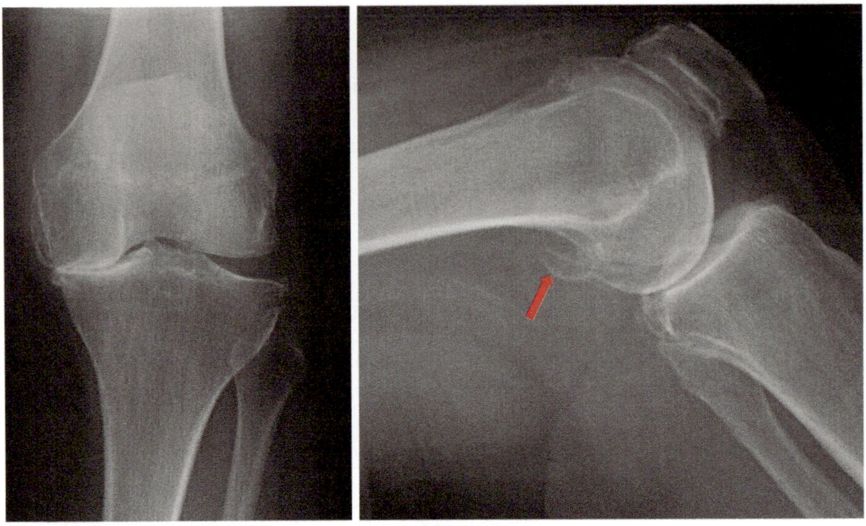

Medial and patellofemoral compartment osteoarthritis with large posterior femoral ostephyte(red arrow), loss of joint space and substantial subchondral sclerosis

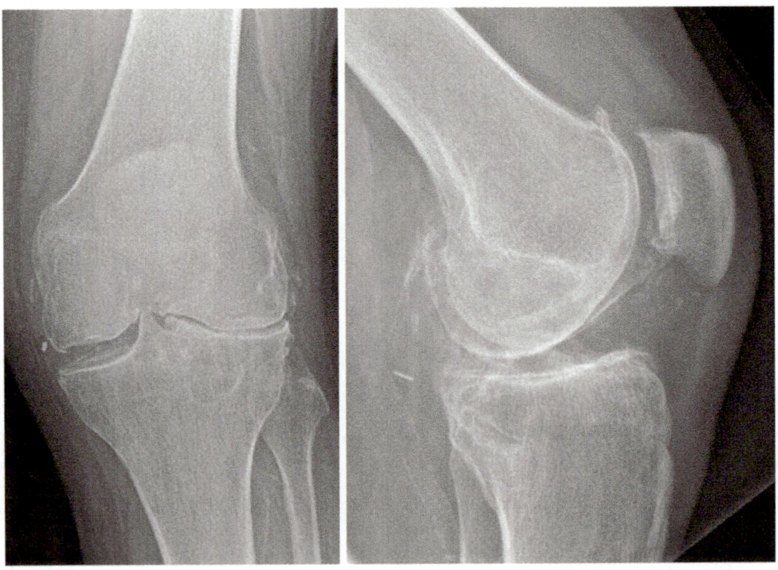

Tibiofemoral and patellofemoral osteoarthritis with joint space loss, ostephyte formation, subchondral sclerosis, large tibial subchondral degenerative cyst and valgus malalignment

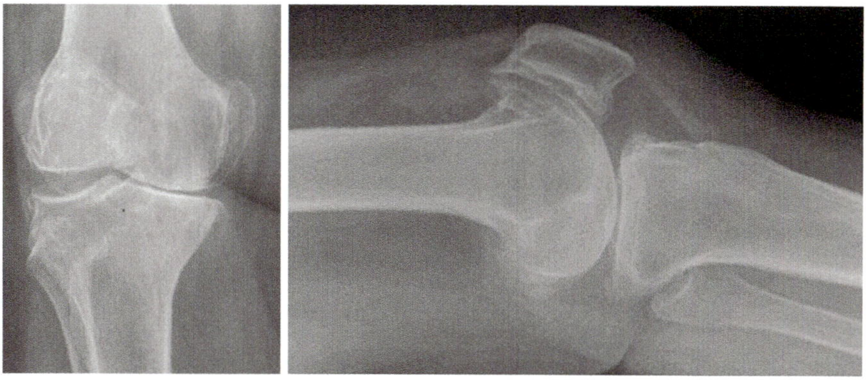

Tibiofemoral and patellofemoral osteoarthritis with large medial femoral osteophyte

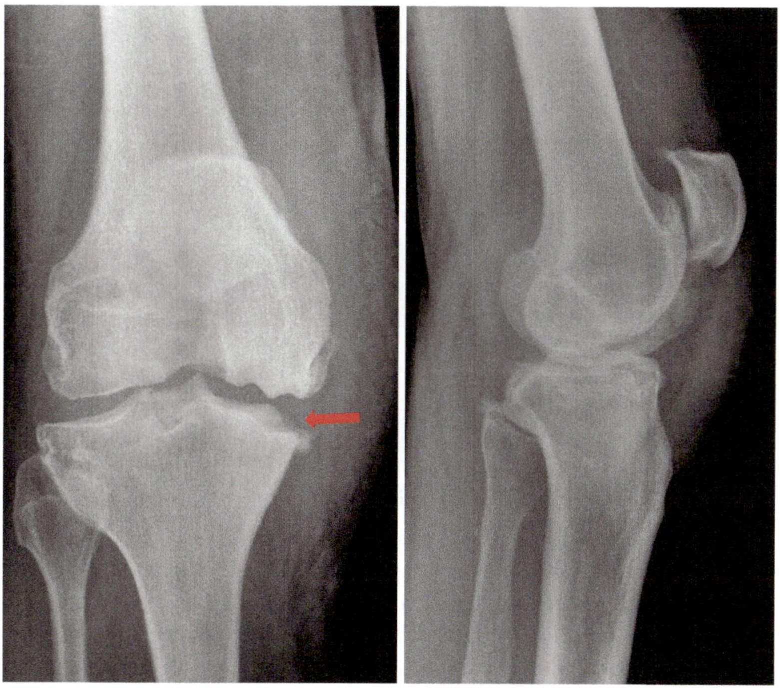

Rheumatoid arthritis with substantial erosions and scalloping of the medial compartment (red arrow)

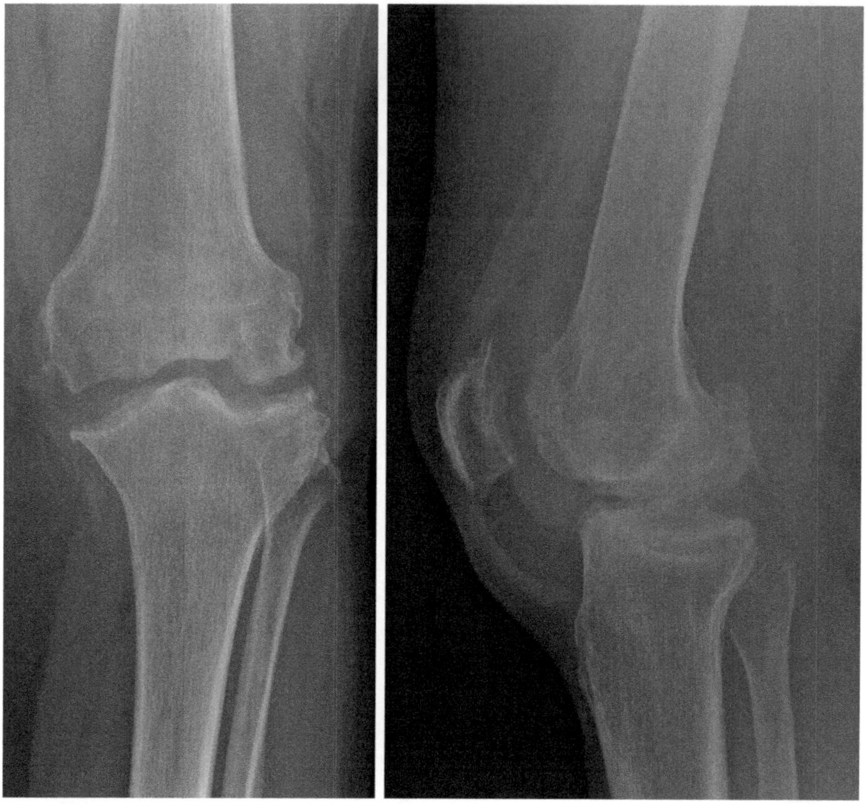

Extensive erosions in psoriatic arthritis

50.7 Clinical Phenotypes of Knee OA

Pan F et al. [13] studied 963 participants (with mean age 63 years) and related their demographics, psychological, lifestyle and comorbidities data to structural pathology of the knee as detected by MRI. This was done to identify knee pain phenotypes. They identified 3 pain phenotypes:

- Class 1: high prevalence of emotional problems and low prevalence of structural damage (25%)
- Class 2: high prevalence of structural damage and low prevalence of emotional problems (20%)
- Class 3: low prevalence of emotional problems and low prevalence of structural damage (55%)

In addition:

- Class 1 and 2 had higher BMI, more comorbidities and a higher prevalence of radiographic knee OA and structural pathology as compared to Class 3
- Class 1 had more pain and more painful sites as compared to class 2 and 3

They concluded that psychological and structural factors interact with each other to exacerbate pain perception, and that an individual approach to treatment is needed.

Knoop J et al. [24] reported 5 different phenotypes in OA:

- "Minimal joint disease phenotype"—minimal radiographic OA
- "Strong muscle phenotype"—strong muscles with severe OA—much as in younger post-traumatic OA cases who continue to be very functional and active
- "Non-obese and weak muscle phenotype"
- "Obese and weak muscle phenotype"
- "Depressive phenotype"

The "depressive phenotype" and "obese and weak muscle phenotype" showed higher pain levels and more severe limitations in activity than the rest.

Dell'Isola A et al. [25], in a systematic analysis, reported 6 potential phenotypes based on the underlying aetiology of OA:

- Chronic pain with prominent central mechanisms (e.g. central sensitisation)
- Inflammatory (with high levels of inflammatory biomarkers)
- Metabolic syndrome (obesity, diabetes, other metabolic alterations)
- Bone and cartilage metabolism (changes in local cartilage metabolism)
- Mechanical overload (due to deranged biomechanics such as varus malalignment)
- Minimal joint disease—minor clinical symptoms and slow progression

Recognising the various phenotypes that may exist, may help guide treatment (e.g. in the strong muscle phenotype use of strengthening exercises may not be beneficial). Similarly, this may also help recognise the variability that exists amongst patients in response to a particular intervention.

50.8 Management of Knee OA

50.8.1 Non-surgical [26–32]

- Leave alone
- Simple analgesia
- Activity modification
- Exercise-physiotherapy to:
  - Strengthen the periarticular muscles of the knee
  - Maintain motion—active
  - Stretch contracted soft tissues to regain motion

- Knee injections—steroid, hyaluronic acid, PRP

50.8.2 Surgical [33–83]

- Arthroscopic debridement, partial meniscectomy, removal of loose bodies
- Realignment procedure—osteotomy
  - Distal femoral
    - Opening wedge
    - Closing wedge
  - Proximal tibial
    - Opening wedge
    - Closing wedge
    - Biplanar
- Knee replacement arthroplasty
  - Unicompartmental (UKR)
    - Medial
    - Lateral
    - PF replacement (PFR)
  - Bicompartmental
  - Total replacement arthroplasty(TKR) (with or without patellar resurfacing)
- Excision arthroplasty
  - Lateral patellar facetectomy in PF OA
- Tibiofemoral fusion arthroplasty in:
  - Instability
  - Neuropathy
  - Infection

Some of the surgical procedures used in OA are discussed next.

50.9 Knee Replacement Arthroplasty for Knee OA

Knee replacement arthroplasty is extensively utilised for knee OA. It may be in the form of TKR (medial and lateral tibiofemoral compartment ± patellar replacement) or in the form of isolated compartment replacement (medial or lateral UKR, PFR).

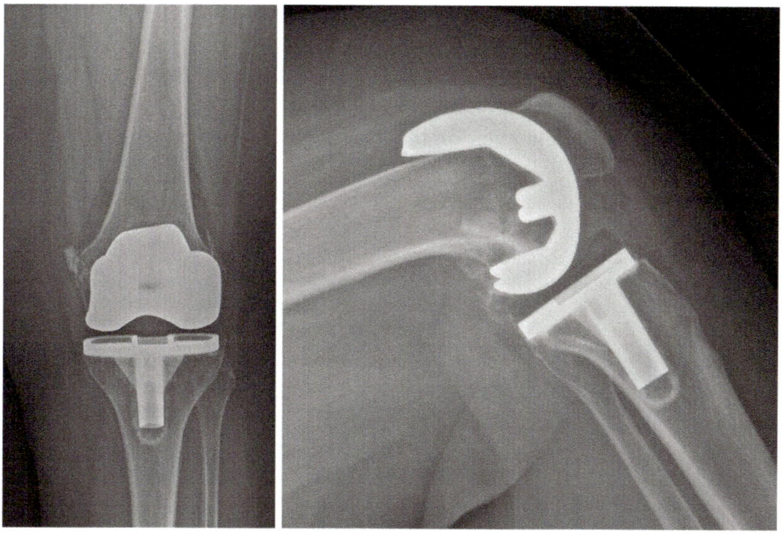

Cruciate retaining total knee arthroplasty, without resurfacing of the patella

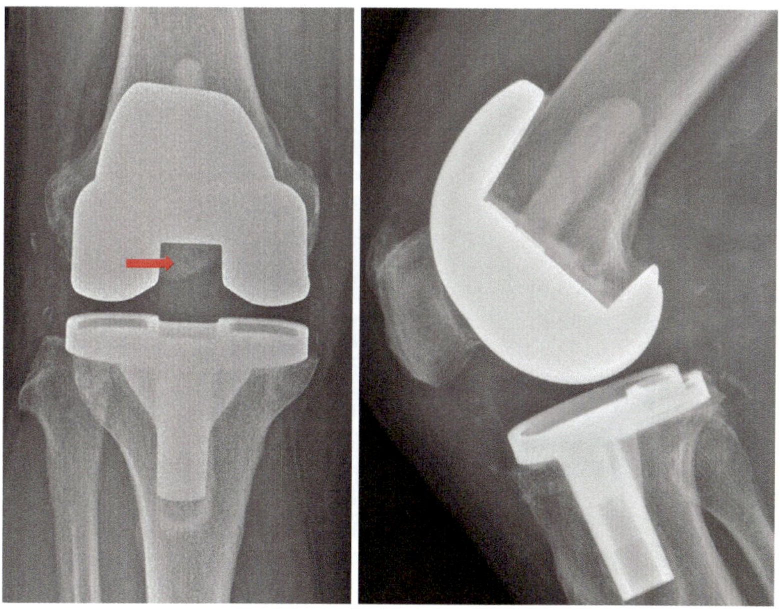

Cruciate sacrificing (as indicated by large central box) knee replacement arthroplasty (patella not replaced)

Multiple factors may be taken into account when considering whether to use a TKR or a UKR/PFR, including:

- Part of the knee which is arthritic

- Likelihood of arthritis progressing to other parts of the knee
- Integrity of soft tissues (ligaments, muscles)
- Technical ability to perform UKR (bone stock, soft tissues, range of motion)
- Patient characteristics—age, sex, BMI
- Clinical and functional outcomes of the prosthesis in the patient population under consideration

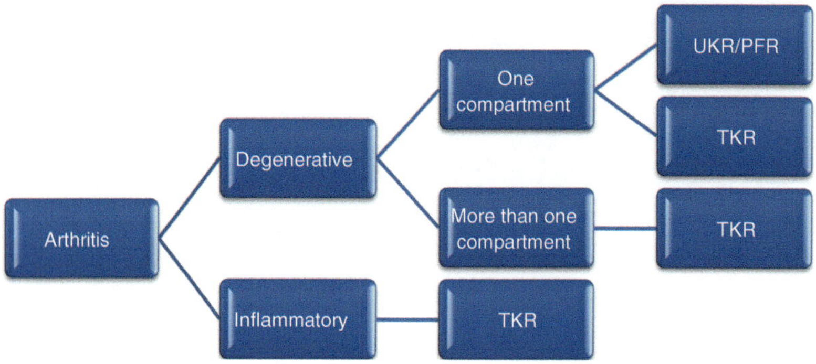

Partial knee replacement arthroplasty may be utilised in osteoarthritis, but not inflammatory arthritis

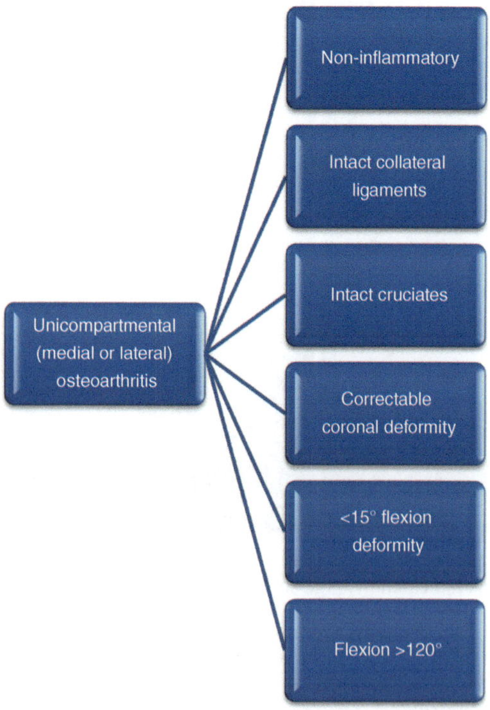

Prerequisites for performing tibiofemoral unicompartmental knee replacement arthroplasty

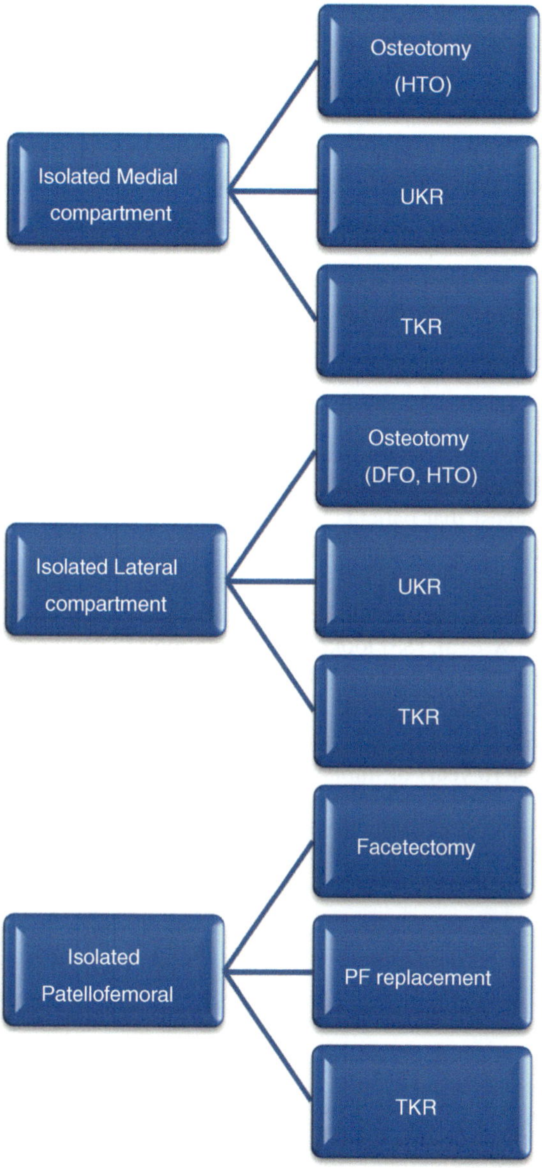

Potential replacement arthroplasty and other options for unicompartmental knee arthritis

50.9.1 *Tibiofemoral UKR*

This replaces the medial (usually) or lateral tibiofemoral compartment in isolation.

The following need to be considered when considering patient suitability for UKR [19–22]:

- Disease limited to one compartment (from which clinically the symptoms originate)
- Likelihood of OA progression to other compartments—inflammatory arthropathy is a process involving all joints hence not suitable for UKR. Progression of disease may be higher following lateral as compared to medial UNA
- Technical ability to implant a unicompartmental prosthesis—requires adequate knee flexion, correctable deformity
- Intact ligaments—to provide knee stability

Contraindications:

- Inflammatory arthritis

Previously described contraindications for tibiofemoral UKR included age < 60, body weight > 82 kg, heavy labour, exposed bone in the PF joint. However, more recent studies suggest that patients with these parameters may do as well or even better than those with no contraindications [23–26].

Furthermore, large osteophytes in the lateral compartment (in the presence of full thickness lateral compartment cartilage) are not a contraindication to medial UKR. Hamilton TW et al. [83] looked at the relation of lateral compartment osteophytes and outcomes in medial UKR. They reported that large osteophytes were associated with a greater degree of macroscopic anterior cruciate ligament (ACL) damage. However, they were not associated with a significant difference in functional outcomes at 10 years or implant survival at 15 years.

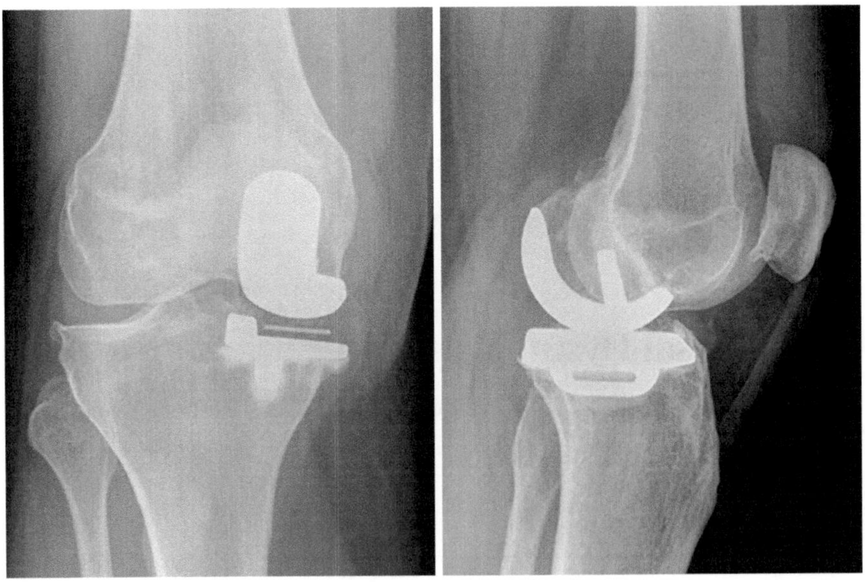

Medial tibiofemoral UKR

50.9.2 Patellofemoral Replacement Arthroplasty

This is indicated for isolated PF arthritis, which is often associated with PF instability. Several prostheses have been described but their results have been inconsistent. Van der List JP et al. [51] evaluated the survivorship and functional outcomes of PFR in a systematic review. They reported 900 revisions in 9619 PFRs giving a 5-, 10-, 15- and 20-year PFR survivorship of 92%, 83%, 75% and 67% respectively. Functional outcomes were reported in 2587 PFRs with an overall score of 82% of the maximum score.

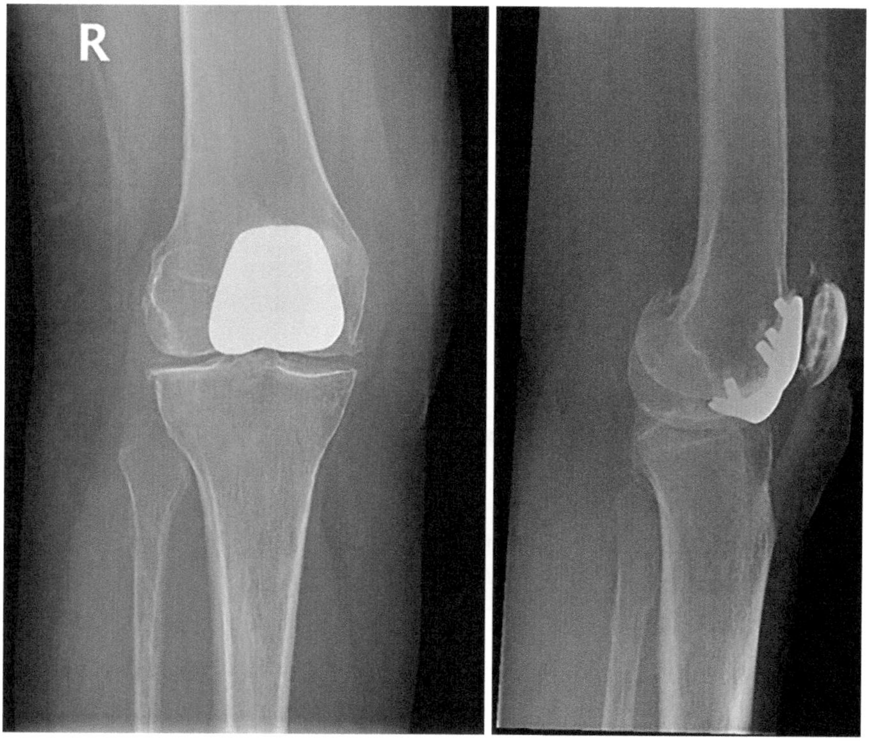

Patellofemoral replacement arthroplasty

Van der List JP et al. [52] in a systematic review showed that PFRs may fail due to:

- OA progression—38%
- Ongoing pain—16%
- Aseptic loosening—14%
- Patellar maltracking—10%

Ongoing pain was responsible for most early failures and OA progression for most late failures. Disease progression following PFR may be lower in those with trochlear dysplasia as compared to those without trochlear dysplasia.

50.9.3 Bicompartmental Knee arthroplasty [53–56]

This arthroplasty concept involves replacement of 2 of the 3 knee compartments. It may be used when OA involves 2 of the 3 knee compartments. It aims to:

- Preserve the cruciate ligaments
- Preserve bone stock
- Preserve normal patellar level and tracking

The above aim to achieve:

- Better joint proprioception
- Better joint kinematics
- Reduce stresses at the implant/bone interface
- Prolong implant longevity
- Improve long term functional outcomes

50.10 Osteotomy for Medial Compartment OA—Varus Knee

Osteotomy for medial compartment OA usually involves the proximal tibia—high tibial osteotomy (HTO). This aims to improve knee alignment and reduce loading of an arthritic medial tibiofemoral compartment.

Indications for HTO:

- Isolated compartment arthritis (from which clinically the symptoms originated)
- Good range of knee motion
- Intact ligaments
- Intra- or extra-articular deformity

Contraindications for HTO:

- Inflammatory arthritis
- Severe obesity
- Smoking
- Severe arthritis

Better outcomes are seen in:

- Primary or secondary isolated medial compartment degenerative arthritis
- Varus deformity <15°
- Good range of motion

- Stable knee

Absolute contraindications:

- Inflammatory arthritis
- Significant lateral tibiofemoral disease

Poorer outcomes may be seen in:

- Severe arthritis (outcomes better with lower degrees of arthritis)
- Advanced PF arthritis
- ≥15° fixed flexion deformity
- >20° fixed varus deformity
- Joint instability—but utilised in ACL, PCL or posterolateral corner (PLC) dysfunction
- Age > 65
- BMI > 27
- Preoperative flexion <120°

Nauide D et al. [56] showed that patients who were younger than 50 and who had preoperative knee flexion greater than 120° had a probability of survival after HTO approaching 95% at 5 years, 80% at 10 years, and 60% at 15 years.

The aim of HTO is to achieve 3–5° valgus from the mechanical axis or 8–10° anatomical valgus. Rudan JF et al. [57] suggested that correction to a femorotibial angle of 6–14° confers better outcomes whereas under correction to less than 5° of femorotibial valgus may confer a high failure rate (62.5%).

50.10.1 HTO Techniques

Opening wedge HTO—this is performed proximal to the tibial tubercle. The osteotomy line runs from a point about 4 cm distal to the tibiofemoral joint line towards the tip of the fibular head. The lateral tibial cortex is preserved, to act as a hinge. The bones are separated to the extent that will allow the deformity correction required. The gap is filled with native or synthetic bone graft.

Closing wedge HTO—this is usually performed proximal to the tibial tubercle. The proximal osteotomy line runs parallel to the tibiofemoral articular surface and about 2.5 cm distal to the tibiofemoral joint line. The distal osteotomy line is oblique and is distal to the proximal line (wedge size) by as much as needed to achieve the required degree of correction. A laterally based wedge is thus removed from between the 2 osteotomy lines. The medial tibial cortex is preserved to act as a hinge around which the distal tibia rotates. The distal part of the tibia is then moved laterally until the osteotomy surfaces are apposed.

A HTO aims to preserve the anatomical anteroposterior tibial slope, unless a change in that slope is required (as in ACL deficiency).

Opening wedge vs. closing wedge HTO

Opening wedge HTO
Advantages:

- Does not require fibular osteotomy or disruption of the proximal tibiofibular joint
- Confers less change in the morphology of the proximal tibia (hence easier conversion to TKR)

Disadvantages:

- Non-union (as it creates a gap that needs to be filled with bone for the osteotomy to unite)
- Need to protect weightbearing until union, as potentially weak construct
- Leg lengthening
- May alter the tibial slope (increase in tibial slope with resultant more anterior tibial translation in relation to the femur—this, however, may be sought for in PCL or PLC disruption)
- May exacerbate patella baja—as the distance between the tibial plateau and tibial tuberosity is lengthened, pulling the patella distally

Closing wedge HTO
Advantages:

- Allows early weightbearing as it is a stronger construct due to apposition of the osteotomy bone surfaces
- Higher union rates

Disadvantages:

- Requires fibular osteotomy, disruption of the proximal tibiofibular joint, or excision of the fibular head—this increases the risk of common peroneal nerve disruption
- Limb shortening
- May change the morphology of the proximal tibia (hence more difficult conversion to TKR)
- Can be used with patellar baja—as the distance between the tibial plateau and tibial tuberosity is shortened allowing the patella to migrate proximally
- Less likely to alter the tibial slope (or may decrease the tibial slope with resultant more posterior tibial translation in relation to the femur overloading the PCL. It may be thus more appropriate in ACL disruption)

50.11 Osteotomy for Lateral Compartment OA—Valgus Knee

Osteotomy for valgus knee deformities is usually done at the distal femur, as valgus malalignment is considered to be a femoral-based deformity (usually a deficiency of the distal femoral condyle). Valgus malalignment may also be due to a tibial deformity or combined tibial and femoral deformities.

Distal femoral osteotomy (DFO)—this may be utilised in:

- Isolated lateral compartment arthritis (but may be also performed in the presence of PF arthritis)
- Clinical valgus deformity
- The aim is for the mechanical axis passing through about 50% of the tibia from medial to lateral

Poor outcomes are seen in:

- BMI > 30 kg/m°
- Inflammatory arthritis
- Age > 65

Ekeland et al. [58] looked at distal femoral opening-wedge osteotomy of knees with lateral compartment OA and reported a survival rate of 88% at 5 years and 74% at 10 years.

50.11.1 DFO Techniques

Opening wedge DFO

- This is performed about 4 cm proximal to the lateral epicondyle with the osteotomy line aiming just proximal to the medial epicondyle, preserving about 1 cm of medial cortical hinge. Bone graft may be used to fill the defect—autograft, allograft, bone substitute. The patient maybe kept non-weightbearing for 6 weeks.

Medial closing wedge DFO

- This is performed on the medial side of the distal femur and is stabilised with plate and screws, staples or just plaster

A lateral opening wedge HTO may also be utilised in cases of articular depression and valgus malunion of the proximal tibia, but in current practise it is rarely performed for valgus knee deformities. However, Eberbach H et al. [59] recently challenged this approach by evaluating the geometry of the valgus knee. They analysed 420 standing full-leg radiographs of patients with valgus malalignment (mechanical femorotibial angle≥4°). They then determined the ideal osteotomy site (distal femur or proximal tibia). They reported that about 41% valgus deformities were tibial based, 24% were femoral based, 27% were femoral and tibial based, and 8% were intra-articular/ligamentary based. In order to obtain a straight-leg axis and an anatomical postoperative joint line with a tolerance of ±4°, the ideal site of a corrective osteotomy was:

- Proximal tibia in 55% of cases
- Distal femur in 20% of cases
- Tibial and femoral (double-level osteotomy) in 25% of cases

If a change in joint line within ±2° was desired, the ideal osteotomy site was:

- Proximal tibia in 41%
- Distal femur in 14%
- Distal femur and proximal tibia (double-level osteotomy) in 45% of cases

Eberbach H et al. [59] thus questioned the widespread belief that valgus malalignment is usually caused by a femoral deformity, as in their study valgus malalignment was attributable to tibial deformity or a combination of femoral- and tibial-based deformity in most cases. Hence, they concluded that varus osteotomies for lateral compartment OA should be done at the tibial site or as a double-level osteotomy in the majority of patients (to avoid an oblique joint line).

50.12 HTO vs. UKR

Santoso MB and Wu L [60] compared HTO to UKR for medial unicompartmental osteoarthritis in a meta-analysis. No significant difference was detected between the 2 groups with regards to:

- Free walking velocity
- Knee functional scores
- Deterioration of the contralateral tibiofemoral or PF compartment
- Revision rate and need for TKR

UKR produced better pain outcomes as well as fewer complications than HTO. They concluded that valgus HTO may provide better physical activity for younger patients whereas UKR is more suitable for older patients due to shorter rehabilitation and faster functional recovery. They were unable to conclude that either method is superior.

However, HTO and UKR share the same indications in only a few selected cases of medial unicompartmental knee arthritis. These indications have been described by Dettoni et al. [61] and include patients who are:

- 55 to 65 years old
- Moderately active
- Non-obese
- Have mild varus malalignment
- Exhibit no joint instability
- Have good range of motion with <5 ° fixed flexion deformity
- Have moderate arthritis involving one compartment

UKR is more appropriate if:

- There is normal knee alignment
- The knee is stable (AP and medial/lateral)
- Patient is low demand and not obese
- Suitable also for more elderly patients to improve overall function

HTO is more appropriate if:

- Varus deformity present
- In younger, higher loading demand patients
- Can be utilised even in presence of anterior/posterior instability

Hence, the ideal patient for HTO is a young, active patient with varus deformity and medial compartment degenerative OA.

Roberston and W-Dahl [62] looked at the results of de-novo TKR, HTO revision to TKR and UKR revision to TKR. The risk of revision was higher after previous UKR and closing wedge HTO but not, opening wedge HTO.

Ekhtiari S et al. [63] evaluated the return to work and sports following HTO in a systematic review. Overall, 85% of patients returned to work postoperatively, and 65% returned at an equal or greater level. About 90% of patients who returned to work or sport did so within 1 year.

An unloading knee brace may be utilised for a short period of time, and its response, guide as to the potential value of performing a HTO. Minzlaff P et al. [64] assessed valgus bracing in symptomatic varus malalignment for testing the expectable "unloading effect" following a valgus HTO. Patients with symptomatic knee varus were fitted with a valgus unloading knee brace for 6–8 weeks. Pain in the affected compartment was monitored before and following bracing and was correlated to pain post HTO. They reported that the temporary use of an unloading valgus knee brace may predict future outcome of HTO surgery in terms of expectable post-operative pain relief.

50.13 UKR vs. Osteotomy vs. TKR

Advantages of tibiofemoral UKR over osteotomy:

- UKR replaces the damaged articular cartilage compartment. In contrast, an osteotomy aims to shift the forces away from the damaged compartment to the healthy compartment
- UKR is easier to revise to a TKR as it does not change the shape of the proximal tibia or distal femur
- May provide better pain relief and function but its longevity may be less in high demand patients (young labourers)

Advantages of tibiofemoral UKR over TKR:

- Better function—the cruciate ligaments and the non-arthritic compartments of the knee are preserved, hence, it is expected that the knee function will be closer to that of the native knee
- Bone preserving—less bone is removed hence it is easier to revise
- UKR has been considered as a time buying procedure (until the patient is older to have a TKR) but is increasingly postulated that UKR may also confer better function. However, this has not be reliably shown in clinical trials [65–67]

Advantages of a TKR vs. UKR and osteotomy:

- Definitive procedure—reduces risk of revision due to arthritis progression
- Can be performed in the presence of substantial motion loss (stiffness), bony deformity, and in the presence of ligamentous disruption, as these can be addressed at the same time

Sun et al. [68] in a systematic review and meta-analysis compared postoperative outcomes between revised UKR and primary TKR. Five studies involving 536 patients were included. The primary TKR group had better function and range of motion than the revised UKR group. Compared with primary TKR, revision of UKR to TKR required more augments, stems, and bone grafts and a thicker polyethylene component. However, there were no significant differences between the 2 groups in revision rate, hospital stay, or complications. They concluded that conversion of UKR to TKR is associated with poorer clinical outcomes and is more complex surgery than primary TKR.

A TKR may be considered to have a certain lifespan. Most TKR implants are expected to last at least 10 years in more than 90% of cases [69, 70]. It is also recognised that some will last much longer than this. However, is also recognised that in some patients the prosthesis may last much less [71–75] such as:

- Younger, high demand patients
- High BMI

Hence, the older the patient the higher the chance they will outlive their prosthesis without needing a revision

Revision surgery is often technically more demanding compared to primary surgery because:

- Soft tissues are scarred from the previous surgery
- There may be associated bone loss—this is equivalent to having a bad tooth which is shaped and covered by a crown. Each time the crown loosens and falls off, some of the tooth substance is lost, until eventually there is not much tooth left to put a crown on and the only option is an extraction or an implant. Similarly, bone loss may mean that specialised implants may be needed (to make up for the lost bone and get anchorage higher up the femur or lower down the tibia). In some cases fusion or even amputation (such as if associated infection) may be necessary
- Revision surgery is associated with higher complication rates than primary surgery

50.14 Complications of Knee Replacement Arthroplasty

These include:

- Infection
- Nerve injury:

  - Infrapatellar branch of saphenous nerve in midline skin incisions
  - Common peroneal nerve injury in the presence of a valgus deformity

- Vascular injury (given the proximity of the popliteal vessels to the knee joint)
- Fracture, during preparation of the bony surfaces
- Knee instability
- Stiffness (loss of knee flexion, extension, both)
- Component loosening
- Component wear
- Polyethylene insert disengagement/dislocation
- Inability to restore alignment
- Complex regional pain syndrome
- Amputation
- Anaesthetic complications

In the UK national joint registry [69] the main reasons for revision of cemented TKRs are (in descending order):

- Aseptic loosening/lysis
- Infection (most likely cause for revision in the first year post-surgery)
- Instability
- Pain and other causes

In the same registry, the rate of revision after primary cemented TKR is higher in:

- Younger patients
- Men as compared to women (if younger than 70 when they had primary surgery)

In contrast, in the same registry, the main reasons for revision for primary UKR (medial and lateral UKR), are:

- Progressive arthritis
- Aseptic loosening /lysis
- Pain

UKR revision is higher in:

- Younger patients
- In women compared to men, except for under the age of 55

50.15 Outcomes of TKR

TKR aims to improve pain, but not necessarily range of motion.

Ritter MA et al. [78] showed that the main predictive factor of the post-surgery range of motion was the preoperative range of motion. Removal of posterior osteophytes and release of the deep medial collateral ligament (MCL), the semimembranosus tendon, and the pes anserinus tendons in patients with large pre-operative varus alignment improved the post-surgery range of motion.

There is evidence that patients with high knee flexion prior to surgery may lose flexion post-surgery. This may be due to the design of the prosthesis and well as changes in the tension of the soft tissues around the knee. In a prospective study [79] it has been shown that:

- In patients with >90° flexion prior to surgery 83% had reduced flexion post-TKR
- In patients with <90° flexion prior to surgery 85% had improved flexion post-TKR

Flexion contractures may be improved with surgery, but residual extension deficit may also be present.

Aderinto et al. [80] investigated the natural history of a fixed flexion deformity (FFD) post TKR. They showed that:

- Pre-operative FFD was a predictor of post-surgery FFD >10° at 1 week and at 6 months (24% of females showing a FFD > 10°, 37% of males)
- However, there was a gradual improvement in knee extension up to 3 years post TKR, by which time residual FFD was mild or absent in most patients, even those who had a severe preoperative FFD

Ritter MA et al. [79] assessed the relationship between flexion contracture and post-TKR outcomes in 5622 knees. They reported that a post-surgery flexion contracture was associated with poorer results. Furthermore, a post-TKR hyperextension deformity of greater than 10° was also associated with an increased risk of worse outcomes.

Evans JT [70] et al. looked at national registry reports of TKR with a systematic review and meta-analysis. They identified 47 case series which reported on 299,291 TKRs, and 5 case series reporting on 7714 UKRs. They estimated a 25 year survival of TKRs (14 registries) of about 82% (95% CI 81–83) and a 25 year survival of UKRs (4 registries) of 70% [68–72]. They concluded that pooled registry data suggests that approximately 82% of TKRs last 25 years and 70% of UKRs last 25 years.

Lankinen P et al. [81] examined patient-related predictive factors that may influence the rate of return to work after TKR in Finnish patients. Of those assessed, 87% returned to work within 1 year after TKR (mean 116 days). Non-manual job and good self-rated general health were associated with a higher rate of return to work.

Skou ST et al. [84] carried out a randomized controlled trial of 100 patients with moderate-to-severe knee OA who were eligible for a TKR. Patients were randomly assigned to TKR followed by 12 weeks of non-surgical treatment (TKR group) or assigned to 12 weeks of non-surgical treatment that included exercise, education, dietary advice, use of insoles, and pain medication (non-surgical treatment group). In the non-surgical-treatment group, 13 patients (26%) underwent TKR before the 12-month follow-up. In the TKR group, 1 patient (2%) received only non-surgical treatment. The TKR had greater functional improvement than the non-surgical treatment group but also had a significantly higher number of serious adverse events than did the non-surgical-treatment group (24 vs. 6).

50.16 Managing Stairs Following TKR

Following TKR the best predictor for ascending or descending stairs without a hand rail was the ability to do so prior to surgery [85].

50.17 Kneeling Following TKR

A substantial proportion of patients (reported rates of 30–80%) have difficulty in kneeling or are not able to kneel on their replaced knee following a TKR and this is one of the "nuisance" factors patients often report. The following may contribute to inability to kneel:

1. Pain—nociceptive, neuropathic
2. Stiffness—limitation of knee flexion
3. Physical inability
4. "Fear of damaging the prosthesis"

However, there is no biomechanical or other contraindication to kneeling following TKR, and kneeling should be encouraged in patients who aim to achieve that ability. Male patients and patients with occupations or hobbies requiring kneeling have been shown to be more likely to kneel after surgery. There is controversy as to whether patellar resurfacing improves or impairs the ability to kneel post surgery [86–89].

50.18 Complex Primary TKR

When assessing a patient with knee arthritis and considering a TKR, several factors which may increase the complexity of the procedure must be considered. In such cases further investigations, adjustment of the surgical technique, or referral to a centre with specialised expertise may be needed. Some of these factors are described below:

50.18.1 Lower Limb Vascular Disease

- Arterial—reduced flow
- Venous—reduced drainage, chronic venous incompetence and leakage with lipodermatosclerosis
- Lymphatic—reduced drainage—elephantiasis like appearance

Management includes:

- Vascular studies—doppler, angiogram
- Revascularisation procedures prior to TKR

50.18.2 Previous Knee Scars

- Surgical
- Traumatic

These may:

- Be associated with soft tissue scarring
- Compromise the vascularity of knee flaps of TKR leading to skin/flap necrosis and wound breakdown

Management includes:

- Assessment by plastics team to:
  - Pre-plan skin incision to minimise risk of necrosis
- Consider soft tissue coverage via local flaps post TKR

50.18.3 Knee Instability

Integrity of the collateral ligaments is assessed—especially the MCL.

Management includes:

- Soft tissue reconstruction procedures
- Use of constrained implants

50.18.4 Lower Limb Malalignment

- Excessive varus or valgus deformity
- Bony deformity vs. soft tissues
  - Integrity of collateral ligaments may be compromised- stretched out at apex of deformity, tight on side of the deformity
- Recurvatum—may be related to:
  - Osseous deformity (valgus)
  - Capsular/ligamentous laxity
  - Neuromuscular disease

Management includes:

- Soft tissue releases
- Altered bone cuts
- Implant augments
- Constrained prostheses

50.18.5 Knee Stiffness

- Flexion/extension deformity

Management includes:

- Extensive soft tissue release
- Altered bone cuts

50.18.6 Bone loss [82]

May be due to:

- Osteonecrosis
- Fractures (traumatic or stress)
- Degenerative or other cysts
- Erosion, in inflammatory arthropathy

Bone loss may be described according to its:

- Depth
- Size
- Location—central vs. peripheral
- Containment—contained vs. not contained, depending on peripheral cortex involvement

Management includes:

- Translating the prosthesis away from the defect
- Cement filling
- Bone grafting:
  - Autograft
  - Allograft
- Utilisation of:
  - Metal augments to replace defect
  - Endoprosthesis
  - Custom made prosthesis

- Stemmed prosthesis to bypass defect

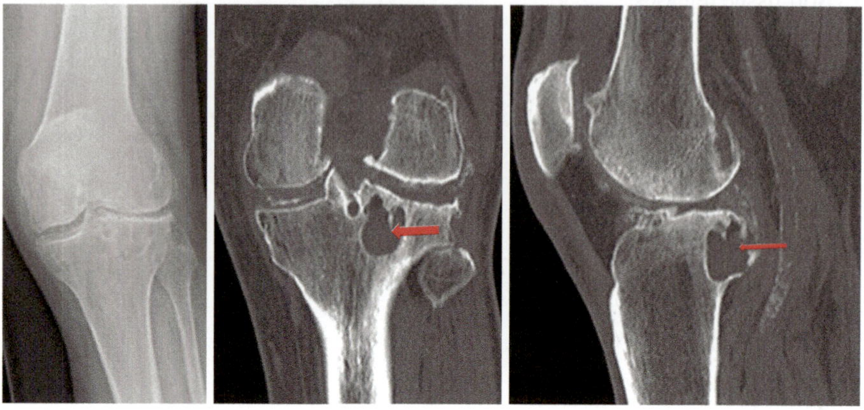

Tibiofemoral and patellofemoral osteoarthritis with large tibial subchondral degenerative cyst (plain radiograph and CT scan)

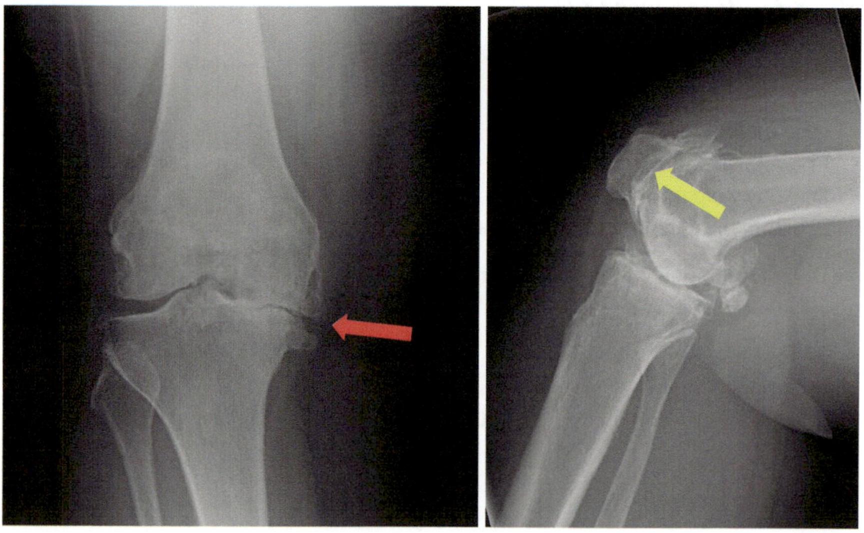

Degenerative changes medial compartment (red arrow) and patellofemoral joint(yellow arrow), with collapse of the medial tibial plateau and medial femoral condyle

50.18.7 Patellofemoral Disruption

- Patellar instability, dislocation
- Previous patellectomy
- Low lying patella

Management includes:

- Patellar stabilisation procedures
- Constrained implants
- Altered bone cuts
- Altered positioning of the patellar resurfacing implant

50.19 Instability in Knee OA [90, 91]

- Knee OA patients often report instability symptoms (shifting, buckling, giving way of the knee)
- In knee OA instability symptoms do not correlate with objectively assessed knee laxity
- Knee instability in OA is associated with poor knee function

Instability of the arthritic knee may lead to over activation of knee muscles, increased compressive loads, with resultant increase in the risk of OA progression, or aggravation of symptoms.

50.20 Acute Flare Ups in Knee OA [92–96]

Patients with knee arthritis may present with an acute flare up of pain. This may be due to:

1. Osteophyte fracture causing:
   (a) Fracture pain
   (b) Resultant loose body
2. Pseudogout attack—due to the deposition of calcium pyrophosphate crystals—more common in the presence of knee OA
3. Tear of the MCL in marked valgus deformity
4. Subchondral stress fracture
5. Inflammatory flare up of arthritis

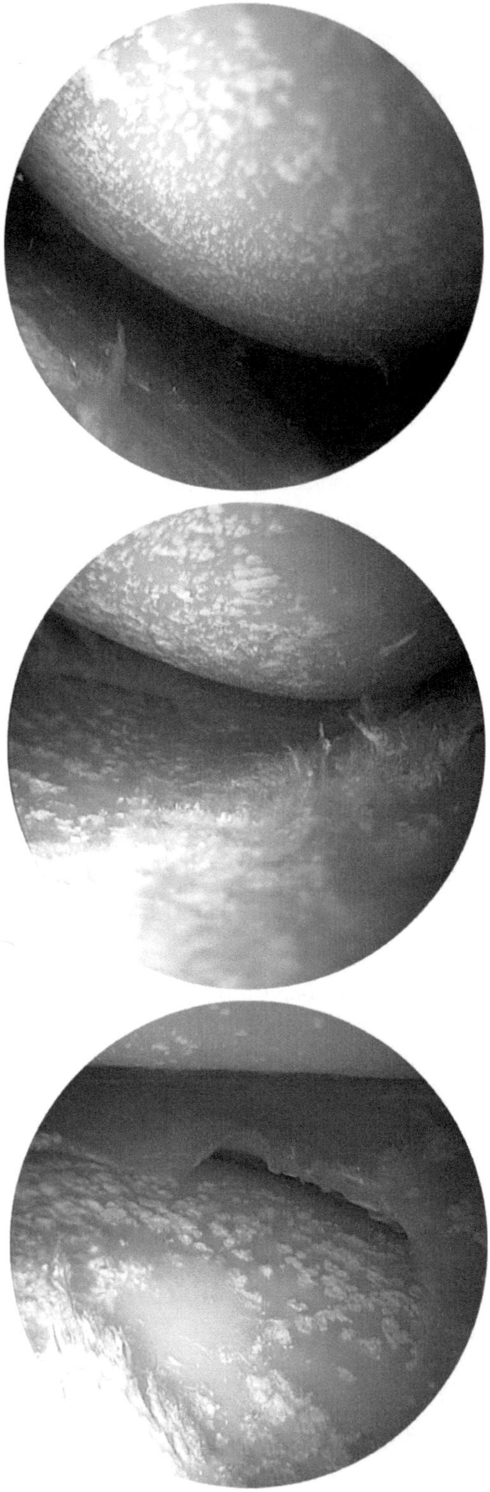

Chondrocalcinosis

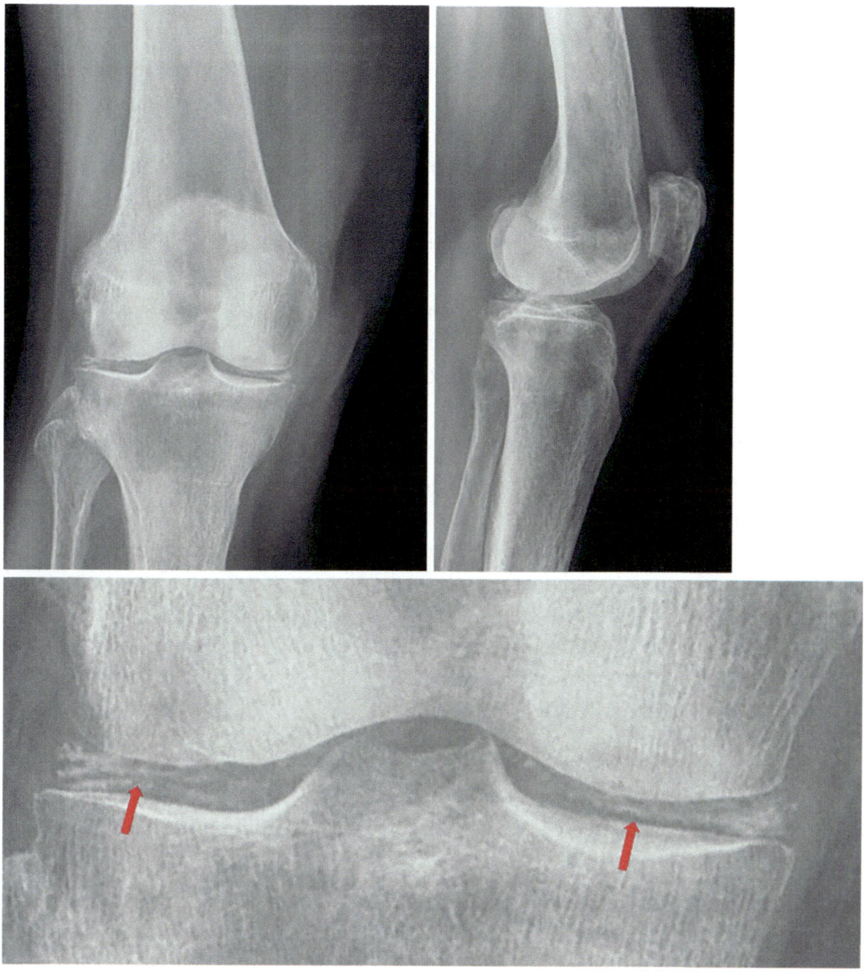

Chondrocalcinosis of both menisci (red arrows)

Murphy SL et al. [93] assessed flare up in patients with symptomatic knee OA. About 80% experienced at least 1 flare up over a 7 day monitoring period with 24% experiencing a flare up on more than 50% of the monitored days.

Learning Pearls

- Patients with knee arthritis may experience pain not just from the joint itself but also form the associated soft tissues which may need addressing in the same way as in the absence of arthritis
- The severity of preoperative radiographic OA is related to post-surgery pain, improvement and satisfaction. Patients with early OA on plain radiographs, have poorer pain relief and outcome following TKR as compared

to those with more advanced OA. Hence, TKR should be used with high caution in patients with early radiographic OA even if their preoperative symptoms are substantial [97–100]. This also needs to be discussed with the patient as part of shared decision making

- Revision rates for knee replacement arthroplasty need to be interpreted with caution as:
  - The decision to revise an unsatisfactory arthroplasty is influenced not only by the objective clinical findings but also subjectively by the decision making of the patient and surgeon
  - A low revision rate may not truly represent the functional and other clinical outcomes of knee arthroplasty. The reported revision rate of TKR is low with 10-year survival rates as high as 95% to 99%. However, a substantial proportion of patients may continue to be symptomatic:
    - Baker PN et al. [101] evaluated TKR in England and Wales and reported a dissatisfaction rate of 18%
    - Bourne RB et al. [102] in a cross-sectional Canadian study of TKR reported a dissatisfaction rate of 19%
    - Price AJ et al. [103] looked at 60 patients younger than 60 years who had a TKR with a minimum 12-year follow-up. They reported that the implant survival rate was 82%, but over 40% of cases continued with pain rated at least as moderate
- Severe joint destruction in the absence of pain raises the possibility of neuropathic arthritis
- Instability arthritis may be seen in instability cases that have been treated surgically or non-surgically
  - Chronic PCL tear has been related to PF arthritis
  - ACL tear has been related to increased risk of OA, including cases who had ACL reconstruction
- In the presence of infective arthritis the initial aim is to treat the infection. Replacement arthroplasty may be considered in joints with previous infective arthritis if the infection has been cured and the inflammatory markers have remained in the normal range, for a substantial period of time (more than a year). Nevertheless, the risk of infection recurring may persist, even in such cases
- Rheumatoid arthritis may exhibit 2 phases:
  - Wet phase—characterised by active inflammation and radiological subarticular erosions
  - Dry phase—where the active inflammation has subsided and radiological features similar to OA (subchondral sclerosis, loss of joint space, subchondral cysts, osteophytes) are seen

- Inflammatory arthritis tends to involve the whole of the joint hence:
  - It may be more difficult to localise the source of a patient's symptoms
  - All diseased areas may need addressing at the time of surgery, such as resurfacing the patella during TKR, to minimise the risk of ongoing symptoms
  - Inflammatory arthritis involves the synovium of the joint and sheaths of periarticular tendons and these may continue causing pain, even after the articular surfaces have been replaced by joint arthroplasty

References

1. Culvenor AG, Øiestad BE, Hart HF, Stefanik JJ, Guermazi A, Crossley KM. Prevalence of knee osteoarthritis features on magnetic resonance imaging in asymptomatic uninjured adults: a systematic review and meta-analysis. Br J Sports Med. 2019;53(20):1268–78.
2. Duncan R, Peat G, Thomas E, Hay EM, Croft P. Incidence, progression and sequence of development of radiographic knee osteoarthritis in a symptomatic population. Ann Rheum Dis. 2011;70:1944–8.
3. Watt FE, Corp N, Kingsbury SR, Frobell R, Englund M, Felson DT, Levesque M, Majumdar S, Wilson C, Beard DJ, Lohmander LS, Kraus VB, Roemer F, Conaghan PG, Mason DJ, Arthritis Research UK Osteoarthritis and Crystal Disease Clinical Study Group Expert Working Group. Towards prevention of post-traumatic osteoarthritis: report from an international expert working group on considerations for the design and conduct of interventional studies following acute knee injury. Osteoarthritis Cartilage. 2019;27(1):23–33.
4. Hinman RS, Crossley KM. Patellofemoral joint osteoarthritis: an important subgroup of knee osteoarthritis. Rheumatology (Oxford). 2007;46:1057–62.
5. Stefanik JJ, Zhu Y, Zumwalt AC, Gross KD, Clancy M, Lynch JA, Frey Law LA, Lewis CE, Roemer FW, Powers CM, Guermazi A, Felson DT. Association between patella alta and the prevalence and worsening of structural features of patellofemoral joint osteoarthritis: the multicenter osteoarthritis study. Arthritis Care Res (Hoboken). 2010;62(9):1258–65.
6. Kalichman L, Zhang Y, Niu J, Goggins J, Gale D, Felson DT, Hunter D. The association between patellar alignment and patellofemoral joint osteoarthritis features--an MRI study. Rheumatology (Oxford). 2007;46(8):1303–8.
7. Ukachukwu V, Duncan R, Belcher J, Shall M, Stefanik J, Crossley K, Thomas MJ, Peat G. Clinical significance of medial versus lateral compartment patellofemoral osteoarthritis: cross-sectional analyses in an adult population with knee pain. Arthritis Care Res (Hoboken). 2017;69(7):943–51.
8. Felson DT, Nevitt MC, Zhang Y, Aliabadi P, Baumer B, Gale D, Li W, Yu W, Xu L. High prevalence of lateral knee osteoarthritis in Beijing Chinese compared with Framingham Caucasian subjects. Arthritis Rheum. 2002;46(5):1217–22.
9. Wise BL, Niu J, Yang M, Lane NE, Harvey W, Felson DT, Hietpas J, Nevitt M, Sharma L, Torner J, Lewis CE, Zhang Y, Multicenter Osteoarthritis (MOST) Group. Patterns of compartment involvement in tibiofemoral osteoarthritis in men and women and in whites and African Americans. Arthritis Care Res (Hoboken). 2012;64(6):847–52.
10. Wang WJ, Sun MH, Palmer J, Liu F, Bottomley N, Jackson W, Qiu Y, Weng WJ, Price A. Patterns of compartment involvement in end-stage knee osteoarthritis in a Chinese orthopedic center: implications for implant choice. Orthop Surg. 2018;10(3):227–34.
11. Atukorala I, Kwoh CK, Guermazi A, Roemer FW, Boudreau RM, Hannon MJ, Hunter DJ. Syitis in knee osteoarthritis: a precursor of disease? Ann Rheum Dis. 2016;75(2):390–5.

12. Felson DT, Niu J, Gross KD, Englund M, Sharma L, Cooke TD, Guermazi A, Roemer FW, Segal N, Goggins JM, Lewis CE, Eaton C, Nevitt MC. Valgus malalignment is a risk factor for lateral knee osteoarthritis incidence and progression: findings from the multicenter osteoarthritis study and the osteoarthritis initiative. Arthritis Rheum. 2013;65(2):355–62.
13. Pan F, Tian J, Cicuttini F, Jones G, Aitken D. Differentiating knee pain phenotypes in older adults: a prospective cohort study. Rheumatology (Oxford). 2019;58(2):274–83.
14. Showery JE, Kusnezov NA, Dunn JC, Bader JO, Belmont PJ Jr, Waterman BR. The rising incidence of degenerative and posttraumatic osteoarthritis of the knee in the United States military. J Arthroplast. 2016;31(10):2108–14.
15. Brown TD, Johnston RC, Saltzman CL, Sh JL, Buckwalter JA. Posttraumatic osteoarthritis: a first estimate of incidence, prevalence, and burden of disease. J Orthop Trauma. 2006;20(10):739–44.
16. Lohmander LS, Englund PM, Dahl LL, Roos EM. The long-term consequence of anterior cruciate ligament and meniscus injuries: osteoarthritis. Am J Sports Med. 2007;35(10):1756–69.
17. Deal CL, Meenan RF, Goldenberg DL, Anderson JJ, Sack B, Pastan RS, Cohen AS. The clinical features of elderly-onset rheumatoid arthritis. A comparison with younger-onset disease of similar duration. Arthritis Rheum. 1985;28(9):987–94.
18. Ferrone C, Andracco R, Cimmino MA. Calcium pyrophosphate deposition disease: clinical manifestations. Reumatismo. 2012;63(4):246–52.
19. Grassi W, De Angelis R. Clinical features of gout. Reumatismo. 2012;63(4):238–45.
20. Bardin T, Richette P. Definition of hyperuricemia and gouty conditions. Curr Opin Rheumatol. 2014;26(2):186–91.
21. Gupta R. A short history of neuropathic arthropathy. Clin Orthop Relat Res. 1993;296:43–9.
22. Elsissy JG, Liu JN, Wilton PJ, Nwachuku I, Gowd AK, Amin NH. Bacterialtic arthritis of the adult native knee joint: a review. JBJS Rev. 2020;8(1):e0059. https://doi.org/10.2106/JBJS.RVW.19.00059.
23. Davis CM, Zamora RA. Surgical options and approaches fortic arthritis of the native hip and knee joint. J Arthroplast. 2020;35(3S):S14–8.
24. Knoop J, van der Leeden M, Thorstensson CA, Roorda LD, Lems WF, Knol DL, Steultjens MP, Dekker J. Identification of phenotypes with different clinical outcomes in knee osteoarthritis: data from the osteoarthritis initiative. Arthritis Care Res (Hoboken). 2011;63(11):1535–42.
25. Dell'Isola A, Allan R, Smith SL, Reiros SS, Steultjens M. Identification of clinical phenotypes in knee osteoarthritis: a systematic review of the literature. BMC Musculoskelet Disord. 2016;17(1):425. https://doi.org/10.1186/s12891-016-1286-2.
26. Gregori D, Giacovelli G, Minto C, Barbetta B, Gualtieri F, Azzolina D, Vaghi P, Rovati LC. Association of pharmacological treatments with long-term pain control in patients with knee osteoarthritis: a systematic review and meta-analysis. JAMA. 2018;320(24):2564–79.
27. Dong R, Wu Y, Xu S, Zhang L, Ying J, Jin H, Wang P, Xiao L, Tong P. Is aquatic exercise more effective than land-based exercise for knee osteoarthritis? Medicine (Baltimore). 2018;97(52):e13823. https://doi.org/10.1097/MD.0000000000013823.
28. Uthman OA, van der Windt DA, Jordan JL, Dziedzic KS, Healey EL, Peat GM, Foster NE. Exercise for lower limb osteoarthritis: systematic review incorporating trial sequential analysis and network meta-analysis. BMJ. 2013;347:f5555. https://doi.org/10.1136/bmj.f5555.
29. Honvo G, Bruyère O, Geerinck A, Veronese N, Reginster JY. Efficacy of chondroitin sulfate in patients with knee osteoarthritis: a comprehensive Meta-analysis exploring inconsistencies in randomized. Placebo-Controlled Trials Adv Ther. 2019;36(5):1085–99.
30. Gohal C, Shanmugaraj A, Tate P, Horner NS, Bedi A, Adili A, Khan M. Effectiveness of valgus offloading knee braces in the treatment of medial compartment knee osteoarthritis: a systematic review. Sports Health. 2018;10(6):500–14. https://doi.org/10.1177/1941738118763913.
31. Zafar AQ, Zamani R, Akrami M. The effectiveness of foot orthoses in the treatment of medial knee osteoarthritis: a systematic review. Gait Posture. 2020;76:238–51.

32. Phillips M, Vannabouathong C, Devji T, Patel R, Gomes Z, Patel A, Dixon M, Bhandari M. Differentiating factors of intra-articular injectables have a meaningful impact on knee osteoarthritis outcomes: a network meta-analysis. Knee Surg Sports Traumatol Arthrosc. 2020;3 https://doi.org/10.1007/s00167-019-05763-1.
33. Palmer JS, Monk AP, Hopewell S, Bayliss LE, Jackson W, Beard DJ, Price AJ. Surgical interventions for symptomatic mild to moderate knee osteoarthritis. Cochrane Database Syst Rev. 2019;7:CD012128. https://doi.org/10.1002/14651858.CD012128.pub2.
34. Liu CY, Li CD, Wang L, Ren S, Yu FB, Li JG, Ma JX, Ma XL. Function scores of different surgeries in the treatment of knee osteoarthritis: a PRISMA-compliant systematic review and network-meta analysis. Medicine (Baltimore). 2018;97(21):e10828. https://doi.org/10.1097/MD.0000000000010828.
35. Hui C, Salmon LJ, Kok A, Williams HA, Hockers N, van der Tempel WM, Chana R, Pinczewski LA. Long-term survival of high tibial osteotomy for medial compartment osteoarthritis of the knee. Am J Sports Med. 2011;39(1):64–70.
36. Howells NR, Salmon L, Waller A, Scanelli J, Pinczewski LA. The outcome at ten years of lateral closing-wedge high tibial osteotomy: determinants of survival and functional outcome. Bone Joint J. 2014;96-B(11):1491–7.
37. Pilone C, Rosso F, Cottino U, Rossi R, Bonasia DE. Lateral opening wedge distal femoral osteotomy for lateral compartment arthrosis/overload. Clin Sports Med. 2019;38(3):351–9.
38. Sherman SL, Thompson SF, Clohisy JCF. Distal Femoral Varus Osteotomy for the Management of Valgus Deformity of the Knee. J Am Acad Orthop Surg. 2018;26(9):313–24.
39. Johal S, Nakano N, Baxter M, Hujazi I, Pandit H, Khanduja V. Unicompartmental knee arthroplasty: the past, current controversies, and future perspectives. J Knee Surg. 2018;31(10):992–8.
40. Siman H, Kamath AF, Carrillo N, Harmsen WS, Pagnano MW, Sierra RJ. Unicompartmental knee arthroplasty vs Total knee arthroplasty for medial compartment arthritis in patients older than 75 years: comparable reoperation, revision, and complication rates. J Arthroplast. 2017;32(6):1792–7.
41. Wilson HA, Middleton R, Abram SGF, Smith S, Alvand A, Jackson WF, Bottomley N, Hopewell S, Price AJ. Patient relevant outcomes of unicompartmental versus total knee replacement: systematic review and meta-analysis. BMJ. 2019;364:l352. https://doi.org/10.1136/bmj.l352.
42. Pisanu G, Rosso F, Bertolo C, Dettoni F, Blonna D, Bonasia DE, Rossi R. Patellofemoral Arthroplasty: Current Concepts and Review of the Literature. Joints. 2017;5(4):237–45.
43. Dahm DL, Kalisvaart MM, Stuart MJ, Slettedahl SW. Patellofemoral arthroplasty: outcomes and factors associated with early progression of tibiofemoral arthritis. Knee Surg Sports Traumatol Arthrosc. 2014;22(10):2554–9.
44. Kinsey TL, Anderson DN, Phillips VM, Mahoney OM. Disease progression after lateral and medial Unicondylar knee arthroplasty. J Arthroplast. 2018;33(11):3441–7. https://doi.org/10.1016/j.arth.2018.07.019.
45. Bae DK, Song SJ, Yoon KH, Noh JH. Long-term outcome of total knee arthroplasty in Charcot joint: a 10- to 22-year follow-up. J Arthroplast. 2009;24(8):1152–6.
46. Vopat BG, Ritterman SA, Kayiaros S, Rubin LE. Primary knee arthrodesis for severe crystalline arthropathy. Am J Orthop (Belle Mead NJ). 2013;42(10):E91–3.
47. Figueiredo A, Ferreira R, Alegre C. Fonseca F Charcot osteoarthropathy of the knee secondary to neurosyphilis: a rare condition managed by a challenging arthrodesis. BMJ Case Rep. 2018;2018 https://doi.org/10.1136/bcr-2018-225337.
48. Gottfriedsen TB, Schrøder HM, Odgaard A. Knee Arthrodesis After Failure of Knee Arthroplasty: A Nationwide Register-Based Study. J Bone Joint Surg Am. 2016;98(16):1370–7.
49. Siller TN, Hadjipavlou A. Knee arthrodesis: long-term results. Can J Surg. 1976;19(3):217–9.
50. van der List JP, Chawla H, Villa JC, Pearle AD. Why do patellofemoral arthroplasties fail today? A systematic review. Knee. 2017;24(1):2–8.

51. van der List JP, Chawla H, Zuiderbaan HA, Pearle AD. Survivorship and functional outcomes of patellofemoral arthroplasty: a systematic review. Knee Surg Sports Traumatol Arthrosc. 2017;25(8):2622–31.
52. Amit P, Singh N, Soni A, Bowman NK, Maden M. Systematic Review of Modular Bicompartmental Knee Arthroplasty for Medio-Patellofemoral Osteoarthritis. J Arthroplasty. 2020;35(3):893–899.e3. https://doi.org/10.1016/j.arth.2019.09.042.
53. Garner A, van Arkel RJ, Cobb J. Classification of combined partial knee arthroplasty. Bone Joint J. 2019;101-B(8):922–8.
54. Ma JX, He WW, Kuang MJ, Sun L, Lu B, Wang Y, Ma XL. Efficacy of bicompartmental knee arthroplasty (BKA) for bicompartmental knee osteoarthritis: a meta analysis. Int J Surg. 2017;46:53–60.
55. Amin NH, Scudday T, Cushner FD. Bicompartmental Knee Arthroplasty. Instr Course Lect. 2017;66:193–9.
56. Naudie D, Bourne RB, Rorabeck CH, Bourne TJ. The install award. Survivorship of the high tibial valgus osteotomy. A 10- to –22-year followup study. Clin Orthop Relat Res. 1999;367:18–27.
57. Rudan JF, Simurda MA. High tibial osteotomy. A prospective clinical and roentgenographic review. Clin Orthop Relat Res. 1990;255:251–6.
58. Ekeland A, Nerhus TK, Dimmen S, Heir S. Good functional results of distal femoral opening-wedge osteotomy of knees with lateral osteoarthritis. Knee Surg Sports Traumatol Arthrosc. 2016;24(5):1702–9.
59. Eberbach H, Mehl J, Feucht MJ, Bode G, Südkamp NP, Niemeyer P. Geometry of the Valgus knee: contradicting the dogma of a femoral-based deformity. Am J Sports Med. 2017;45(4):909–14.
60. Santoso MB, Wu L. Unicompartmental knee arthroplasty, is it superior to high tibial osteotomy in treating unicompartmental osteoarthritis? A meta-analysis and systemic review. J Orthop Surg Res. 2017;12(1):50. https://doi.org/10.1186/s13018-017-0552-9.
61. Dettoni F, Bonasia DE, Castoldi F, Bruzzone M, Blonna D, Rossi R. High tibial osteotomy versus unicompartmental knee arthroplasty for medial compartment arthrosis of the knee: a review of the literature. Iowa Orthop J. 2010;30:131–40.
62. Robertsson O, W-Dahl A. The risk of revision after TKA is affected by previous HTO or UKA. Clin Orthop Relat Res. 2015;473(1):90–3.
63. Ekhtiari S, Haldane CE, de Sa D, Simuic N, Musahl V, Ayeni OR. Return to Work and Sport Following High Tibial Osteotomy: A Systematic Review. J Bone Joint Surg Am. 2016;98(18):1568–77.
64. Minzlaff P, Saier T, Brucker PU, Haller B, Imhoff AB, Hinterwimmer S. Valgus bracing in symptomatic varus malalignment for testing the expectable "unloading effect" following valgus high tibial osteotomy. Knee Surg Sports Traumatol Arthrosc. 2015;23(7):1964–70.
65. Beard DJ, Davies LJ, Cook JA, MacLennan G, Price A, Kent S, Hudson J, Carr A, Leal J, Campbell H, Fitzpatrick R, Arden N, Murray D, Campbell MK, TOPKAT Study Group. The clinical and cost-effectiveness of total versus partial knee replacement in patients with medial compartment osteoarthritis (TOPKAT): 5-year outcomes of a randomised controlled trial. Lancet. 2019;394(10200):746–56.
66. Blevins JL, Carroll KM, Burger JA, Pearle AD, Bostrom MP, Haas SB, Sculco TP, Jerabek SA, Mayman DJ. Postoperative outcomes of total knee arthroplasty compared to unicompartmental knee arthroplasty: A matched comparison. Knee. 2020;31 https://doi.org/10.1016/j.knee.2019.12.005.
67. Casper DS, Fleischman AN, Papas PV, Grossman J, Scuderi GR, Lonner JH. Unicompartmental knee arthroplasty provides significantly greater improvement in function than Total knee

arthroplasty despite equivalent satisfaction for isolated medial compartment osteoarthritis. J Arthroplast. 2019;34(8):1611–6.
68. Sun X, Su Z. A meta-analysis of unicompartmental knee arthroplasty revised to total knee arthroplasty versus primary total knee arthroplasty. J Orthop Surg Res. 2018;13(1):158. https://doi.org/10.1186/s13018-018-0859-1.
69. 16th Annual Report, National Joint Registry for England, Wales, Northern Ireland and the Isle of Man. Accessed 04 May 20. https://reports.njrcentre.org.uk/Portals/0/PDFdownloads/NJR%2016th%20Annual%20Report%202019.pdf
70. Evans JT, Walker RW, Evans JP, Blom AW, Sayers A, Whitehouse MR. How long does a knee replacement last? A systematic review and meta-analysis of case series and national registry reports with more than 15 years of follow-up. Lancet. 2019;393(10172):655–63.
71. Karas V, Calkins TE, Bryan AJ, Culvern C, Nam D, Berger RA, Rosenberg AG, Della Valle CJ. Total knee arthroplasty in patients less than 50 years of age: results at a mean of 13 years. J Arthroplast. 2019;34(10):2392–7.
72. Niemeläinen M, Moilanen T, Huhtala H, Eskelinen A. Outcome of knee arthroplasty in patients aged 65 years or less: a prospective study of 232 patients with 2-year follow-up. Scand J Surg. 2019;108(4):313–20.
73. Lange JK, Lee YY, Spiro SK, Haas SB. Satisfaction rates and quality of life changes following Total knee arthroplasty in age-differentiated cohorts. J Arthroplast. 2018;33(5):1373–8.
74. Shearer J, Agius L, Burke N, Rahardja R, Young SW. BMI is a Better Predictor of Periprosthetic Joint Infection Risk Than Local Measures of Adipose Tissue After TKA. J Arthroplasty. 2020;24 https://doi.org/10.1016/j.arth.2020.01.048.
75. DeMik DE, Bedard NA, Dowdle SB, Elkins JM, Brown TS, Gao Y, Callaghan JJ. Complications and obesity in arthroplasty-a hip is not a knee. J Arthroplast. 2018;33(10):3281–7.
76. Sundaram K, Udo-Inyang I, Mont MA, Molloy R, Higuera-Rueda C, Piuzzi NS. Vascular injuries in Total knee arthroplasty: a systematic review and Meta-analysis. JBJS Rev. 2020;8(1):e0051. https://doi.org/10.2106/JBJS.RVW.19.00051.
77. Lewis GN, Rice DA, McNair PJ, Kluger M. Predictors of persistent pain after total knee arthroplasty: a systematic review and meta-analysis. Br J Anaesth. 2015;114(4):551–61.
78. Ritter MA, Campbell ED. Effect of range of motion on the success of a total knee arthroplasty. J Arthroplast. 1987;2(2):95–7.
79. Ritter MA, Lutgring JD, Davis KE, Berend ME, Pierson JL, Meneghini RM. The role of flexion contracture on outcomes in primary total knee arthroplasty. J Arthroplast. 2007;22(8):1092–6.
80. Aderinto J, Brenkel IJ, Chan P. Natural history of fixed flexion deformity following total knee replacement: a prospective five-year study. J Bone Joint Surg Br. 2005;87(7):934–6.
81. Lankinen P, Laasik R, Kivimäki M, Aalto V, Saltychev M, Vahtera J, Mäkelä K. Are patient-related pre-operative factors influencing return to work after total knee arthroplasty. Knee. 2019;26(4):853–60.
82. Fosco, Matteo & Ayad, Razan & Amendola, Luca & Dallari, Dante & Tigani, Domenico (2012) Management of Bone Loss in Primary and Revision Knee Replacement Surgery. 10.5772/26995. In Recent Advances in Arthroplasty.
83. Hamilton TW, Choudhary R, Jenkins C, Mellon SJ, Dodd CAF, Murray DW, Pandit HG. Lateral osteophytes do not represent a contraindication to medial unicompartmental knee arthroplasty: a 15-year follow-up. Knee Surg Sports Traumatol Arthrosc. 2017;25(3):652–9.
84. Skou ST, Roos EM, Laursen MB, Rathleff MS, Arendt-Nielsen L, Simonsen O, Rasmussen S. A Randomized, Controlled Trial of Total Knee Replacement. N Engl J Med. 2015;373(17):1597–606.

85. Zeni JA Jr, Snyder-Mackler L. Preoperative predictors of persistent impairments during stair ascent and descent after total knee arthroplasty. J Bone Joint Surg Am. 2010;92(5):1130–6. https://doi.org/10.2106/JBJS.I.00299.
86. Wylde V, Artz N, Howells N, Blom AW. Kneeling ability after total knee replacement. EFORT Open Rev. 2019;4(7):460–7.
87. Smith JRA, Mathews JA, Osborne L, Bakewell Z, Williams JL. Why do patients not kneel after total knee replacement? Is neuropathic pain a contributing factor? Knee. 2019;26(2):427–34.
88. Tsukada S, Kurosaka K, Nishino M, Hirasawa N. Cutaneous Hypesthesia and kneeling ability after Total knee arthroplasty: a randomized controlled trial comparing anterolateral and anteromedial skin incision. J Arthroplast. 2018;33(10):3174–80.
89. White L, Stockwell T, Hartnell N, Hennessy M, Mullan J. Factors preventing kneeling in a group of pre-educated patients post total knee arthroplasty. J Orthop Traumatol. 2016;17(4):333–8.
90. Wallace DT, Riches PE, Picard F. The assessment of instability in the osteoarthritic knee. EFORT Open Rev. 2019;4(3):70–6.
91. Neelapala YVR. Self-reported instability in knee osteoarthritis: a scoping review of literature. Curr Rheumatol Rev. 2019;15(2):110–5.
92. Parry EL, Thomas MJ, Peat G. Defining acute flares in knee osteoarthritis: a systematic review. BMJ Open. 2018;8(7):e019804. https://doi.org/10.1136/bmjopen-2017-019804.
93. Murphy SL, Lyden AK, Kratz AL, Fritz H, Williams DA, Clauw DJ, Gammaitoni AR, Phillips K. Characterizing pain flares from the perspective of individuals with symptomatic knee osteoarthritis. Arthritis Care Res (Hoboken). 2015;67(8):1103–11.
94. Parry E, Ogollah R, Peat G. 'Acute flare-ups' in patients with, or at high risk of, knee osteoarthritis: a daily diary study with case-crossover analysis. Osteoarthr Cartil. 2019;27(8):1124–8.
95. Fam AG, Topp JR, Stein HB, Little AH. Clinical and roentgenographic aspects of pseudogout: a study of 50 cases and a review. Can Med Assoc J. 1981;124(5):545–51.
96. Bennett RM, Lehr JR, McCarty DJ. Crystal shedding and acute pseudogout. An hypothesis based on a therapeutic failure. Arthritis Rheum. 1976;19(1):93–7.
97. Peck CN, Childs J, McLauchlan GJ. Inferior outcomes of Total knee replacement in early radiological stages of osteoarthritis. Knee. 2014;21(6):1229–32.
98. Riis A, Rathleff MS, Jensen MB, Simonsen O. Low grading of the severity of knee osteoarthritis pre-operatively is associated with a lower functional level after total knee replacement: a prospective cohort study with 12 months' follow-up. Bone Joint J. 2014;96-B(11):1498–502.
99. Scott CE, Oliver WM, MacDonald D, Wade FA, Moran M, Breusch SJ. Predicting dissatisfaction following total knee arthroplasty in patients under 55 years of age. Bone Joint J. 2016;98-B(12):1625–34.
100. Youlden DJ, Dannaway J, Enke O. Radiographic severity of knee osteoarthritis and its relationship to outcome post total knee arthroplasty: a systematic review. ANZ J Surg. 2020;90(3):237–42.
101. Baker PN, van der Meulen JH, Lewsey J, Gregg PJ, National Joint Registry for England and Wales. The role of pain and function in determining patient satisfaction after total knee replacement. Data from the National Joint Registry for England and Wales. J Bone Joint Surg Br. 2007;89(7):893–900.
102. Bourne RB, Chesworth BM, Davis AM, Mahomed NN, Charron KD. Patient satisfaction after total knee arthroplasty: who is satisfied and who is not? Clin Orthop Relat Res. 2010;468(1):57–63.
103. Price AJ, Longino D, Rees J, Rout R, Pandit H, Javaid K, Arden N, Cooper C, Carr AJ, Dodd CA, Murray DW, Beard DJ. Are pain and function better measures of outcome than revision rates after TKR in the younger patient? Knee. 2010;17(3):196–9.

Chapter 51
Painful Knee Replacement Arthroplasty

This is a condition whereby a knee replacement arthroplasty (partial or total) causes pain. This may be substantial and limiting patient's function.

It may be due to several causes including [1–19]:

- Intra-articular/Extra-articular
- Soft tissue/Bony
- Neuropathic
- Progression/development of knee arthritis in non-replaced compartments
- Arthroplasty specific including:
  - Instability
  - Patellar maltracking
  - Wear
  - Fixation loosening
  - Peri-prosthetic infection
  - Stiffness
  - Soft tissue impingement

51.1 Differential Diagnosis of Painful Knee Arthroplasty

- Referred pain–hip, spine
- Metabolic bone disease
- Psychological factors

In addition to the above, other causes of pain need to be considered as they would be in a native knee that has not been replaced. These include:

- Tendinopathy
- Bursitis

C. Panayiotou Charalambous, *The Knee Made Easy*,
https://doi.org/10.1007/978-3-030-54506-2_51

- Inflammatory/crystal arthropathy
- Synovial disorders
- Neoplasia

Lim et al. [20] looked at 178 cases of primary total knee replacement arthroplasty (TKR) with persistent pain not resolved after 1 year post surgery for causes other than infection. These causes included:

Intra-articular causes-83:
- Aseptic loosening-40
- Polyethylene wear-16
- Instability-10
- Recurrent haemarthrosis-5
- Patellar maltracking-4
- Tendon tears-4
- Stiffness-2

Extra-articular causes-39:
- Spinal nerve entrapment-10
- Hip OA/AVN-6

Unexplained-23

51.2 Clinical Symptoms of Painful Knee Replacement Arthroplasty

Pain nature, location and other characteristics of pain is obtained:

- Pain occurrence—continuous or intermittent, at rest or only on activity
- Timing of onset of pain
  - Pain is same as prior to replacement surgery, no improvement
  - Pain is different to that experienced prior to surgery, but is present since surgery
  - Pain free period post-surgery, followed by new onset of pain
- Speed of pain onset
  - Acute/gradual
- Precipitating event
  - No precipitating factor
  - Post injury
  - Post wound healing problems/wound infection
- Associated stiffness or instability that confer substantial functional loss

51.3 Clinical Signs

- Look, feel, move
- Knee swelling–effusion, synovitis
- Assess muscle strength
- Assess knee stability

51.4 Investigations for the Painful Knee Replacement Arthroplasty

- Plain radiographs of the knee–anteroposterior, lateral and skyline views to:
  - Assess the position of the prosthesis, determine if any change compared to immediate post-surgical radiographs (suggestive of loosening)
  - Determine if there has been any further arthritis development/progression (if unicompartmental arthroplasty in situ or if not all articulating surfaces have been replaced)
- Plain radiographs of the hip and lumbosacral spine to exclude referred pain
- Plain radiographs –long leg film to assess alignment
- CT scan with 3D reconstruction to:
  - Assess rotational, sagittal and coronal profile of the prosthesis and overall alignment of the lower limb
  - Look for early arthritis in non-replaced compartments
- MRI to look for associated soft tissue lesions (ligamentous, tendons)
- Bone scan–to look for:
  - Prosthesis infection
  - Aseptic loosening
  - Abnormal loading of underlying bone
- SPECT/CT to anatomically localise hot spots to help determine origin of pain
- Nerve conduction studies/electromyography
- Examination under anaesthesia–to assess range of motion, stability
- Knee Aspiration –
  - Fluid sent for:
    - Culture and sensitivity to look for infection
    - Microscopy to look for crystal arthropathy- gout/pseudogout

- Arthroscopic evaluation
  - Look for:
    - Insert wear
    - Metallosis
    - Synovitis
    - Soft tissue entrapment between articulating surfaces
    - Soft tissue impingement–such as synovium, fat pad
  - Biopsy of synovium for:
    - Culture and sensitivity to look for infection
    - Histology–exclude neoplastic cause (e.g. PVNS)

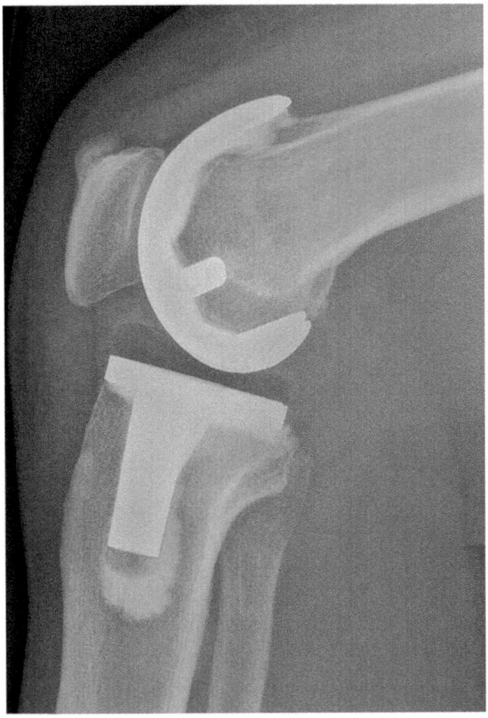

Painfull TKR due to quadriceps tendinopathy (associated with patellar superior pole spur)

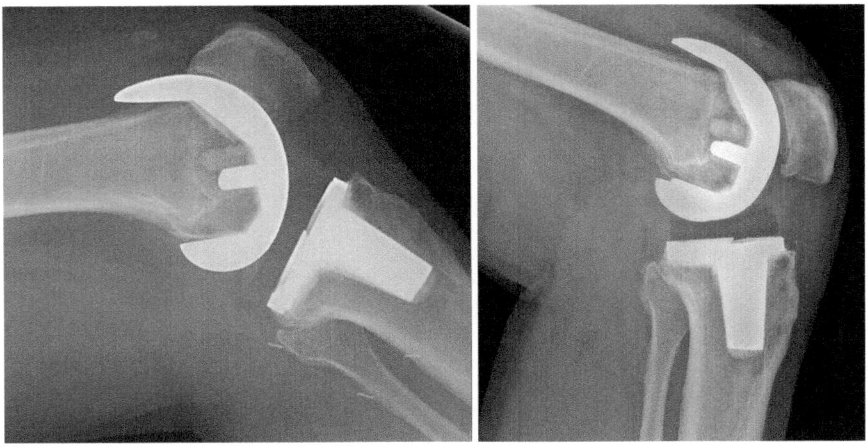

Cruciate retaining knee arthroplastry (patella not replaced) - patient presented with ongoing pain and limited knee flexion

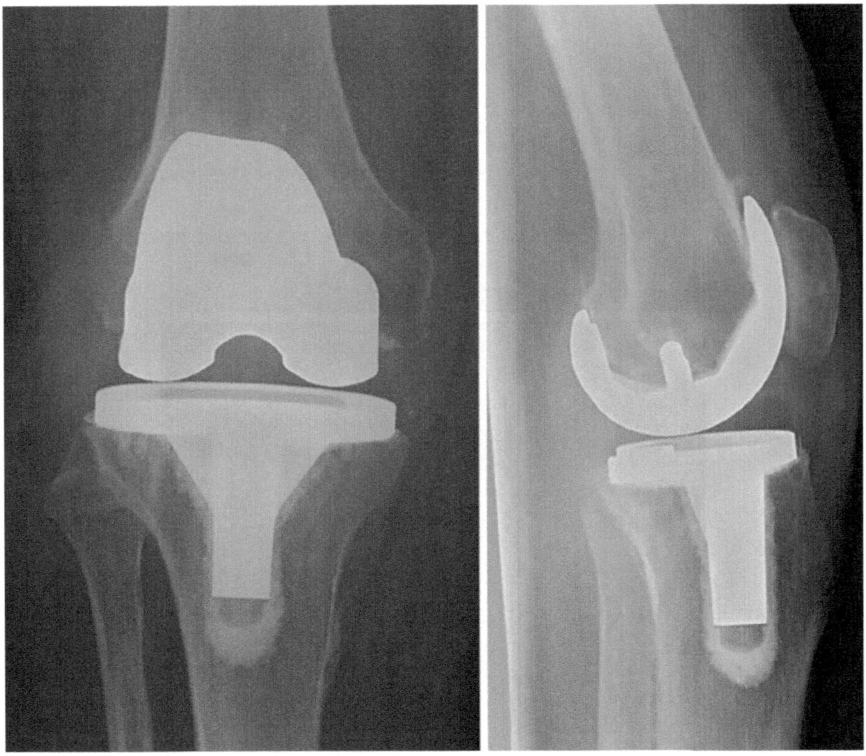

Loosening of the femoral component with associated osteolysis

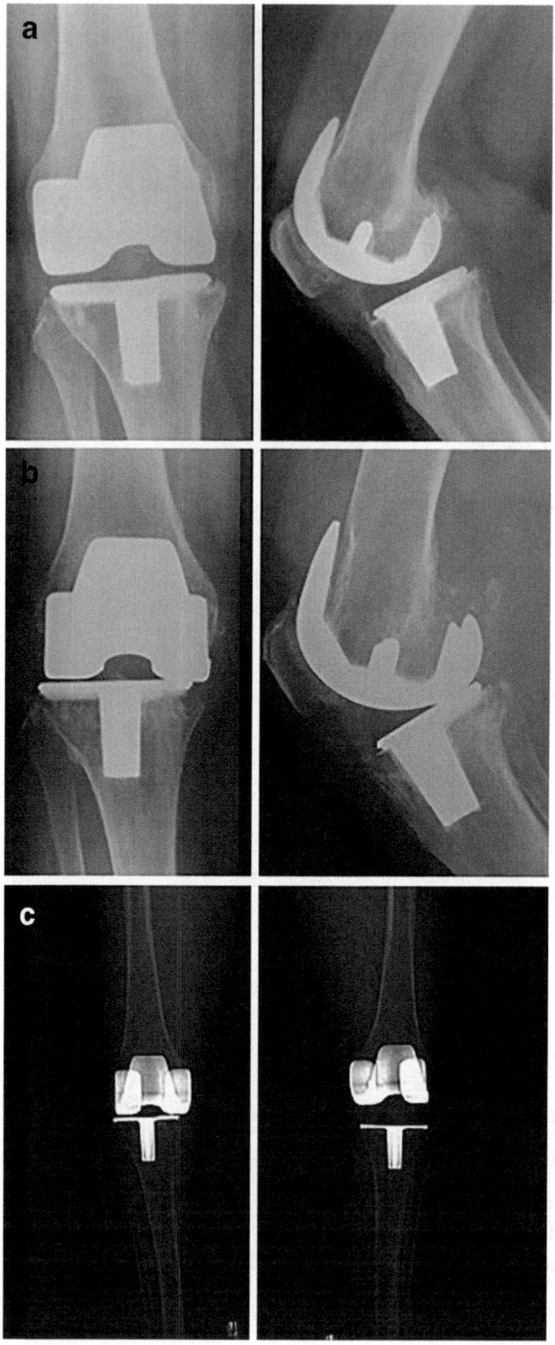

Wear of the polyethylene insert and tibial loosening in knee replacement arthroplasty (a) initial postoperative radiographs, (b) radiographs 15 years post surgery, (c) CT of ipsilateral and contralateral knee replacements of same patient

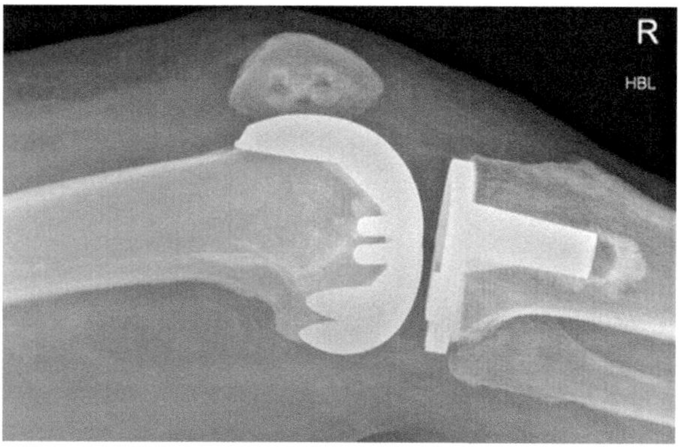

TKR with intact component fixation, but with substantial residual flexion deformity causing chronic pain

51.5 Management of Painful Knee Replacement Arthroplasty

Management of the painful knee arthroplasty aims to:

- Improve pain
- Address the underlying cause leading to pain

In some cases it is accepted that symptomatic control of pain may be all that can be achieved, without addressing the underlying cause of pain.

51.5.1 Non-surgical

Pain and associated symptoms are addressed as follows:

Pain:

- Oral analgesia, non-steroidal anti-inflammatories (oral, topical)
- Physiotherapy (localised ultrasound, megapulse, acupuncture)
- Knee steroid injection (for extra-articular lesions)

Stiffness

- Physiotherapy–stretching exercises that aim to elongate the contracted, shrunk capsule and ligaments
- Adequate pain control is essential for stretching exercises to be performed

Instability:

- Muscle strengthening, proprioception training
- Bracing:
  - To provide mechanical support
  - Aid proprioception

Infection:

- Superficial
  - Antibiotic therapy
  - Wound debridement
- Deep
  - Antibiotic therapy
    - Short term
    - Chronic suppression therapy

51.5.2 *Surgical [14–30]*

51.5.2.1 Stiffness

Persistent stiffness may be treated with surgery:

- Manipulation of the knee–under general anaesthesia the knee is moved by the surgeon and stretched, to tear the contracted tissue and regain movement.
- Arthroscopic release–for arthrofibrosis, removal of any obstructing intra-articular structures.
- Open arthrolysis–the contracted tissue is divided, adhesions are excised. Hardware used for fracture fixation, and which may be providing a mechanical block to movement are removed.
- Tendon lengthening

51.5.2.2 Instability

- Ligament reconstruction of deficient ligaments
- Revision surgery –
  - Insert exchange
  - Constrained implants that can compensate for deficient ligaments

51.5.2.3 Infection

- Superficial
  - Infected wound debridement
- Deep

- Arthroscopic washout
- Open washout ± synovectomy ±liner exchange
- Revision surgery
  - Single stage
  - Two stage

Revision surgery for infection may be carried in a single or 2 stages:

- Single stage–the implants are removed, the bone is debribed and a new prosthesis is inserted in 1 operation. Multiple biopsies are obtained for culture and sensitivity which help to guide as to post-surgery antibiotic treatment.
  - Two stage–the implants are removed, the bone is debribed and a spacer that contains antibiotics (off the shelf or cement made) is inserted. This aims to maintain the knee ligaments at length and prevent contracture, as well as release locally antibiotics to help eradicate any residual infection. Multiple biopsies are obtained for culture and sensitivity which help to guide as to post-surgery antibiotic treatment. Once the infection is clinically settled, and the haematological markers of infection (ESR, CRP) have returned to within normal range, the second stage is carried out whereby the spacer is removed and a new prosthesis is inserted.

51.5.2.4 Arthritis Progression

- Revision surgery to replace the knee compartments showing arthritis progression

51.5.2.5 Loosening/Wear

- Revision surgery
  - Partial–of loose/worn prosthesis components
  - Total–of all prosthesis components

Learning Pearls

- Not all pain following a joint arthroplasty may be attributed to the arthroplasty per se. Many of the other causes of pain encountered in the native knee may still be the cause of the patient's symptoms following replacement arthroplasty. In the absence of a specific source of pain attributed to the joint arthroplasty, revision surgery is not advised as it is likely that the patient will continue with ongoing pain.
- The timing of pain onset may guide as to its underlying cause:
  - If the pain is similar to the pain that the patient experienced prior to surgery the possibility of another source of pain (other than the knee–such as referred hip or lumbosacral spine pain) needs to be considered.

- Pain present since the time of surgery may point towards the possibility of low grade peri-prosthetic infection
- Pain starting after a period of pain relief following the arthroplasty procedure may point towards arthritis progression, prosthesis wear or aseptic loosening

- Lewis GN et al. [21] carried out a systematic review and meta-analysis of predictor variables associated with persistent pain after TKR. They included 32 studies involving almost 30,000 patients and reported that catastrophizing, mental health, preoperative knee pain, and pain at other sites, are the strongest independent predictors of persistent pain following TKR.

References

1. Toms AD, Mandalia V, Haigh R, Hopwood B. The management of patients with painful total knee replacement. J Bone Joint Surg Br. 2009;91(2):143–50.
2. Elson DW, Brenkel IJ. A conservative approach is feasible in unexplained pain after knee replacement: a selected cohort study. J Bone Joint Surg Br. 2007;89(8):1042–5.
3. Momoli A, Giarretta S, Modena M, Micheloni GM. The painful knee after total knee arthroplasty: evaluation and management. Acta Biomed. 2017;88(2S):60–7.
4. McDowell M, Park A, Gerlinger TL. The painful Total knee Arthroplasty. Orthop Clin North Am. 2016;47(2):317–26.
5. Cercek R, Bassett R, Myerthall S. Evaluation of the painful total knee arthroplasty. J Knee Surg. 2015;28(2):113–8.
6. Park CN, Zuiderbaan HA, Chang A, Khamaisy S, Pearle AD, Ranawat AS. Role of magnetic resonance imaging in the diagnosis of the painful unicompartmental knee arthroplasty. Knee. 2015;22(4):341–6.
7. Citak M, Cross MB, Gehrke T, Dersch K, Kendoff D. Modes of failure and revision of failed lateral unicompartmental knee. Arthroplasties Knee. 2015;22(4):338–40.
8. van der List JP, Zuiderbaan HA, Pearle AD. Why do medial Unicompartmental knee Arthroplasties fail today? J Arthroplast. 2016;31(5):1016–21.
9. van der List JP, Chawla H, Villa JC, Pearle AD. Why do patellofemoral arthroplasties fail today? A systematic review. Knee. 2017;24(1):2–8.
10. Bendixen NB, Eskelund PW, Odgaard A. Failure modes of patellofemoral arthroplasty-registries vs. clinical studies: a systematic review. Acta Orthop. 2019;90(5):473–8.
11. Le DH, Goodman SB, Maloney WJ, Huddleston JI. Current modes of failure in TKA: infection, instability, and stiffness predominate. Clin Orthop Relat Res. 2014;472(7):2197–200.
12. Parvizi J, Fassihi SC, Enayatollahi MA. Diagnosis of Periprosthetic joint infection following hip and knee Arthroplasty. Orthop Clin North Am. 2016;47(3):505–15.
13. Shohat N, Goswami K, Fillingham Y, Tan TL, Calkins T, Della Valle CJ, George J, Higuera C, Parvizi J. Diagnosing Periprosthetic joint infection in inflammatory arthritis: assumption is the enemy of true understanding. J Arthroplast. 2018;33(11):3561–6.
14. Ting NT, Della Valle CJ. Diagnosis of Periprosthetic joint infection-an algorithm-based approach. J Arthroplast. 2017;32(7):2047–50.
15. Cottino U, Sculco PK, Sierra RJ, Abdel MP. Instability after Total knee Arthroplasty. Orthop Clin North Am. 2016;47(2):311–6.
16. Song SJ, Detch RC, Maloney WJ, Goodman SB, Huddleston JI 3rd. Causes of instability after total knee arthroplasty. J Arthroplast. 2014;29(2):360–4.

17. Abdel MP, Haas SB. The unstable knee: wobble and buckle. Bone Joint J. 2014;96-B(11 Supple A):112–4.
18. Potty AG, Tzeng TH, Sams JD, Lovell ME, Mihalko WM, Thompson KM, Parke J, Manning BT, Dennis DA, Goodman SB, Saleh KJ. Diagnosis and Management of Intra-articular Causes of pain after Total knee Arthroplasty. Instr Course Lect. 2015;64:389–401.
19. Manning BT, Lewis N, Tzeng TH, Saleh JK, Potty AG, Dennis DA, Mihalko WM, Goodman SB, Saleh KJ. Diagnosis and Management of Extra-articular Causes of pain after Total knee Arthroplasty. Instr Course Lect. 2015;64:381–8.
20. Lim HA, Song EK, Seon JK, Park KS, Shin YJ, Yang HY. Causes of aseptic persistent pain after Total knee Arthroplasty. Clin Orthop Surg. 2017;9(1):50–6.
21. Lewis GN, Rice DA, McNair PJ, Kluger M. Predictors of persistent pain after total knee arthroplasty: a systematic review and meta-analysis. Br J Anaesth. 2015;114(4):551–61.

Chapter 52
Instability in Knee Replacement Arthroplasty

This is a condition where there is symptomatic translation of one articulating surface in relation to another following knee replacement arthroplasty (partial or total). The patient may complain of pain, apprehension or the knee giving way. Such instability may involve the tibiofemoral or patellofemoral(PF) articulations. Many of the principles applying to the native knee also apply to knee replacement arthroplasty [1–15].

52.1 Describing Knee Instability

Knee instability may be described in various ways and some of these are presented below:

According to the Joint Involved
One or more joints may be simultaneously affected by instability.

C. Panayiotou Charalambous, *The Knee Made Easy*,
https://doi.org/10.1007/978-3-030-54506-2_52

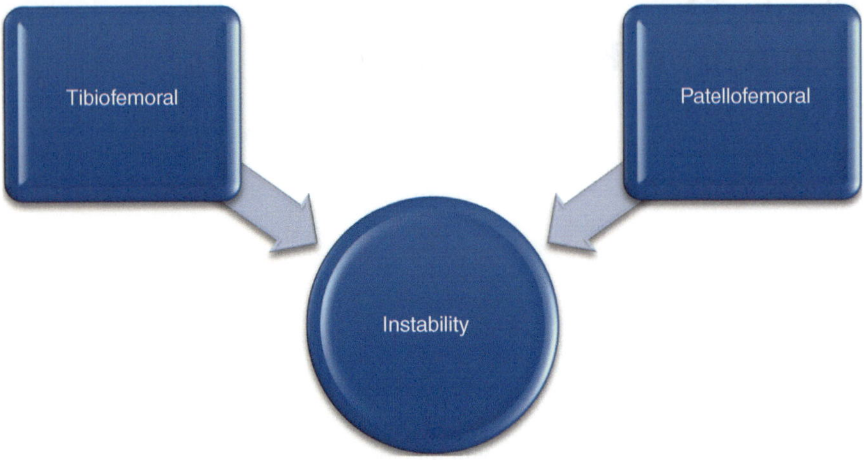

Instability of a TKR may be described according to the articulation involved

Number of Instability Episodes

- First time instability—refers to the first episode of instability
- Recurrent instability—refers to more than one episode of instability

Degree of Translation

- Subluxation
- Dislocation

One articulating surface may sublux (displace but still remain in partial contact with the opposite articulating surface). Alternatively, a joint may dislocate (with loss of all articular contact).

Reducibility

- Spontaneously reducible
- Spontaneously irreducible

Following dislocation the articulating surfaces may either relocate spontaneously or need to be reduced medically.

According to the Direction of Translation of One Articulating Surface to the Other

- PF joint—translation of the patella in relation to the femoral trochlea
  - Lateral
  - Medial

- Tibiofemoral joint—translation of the tibia in relation to the femur:
  - Sagittal—Anterior/posterior
  - Rotational
  - Coronal
    - Varus
    - Valgus
  - Multidirectional—instability occurs in two or more directions

  The direction of instability can be determined by:

- Clinical history—identifying the position that reproduces instability symptoms
- Clinical examination
  - Visual inspection
  - Assessment of:
  - Varus/valgus laxity
  - Flexion/extension laxity
  - Rotational laxity
- Radiographs or other radiological investigations

According to the Initiating Event
- Iatrogenic—present since replacement surgery
- Traumatic—as a result of a further specific, substantial trauma
- Atraumatic—occurring gradually with no precipitating substantial trauma

According to the Frequency of Instability
- First time—the first episode of instability
- Recurrent—the second or subsequent episode of instability
- Permanent—present all time
- Intermittent—alternating instability with stability
- Habitual—occurring with each flexion/extension cycle of the knee

According to the Degree of Knee Flexion at which Instability Occurs
- Extension
- 90° flexion
- Midflexion
- Hyperextension

52.2 Causes of Knee Instability

Instability may be due to disruption or inefficiency of dynamic or static stabilisers:

52.2.1 *Static*

- Ligaments
  - Detached
  - Torn
  - Stretched
- Replacement insert
  - Inadequate thickness
  - Wear

52.2.2 *Dynamic*

- Weak
- Discoordinated
- Lack of stable platform to act upon
- Abnormal muscle activation
- Defective proprioception
- Excessive joint laxity
- Insufficient core control
- Insufficient hip control
- Insufficient ankle and foot control

Song SJ et al. [5] described 6 categories of instability following TKR:

1. Flexion/extension gap mismatch
2. Component malposition
3. Isolated ligament dysfunction (collaterals/posterior cruciate ligament(PCL))
4. Extensor mechanism dysfunction
5. Component loosening
6. Global instability

In the series reported by Song SJ et al. [5] 30% of cases had multifactorial instability.

Flexion instability occurs with the knee in flexion. It may be due to:

- Loose flexion gap (this is the space between the distal femur and proximal tibia with the knee in flexion)—the thickness of the replacement implants may be inadequate in relation to the gap created following resection of the articular surfaces, leading to a loose flexion gap
- PCL deficiency:

- Present prior to surgery, or occurring at the time of surgery but not addressed during the replacement arthroplasty (such as by the use of implants utilised in the PCL deficient knee)
- Occurring subsequent to the replacement arthroplasty

Extension instability occurs with the knee in extension. It may be due to:

- Loose extension gap (this is the space between the distal femur and proximal tibia with the knee in extension)—the thickness of the replacement implants may be inadequate in relation to the gap created following resection of the articular surfaces, leading to a loose extension gap.
- Collateral ligament deficiency (medial or lateral) with:
  - Present prior to surgery, or occurring at the time of surgery, but not addressed during the replacement arthroplasty (such as by soft tissue repair/reconstruction or by the use of implants utilised in the collateral ligament deficient knee)
  - Occurring subsequent to the replacement arthroplasty

52.3 Clinical Symptoms of Knee Replacement Arthroplasty Instability

- Feeling of abnormal displacement—this may range from:
  - Feeling "wobbly" to
  - "Popping in and out" to
  - "Giving way"
  - "Falling down"
- Locking/catching
- Pain, vague, leg heaviness
- Recurrent effusion/synovitis
- Leg weakness
- Clicking, clunking
- Dead leg syndrome, paraesthesia
- Subluxation
- Dislocation (rare)

Symptoms may be aggravated by leg or knee position or motion:

- Rotational instability—as when turning or twisting
- Flexion instability—as when descending stairs
- Extension instability—upon weightbearing
- PF instability—straightening the knee from full flexion, flexing knee from full extension

52.4 Clinical Signs of Knee Replacement Arthroplasty Instability

These aim to assess:

- Apprehension, subluxation, dislocation and relocation of the examined joint
- Laxity of the tibiofemoral joint (flexion/extension, varus/valgus)—stress testing, Posterior tibial sag in knee flexion
- Laxity of the PF joint (lateral, medial)
- Neurological deficit
- Abnormal muscle activation
- Core/hip weakness/imbalance
- Ankle/foot weakness/imbalance

52.5 Investigations for Knee Replacement Arthroplasty Instability

Investigations of the unstable knee aim to confirm the presence of instability and determine its likely cause. These include:

- Radiological
  - Plain radiographs: Anteroposterior, lateral, skyline
  - Stress views
  - Long leg film to assess alignment
  - CT Scan- to assess prosthesis alignment, including rotational
  - MRI/Ultrasound—to assess the integrity of peri-articular ligaments and tendons
- Neurophysiological
  - Nerve conduction studies
  - Electromyography

- Inflammatory markers, knee fluid aspiration and/or synovial biopsy for microbiological examination to exclude infection
- Examination under general anaesthesia
- Arthroscopic evaluation—assess insert wear

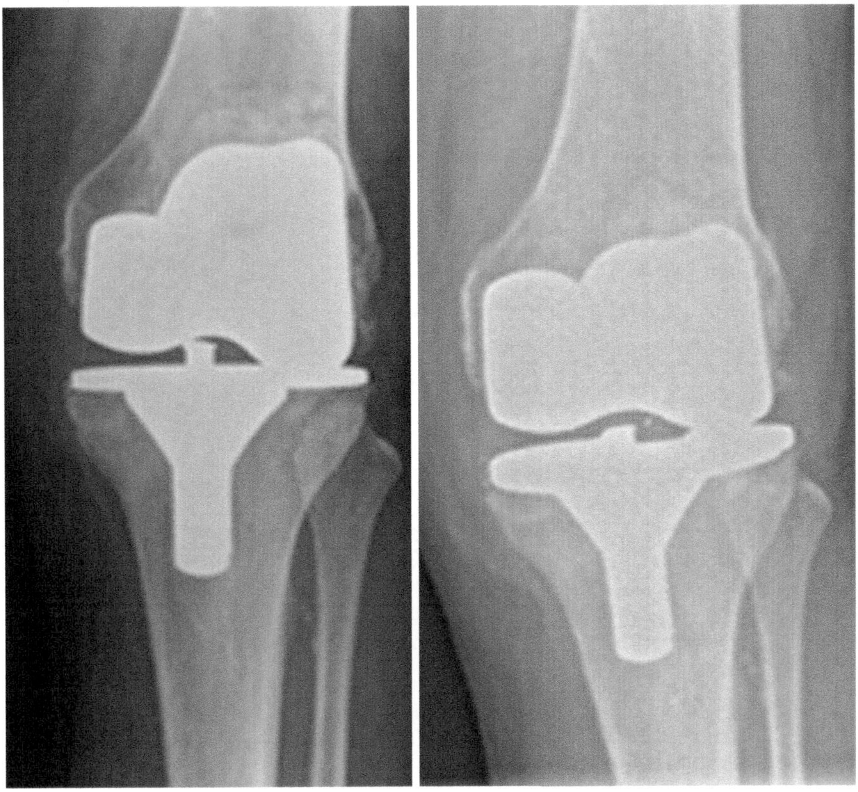

Medial Instability in TKR following MCL disruption due to a further acute traumatic injury

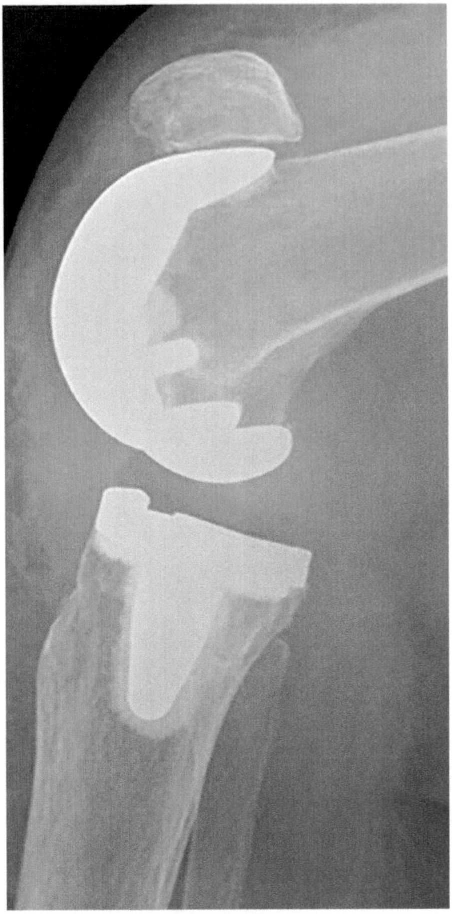

Knee replacement arthroplasty instability in sagittal plane

52.6 Management of Knee Replacement Arthroplasty Instability

Management depends on:

- Symptoms—severity, frequency
- Underlying cause
- Direction of instability
- Functional impairment

Management aims to improve joint stability and reduce further subluxations or dislocations. In doing so, surgery may help to improve associated functional loss, apprehension, or pain.

52.6.1 *Non-surgical*

- Activity modification, avoiding unstable leg/knee positions
- External devices—taping, bracing, ankle foot orthotics
- Physiotherapy to address deficits in:
  - Core imbalance—core strengthening
  - Poor pelvic control—strengthening of pelvic muscles
  - Poor hip control—weakness of abductors, extensors, external rotators
  - Foot and ankle control/position
  - Proprioception—proprioceptive training
  - Quadriceps and hamstring weakness- muscle strengthening, balance
- Antibiotics if underlying infection

52.6.2 *Surgical*

If symptoms do not improve with non-surgical intervention and patient has structural lesions that are amenable to surgery, surgery may be considered. Surgery may also be considered early if the underlying cause is infection.

Surgical interventions for stability may be described according to the articulation involved and the structures addressed:

52.6.3 *Tibiofemoral Instability Following Knee Replacement Arthroplasty*

Surgical options include:

- Soft tissue procedure (ligament reconstruction, release of tight structures)
- Implant procedure—
  - Revision surgery:
    - Alter insert thickness
    - Reposition implants (alter alignment)
    - Constrained implants
- Combined

52.6.4 *Patellofemoral Instability Following Knee Replacement Arthroplasty*

PF instability is usually in a lateral direction, and may be due to retinacula imbalance, femoral or tibial component malposition (placed in excessive internal rotation or in excessive medialisation), failure to medialize the patellar button (if patella resurfaced), too thick resurfaced patella, residual valgus alignment of the knee, and surgery aims to address these:

- Soft tissue procedure (release of tight lateral retinaculum, release of collaterals to improve knee alignment, medial PF ligament reconstruction)
- Bony procedure—distal extensor mechanism realignment (tibial tubercle transfer)
- Implant procedure—
  - Revision surgery:
    - Reposition implants (alter alignment/implant position)
    - Alter implant size
- Combined

Learning Pearls

- A wide spectrum of knee laxity may occur following TKR and this may not correlate with patient's subjective satisfaction. Hence, clinical laxity should be interpreted with caution.
- The timing of instability onset may guide as to its underlying cause:
  - If the instability is similar to instability experienced prior to surgery, the following potential causes need to be considered:
    - A cause local to the knee not addressed at the time of surgery
    - A cause not directly attributable to the knee or the replacement prosthesis (such as neurological disruption)
  - Instability present only since the time of surgery may point towards:
    - A surgical cause
  - Instability starting after a long period of stability following the arthroplasty procedure may point towards:
    - Insert wear, implant loosening, PCL disruption, infection
- Results of revision surgery for instability are often unpredictable (such as for flexion, midflexion instability) and should be approached with caution. Non-surgical management options may be extensively utilised.

References

1. Cottino U, Sculco PK, Sierra RJ, Abdel MP. Instability after Total knee arthroplasty. Orthop Clin North Am. 2016;47(2):311–6.
2. Wautier D, Thienpont E. Changes in anteroposterior stability and proprioception after different types of knee arthroplasty. Knee Surg Sports Traumatol Arthrosc. 2017;25(6):1792–800.
3. di Laura FG, Zaffagnini S, Filardo G, Romandini I, Fusco A, Candrian C. Total knee arthroplasty in patients with knee osteoarthritis: effects on proprioception. A systematic review and best evidence synthesis. J Arthroplast. 2019;34(11):2815–22.
4. Bragonzoni L, Rovini E, Barone G, Cavallo F, Zaffagnini S, Benedetti MG. How proprioception changes before and after total knee arthroplasty: a systematic review. Gait Posture. 2019;72:1–11.
5. Song SJ, Detch RC, Maloney WJ, Goodman SB, Huddleston JI 3rd. Causes of instability after total knee arthroplasty. J Arthroplast. 2014;29(2):360–4.
6. Abdel MP, Haas SB. The unstable knee: wobble and buckle. Bone Joint J. 2014;96-B(11 Supple A):112–4.
7. Nam D, Abdel MP, Cross MB, LE LM, Reinhardt KR, BA MA, Man DJ, Hanssen AD, Sculco TP. The management of extensor mechanism complications in total knee arthroplasty. AAOS exhibit selection. J Bone Joint Surg Am. 2014;96(6):e47. https://doi.org/10.2106/JBJS.M.00949.
8. Tsubosaka M, Matsumoto T, Takayama K, Nakano N, Kuroda R. Two cases of late medial instability of the knee due to hip disease after total knee arthroplasty. Int J Surg Case Rep. 2017;37:200–4.
9. Green CC, Haidukewych GJ. Isolated Polyethylene Insert Exchange for Flexion Instability After Primary Total Knee Arthroplasty Demonstrated Excellent Results in Properly Selected Patients. J Arthroplasty. 2020; https://doi.org/10.1016/j.arth.2020.01.006.
10. Jin C, Zhao JY, Santoso A, Song EK, Chan CK, Jin QH, Ko JW, Seon JK. Primary repair for injury of medial collateral ligament during total-knee arthroplasty. Medicine (Baltimore). 2019;98(39):e17134.
11. Bohl DD, Wetters NG, Del Gaizo DJ, Jacobs JJ, Rosenberg AG, Della Valle CJ. Repair of Intraoperative Injury to the Medial Collateral Ligament During Primary Total Knee Arthroplasty. J Bone Joint Surg Am. 2016;98(1):35–9.
12. Ramappa M. Midflexion instability in primary total knee replacement: a review. SICOT J. 2015;1:24. https://doi.org/10.1051/sicotj/2015020.
13. Petrie JR, Haidukewych GJ. Instability in total knee arthroplasty: assessment and solutions. Bone Joint J. 2016;98-B(1 Suppl A):116–9.
14. Stambough JB, Edwards PK, Mannen EM, Barnes CL, Mears SC. Flexion Instability After Total Knee Arthroplasty. J Am Acad Orthop Surg. 2019;27(17):642–51.
15. Meding JB, Keating EM, Ritter MA, Faris PM, Berend ME. Genu recurvatum in total knee replacement. Clin Orthop Relat Res. 2003;416:64–7.

Chapter 53
Synovial Chondromatosis of the Knee

This is a condition where cartilaginous loose bodies form in the knee (which is a joint lined by synovium) [1–28]. This may be:

- Primary—the synovial cells undergo primary metaplasia to chondrocytes, which go on to form cartilaginous bodies that enlarge and may become calcified or ossified. The nodules may be seen within the synovium or be loosely attached to it, or be completely free.
- Secondary—osteochondral fractures of the knee, degenerative arthritis or osteonecrosis cause fragmentation of the joint surface or detachment of osteophytes which form loose bodies. These loose bodies provide a central nidus which can then become covered with cartilage and may grow in size. There is proliferation of connective tissue cells and subsequent cartilaginous metaplasia.

Primary synovial chondromatosis may show three stages:

1. Confined to the synovium
2. Active synovium with loose bodies
3. Inactive synovium with residual loose bodies

Synovial chondromatosis usually affects one joint (often the knee) and is intra-articular. However, it may also involve extra-articular tissues such as tendon sheaths or bursae. It may also involve the infrapatellar fat pad. Synovial chondromatosis has been described following total knee replacement arthroplasty(TKR), arising from residual synovium.

53.1 Clinical Symptoms of Synovial Chondromatosis

- Knee pain
- Clicking/clunking/crepitus
- Locking

C. Panayiotou Charalambous, *The Knee Made Easy*,
https://doi.org/10.1007/978-3-030-54506-2_53

- Stiffness
- Visible or palpable swelling

53.2 Clinical Signs of Synovial Chondromatosis

- Visible swelling
- Localised tenderness
- Reduced knee motion—active and passive

53.3 Investigations for Synovial Chondromatosis [12–14]

- Plain radiographs—aberrant calcified bodies
- MRI—can demonstrate non-calcified cartilaginous bodies (that are not visible on plain radiographs)
- Biopsy and histological examination

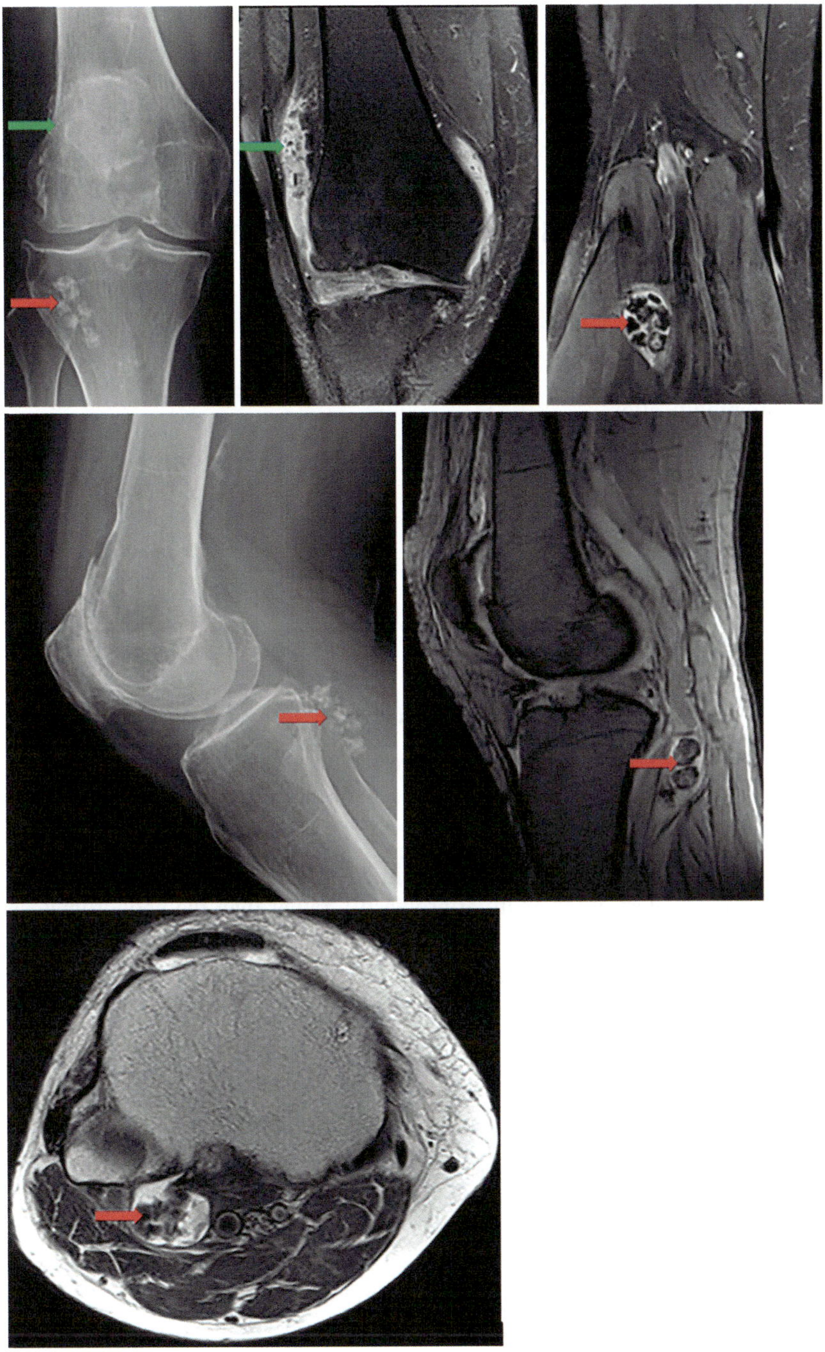

Synovial chondromatosis of cyst related to tibiofibular joint (red arrow) and suprapatellar pouch (green arrow), with associated patellofemoral and tibiofemoral degenerative changes

53.4 Differential Diagnosis of Synovial Chondromatosis

- Osteochondral lesions—traumatic, OCD
- Neoplastic lesions (e.g. synovial sarcoma, periosteal chondroma)

53.5 Management of Synovial Chondromatosis

53.5.1 Non-surgical

- Leave alone
- Activity modification
- Analgesia
- Physiotherapy:
  - Improve passive motion

53.5.2 Surgical

- Surgical removal of loose bodies (arthroscopic/open) + knee synovectomy

If only the loose bodies are removed the residual synovium may produce further loose bodies. However, progression may not occur if the synovium becomes inactive.

- In synovial chondromatosis associated with knee arthritis, the latter may be the main focus of intervention (with arthroplasty), rather than the chondromatosis per se. TKR in the background of synovial chondromatosis helps improve pain but may be associated with a high risk of recurrence (25%) and other complications (stiffness, need of revision surgery)

Learning Pearls

- Intra-articular loose bodies of the knee may lead to secondary arthritis due to third body wear (caught between the articular surfaces causing damage)
- In the absence of obvious degenerative changes, a history of injury should be sought as what looks as primary synovial chondromatosis may be a secondary condition.
- Malignant transformation to synovial chondrosarcoma is a rare but recognised complication, to be considered when aggressive clinical or radiological features are encountered (such as periarticular soft tissue involvement or bone infiltration by a cartilaginous mass), or in the presence of rapid

deterioration of clinical findings, or when there is a rapid recurrence following surgical synovectomy.

- Synovial chondromatosis may occur after TKR and should be considered in the differential diagnosis of pain, swelling, or limitation of motion [2].

References

1. Neumann JA, Garrigues GE, Brigman BE, Eward WC. Synovial Chondromatosis. JBJS Rev. 2016;4(5) https://doi.org/10.2106/JBJS.RVW.O.00054.
2. Majima T, Kamishima T, Susuda K. Synovial chondromatosis originating from the synovium of the anterior cruciate ligament: a case report. Sports Med Arthrosc Rehabil Ther Technol. 2009;1(1):6.
3. Kyung BS, Lee SH, Han SB, Park JH, Kim CH, Lee DH. Arthroscopic treatment of synovial chondromatosis at the knee posteriortum using a trans-septal approach: report of two cases. Knee. 2012;19(5):732–5.
4. Sebaaly A, Maalouf G, Bayyoud W, Bachour F. Synovial chondromatosis of the posterior compartment of the knee: A Case Report & Literature Review Focusing on Arthroscopic Treatment. J Med Liban. 2016;64(1):43–6.
5. Lee DH, Jeong TW. Uncommon primary synovial Chondromatosis involving only the infrapatellar fat pad in an elderly patient. Knee Surg Relat Res. 2016;28(1):79–82.
6. Maljanovič M, Ristič V, Rasovič P, Matijevič R, Milankov V. Solitary synovial chondromatosis as a cause of Hoffa's fat pad impingement. Med Pregl. 2015;68(1–2):49–52.
7. Shah DP, Diwakar M, Dargar N. Bakers cyst with synovial chondromatosis of knee—a rare case report. J Orthop Case Rep. 2016;6(1):17–9.
8. Ho SW, Hoa LM, Lee KT. A rare case of concomitant intra-articular and extra-articular synovial Chondromatosis of the knee joint. Ann Acad Med Singap. 2019;48(5):161–4.
9. Lin RC, Lue KH, Lin ZI, Lu KH. Primary synovial chondromatosis mimicking medial meniscal tear in a young man. Arthroscopy. 2006;22(7):803.e1–3.
10. Sim FH, Dahlin DC, Ivins JC. Extra-articular synovial chondromatosis. J Bone Joint Surg Am. 1977;59(4):492–5.
11. Choi JK, Jeong JH, Lee CT, Kim SJ. Synovial chondromatosis in the quadriceps tendon. Arthroscopy. 2003;19(4):E36.
12. Crotty JM, Monu JU, Pope TL Jr. Synovial osteochondromatosis. Radiol Clin N Am. 1996;34(2):327–42.
13. Boninsegna E, Fassio A, Testoni M, Gatti D, Viapiana O, Mansueto G, Rossini M. Radiological features of knee joint synovial chondromatosis. Reumatismo. 2019;71(2):81–4.
14. Maghear L, Serban O, Papp I, Otel O, Manole S, Botan E, Fodor D. Multimodal ultrasonographic evaluation in a case with unossified primary synovial osteochondromatosis. Med Ultrason. 2018;20(4):527–30.
15. Houdek MT, Wyles CC, Rose PS, Stuart MJ, Sim FH, Taunton MJ. High rate of local recurrence and complications following Total knee arthroplasty in the setting of synovial Chondromatosis. J Arthroplast. 2017;32(7):2147–50.
16. Deinum J, Nolte PA. Total knee arthroplasty in severe synovial osteochondromatosis in an osteoarthritic knee. Clin Orthop Surg. 2016;8(2):218–22. https://doi.org/10.4055/cios.2016.8.2.218.
17. Crawford MD, Kim HT. New-onset synovial chondromatosis after total knee arthroplasty. J Arthroplasty. 2013;28(2):375.e1–4.
18. McCarthy C, Anderson WJ, Vlychou M, Inagaki Y, Whitwell D, Gibbons CL, Athanasou NA. Primary synovial chondromatosis: a reassessment of malignant potential in 155 cases. Skelet Radiol. 2016;45(6):755–62.

19. Perry BE, McQueen DA, Lin JJ. Synovial chondromatosis with malignant degeneration to chondrosarcoma. Report of a case. J Bone Joint Surg Am. 1988;70(8):1259–61.
20. Hallam P, Ashwood N, Cobb J, Fazal A, Heatley W. Malignant transformation in synovial chondromatosis of the knee? Knee. 2001;8(3):239–42.
21. Jonckheere J, Shahabpour M, Willekens I, Pouliart N, Dezillie M, Vanhoenacker F, De Mey J. Rapid malignant transformation of primary synovial chondromatosis into chondrosarcoma. JBR-BTR. 2014;97(5):303–7.
22. Yao MS, Chang CM, Chen CL, Chan WP. Synovial chondrosarcoma arising from synovial chondromatosis of the knee. JBR-BTR. 2012;95(6):360–2.
23. Samson L, Mazurkiewicz S, Treder M, Wiśniewski P. Outcome in the arthroscopic treatment of synovial chondromatosis of the knee. Ortop Traumatol Rehabil. 2005;7(4):391–6.
24. Pengatteeri YH, Park SE, Lee HK, Lee YS, Gopinathan P, Han CW. Synovial chondromatosis of the posterior cruciate ligament managed by a posterior-posterior triangulation technique. Knee Surg Sports Traumatol Arthrosc. 2007;15(9):1121–4.
25. Jesalpura JP, Chung HW, Patnaik S, Choi HW, Kim JI, Nha KW. Arthroscopic treatment of localized synovial chondromatosis of the posterior knee joint. Orthopedics. 2010;33(1):49–51. https://doi.org/10.3928/01477447-20091124-22.
26. Ogilvie-Harris DJ, Saleh K. Generalized synovial chondromatosis of the knee: a comparison of removal of the loose bodies alone with arthroscopic synovectomy. Arthroscopy. 1994;10(2):166–70.
27. Coolican MR, Dandy DJ. Arthroscopic management of synovial chondromatosis of the knee. Findings and results in 18 cases. J Bone Joint Surg Br. 1989;71(3):498–500.
28. Dorfmann H, De Bie B, Bonvarlet JP, Boyer T. Arthroscopic treatment of synovial chondromatosis of the knee. Arthroscopy. 1989;5(1):48–51.

Chapter 54
Pigmented Villonodular Synovitis of the Knee

This is a condition where there is hyperplasia of the synovium, synovial giant cell accumulation and intracellular and extracellular hemosiderin deposition. This may involve the lining of synovial joints, tendon sheaths or bursae. Pigmented villonodular synovitis (PVNS) usually affects one joint and is intra-articular, usually involving the knee. However, it may also involve extra-articular tissues such as tendon sheaths or bursae. PVNS has also been described following total knee replacement arthroplasty (TKR), arising from residual synovium. It has also been reported following the implantation of fracture fixation devices.

Although initially limited to synovium, PVNS may lead to bone and articular cartilage changes due to pressure effects or the release of inflammatory mediators by macrophages and osteoclast like giant cells, leading to erosion and osteolysis [1–14]. Similarly, it may invade and destroy adjacent soft tissue. Colony-stimulating factor −1 has been implicated in its pathogenesis.

PVNS most commonly affects females in the 20–40 age group. The most common joint involved is the knee followed by the hip.

Intra-articular PVNS involving the knee may be 1 of 2 growth patterns:

- Localised nodular—usually involving the anterior part of the knee
- Diffuse villous—involving multiple parts of the knee

The pathogenesis of PVNS is uncertain but may be related to:

- Injury induced synovial inflammation and proliferation
- Neoplasia (benign)—most likely

C. Panayiotou Charalambous, *The Knee Made Easy*,
https://doi.org/10.1007/978-3-030-54506-2_54

54.1 Clinical Symptoms of Pigmented Villonodular Synovitis

- Knee pain
- Clicking/clunking
- Recurrent swelling
- Locking
- Stiffness
- Visible or palpable swelling

54.2 Clinical Signs of Pigmented Villonodular Synovitis

- Visible/palpable swelling
- Localised tenderness
- Reduced knee motion—active and passive

54.3 Investigations for Pigmented Villonodular Synovitis

- Plain radiographs:
  - Periarticular erosions
  - Degenerative changes in advanced disease
- MRI—low or intermediate signal intensity on T1-weighted and low signal intensity on T2-weighted images. Findings on MRI are mainly attributable to the hemosiderin deposition in the affected tissues due to its magnetic susceptibility properties.
- Arthroscopic evaluation/biopsy and histological examination—macroscopically rust coloured synovial hypertrophy/rusty effusion

54.4 Differential Diagnosis of Pigmented Villonodular Synovitis

- Inflammatory arthropathy
- Haemophilic arthropathy
- Hemochromatosis
- Hemosiderosis
- Synovitis due to intra-articular bleeding
- Uncalcified synovial chondromatosis
- Tuberculous arthritis
- Neoplastic lesions (e.g. synovial sarcoma)

54.5 Management of Pigmented Villonodular synovitis [15–26]

54.5.1 *Non-surgical*

- Leave alone
- Activity modification
- Analgesia
- Physiotherapy:
  - Improve passive motion

54.5.2 *Surgical*

- Surgical removal of the synovium (arthroscopic+/−open synovectomy)
- Intra-articular radio-isotope injection or external beam radiation used as adjuvant therapy following surgical excision to minimise risk of recurrence
- High recurrence rates (up to 48%) has been reported with diffuse PVNS, but this is much lower with localised PVNS (9%).
- In cases of PVNS associated with knee degeneration or arthritis, the latter may be the main focus of intervention (with arthroplasty), along with synovectomy, rather than sole synovectomy. TKR in the presence of PVNS has been shown to be associated with a higher risk of post-surgical stiffness and infection.

Learning Pearls

- Malignant transformation of PVNS is a very rare but a recognised entity, and needs to be considered when aggressive clinical or radiological features are encountered (such as periarticular soft tissue involvement or bone infiltration). It may arise concomitantly with benign PVNS or follow a previously documented benign PVNS at the same site. Such neoplasms may be locally aggressive or metastasize [4, 14].
- PVNS following implantation of orthopaedic devices (replacement or fixation devices) has been reported

References

1. Taylor R, Kashima TG, Knowles H, Gibbons CL, Whitwell D, Athanasou NA. Osteoclast formation and function in pigmented villonodular synovitis. J Pathol. 2011;225(1):151–6.
2. Molena B, Sfriso P, Oliviero F, Pagnin E, Teramo A, Lunardi F, Stramare R, Scanu A, Nardacchione R, Rubaltelli L, Calabrese F, Punzi L, Fiocco U. Synovial colony-stimulating factor-1 mRNA expression in diffuse pigmented villonodular synovitis. Clin Exp Rheumatol. 2011;29(3):547–50.

3. Tyler WK, Vidal AF, Williams RJ, Healey JH. Pigmented villonodular synovitis. J Am Acad Orthop Surg. 2006;14(6):376–85.
4. Patel KH, Gikas PD, Pollock RC, Carrington RW, Cannon SR, Skinner JA, Briggs TW, Aston WJS. Pigmented villonodular synovitis of the knee: a retrospective analysis of 214 cases at a UK tertiary referral Centre. Knee. 2017;24(4):808–15.
5. Gokhale N, Purohit S, Bhosale PB. Pigmented Villonodular Synovitis Presenting as a Popliteal Cyst. J Orthop Case Rep. 2015;5(3):63–5.
6. Willimon SC, Busch MT, Perkins CA. Pigmented Villonodular synovitis of the knee: an underappreciated source of pain in children and adolescents. J Pediatr Orthop. 2018;38(8):e482–5.
7. Yamashita H, Endo K, Enokida M, Teshima R. Multifocal localized pigmented villonodular synovitis arisingarately from intra- and extra-articular knee joint: case report and literature review. Eur J Orthop Surg Traumatol. 2013;23(Suppl 2):S273–7.
8. Galli M, Ciriello V, Menghi A, Perisano C, Maccauro G, Zetti E. Localized pigmented villonodular synovitis of the anterior cruciate ligament of the knee: an exceptional presentation of a rare disease with neoplastic and inflammatory features. Int J Immunopathol Pharmacol. 2012;25(4):1131–6.
9. Rajani R, Ogden L, Matthews CJ, Gibbs CP. Diffuse Pigmented Villonodular Synovitis as a Rare Cause of Graft Failure Following Anterior Cruciate Ligament Reconstruction. Orthopedics. 2018;41(1):e142–4. https://doi.org/10.3928/01477447-20170719-06.
10. Xie GP, Jiang N, Liang CX, Zeng JC, Chen ZY, Xu Q, Qi RZ, Chen YR, Yu B. Pigmented villonodular synovitis: a retrospective multicenter study of 237 cases. PLoS One. 2015;10(3):e0121451. https://doi.org/10.1371/journal.pone.0121451.
11. Ryan RS, Louis L, O'Connell JX, Munk PL. Pigmented villonodular synovitis of the proximal tibiofibular joint. Australas Radiol. 2004;48(4):520–2.
12. Jobe CM, Raza A, Zuckerman L. Pigmented villonodular synovitis: extrasynovial recurrence. Arthroscopy. 2011;27(10):1449–51.
13. Kia C, O'Brien DF, Ziegler C, Pacheco R, Forouhar F, Williams V. An unusual case of pigmented villonodular synovitis after total knee arthroplasty presenting with recurrent hemarthrosis. Arthroplast Today. 2018;4(4):426–30.
14. Sistla R, JVSV, Afroz T. Malignant Pigmented Villonodular Synovitis-A Rare Entity. J Orthop Case Rep. 2014;4(4):9–11.
15. Rhee PC, Sassoon AA, Sayeed SA, Stuart MS, Dahm DL. Arthroscopic treatment of localized pigmented villonodular synovitis: long-term functional results. Am J Orthop (Belle Mead NJ). 2010;39(9):E90–4.
16. Keyhani S, Kazemi SM, Ahn JH, Verdonk R, Soleymanha M. Arthroscopic treatment of diffuse pigmented Villonodular synovitis of the knee: complete synovectomy andtum removal-midterm results. J Knee Surg. 2019;32(5):427–33.
17. Loriaut P, Djian P, Boyer T, Bonvarlet JP, Delin C, Makridis KG. Arthroscopic treatment of localized pigmented villonodular synovitis of the knee. Knee Surg Sports Traumatol Arthrosc. 2012;20(8):1550–3.
18. Chang JS, Higgins JP, Kosy JD, Theodoropoulos J. Systematic Arthroscopic Treatment of Diffuse Pigmented Villonodular Synovitis in the Knee. Arthrosc Tech. 2017;6(5):e1547–51.
19. Lui TH. Arthroscopic treatment of pigmented villonodular synovitis of the proximal tibiofibular joint. Knee Surg Sports Traumatol Arthrosc. 2015;23(8):2278–82.
20. Gu HF, Zhang SJ, Zhao C, Chen Y, Bi Q. A comparison of open and arthroscopic surgery for treatment of diffuse pigmented villonodular synovitis of the knee. Knee Surg Sports Traumatol Arthrosc. 2014;22(11):2830–6.
21. Casp AJ, Browne JA, Durig NE, Werner BC. Complications after Total knee arthroplasty in patients with pigmented Villonodular synovitis. J Arthroplast. 2019;34(1):36–9.
22. Houdek MT, Scorianz M, Wyles CC, Trousdale RT, Sim FH, Taunton MJ. Long-term outcome of knee arthroplasty in the setting of pigmented villonodular synovitis. Knee. 2017;24(4):851–5.

23. Su W, Zhou Y, Lu W, Zeng M, Hu Y, Xie J. Short-term outcomes of synovectomy and Total knee replacement in patients with diffuse-type pigmented Villonodular synovitis. J Knee Surg. 2019;21 https://doi.org/10.1055/s-0039-1694736.
24. Duan Y, Qian J, Chen K, Zhang Z. Necessity of adjuvant postoperative radiotherapy for diffuse pigmented villonodular synovitis of the knee: a case report and literature review. Medicine (Baltimore). 2018;97(3):e9637. https://doi.org/10.1097/MD.0000000000009637.
25. Mollon B, Lee A, Busse JW, Griffin AM, Ferguson PC, Wunder JS, Theodoropoulos J. The effect of surgical synovectomy and radiotherapy on the rate of recurrence of pigmented villonodular synovitis of the knee: an individual patient meta-analysis. Bone Joint J. 2015;97-B(4):550–7.
26. Park G, Kim YS, Kim JH, Lee SW, Song SY, Choi EK, Yi SY, Ahn SD. Low-dose external beam radiotherapy as a postoperative treatment for patients with diffuse pigmented villonodular synovitis of the knee: 4 recurrences in 23 patients followed for mean 9 years. Acta Orthop. 2012;83(3):256–60.

Chapter 55
Proximal Tibiofibular Joint Arthropathy

This refers to the presence of a diseased proximal tibiofibular joint. As this is a synovial joint, it may be affected by any of the disorders involving synovial joints [1–14]. These may occur in isolation or in association with similar involvement of the ipsilateral tibiofemoral joint. They include:

- Osteoarthritis—degeneration of the articular cartilage of the tibiofibular joint
  - Often coexists with tibiofemoral joint arthritis
  - May be associated with hamstring tightness
  - May be post-traumatic
- Inflammatory arthritis
- Infective arthritis
- Crystal arthropathy
  - Gout
  - Pseudogout
- Neoplastic causes
- Synovial conditions
  - Synovial cysts
  - Synovial chondromatosis
  - PVNS

55.1 Clinical Symptoms of Tibiofibular Joint Arthropathy

Proximal tibiofibular joint disease often causes similar clinical symptoms despite the underlying causative disorder:

C. Panayiotou Charalambous, *The Knee Made Easy*,
https://doi.org/10.1007/978-3-030-54506-2_55

- Pain over or in the joint:
  - Worse on weightbearing or twisting the leg
- Gradual onset of symptoms or post-traumatic
- Common peroneal nerve symptoms due to irritation or mass lesion pressure effect

55.2 Clinical Signs of Tibiofibular Joint Arthropathy

Proximal tibiofibular joint disease often causes similar clinical signs despite the underlying causative disorder:

- Tenderness localised to the proximal tibiofibular joint
- Proximal tibiofibular joint crepitus
- Swelling related to the proximal tibiofibular joint
- Neurological signs related to the common peroneal nerve

55.3 Investigations for Tibiofibular Joint Arthropathy

- Plain radiographs
- MRI
- CT

55.4 Management of Tibiofibular Joint Arthropathy

Several management options are available for managing arthropathy of the proximal tibiofibular joint [6, 9, 15–18] and include:

55.4.1 Non-surgical

- Leave alone
- Activity modification
- Analgesia
- Physiotherapy
  - Local treatment—cold or heat therapy
  - Passive joint mobilisation

  - Knee muscle strengthening, stretching
  - Hamstring tendon stretching
  - Addressing motion deficits in the tibiofemoral joint
- Proximal tibiofibular joint intra-articular steroid injections

55.4.2 *Surgical*

- Proximal tibiofibular joint excision ± stabilisation of the fibula
- Arthrodesis of the proximal tibiofibular joint
- Stabilisation of the proximal tibiofemoral joint ± interposition arthroplasty

References

1. Curatolo CM, Bach G, Mutty CE, Zo JM. Review of Common Clinical Conditions of the Proximal Tibiofibular Joint. Am J Orthop (Belle Mead NJ). 2018;47(12) https://doi.org/10.12788/ajo.2018.0105.
2. Nadaud MC, Ewing JW. Proximal tibiofibular arthritis: an unusual cause of lateral knee pain. Orthopedics. 2001;24(4):397–8.
3. Eichenblat M, Nathan H. The proximal tibio fibular joint. An anatomical study with clinical and pathological considerations. Int Orthop. 1983;7(1):31–9.
4. Ozcan O, Boya H, Oztekin HH. Clinical evaluation of the proximal tibiofibular joint in knees with severe tibiofemoral primary osteoarthritis. Knee. 2009;16(4):248–50.
5. Oztuna V, Yildiz A, Ozer C, Milcan A, Kuyurtar F, Turgut A. Involvement of the proximal tibiofibular joint in osteoarthritis of the knee. Knee. 2003;10(4):347–9.
6. Bozkurt M, Yilmaz E, Akseki D, Havitcioğlu H, Günal I. The evaluation of the proximal tibiofibular joint for patients with lateral knee pain. Knee. 2004;11(4):307–12.
7. Wakabayashi H, Nakamura T, Nishimura A, Hagi T, Hasegawa M, Sudo A. Isolated proximal tibiofibular joint arthritis in a patient with juvenile idiopathic arthritis: a case report. Mod Rheumatol. 2018;28(1):203–6.
8. Ben Taarit C, Kaffel D, Zribi S, Khiari K, Ben Abdallah N, Ben Maiz H, Khedhe A. An exceptional manifestation of spondylarthropathy: destructive proximal tibio-fibular arthritis. Joint Bone Spine. 2008;75(3):368–70.
9. Weiss C, Averbuch PF, Steiner GC, Rusoff JH. Synovial chondromatosis and instability of the proximal tibiofibular joint. Clin Orthop Relat Res. 1975;108:187–90.
10. Alsahhaf A, Renno W. Ganglion Cyst at the Proximal Tibiofibular Joint in a Patient with Painless Foot Drop. Pain Physician. 2016;19(8):E1147–60.
11. Pagnoux C, Lhotellier L, Ek JJ, Ballard M, Chazerain P, Ziza JM. Synovial cysts of the proximal tibiofibular joint: three case reports. Joint Bone Spine. 2002;69(3):331–3.
12. Lui TH. Arthroscopic treatment of pigmented villonodular synovitis of the joint. Knee Surg Sports Traumatol Arthrosc. 2015;23(8):2278–82.
13. Ryan RS, Louis L, O'Connell JX, Munk PL. Pigmented villonodular synovitis of the proximal tibiofibular joint. Australas Radiol. 2004;48(4):520–2.
14. Cain ME, Doornberg JN, Duit R, Clarnette J, Jaarsma R, Jadav B. High incidence of screw penetration in the proximal and distal tibiofibular joints after intramedullary nailing of tibial fractures-a prospective cohort and mapping study. Injury. 2018;49(4):871–6.

15. Kapoor V, Theruvil B, Britton JM. Excision arthroplasty of superior tibiofibular joint for recurrent proximal tibiofibular cyst. A report of two cases. Joint Bone Spine. 2004;71(5):427–9.
16. Miskovsky S, Kaeding C, Weis L. Proximal tibiofibular joint ganglion cysts: excision, recurrence, and joint arthrodesis. Am J Sports Med. 2004;32(4):1022–8.
17. Yaniv M, Koenig U, Imhoff AB. A technical solution for secondary arthritis due to chronic proximal tibiofibular joint instability. Knee Surg Sports Traumatol Arthrosc. 1999;7(5):334–6.
18. Lateur G, Pailhé R, Refaie R, Rubens-Duval B, Morin V, Boudissa M, Saragaglia D. Ganglion cysts of the proximal tibiofibular articulation: the role of arthrodesis and combined partial fibula excision. Int Orthop. 2018;42(6):1233–9.

Chapter 56
Anterior Cruciate Ligament Knee Instability

This is a condition where there is symptomatic instability of the tibiofemoral articulation due to dysfunction of the anterior cruciate ligament (ACL).

56.1 Causes of ACL Instability [1–16]

Disruption of the ACL may be:

- Congenital/developmental
- Acquired
  - Acute substantial trauma (most common)
  - Spontaneous (rare):
    - Anabolic steroids misuse
    - Chronic repetitive microtrauma—this may be see in athletes that repetitively stretch the ACL

  Disruption of the ACL may be:

- Isolated, single ligament
- Associated with other ligamentous dysfunction/injuries
- Associated with bony abnormalities—developmental, traumatic, degenerative

Although ACL instability may be part of multiligament instability and may be congenital or developmental, isolated post-traumatic anterior instability is considered in this chapter.

Traumatic ACL disruption may be described:

C. Panayiotou Charalambous, *The Knee Made Easy*,
https://doi.org/10.1007/978-3-030-54506-2_56

According to the Type of Disruption

- Avulsion of the ACL from its femoral origin
  - Soft tissue avulsion
  - Bony avulsion
- Avulsion of the ACL tibial insertion
  - Soft tissue avulsion
  - Bony avulsion (tibial spine avulsion fracture)
- Intra-substance tear

According to the Completeness of Disruption

- Complete—both bundles
- Partial:
  - One bundle
  - Proportion of fibres

According to the Mechanism of Injury Leading to Disruption

- Contact—with another player or a surface/object
- Non-contact—most ACL injuries occur secondary to non-contact injuries

56.2 Risk Factors for ACL Disruption

- Activity related: Sports predisposing to non-contact or contact injuries—skiing with cleats
- Patient related: Female sex, narrow femoral notch, larger knee valgus angle, weaker quadriceps/hamstrings, extension landing patterns

56.3 Intra-articular Disruptions Associated with ACL Tears

Cimino PM et al. [28] looked at the incidence of meniscal tears associated with acute ACL disruption in a series of 328 cases secondary to snow skiing accidents and reported:

- 75 (23%) coexistent meniscal injuries:
  - 43 (13%) lateral meniscus
  - 32 (10%) medial meniscus
  - 32 (43%) of the 75 meniscal tears were peripheral detachments from the capsule (red-red tears)

In other sports activities, reported meniscal tears range from 53% to 65%, in previous studies.

Chen G et al. [51] evaluated the rate of meniscal and chondral injuries accompanying 66 acute ACL tears in young adult patients within 1 month from injury and reported:

- Meniscal tears in 30 (46%)
  - Lateral meniscal tear 19 (29%)
  - Medial meniscal tear 8 (12%)
  - Both 3 (5%)
- Chondral injury in 28 (42%), classified using the Outerbridge classification as:
  - 17 (26)–I
  - 11 (17) –II

Such associated intra-articular injuries are important to recognise as they may:

- Account for ongoing symptoms which may be wrongly attributed to the ACL disruption
- Need specific intervention in isolation or in addition to intervention for the ACL
- Influence long term prognosis

56.4 Effects of ACL Disruption

A ligament is taut only when it is firmly attached at its two ends. This is analogous to hanging from a rope. The rope may lose part of its substance (partial tear) but still provide support, but if completely gone then one may fall down. Similarly, if the ACL is disrupted it may compromise its ability to maintain the position of the tibia relative to the femur. With ACL dysfunction the following exaggerated displacements of the tibia in relation to the femur (subluxation of the tibiofemoral articulation) may occur:

- Anterior displacement of the tibia relative to the femur
- Internal rotation of the tibia relative to the femur

56.5 Clinical History of a Traumatic Event

The following characteristics of the injury that led to the onset of symptoms may suggest an ACL disruption:

- A history of a substantial traumatic event (an event the patient can easily recall):
- Patient felt/heard "pop" in the knee
- Unable to get up and stand/walk/continue game

- Knee swell up straight away
- Mechanism of injury consistent with an ACL tear
  - Contact (hyperextension, valgus)/non-contact –most common (hyperextension, valgus, rotation)
  - Pivoting—tibia forced into valgus and internal rotation
- Required medical attention

56.6 Clinical Symptoms of ACL Instability

- Acute presentation
  - Painful, swollen knee, diffusely tender knee
  - Loss of knee motion, movements painful, difficult to weight bear
- Chronic presentation
  - Clicking, clunking due to abnormal translation of the knee
  - Feeling of abnormal displacement—"giving way", feeling "wobbly" to "popping in and out"
  - Apprehension in turning or twisting (scared that the knee may come out)
  - Vague knee pain
  - Dead leg syndrome, heavy leg, paraesthesia
  - Intermittent swelling
  - Symptoms brought on/aggravated by turning/twisting activities

Following the acute injury, the acute pain may improve, knee motion restored, and the patient may be left with feeling of instability or other symptoms.

56.7 Clinical Signs of ACL Instability

- Anterior knee laxity—Lachman test, anterior drawer test
- Pivot shift test
- Generalised ligamentous laxity with high Beighton score

56.8 Investigations for ACL Instability

Investigations of ACL instability aim to confirm the ACL disruption, determine the type of ACL disruption, identify any associated structural lesions (ligamentous, bony, meniscal, chondral). These include:

- Radiological
  - Plain radiographs—may demonstrate avulsion fracture of the ACL origin or insertion
  - Segond fracture—this is an avulsion fracture of the tibial insertion of the anterolateral ligament/capsule
  - MRI Scan
    - Assess the integrity of the ACL
    - Bone bruising—in ACL tears this is usually found in the posterior part of the proximal tibia
  - CT scan if tibial spine avulsion fracture (to define extent of bony fragment, look for comminution, and for other associated proximal tibial fractures)
- Examination under general anaesthesia—joint translation and laxity is assessed with the patient under general anaesthesia to abolish pain, apprehension, and allow muscle relaxation
- Arthroscopic evaluation—direct visualisation of the ACL

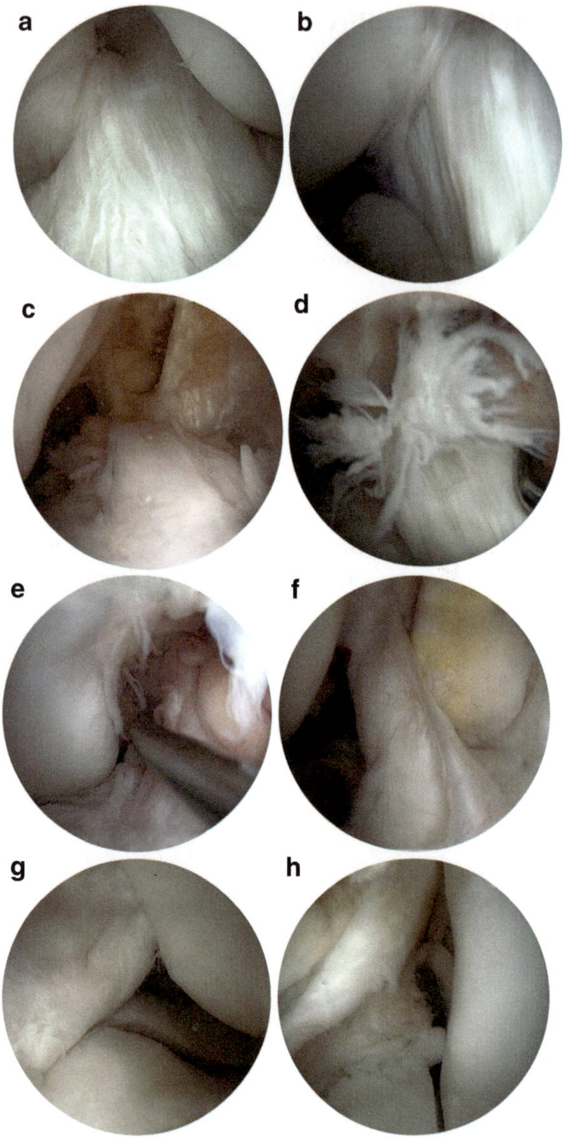

(**a**, **b**) Intact ACL in right knee. (**c**–**f**) disrupted ACL in right knee. (**g**) Intact ACL in left knee. (**h**) disrupted ACL in left knee

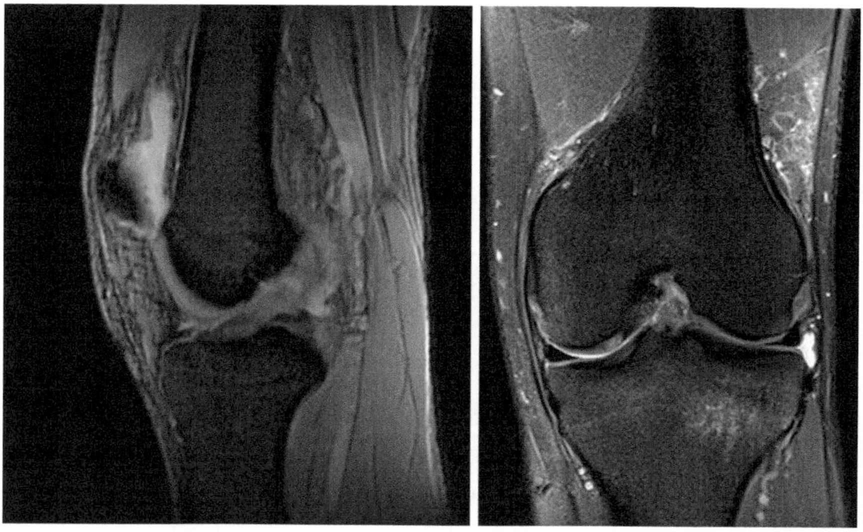

Ruptured ACL (MRI scan)

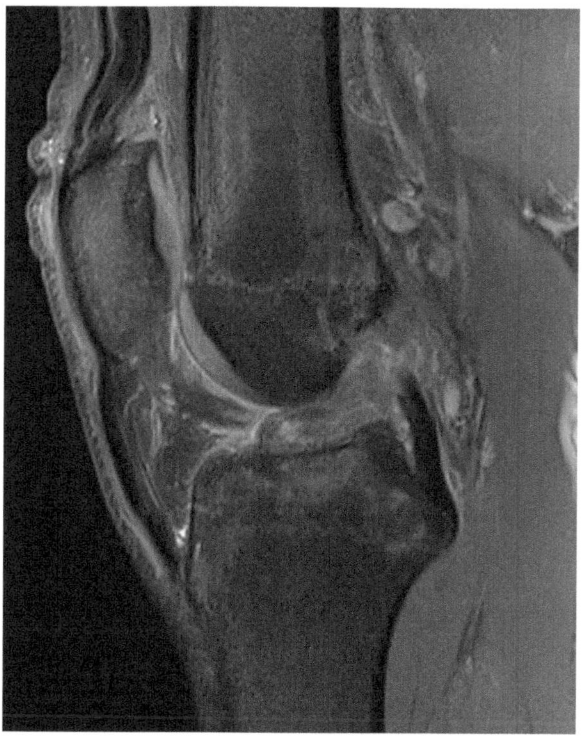

ACL rupture with ACL healed onto the PCL

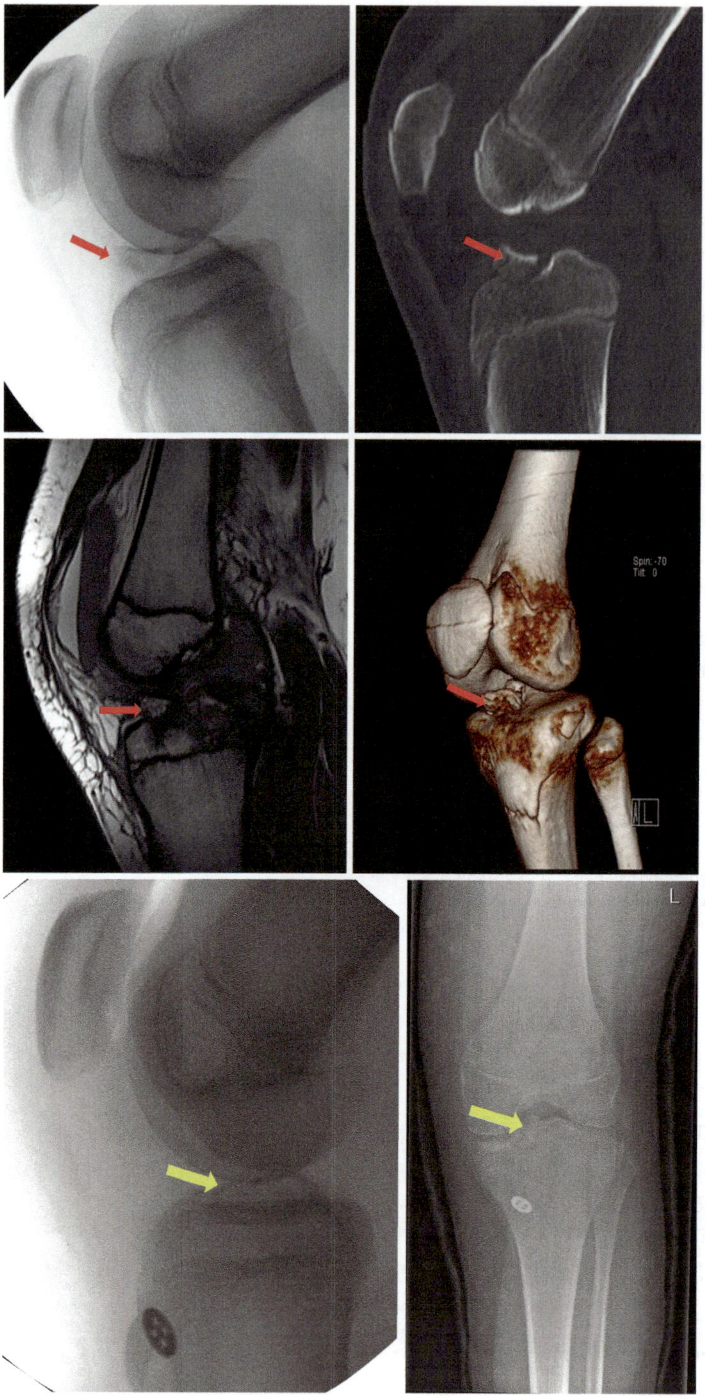

Avulsion of the ACL attachment onto the proximal tibia (red arrows) reattached with sutures tied over of tibial button (yellow arrows)

56.9 Management of ACL instability [17–38]

Initial management aims at:

- Reducing the acute inflammation of the knee using the Rest, Ice, Compression, Elevation (RICE) principles
- Restore motion (tibiofemoral/patellofemoral(PF))
- Quadriceps/hamstring activation
- Proprioception training
- Activity specific mobilisation

Further management aims at improving ongoing symptoms of instability and hence, improve a patient's function or reducing the risk of further instability. This depends on:

- Symptoms—severity, frequency
- Underlying cause
- Functional demand of the patient

56.9.1 Non-surgical

- Leave alone
- Activity modification, avoiding unstable positions
- Physiotherapy to address:
  - Core imbalance—core strengthening
  - Hip muscle weakness —strengthening of hip muscles
  - Proprioception—proprioceptive training
  - Hamstring weakness—hamstring muscle strengthening
- External knee devices—ACL bracing

It should be noted that non-surgical management does not specifically address the ACL disruption but aims to improve stability by enhancing the function of dynamic stabilisers (through strengthening, better control and coordination).

56.9.2 Surgical

- Reconstruction—using a graft that is secured in bone tunnels in the femur and tibia. Fixation is achieved by multiple means including suspensory (e.g. suture button) and non-suspensory devices (e.g. interference screw fixation). Various graft types and techniques may be utilised:

- Autograft—hamstring tendons, patellar tendon with a bone block from its patellar origin and tibial tubercle insertion, quadriceps tendon
- Allograft
- Synthetic graft
- Single bundle vs. double bundle

- Repair
  - Tibial spine avulsion fracture
  - Femoral soft tissue avulsion (repair ± internal bracing)

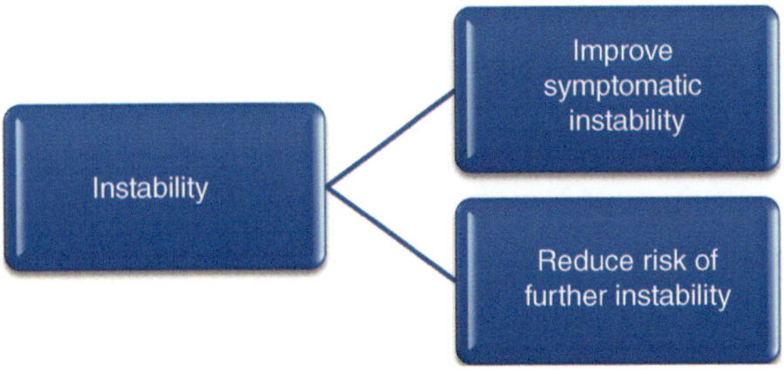

Aim of managing the ACL deficient knee

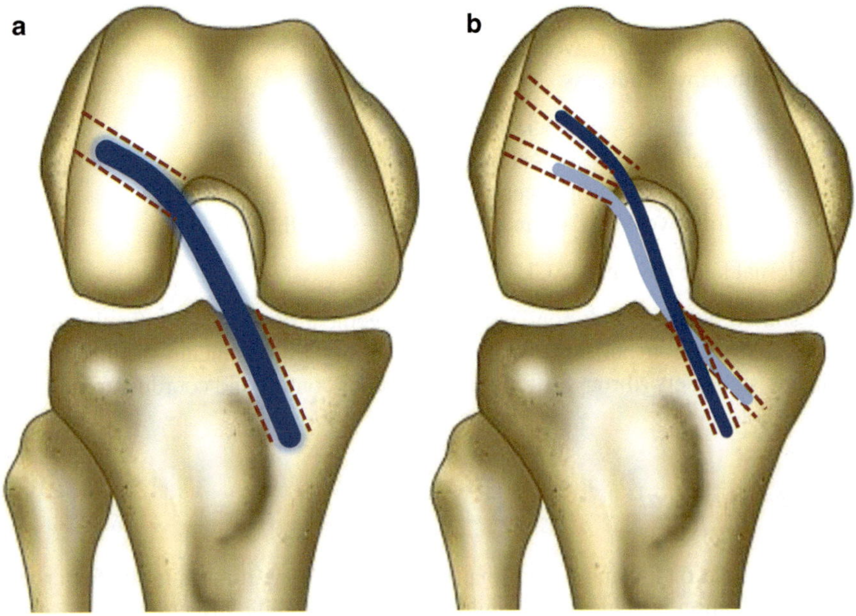

(a) Single bundle, (b) double bundle ACL reconstruction

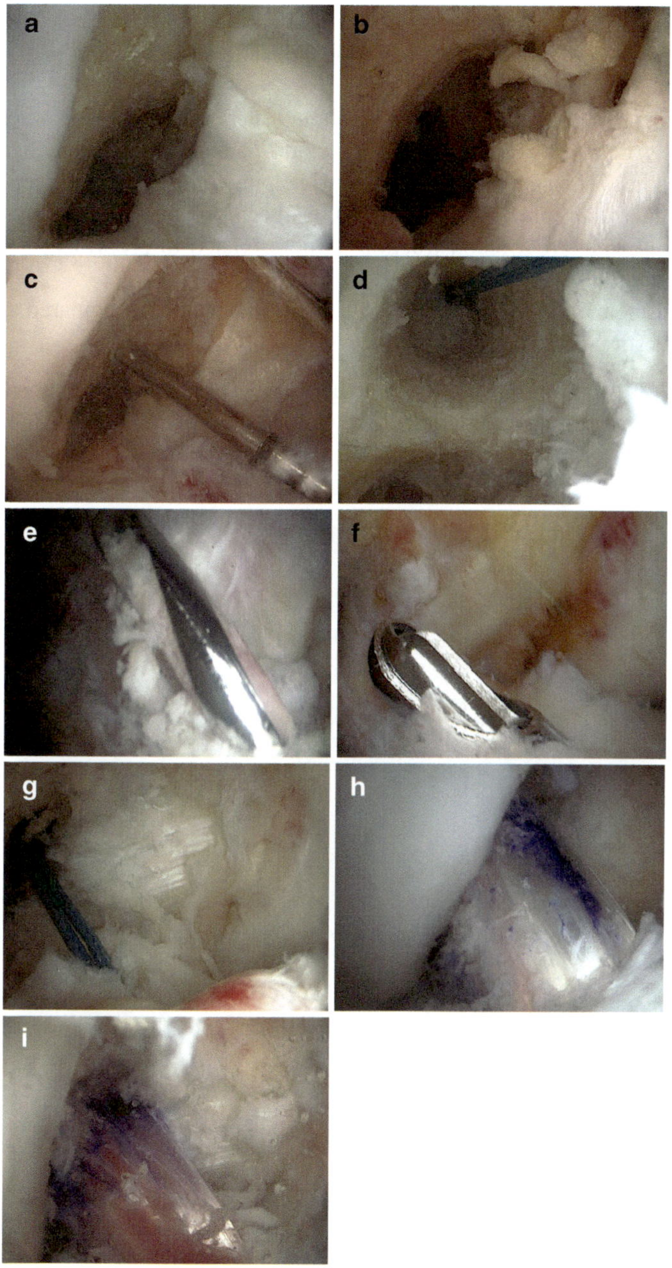

ACL single bundle reconstruction with semitendinosus and gracilis. (a) Debridement of the lateral wall of the femoral notch; (b) Lateral wall notchplasty; (c) Femoral guidewire is inserted which is over reamed to create the femoral tunnel; (d) Femoral tunnel (suture is used to pull the graft through); (e) Tibial tunnel drilled antegrade (from the outer tibial surface to the tibial plateau; (f) Residual ACL stump at the level of the tibial tunnel aperture is excised; (g) Graft is pulled through, through the tibial tunnel and into the femoral tunnel; (h, i) ACL graft in situ

ACL reconstruction surgery may work by:

- Mechanical effect—physically limiting anterior translation and rotation of the tibia in relation to the femur
- Proprioceptive mechanism—it is of note that although a graft used to reconstruct the ACL (usually hamstring graft) may stretch out, patients continue with a clinically stable knee. This may be due to the graft helping to restore proprioception and hence muscular control of the knee. It has been shown that functional knee stability following ACL reconstruction is more related to proprioceptive control rather than graft tightness
- A tight graft limiting motion may cause much trouble to the patient, compared to a graft which has stretched out

Higuchi H et al. [39] showed that there was no correlation between static passive stability on Lachman testing and functional knee score levels post-ACL reconstruction.

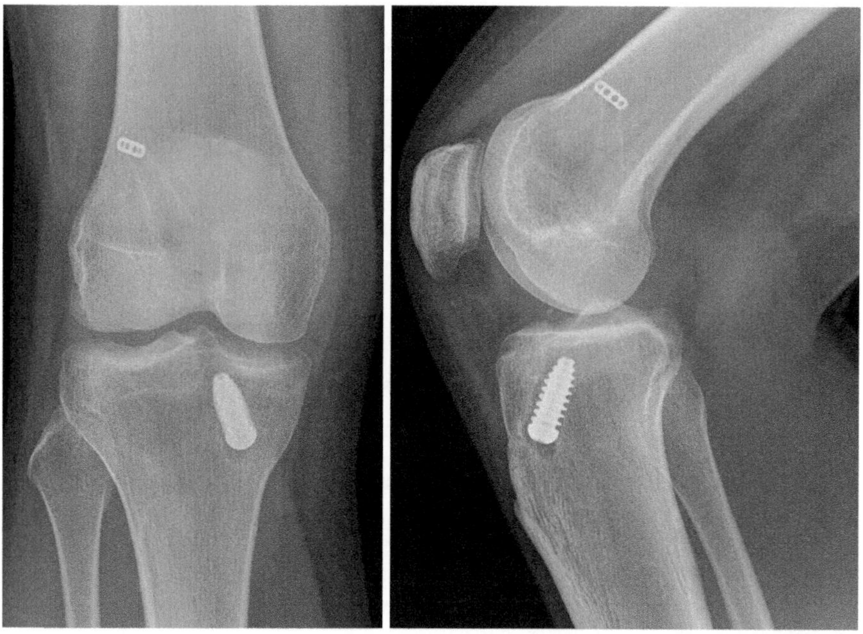

Single bundle ACL reconstruction with ipsilateral hamstring tendons secured to the tibial tunnel with a metallic interference screw and to the femoral tunnel with a suspensory suture button

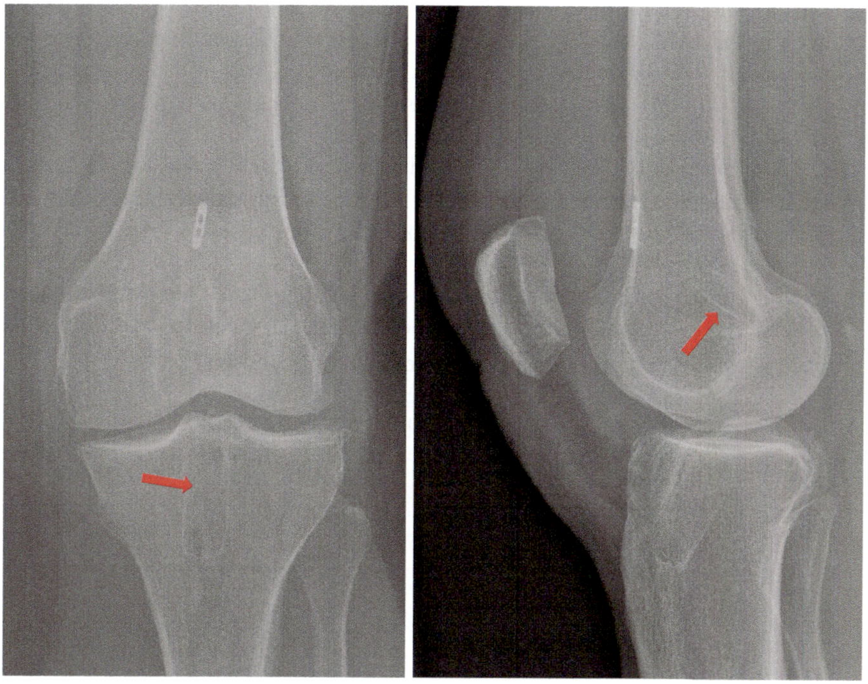

Post single bundle ACL reconstruction. Tibial fixation with a non-metallic (hence radiolucent) interference screw, and femoral tunnel fixation with a suspensory suture button. The walls of the tibial and femoral tunnels appear corticated (red arrows)

56.10 ACL Extra-Articular Procedures [40–43]

When the ACL tears there may be additional disruption of extra-articular structures that act as a restraint to rotation of the tibia on the femur. As a result there has been suggestion that reconstructing these extra-articular restraints in addition to reconstructing the ACL may help further improve rotational stability. Although such additional extra-articular reconstruction may not be essential in all cases of intra-articular ACL reconstruction, it may be considered in:

- Revision cases where ACL failed despite good graft positioning and not a substantial reinjury
- Knee hyperlaxity
- Chronic ACL tears with associated damage to the anterolateral structures (radiologically identified

Several extra-articular procedures have been described [44] including:

1. MacIntosh—A strip of iliotibial band (ITB) is detached proximally and passed deep to the LCL, and then through an osteoperiosteal tunnel, posterior to the lateral collateral ligament (LCL) femoral attachment. The graft is looped posteriorly through the lateral intermuscular septum, brought down deep to the LCL and sutured back onto itself at Gerdy's tubercle.
2. Lemaire procedure—A strip of ITB is detached proximally and passed deep to the LCL and through a femoral tunnel at the attachment of the head of the lateral gastrocnemius. The graft is then brought distally, passed again deep to the LCL and fixed to the ITB.
3. Lateral 1/3 of patellar tendon tenodesis—the lateral 1/3rd of the patellar tendon is harvested proximally with a patellar bone block, passed deep to the LCL, and fixed within a bony groove deep to the femoral origin of the LCL.

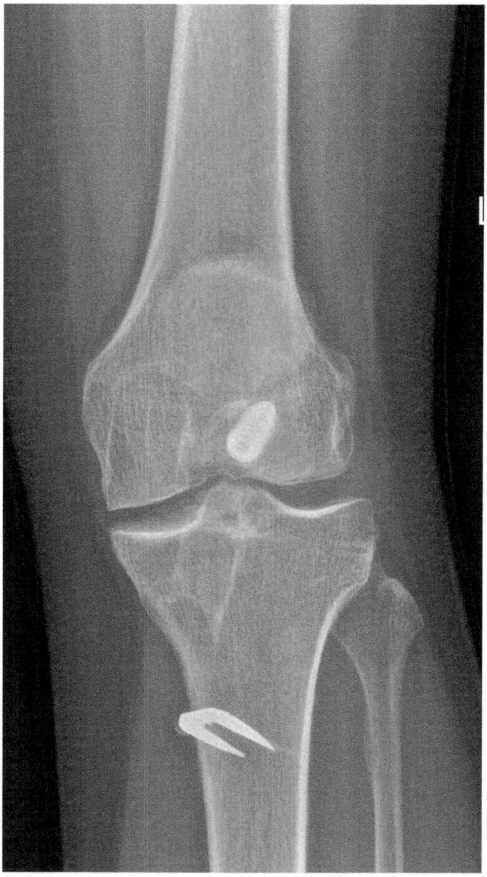

Single bundle ACL reconstruction with ipsilateral hamstring tendons secured to the tibial tunnel with a non-metallic interference screw and a metallic staple, and to the femoral tunnel with a metallic interference screw

56.11 Considerations in the Management of Post-Traumatic ACL Deficiency

In considering the definitive management of ACL disruption several considerations must be taken into account some of which are described below.

56.11.1 Natural History

It is recognised that:

- A substantial proportion of patients who do not have ACL surgery manage to function without any debilitating knee instability. Noyes et al. [45] examined the effect of ACL disruption on individuals who were active in sports and described 3 groups with regards to their outcome (known as the rule of thirds):
  - Copers (about 1/3rd)—compensate well with no surgical intervention, and go back to strenuous sports
  - Adapters (about 1/3rd) –compensate by modifying their activities (but with symptoms during recreational sports)
  - Non-copers (about 1/3rd)—don't manage, and continue with instability (including instability during walking activities) that requires further intervention
- In a subsequent study [46] they looked at patients with chronic ACL laxity who underwent a rehabilitation program. More than 1/3rd of patients improved with no or minimal symptoms during daily activities or during recreational activities, but had some symptoms during strenuous sports activity. One-third of patients became worse and failed the program, complaining of symptoms of pain, swelling or giving-way that prevented any recreational activities and were often present with daily activities. More than 1/3rd of patients (36%) did not benefit from the rehabilitation program and required ACL reconstruction
- Persistent instability may:
  - Limit ability of an individual to achieve high level functional potential
  - Predispose to further meniscal tears or further chondral damage both of which are related to the development of knee arthritis

A substantial proportion of patients sustaining an ACL tear will develop secondary degenerative changes (arthritis) [47–49]. Cinque ME [47] et al. carried out a meta-analysis of the prevalence of radiographic osteoarthritis(OA) following ACL reconstruction, including 38 studies (4108 patients). The prevalence of OA after an ACL reconstruction significantly increased with time from surgery, with estimated rates of about:

- 11% (6%–19%) at 5 years
- 21% (15%–28%) at 10 years
- 52% (29%–74%) at 20 years post-surgery

Increased chronicity of the ACL tear prior to surgery and older patient age were also associated with greater OA rates.

Lie MM et al. [48] in a systematic review on the prevalence and risk factors for knee OA more than 10 years after ACL tear, reported that the radiographic OA prevalence varied between 0% and 100%. One study reported a 35% rate of symptomatic knee OA for the tibiofemoral joint and one study a 15% symptomatic OA for the PF joint (15%). Across studies meniscectomy was a consistent risk factor for OA.

Along similar lines, Claes S et al. [49] systematically analysed the prevalence of OA following ACL reconstruction with a minimum follow-up of 10 years. They included 16 studies (1554 reconstructions). Of these 453 (28%) showed radiological signs of OA. 50% of patients with meniscectomy had OA versus 16% of those without meniscectomy.

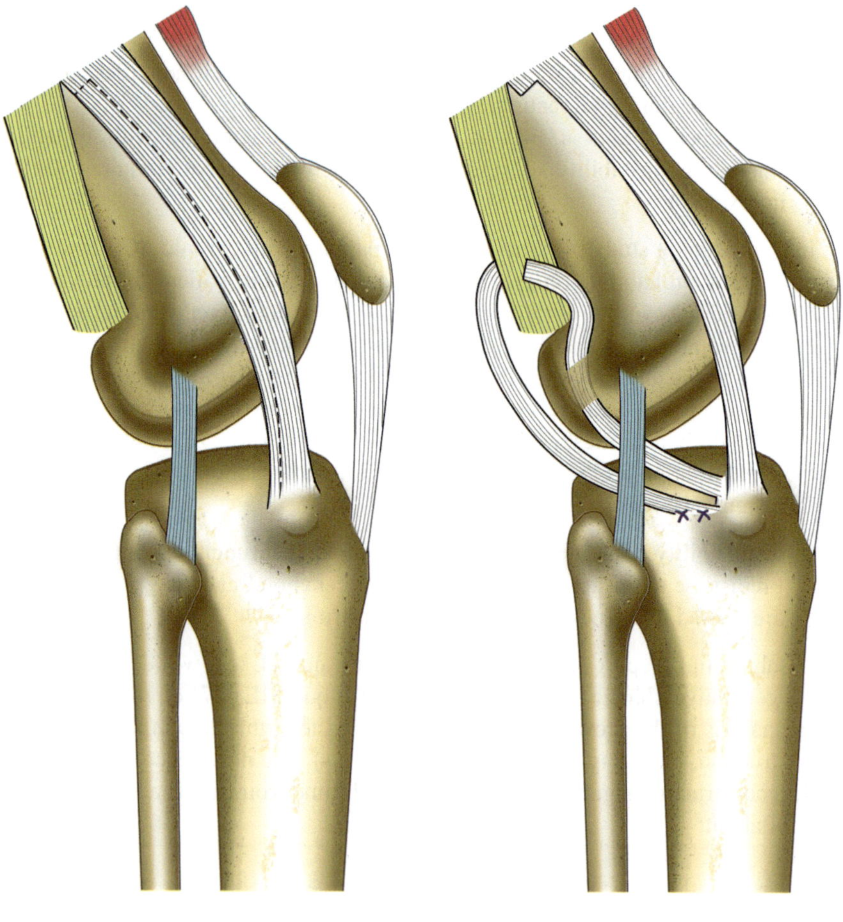

MacIntosh reconstruction of the anterolateral ligament of the knee

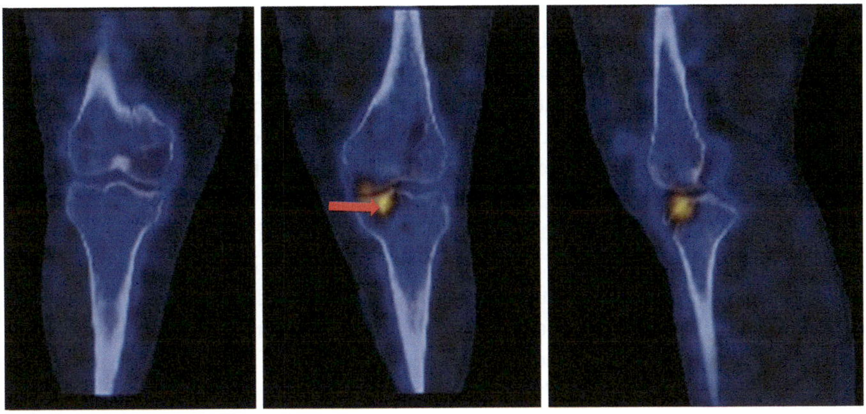

SPECT showing increased uptake (red arrow) on the medial compartment associated with overloading, in a patient presenting with pain several years post anterior cruciate ligament reconstruction

56.11.2 Timing of Encountering the ACL Instability Patient

The patient may present at different stages following ACL disruption to the clinician:

- Acute—just after the injury
- Sub-acute—after the acute injury has settled and patient has had a course of physiotherapy but continues with substantial instability which is limiting day to day activities or more strenuous activities/sports
- Chronic—after a long period of managing day to day activities and more strenuous activities, patient may experience a substantial instability episode leading a knee flare up or further associated injury(meniscal/chondral)

Hence, the approach on how to deal with the underlying ACL disruption may differ according to the above.

56.11.3 Timing of ACL Reconstruction

ACL reconstruction may be:

- Acute —in the very first few days post injury
- Subacute—once the acute inflammation settles and joint motion including knee extension is restored
- Chronic—patient returns to usual function and is only considered for surgical intervention if further substantial instability episodes occur

Acute and subacute ACL reconstruction aim to reduce the risk of further instability episodes and resultant further meniscal injuries or chondral injuries, whereas chronic reconstruction aims to address on-going instability symptoms [28, 50, 51].

Given the natural history of ACL reconstruction, if surgery is offered to all individuals with an ACL disruption, then a substantial proportion may undergo unnecessary surgery. Furthermore, the concern with very early ACL reconstruction is that it may act as a second insult on the injured knee, predisposing to intra-articular adhesions (arthrofibrosis) and loss of knee motion (although this has been questioned by recent studies which failed to show an association between early surgery and increased risk of arthrofibrosis). In addition, if ACL reconstruction is performed prior to restoration of normal range of motion (particularly extension) this may lead to chronic motion loss. Acute reconstruction is however not practically possible in many healthcare settings due to delays in initial assessment by a knee specialist and also waiting list delays.

The concern with chronic reconstruction is that the knee may continue with instability that predisposes to further meniscal and chondral injuries.

Clinical decision is thus challenging, and at the moment there is no way of reliably predicting whether an individual will cope with an ACL deficient knee, and hence which patients would benefit from an early reconstruction once the acute inflammation settles and the range of motion is restored.

Patients that may be at an increased risk of persistent instability (although not absolute) and who may thus be offered early surgery include:

- Young, high demand patients who plan to return to activities that involve substantial pivoting
- Those that continue with substantial knee instability early on, despite a trial period of physiotherapy

56.11.4 ACL Disruption in Older Age

ACL injuries may occur in older age. Older patients may be able to tolerate ACL disruptions better than younger patients and hence a higher threshold for intervening may be needed. However, in the presence of ongoing instability, surgical intervention is appropriate despite the patient's age [52–55].

Kim KT [52] compared the results of ACL reconstruction in those over 40 with those under 40 years of age in a meta-analysis. They showed that following ACL reconstruction, there was no significant difference in clinical, functional and laxity measurement outcomes between the 2 groups.

56.11.5 ACL Disruption Associated with a Meniscal Tear

In such cases there are several considerations [56–60]:

- Meniscal repair healing rates are higher when combined with ACL reconstruction as compared to isolated meniscal repairs
- Meniscectomy is associated with better outcomes and less reoperation rates than meniscal repairs
- Meniscal repair plus ACL reconstruction is associated with better outcomes as compared to isolated meniscal repair

One option is to address both the meniscal tear and ACL tear on the same occasion. There is evidence that the rate of healing of meniscal repairs done at the time of ACL reconstruction may be higher than of those done in isolation. Furthermore, stabilising the knee may limit excessive shear forces and thus failure of the meniscal repair.

However, in some cases it may be that the meniscal tear is causing most of the symptoms rather than the ACL disruption per se. It may be difficult to distinguish between symptoms of instability and intermittent catching or locking due to an associated meniscal tear (such as bucket handle tear). Dealing with the meniscal tear with arthroscopic surgery without an ACL reconstruction (which is more extensive surgery) may allow most symptoms to settle and thus avoid the need for a more extensive surgical procedure. This approach may be preferable in cases where partial meniscectomy rather than meniscal repair is likely to be performed.

56.11.6 ACL Disruption Associated with Malalignment

Malalignment may put excessive forces on an ACL reconstruction graft, leading to dysfunction of the reconstruction. Hence, in such cases combination of ACL reconstruction with a proximal tibial osteotomy may be considered [61–64].

- Varus malalignment—opening wedge high tibial osteotomy
- Increased tibial slope—anterior closing wedge proximal tibial osteotomy

Kim SJ et al. [64] evaluated whether a valgus high tibial osteotomy is essential in primary varus knees undergoing ACL reconstruction. They reported that stability and functional scores after ACL reconstruction were not adversely altered by primary varus alignment. Thus, they recommended that if there is no medial compartment arthritis or varus thrust, a correctional tibial osteotomy is not crucial in primary varus knees undergoing ACL reconstruction.

56.11.7 ACL Disruption Associated with Osteoarthritis

On occasions, ACL disruption may occur in association with OA. This may be isolated compartment arthritis or more extensive arthritis. In this scenario it is important to determine:

1. What is the main cause of the patient's symptoms—the arthritis, or the ACL instability?

A trial of bracing to help instability may help distinguish between the two. Similarly, addressing the pain of arthritis may help distinguish as to which is the main source of the patient's troubles.

In such cases surgical intervention may be in the form of:

- Total knee replacement arthroplasty (TKR)

- Unicompartmental replacement arthroplasty along with ACL reconstruction surgery [65, 66]
- Tibial osteotomy along with ACL reconstruction surgery

56.12 Return to Sports Following ACL Reconstruction [37, 67]

Mohtadi NG and Chan DS [67] systematically reviewed 15 prognostic studies evaluating sport-specific performance outcomes and/or return to play after arthroscopic ACL reconstruction for athletes participating in competitive sports (soccer, football, ice hockey, basketball, alpine ski, ski snowboarding, and baseball). They reported that most high-performance or professional athletes returned to their preinjury level of sport after ACL reconstruction. They also suggested that there is a measurable decrease in performance but this sport-specific.

One of the concerns about returning to sports is the risk of further ACL injury This risk is greatest within the first 2 years following ACL reconstruction, with up to 1/3rd of younger athletes sustaining a second ACL injury within this time. The incidence rate of a further ACL injury is much greater in the first as compared to the second year. Nagelli CV and Hewett TE [37] in an evidence synthesis assessing the timing of return to sports, reported that athletes achieve baseline joint health and function at about 2 years after ACL reconstruction. On the basis of this they suggested that a delay in returning to sports for nearly 2 years may substantially reduce the incidence of second ACL injuries. This however, must be balanced with the demands and aspirations of the athlete but is an important issue to consider in discussions with the patient.

Learning Pearls

- A thorough clinical history is essential in order to determine the exact symptoms of the patient with a disrupted ACL. ACL disruption may cause pain or locking (due to the mechanical effect of the ACL stump) or limitation of movement due to the development of arthrofibrosis, which will not be helped by surgical interventions aimed at addressing instability
- An ACL which has avulsed from its femoral origin may heal onto the posterior cruciate ligament (PCL). This may make the diagnosis of ACL tear more difficult because:
  - It may result in an end point being present on clinical examination when applying an anterior force to the tibia (in the Lachman or anterior drawer test)
  - The femoral avulsion and resultant empty lateral wall may not be easily visible arthroscopically with the knee in flexion, and may become apparent only on probing or on positioning the leg in the figure of four
- In considering surgical intervention, it is important to recognise that the aim is to improve knee stability rather than improve pain, and for this to be communicated to the patient as part of shared decision making

- There is no strong clinical evidence that double-bundle reconstruction offers a functional advantage over single-bundle reconstruction
- Hamstring and patellar tendon grafts have been shown to confer similar long term outcomes
- There is very limited evidence as to the role of femoral soft tissue ACL repairs (± internal bracing), hence this should be viewed with high caution
- Hyperlaxity may confer poorer outcomes following ACL reconstruction. Magnussen RA et al. [68] assessed the effect of high-grade pre-surgery knee laxity on the outcomes of primary isolated ACL reconstruction in 2325 patients. Patients with high laxity on Lachman, anterior drawer, or pivot shift tests were classified as having a high-grade laxity. 32% of cases had high-grade laxity on at least 1 examination test:
  - High-grade Lachman—14.4%
  - High-grade pivot shift—26.5%
  - High-grade anterior drawer—10.0%
  - At a follow up of 6 years high-grade pre-reconstruction Lachman and pivot shift test were associated with significantly increased odds of ACL graft revision. Poorer patient-reported outcome scores in the high-grade laxity group were also noted, but this did not reach clinical relevance
- In a related study Magnussen RA et al. [69] showed that chronic tears(>6 months), generalised ligamentous laxity, and the presence of a lateral or medial meniscal tears were associated with increased laxity on the Lachman, pivot shift and anterior drawer testing

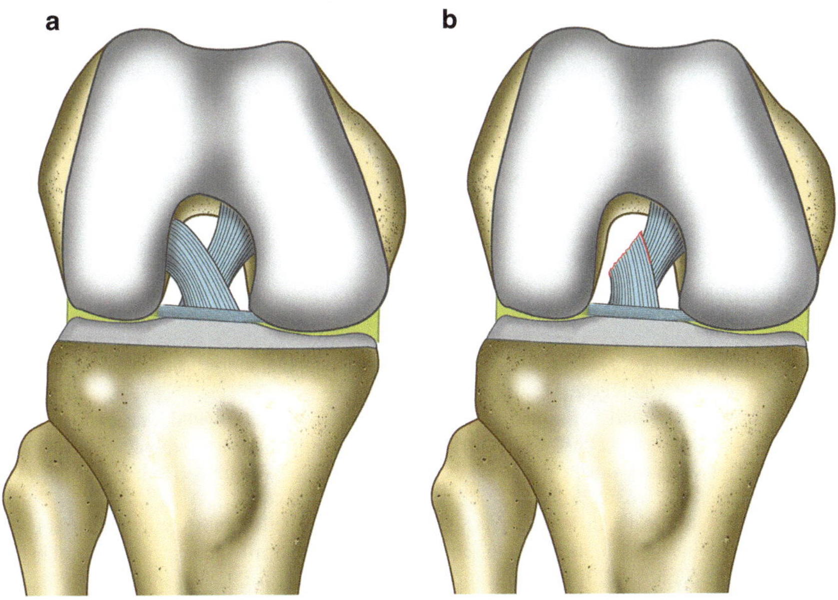

(a) Intact ACL (b) ACL avulsed from its femoral origin and healed onto the PCL

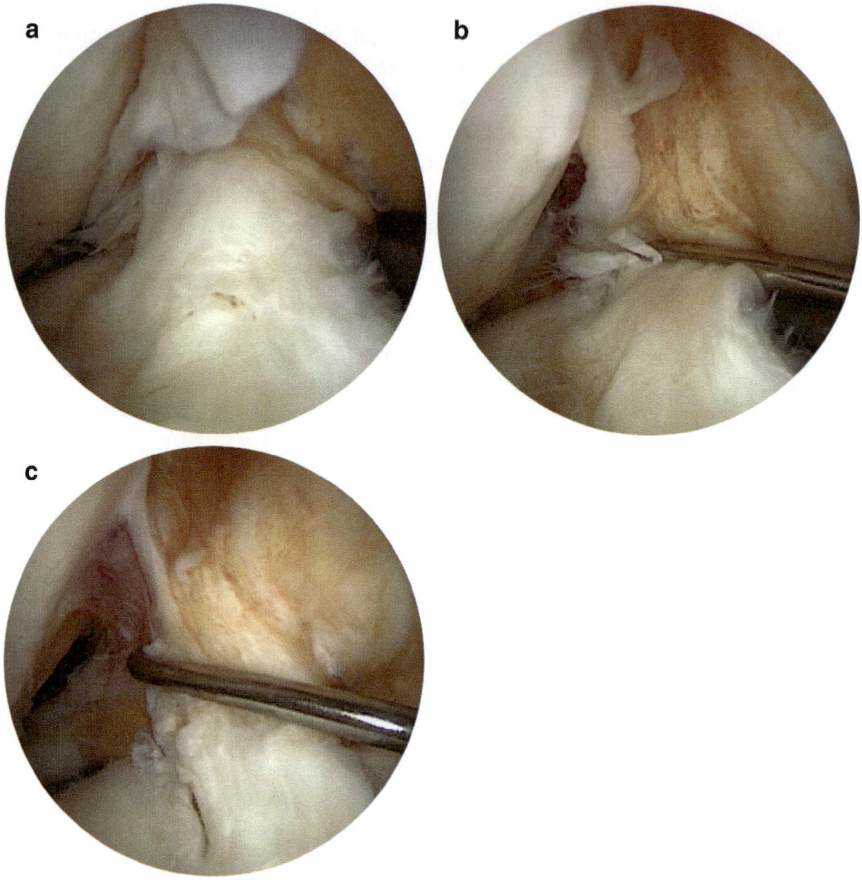

The ACL may avulse from its femoral origin and heal onto the PCL. (a) When visualised with the knee in flexion, this avulsion may not be obvious and may be mistaken for an intact ACL. (b) Probing the ACL may help identify an empty lateral wall of the femoral notch. (c) Placing the leg in the figure of four position and probing the ACL stump makes the tear more easily identifiable

References

1. Murali J, Monchik K, Fadale P. Congenital absence of the anterior cruciate ligament. Am J Orthop (Belle Mead NJ). 2015;44(8):E283–5.
2. Davanzo D, Fornaciari P, Barbier G, Maniglio M, Petek D. Review and long-term outcomes of cruciate ligament reconstruction versus conservative treatment in siblings with congenital anterior cruciate ligament aplasia. Case Rep Orthop. 2017;2017:1636578. https://doi.org/10.1155/2017/1636578.
3. Takahashi S, Nagano Y, Ito W, Kido Y, Okuwaki T. A retrospective study of mechanisms of anterior cruciate ligament injuries in high school basketball, handball, judo, soccer, and volleyball. Medicine (Baltimore). 2019;98(26):e16030. https://doi.org/10.1097/MD.0000000000016030.

4. Pfeifer CE, Beattie PF, Sacko RS, Hand A. Risk factors associated with non-contact anterior cruciate ligament injury: a systematic review. Int J Sports Phys Ther. 2018;13(4):575–87.
5. Volpi P, Bisciotti GN, Chamari K, Cena E, Carimati G, Bragazzi NL. Risk factors of anterior cruciate ligament injury in football players: a systematic review of the literature. Muscles Ligaments Tendons J. 2016;6(4):480–5.
6. Salem HS, Shi WJ, Tucker BS, Dodson CC, Ciccotti MG, Freedman KB, Cohen SB. Contact versus noncontact anterior cruciate ligament injuries: is mechanism of injury predictive of concomitant knee pathology? Arthroscopy. 2018;34(1):200–4.
7. Bouras T, Fennema P, Burke S, Bosman H. Stenotic intercondylar notch type is correlated with anterior cruciate ligament injury in female patients using magnetic resonance imaging. Knee Surg Sports Traumatol Arthrosc. 2018;26(4):1252–7.
8. Kaeding CC, Léger-St-Jean B, Magnussen RA. Epidemiology and diagnosis of anterior cruciate ligament injuries. Clin Sports Med. 2017;36(1):1–8. https://doi.org/10.1016/j.csm.2016.08.001.
9. Huang YL, GJ, Mulligan CMS, Oh J, Norcross MF. A Majority of Anterior Cruciate Ligament Injuries Can Be Prevented by Injury Prevention Programs: A Systematic Review of Randomized Controlled Trials and Cluster-Randomized Controlled Trials With Meta-analysis. Am J Sports Med. 2019;363546519870175 https://doi.org/10.1177/0363546519870175.
10. Peterson JR, Krabak BJ. Anterior cruciate ligament injury: mechanisms of injury and strategies for injury prevention. Phys Med Rehabil Clin N Am. 2014;25(4):813–28.
11. Smith HC, Vacek P, Johnson RJ, Slauterbeck JR, Hashemi J, Shultz S, Beynnon BD. Risk factors for anterior cruciate ligament injury: a review of the literature - part 1: neuromuscular and anatomic risk. Sports Health. 2012;4(1):69–78.
12. Gagnier JJ, Morgenstern H, Chess L. Interventions designed to prevent anterior cruciate ligament injuries in adolescents and adults: a systematic review and meta-analysis. Am J Sports Med. 2013;41(8):1952–62.
13. Marshall SW. Recommendations for defining and classifying anterior cruciate ligament injuries in epidemiologic studies. J Athl Train. 2010;45(5):516–8.
14. Boden BP, Sheehan FT, Torg JS, Hewett TE. Noncontact anterior cruciate ligament injuries: mechanisms and risk factors. J Am Acad Orthop Surg. 2010;18(9):520–7.
15. Webster KE, Hewett TE. Meta-analysis of meta-analyses of anterior cruciate ligament injury reduction training programs. J Orthop Res. 2018;36(10):2696–708.
16. Zhang L, Hacke JD, Garrett WE, Liu H, Yu B. Bone bruises associated with anterior cruciate ligament injury as indicators of injury mechanism: a systematic review. Sports Med. 2019;49(3):453–62.
17. Monk AP, Davies LJ, Hopewell S, Harris K, Beard DJ, Price AJ. Surgical versus conservative interventions for treating anterior cruciate ligament injuries. Cochrane Database Syst Rev. 2016;4:CD011166. https://doi.org/10.1002/14651858.CD011166.pub2.
18. van der List JP, Vermeijden HD, Sierevelt IN, DiFelice GS, van Noort A, Kerkhoffs GMMJ. Arthroscopic primary repair of proximal anterior cruciate ligament tears seems safe but higher level of evidence is needed: a systematic review and meta-analysis of recent literature. Knee Surg Sports Traumatol Arthrosc. 2019;5:1946–57. https://doi.org/10.1007/s00167-019-05697-8.
19. Mouarbes D, Menetrey J, Ot V, Courtot L, Berard E, Cavaignac E. Anterior cruciate ligament reconstruction: a systematic review and meta-analysis of outcomes for quadriceps tendon autograft versus bone-patellar tendon-bone and hamstring-tendon autografts. Am J Sports Med. 2019;47(14):3531–40.
20. Salem HS, Varzhapetyan V, Patel N, Dodson CC, Tjoumakaris FP, Freedman KB. Anterior cruciate ligament reconstruction in young female athletes: patellar versus hamstring tendon autografts. Am J Sports Med. 2019;47(9):2086–92.
21. Wang S, Zhang C, Cai Y, Lin X. Autograft or allograft? Irradiated or not? A contrast between autograft and allograft in anterior cruciate ligament reconstruction: a meta-analysis. Arthroscopy. 2018;34(12):3258–65.

22. van der List JP, Jonkergouw A, van Noort A, Kerkhoffs GMMJ, DiFelice GS. Identifying candidates for arthroscopic primary repair of the anterior cruciate ligament: a case-control study. Knee. 2019;26(3):619–27.
23. Chen H, Chen B, Tie K, Fu Z, Chen L. Single-bundle versus double-bundle autologous anterior cruciate ligament reconstruction: a meta-analysis of randomized controlled trials at 5-year minimum follow-up. J Orthop Surg Res. 2018;13(1):50. https://doi.org/10.1186/s13018-018-0753-x.
24. Kay J, Memon M, XRG, Peteerson D, Simunovic N, Ayeni OR. Over 90% of children and adolescents return to sport after anterior cruciate ligament reconstruction: a systematic review and meta-analysis. Knee Surg Sports Traumatol Arthrosc. 2018;26(4):1019–36.
25. Devitt BM, Bell SW, Ardern CL, Hartwig T, Porter TJ, Feller JA, Webster KE. The Role of Lateral Extra-articular Tenodesis in Primary Anterior Cruciate Ligament Reconstruction: A Systematic Review With Meta-analysis and Best-Evidence Synthesis. Orthop J Sports Med. 2017;5(10):2325967117731767. https://doi.org/10.1177/2325967117731767.
26. Volpin A, Kini SG, Meuffels DE. Satisfactory outcomes following combined unicompartmental knee replacement and anterior cruciate ligament reconstruction. Knee Surg Sports Traumatol Arthrosc. 2018;26(9):2594–601.
27. Anderson CN, Anderson AF. Management of the Anterior Cruciate Ligament-Injured Knee in the skeletally immature athlete. Clin Sports Med. 2017;36(1):35–52.
28. Kwok CS, Harrison T, Servant C. The optimal timing for anterior cruciate ligament reconstruction with respect to the risk of postoperative stiffness. Arthroscopy. 2013;29(3):556–65.
29. Dunn KL, Lam KC, Valovich McLeod TC. Early operative versus delayed or nonoperative treatment of anterior cruciate ligament injuries in pediatric patients. J Athl Train. 2016;51(5):425–7.
30. Sanders TL, Kremers HM, Bryan AJ, Fruth KM, Larson DR, Pareek A, Levy BA, Stuart MJ, Dahm DL, Krych AJ. Is anterior cruciate ligament reconstruction effective in preventing secondary meniscal tears and osteoarthritis? Am J Sports Med. 2016;44(7):1699–707. https://doi.org/10.1177/0363546516634325.
31. Ralles S, Agel J, Obermeier M, Tompkins M. Incidence of secondary intra-articular injuries with time to anterior cruciate ligament reconstruction. Am J Sports Med. 2015;43(6):1373–9.
32. Mascarenhas R, Cvetanovich GL, Sayegh ET, Verma NN, Cole BJ, Bush-Joseph C, Bach BR Jr. Does double-bundle anterior cruciate ligament reconstruction improve postoperative knee stability compared with single-bundle techniques? A systematic review of overlapping meta-analyses. Arthroscopy. 2015;31(6):1185–96.
33. Björnsson H, Desai N, Musahl V, Alentorn-Geli E, Bhandari M, Fu F, Samuelsson K. Is double-bundle anterior cruciate ligament reconstruction superior to single-bundle? A comprehensive systematic review. Knee Surg Sports Traumatol Arthrosc. 2015;23(3):696–739.
34. Magnussen RA, Duthon V, Servien E, Neyret P. Anterior cruciate ligament reconstruction and osteoarthritis: evidence from long-term follow-up and potential solutions. Cartilage. 2013;4(3 Suppl):22S–6S.
35. Hoogeslag RAG, Brouwer RW, Boer BC, de Vries AJ. Huis in 't veld R. acute anterior cruciate ligament rupture: repair or reconstruction? Two-year results of a randomized controlled clinical trial. Am J Sports Med. 2019;47(3):567–77.
36. Kruse LM, Gray B, Wright RW. Rehabilitation after anterior cruciate ligament reconstruction: a systematic review. J Bone Joint Surg Am. 2012;94(19):1737–48.
37. Nagelli CV, Hewett TE. Should return to sport be delayed until 2 years after anterior cruciate ligament reconstruction? Biological and Functional Considerations Sports Med. 2017;47(2):221–32.
38. Secrist ES, Frederick RW, Tjoumakaris FP, Stache SA, Hammoud S, Freedman KB. A Comparison of Operative and Nonoperative Treatment of Anterior Cruciate Ligament Injuries. JBJS Rev. 2016;4(11) https://doi.org/10.2106/JBJS.RVW.15.00115.
39. Higuchi H, Terauchi M, Kimura M, Kobayashi A, Takeda M, Watanabe H, Takagishi K. The relation between static and dynamic knee stability after ACL reconstruction. Acta Orthop Belg. 2003;69(3):257–66.

40. Ferretti A, Monaco E, Ponzo A, Basiglini L, Iorio R, Caperna L, Conteduca F. Combined intra-articular and extra-articular reconstruction in anterior cruciate ligament-deficient knee: 25 years later. Arthroscopy. 2016;32(10):2039–47.
41. Carr JB 2nd, Yildirim B, Richter D, Etier BE, Anderson MW, Pierce J, Diduch DR. Primary anterolateral ligament rupture in patients requiring revision anterior cruciate ligament reconstruction: a retrospective case-control magnetic resonance imaging review. Arthroscopy. 2018;34(11):3055–62.
42. Getgood A, Hewsion C, Bryant D, Litchfield R, Heard M, Buchko G, Hiemstra LA, Willits KR, Firth A, MacDonald P, Stability Study Group CANADA & EUROPE. No Difference in Functional Outcomes When Lateral Extra-articular Tenodesis is Added to Anterior Cruciate Ligament Reconstruction in young active patients: The Stability Study. Arthroscopy. 2020;5 https://doi.org/10.1016/j.arthro.2020.02.015.
43. Ra HJ, Kim JH, Lee DH. Comparative clinical outcomes of anterolateral ligament reconstruction versus lateral extra-articular tenodesis in combination with anterior cruciate ligament reconstruction: systematic review and meta-analysis. Arch Orthop Trauma Surg. 2020;5:923–31. https://doi.org/10.1007/s00402-020-03393-8.
44. Slette EL, Mikula JD, Schon JM, Chetti DC, Kheir MM, Turnbull TL, RF LP. Biomechanical results of lateral extra-articular Tenodesis procedures of the knee: a systematic review. Arthroscopy. 2016;32(12):2592–611.
45. Noyes FR, Mooar PA, Matthews DS, Butler DL. The symptomatic anterior cruciate-deficient knee. Part I: the long-term functional disability in athletically active individuals. J Bone Joint Surg Am. 1983;65(2):154–62.
46. Noyes FR, Matthews DS, Mooar PA, Grood ES. The symptomatic anterior cruciate-deficient knee. Part II: the results of rehabilitation, activity modification, and counseling on functional disability. J Bone Joint Surg Am. 1983;65(2):163–74.
47. Cinque ME, Dornan GJ, Chahla J, Moatshe G, LaPrade RF. High rates of osteoarthritis develop after anterior cruciate ligament surgery: an analysis of 4108 patients. Am J Sports Med. 2018;46(8):2011–9.
48. Lie MM, Risberg MA, Storheim K, Engebretsen L, Øiestad BE. What's the rate of knee osteoarthritis 10 years after anterior cruciate ligament injury? An updated systematic review. Br J Sports Med. 2019;53(18):1162–7.
49. Claes S, Hermie L, Verdonk R, Bellemans J, Verdonk P. Is osteoarthritis an inevitable consequence of anterior cruciate ligament reconstruction? A meta-analysis. Knee Surg Sports Traumatol Arthrosc. 2013;21(9):1967–76.
50. Chen KH, Chiang ER, Wang HY, Ma HL. Correlation of meniscal tear with timing of anterior cruciate ligament reconstruction in patients without initially concurrent meniscal tear. J Knee Surg. 2019;32(11):1128–32.
51. Shelbourne KD, Wilckens JH, Mollabashy A, Arlo M. Arthrofibrosis in acute anterior cruciate ligament reconstruction. The effect of timing of reconstruction and rehabilitation. Am J Sports Med. 1991;19(4):332–6.
52. Kim KT, Kim HJ, Lee HI, Park YJ, Kang DG, Yoo JI, Moon DK, Cho SH, Hwang SC. A Comparison of Results after Anterior Cruciate Ligament Reconstruction in over 40 and under 40 Years of Age: A Meta-Analysis. Knee Surg Relat Res. 2018;30(2):95–106.
53. Weng CJ, Yeh WL, Hsu KY, Chiu CH, Chang SS, Chen AC, Chan YS. Clinical and functional outcomes of anterior cruciate ligament reconstruction with autologous hamstring tendon in patients aged 50 years or older. Arthroscopy. 2020;36(2):558–62.
54. Toanen C, Demey G, Ntagiopoulos PG, Ferrua P, Dejour D. Is there any benefit in anterior cruciate ligament reconstruction in patients older than 60 years? Am J Sports Med. 2017;45(4):832–7.
55. Mall NA, Frank RM, Saltzman BM, Cole BJ, Bach BR Jr. Results After Anterior Cruciate Ligament Reconstruction in Patients Older Than 40 Years: How Do They Compare With Younger Patients? A Systematic Review and Comparison With Younger Populations. Sports Health. 2016;8(2):177–81.

56. Cimino PM. The incidence of meniscal tears associated with acute anterior cruciate ligament disruption secondary to snow skiing accidents. Arthroscopy. 1994;10(2):198–200.
57. Chen G, Tang X, Li Q, Zheng G, Yang T, Li J. The evaluation of patient-specific factors associated with meniscal and chondral injuries accompanying ACL rupture in young adult patients. Knee Surg Sports Traumatol Arthrosc. 2015;23(3):792–8.
58. Toman CV, Dunn WR, Spindler KP, Amendola A, Andrish JT, Bergfeld JA, Flanigan D, Jones MH, Kaeding CC, Ge XR, Matava MJ, EC MC, Parker RD, Wolcott M, Vidal A, Wolf BR, Huston LJ, Harrell FE Jr, Wright RW. Success of meniscal repair at anterior cruciate ligament reconstruction. Am J Sports Med. 2009;37(6):1111–5. https://doi.org/10.1177/0363546509337010.
59. Wasserstein D, Dwyer T, Gandhi R, Austin PC, Mahomed N, Ogilvie-Harris D. A matched-cohort population study of reoperation after meniscal repair with and without concomitant anterior cruciate ligament reconstruction. Am J Sports Med. 2013;41(2):349–55.
60. Sarraj M, Coughlin RP, Solow M, Ekhtiari S, Simunovic N, Krych AJ, MacDonald P, Ayeni OR. Anterior cruciate ligament reconstruction with concomitant meniscal surgery: a systematic review and meta-analysis of outcomes. Knee Surg Sports Traumatol Arthrosc. 2019;27(11):3441–52.
61. Jin C, Song EK, Jin QH, Lee NH, Seon JK. Outcomes of simultaneous high tibial osteotomy and anterior cruciate ligament reconstruction in anterior cruciate ligament deficient knee with osteoarthritis. BMC Musculoskelet Disord. 2018;19(1):228. https://doi.org/10.1186/s12891-018-2161-0.
62. Crawford MD, Diehl LH, Amendola A. Surgical management and treatment of the anterior cruciate ligament-deficient knee with Malalignment. Clin Sports Med. 2017;36(1):119–33.
63. Vaishya R, Vijay V, Jha GK, Agarwal AK. Prospective study of the anterior cruciate ligament reconstruction associated with high tibial opening wedge osteotomy in knee arthritis associated with instability. J Clin Orthop Trauma. 2016;7(4):265–71.
64. Kim SJ, Moon HK, Chun YM, Chang WH, Kim SG. Is correctional osteotomy crucial in primary varus knees undergoing anterior cruciate ligament reconstruction? Clin Orthop Relat Res. 2011;469(5):1421–6.
65. Tian S, Wang B, Wang Y, Ha C, Liu L, Sun K. Combined unicompartmental knee arthroplasty and anterior cruciate ligament reconstruction in knees with osteoarthritis and deficient anterior cruciate ligament. BMC Musculoskelet Disord. 2016;17:327.
66. Ventura A, Legnani C, Terzaghi C, Iori S, Borgo E. Medial unicondylar knee arthroplasty combined to anterior cruciate ligament reconstruction. Knee Surg Sports Traumatol Arthrosc. 2017;25(3):675–80.
67. Mohtadi NG, Chan DS. Return to sport-specific performance after primary anterior cruciate ligament reconstruction: a systematic review. Am J Sports Med. 2018;46(13):3307–16.
68. Magnussen RA, Reinke EK, Huston LJ, MOON Group, Hewett TE, Spindler KP. Effect of high-grade preoperative knee laxity on anterior cruciate ligament reconstruction outcomes. Am J Sports Med. 2016;44(12):3077–82.
69. Magnussen RA, Reinke EK, Huston LJ, MOON Group, Hewett TE, Spindler KP. Factors associated with high-grade Lachman, pivot shift, and anterior drawer at the time of anterior cruciate ligament reconstruction. Arthroscopy. 2016;32(6):1080–5.

Chapter 57
Posterior Cruciate Ligament Knee Instability

This is a condition whereby there is symptomatic instability of the tibiofemoral articulation due to dysfunction of the posterior cruciate ligament (PCL).

57.1 Causes of PCL Instability [1–9]

Disruption of the PCL may be:

- Congenital/developmental
- Acquired
  - Spontaneous (rare)

    Chronic repetitive microtrauma—This may be seen in athletes that repetitively stretch the PCL
  - Acute substantial trauma (most common)

  Disruption of the PCL may be:

- Isolated, single ligament
- Associated with other ligamentous dysfunction/injuries
- Associated with bony abnormalities—developmental, traumatic, degenerative

Although PCL instability may be part of multiligament instability and may congenital or developmental, isolated post-traumatic PCL instability is considered in this chapter.

Traumatic PCL disruption may be described:

C. Panayiotou Charalambous, *The Knee Made Easy*,
https://doi.org/10.1007/978-3-030-54506-2_57

According to the Type of Disruption

- Avulsion of the PCL from its femoral origin
  - Soft tissue avulsion
  - Bony avulsion
- Avulsion of the PCL tibial insertion
  - Soft tissue avulsion
  - Bony avulsion
- Intra-substance tear

According to the Completeness of Disruption

- Complete—both bundles
- Partial:
  - One bundle
  - Proportion of fibres

According to the Mechanism of Injury Leading to Disruption

- Contact—with another player or a surface/object of the flexed knee that leads to posterior displacement of the tibia in relation to the femur (dashboard injuries—driver sat with knee flexed and dashboard forces tibia posteriorly, athlete falling down with knee flexed and with tibia forced posteriorly). Most PCL injuries are contact injuries
- Non-contact—forced flexion plus internal rotation, forced varus or valgus with rotation are also associated with PCL tears

57.2 Effects of PCL Disruption

A ligament is taut only when it is firmly attached at its two ends. This is analogous to hanging from a rope. The rope may lose part of its substance (partial tear) but still provide support, but if completely gone then one may fall down. Similarly, if the PCL is disrupted it may compromise its ability to maintain the position of the tibia relative to the femur. With PCL dysfunction the following exaggerated displacements of the tibia in relation to the femur (subluxations of the tibiofemoral articulation) may occur:

- Posterior displacement of the tibia relative to the femur
- External rotation of the tibia relative to the femur

57.2.1 *Intra-articular Disruptions Associated with a PCL Tear*

Hamada et al. [10] looked at the cartilaginous damage associated with acute isolated PCL injury, arthroscopically, in 61 consecutive patients and found:

- 17 (28%) had a meniscal tear
  - 3 medial meniscal tear
  - 11 lateral meniscal tear
  - 3 both medial and lateral meniscal tears
  - Most (10) of these were longitudinal tears of the anterior segment of the lateral meniscus
- 32 (52%) had articular cartilage injury
  - 7 greater than one half of the thickness of the articular cartilage
  - 3 involving erosion to the subchondral bone
  - Most involved the medial femoral condyle—19 cases (31%)

Ringler et al. [11] evaluated the prevalence of intra-articular pathology associated with isolated PCL tear using MRI in 48 knees and reported:

- 69% of isolated PCL tears were mid-substance
- 27% were proximal avulsions
- 25% had meniscal tears
- 23% had focal cartilage lesions, usually affecting the central third medial femoral condyle and medial trochlea

57.3 Clinical History of a Traumatic Event

The following characteristics of the injury that led to the onset of symptoms may suggest a PCL disruption:

- A history of a substantial traumatic event (an event a patient can easily recall)
- Patient felt/heard pop in the knee
- Mechanism of injury whereby knee was flexed and tibia pushed backwards
- Patient unable to get up and stand/ walk
- Knee swelling
- Required medical attention

57.4 Clinical Symptoms of PCL Instability

- Acute presentation
  - Painful, swollen knee, diffusely tender knee
- Chronic presentation
  - Feeling of abnormal displacement—"giving way", feeling "wobbly"
  - Instability upon decelerating activities (going down stairs or downhill, decelerating after running in straight line), not much instability on twisting activities
  - Clicking, clunking due to abnormal translation of the knee
  - Patellofemoral (PF) pain- anterior knee pain, pain felt at the back of the knee
  - Dead leg syndrome, heavy leg, paraesthesia
  - Intermittent swelling

Following the acute injury, the acute pain, may improve, knee motion restored and the patient is left with feeling of instability or other symptoms.

57.5 Clinical Signs of PCL Instability

- Posterior sag of the tibia in relation to the femur, reduction/loss of medial tibial condyle step off
- Posterior knee laxity—posterior drawer test
- Reverse pivot shift test

57.6 Investigations for PCL Instability [12–18]

Investigations for PCL instability aim to confirm the PCL disruption, determine the type of PCL disruption, and identify any associated structural lesions (ligamentous, bony, meniscal, chondral). These include:

- Radiological
  - Plain radiographs:

    Stress view, tunnel view, AP, lateral may demonstrate avulsion fracture, medial "Segond fracture", assess malalignment, posterior tibial slope, or the presence of osteoarthritis (OA) in the medial and PF compartments in chronic injuries

– MRI Scan:

As the knee is placed in extension during MRI, the intact PCL appears curved and lax whereas the anterior cruciate ligament (ACL) looks taut and straight

Bone bruising—in PCL tears this is usually found in the anterior part of the proximal tibia

In chronic PCL disruptions the PCL may appear intact but the knee is unstable as MRI gives only a static assessment. The following may suggest a disrupted PCL:

Discontinuity of the PCL substance
PCL soft tissue avulsion
Thickened PCL > 7 mm

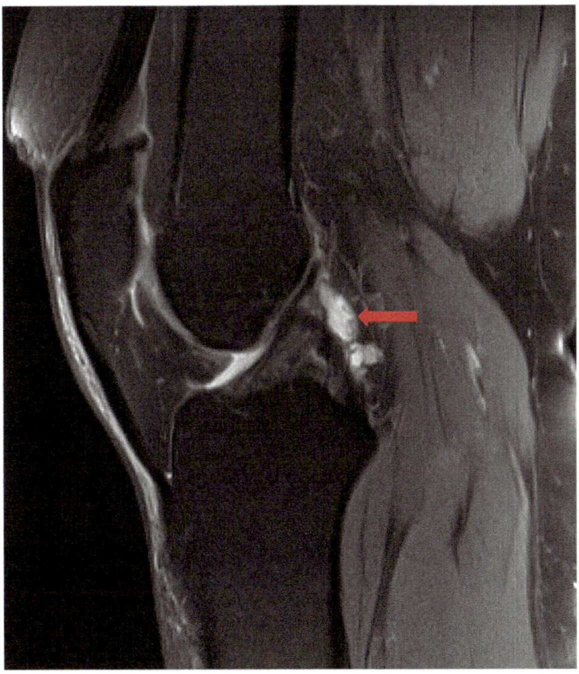

PCL tear with cystic changes

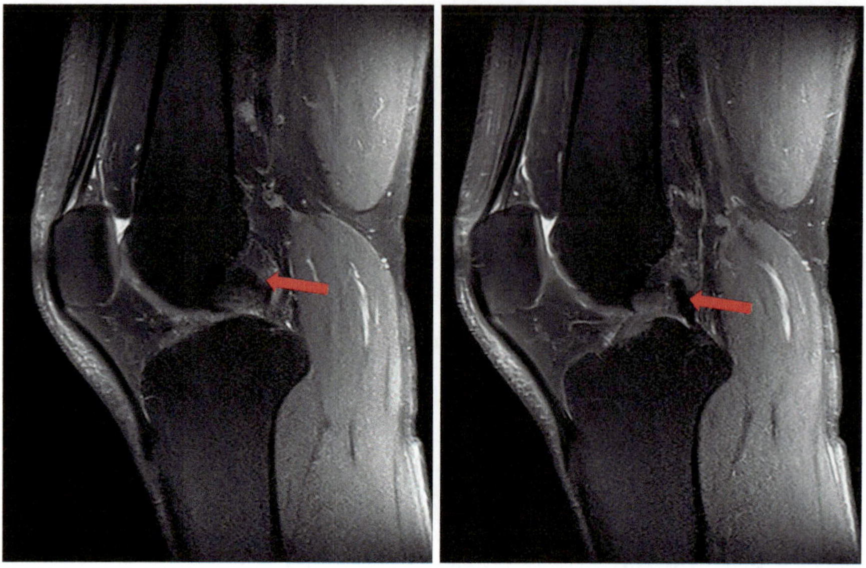

Buckling of PCL due to tear (red arrow)

Ligament continuity is often seen in chronic PCL tears. Jung YB et al. [16] reported continuity in 72% of cases, with a higher continuity rate at more than 6 months post injury. However, continuity does not equate function, as the PCL may have healed in a lengthened position and thus be dysfunctional.

- CT scan—in the presence of tibial avulsion fracture to define the extent of bony fragment and other associated proximal tibial fractures
  - Examination under general anaesthesia—joint translation and laxity is assessed with the patient under general anaesthesia to abolish pain and allow muscle relaxation
  - Arthroscopic evaluation

57.7 Management of PCL Instability [19–27]

Initial management aims at:

- Reducing the acute inflammation of the knee using the Rest, Ice, Compression, Elevation (RICE) principles
- Restore motion (tibiofemoral/PF)
- Quadriceps/hamstring activation
- Proprioception training
- Activity specific mobilisation

Further management aims at improving ongoing symptoms of instability and hence improve a patient's function or reducing the risk of further instability. This depends on:

- Symptoms—severity, frequency
- Underlying cause
- Functional demand of individual

57.7.1 Non-surgical

- Leave alone
- Activity modification, avoiding unstable positions
- Physiotherapy to address:
  - Core imbalance—core strengthening
  - Hip muscle weakness —strengthening of hip muscles
  - Proprioception—proprioceptive training
  - Quadriceps weakness—Quadriceps muscle strengthening to pull the tibia forwards
- External knee devices—PCL bracing

It should be noted that non-surgical management does not specifically address the PCL disruption but aims to improve stability by enhancing the function of dynamic stabilisers (through strengthening, better control and coordination).

57.7.2 Surgical

- Repair
  - Avulsion fracture fixation
  - Femoral soft tissue avulsion
- Reconstruction—using a graft that is secured in bone tunnels of the femur and tibia. Fixation is achieved by multiple means including suspensory (e.g. suture button) and non-suspensory devices (e.g. interference screw fixation). Several grafts and techniques may be utilised:
  - Autograft—hamstring tendons, patellar tendon with a bone block from its patellar origin and tibial tubercle insertion, quadriceps tendon
  - Allograft
  - Synthetic graft
  - Single bundle vs. double bundle

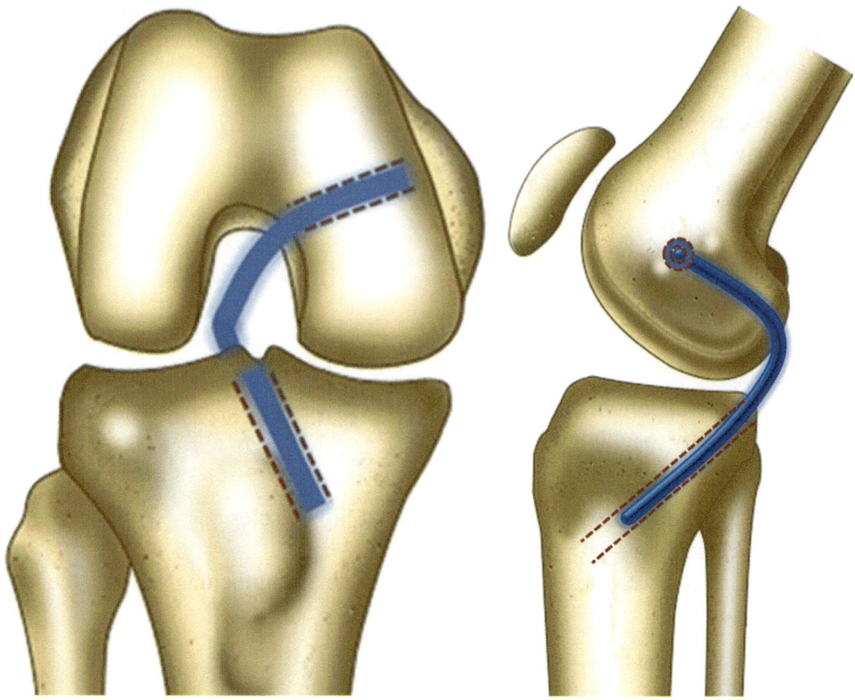

PCL single bundle reconstruction

PCL reconstruction surgery may work by:

- Mechanical effect—limiting translation of the tibia in relation to the femur
- Proprioceptive mechanism

57.8 Considerations in the Management of Post-Traumatic PCL Deficiency

In considering the definitive management of PCL disruption several considerations must be taken into account some of which are described below.

57.8.1 Natural History of PCL Disruption

It is recognised that:

- A substantial proportion of patients who do not have PCL surgery manage to function without any debilitating knee instability

- Persistent instability may:
  - Limit ability of an individual to achieve high level functional potential
- A substantial proportion of patients sustaining an PCL tear will develop secondary degenerative changes (arthritis)

Jung YB et al. [16] assessed the healing process of the injured PCL using instability measurements and MRI findings in 46 cases of complete PCL tear. They reported:

- 13 (28%) showed nearly normal PCL contour
- 20 (44%) showed continuity but deformed PCL contour
- 13 (28%) showed PCL discontinuity
- The group that had the MRI more than 6 months after injury showed more continuity than the group that obtained MRI within 6 months of the injury
- Cases with nearly normal continuity on MRI showed better stability results in the KT-1000 arthrometer and stress radiographs than those with discontinuity
- The presence of other combined ligament injuries had a statistically significant negative effect on regaining PCL continuity

Shelbourne KD et al. [28] assessed 68 patients with an acute, isolated PCL injury treated non-surgically. Forty four patients were available for both objective and subjective evaluations at a mean of 14.3 years (range, 10–21 years) after injury. All 68 patients underwent subjective follow-up at a mean of 17.6 years after injury. They showed that:

- The mean quadriceps muscle strength was 97% of the non-involved leg
- All patients had normal knee range of motion
- The overall grade of radiographs was rated as:
  - Normal in 26 patients (59%)
  - Nearly normal in 13 patients (30%)
  - Abnormal in 4 patients (9%)
  - Severely abnormal in 1 patient (2%)
- The grade of osteoarthritis (OA) on radiographs was not different in any knee compartment based on PCL laxity grade. Five patients (11%) had medial joint space narrowing greater than 2 mm
- High scores were seen on subjective functional ratings at a mean of 17 years post-injury
- There was no difference in subjective scores between PCL laxity grades

They concluded that long-term results after an isolated PCL injury show that patients remain active, have good strength and full knee range of motion, and report good subjective scores. The prevalence of moderate to severe OA was 11%. Results were not influenced by PCL laxity grade.

Torg JS et al. [29] assessed the natural history of the PCL. Forty three patients with an average interval of 6.3 years (range, one to 37 years) between injury and evaluation were included in their study. Fourteen patients had a straight unidirectional posterior instability and 29 had a combined multidirectional instability. It was established that PCL disruption associated with combined abnormalities (chondromalacia of the patella, meniscal derangement, quadriceps atrophy, or degenerative changes) gave a worse functional outcome.

57.8.2 Timing of Encountering the Patient

The patient may present at different stages following PCL disruption to the clinician:

- Acute—just after the injury
- Subacute—after the acute injury has settled and has had a course of physiotherapy but continues with substantial instability which is limiting day to day activities
- Chronic—after the patient returned to normal activities but has experienced further instability
- Chronic—after a long period of managing, the patient experiences a substantial instability episode leading a knee flare up or further associated injury(meniscal/chondral)

Hence the approach on how to deal with the underlying PCL disruption may differ according to the above.

57.8.3 Timing of PCL Reconstruction

PCL reconstruction may be:

- Acute—in the very first few days post injury
- Subacute—once the acute inflammation settles and joint motion including knee extension is restored
- Chronic—patient returns to usual function and is only considered for surgical intervention if further substantial instability episodes occur

Given the natural history of PCL reconstruction, if surgery is offered to all individuals with a PCL disruption, then a substantial proportion may undergo unnecessary surgery.

57.8.4 Associated Injuries

It is recognised that a substantial proportion of acute trauma in PCL disruptions are associated with other intra-articular injuries [10, 11].

Such associated injuries are important to recognise as they may:

- Account for ongoing symptoms which may be wrongly attributed to the PCL
- Need specific intervention in isolation or in addition to intervention for the PCL disruption
- Determine long term prognosis

Wang SH et al. [30] studied 4169 patients diagnosed with PCL tear and reported that there was a statistically significant higher cumulative incidence of meniscus tear (1.1%), OA (2.7%) and subsequent TKR (0.9%) amongst patients with a PCL tear than those without a tear. PCL reconstruction patients had a significantly lower cumulative incidence of meniscus tear (0.4%), OA (2.3%) and subsequent TKR (0.5%) compared with non-reconstructed patients (2.4%, 3.5%, 1.7% $p < 0.05$). After adjusting for covariates, PCL-injured patients who underwent reconstruction within 1 year after PCL injury showed a significantly lower risk of subsequent sequelae than those who did not undergo reconstruction.

57.8.5 PCL Disruption Associated with Arthritis

PCL instability may predispose to further meniscal tears, increase compartmental pressures (mainly medial and PF compartments) increasing the risk of degeneration and thus OA [31–33].

Hence, PCL disruption may present in association with OA. This may be isolated compartment arthritis or more extensive arthritis. PCL injuries have been related to an increased risk of developing PF and medial compartment arthritis.

In this scenario is important to determine:

- What is the main cause of the patient's symptoms—the arthritis or the PCL instability

A trial of PCL bracing to help instability may help distinguish between the two. Similarly, addressing the pain of the arthritis may help distinguish between the two.

57.8.6 PCL Disruption Associated with Malalignment [34–37]

Malalignment may put excessive forces on a PCL reconstructed graft, leading to dysfunction of the reconstruction. Hence, in such cases, combination of PCL reconstruction with a proximal tibial osteotomy may be considered.

- Varus malalignment—opening wedge high tibial osteotomy
  Reduced/reverse tibial slope—anterior opening wedge proximal tibial osteotomy

57.9 Return to Sports Following PCL Non-surgical and Surgical Management

- Agolley D et al. [38] evaluated prospectively 46 consecutive athletes with an MRI-confirmed isolated PCL injury presenting within 4 weeks of injury (grade II or III injury). Management involved initial bracing followed by an individualised rehabilitation programme. The reported that:
  - Mean time to return to sports-specific training was 10.6 weeks
  - Mean time to return to full competitive sport was 16.4 weeks (10 to 40)
  - 42 (91%) were playing at the same/higher sport level at 2 years post-injury
  - 32 (70%) were playing at the same/higher sport level at 5 years post-injury
  - 38 (83%) were playing at a competitive sports level at 5 years post-injury
- Lee DW et al. [39] evaluated the clinical outcomes of transtibial PCL reconstruction with fresh frozen allograft and remnant preservation in 52 patients, with a mean follow-up of 29.5 ± 8.6 months. The subjective assessments and functional tests significantly improved postoperatively. Mean time to return to full sports activity was 9.7 ± 5.1 months. Thirty-eight (73.1%) and 45 (86.5%) patients could return to previous sports activities at 9 and 24 months, respectively. A sports-experience questionnaire indicated that 48% and 69.2% of the patients were participating with unlimited effort and performance, respectively, and no pain at 9 and 24 months
- Devitt BM et al. [40] systematically reviewed the literature to determine the rates of return to sport and functional outcomes of patients after isolated PCL reconstruction. They included 14 studies. The median time from injury to surgery was 10.6 months (range, 6 weeks-21 years). Subjective and objective scores improved substantially as did knee laxity. However, there was a low rate of return to preinjury level of sport of only 44% (95% CI, 23%–66%)

Learning Pearls

- As successful outcomes are often seen with non-surigical management of PCL injuries, this may be the preferred approach for most cases
- There is no strong clinical evidence that double-bundle reconstruction offers a functional advantage over single-bundle reconstruction with equivalent long term outcomes reported for both [41]
- Equivalent outcomes have been reported with different grafts (hamstring tendons, patellar tendon, quadriceps tendon and allografts) [42]
- Acute surgery is considered in displaced PCL bony avulsion (usually involves the tibial insertion)
- In considering surgical intervention it is important to recognise that the aim is to improve knee stability rather than improving pain

References

1. Chahla J, Williams BT, LaPrade RF. Posterior Cruciate Ligament. Arthroscopy. 2020;36(2):333–5.
2. Janousek AT, Jones DG, Clatworthy M, Higgins LD, Fu FH. Posterior cruciate ligament injuries of the knee joint. Sports Med. 1999;28(6):429–41.
3. Petrigliano FA, McAllister DR. Isolated posterior cruciate ligament injuries of the knee. Sports Med Arthrosc Rev. 2006;14(4):206–12.
4. Miller MD, Bergfeld JA, Fowler PJ, Harner CD, Noyes FR. The posterior cruciate ligament injured knee: principles of evaluation and treatment. Instr Course Lect. 1999;48:199–207.
5. García N, Debandi A, Delgado G, Rosales J, Verdugo M. Isolated posterior cruciate ligament aplasia: a case report. Skelet Radiol. 2019;48(9):1439–42.
6. da Gama MM, Bruno AA, Grisone B, Bernardelli G, Pietrogrande L. Isolated congenital absence of posterior cruciate ligament? A case report. Chir Organi Mov. 2008;92(2):105–7.
7. Iwata S, Suda Y, Nagura T, Matsumoto H, Otani T, Andriacchi TP, Toyama Y. Clinical disability in posterior cruciate ligament deficient patients does not relate to knee laxity, but relates to dynamic knee function during stair descending. Knee Surg Sports Traumatol Arthrosc. 2007;15(4):335–42.
8. Katsman A, Strauss EJ, Campbell KA, Alaia MJ. Posterior cruciate ligament avulsion fractures. Curr Rev Musculoskelet Med. 2018;11(3):503–9.
9. Goyal K, Tashman S, Wang JH, Li K, Zhang X, Harner C. In vivo analysis of the isolated posterior cruciate ligament-deficient knee during functional activities. Am J Sports Med. 2012;40(4):777–85.
10. Hamada M, Shino K, Mitsuoka T, Toritsuka Y, Natsu-Ume T, Horibe S. Chondral injury associated with acute isolated posterior cruciate ligament injury. Arthroscopy. 2000;16(1):59–63.
11. Ringler MD, Shotts EE, Collins MS, Howe BM. Intra-articular pathology associated with isolated posterior cruciate ligament injury on MRI. Skelet Radiol. 2016;45(12):1695–703.
12. Kim SG, Kim SH, Choi WS, Bae JH. Supine lateral radiographs at 90° of knee flexion have a similar diagnostic accuracy for chronic posterior cruciate ligament injuries as stress radiographs. Knee Surg Sports Traumatol Arthrosc. 2019;27(8):2433–9.
13. Servant CT, Ramos JP, Thomas NP. The accuracy of magnetic resonance imaging in diagnosing chronic posterior cruciate ligament injury. Knee. 2004;11(4):265–70.
14. Xu B, Zhang H, Li B, Wang W. Comparison of magnetic resonance imaging for patients with acute and chronic anterior cruciate ligament tears. Medicine (Baltimore). 2018;97(10):e0001. https://doi.org/10.1097/MD.0000000000010001.
15. Kam CK, Chee DW, Peh WC. Magnetic resonance imaging of cruciate ligament injuries of the knee. Can Assoc Radiol J. 2010;61(2):80–9.
16. Jung YB, GHJ, Yang JJ, Yang DL, Lee YS, Song IS, Lee HJ. Characterization of spontaneous healing of chronic posterior cruciate ligament injury: analysis of instability and magnetic resonance imaging. J Magn Reson Imaging. 2008;27(6):1336–40.
17. Kose O, Ozyurek S, Turan A, Guler F. Reverse Segond fracture and associated knee injuries: a case report and review of 13 published cases. Acta Orthop Traumatol Turc. 2016;50(5):587–91.
18. Yazdi H, Gomrokchi AY, Aminizade S, Sohrabi S. Reverse Segond fracture without posterior cruciate ligament injury—a report of two cases and review of the literature. J Orthop Case Rep. 2019;9(3):90–2.
19. Safran MR, Allen AA, Lephart SM, Borsa PA, Fu FH, Harner CD. Proprioception in the posterior cruciate ligament deficient knee. Knee Surg Sports Traumatol Arthrosc. 1999;7(5):310–7.
20. LaPrade RF, Smith SD, Wilson KJ, Wijdicks CA. Quantification of functional brace forces for posterior cruciate ligament injuries on the knee joint: an in vivo investigation. Knee Surg Sports Traumatol Arthrosc. 2015;23(10):3070–6.
21. Song JG, Nha KW, Lee SW. Open Posterior Approach versus Arthroscopic Suture Fixation for Displaced Posterior Cruciate Ligament Avulsion Fractures: Systematic Review. Knee Surg Relat Res. 2018;30(4):275–83.
22. Zhao X, Kuang SD, Su C, Xiao WF, Lei GH, Gao SG. Arthroscopic treatment of femoral avulsion fracture of the posterior cruciate ligament in association with meniscus tear. Orthop Surg. 2020;10:692–7. https://doi.org/10.1111/os.12636.

23. Vermeijden HD, van der List JP, DiFelice GS. Arthroscopic posterior cruciate ligament primary repair. Sports Med Arthrosc Rev. 2020;28(1):23–9.
24. van der List JP, Di Felice GS. Arthroscopic Primary Posterior Cruciate Ligament Repair With Suturementation. Arthrosc Tech. 2017;6(5):e1685–90. https://doi.org/10.1016/j.eats.2017.06.024. eCollection 2017
25. Hopper GP, Heusdens CHW, Dossche L, Mackay GM. Posterior Cruciate Ligament Repair With Suture Tapementation. Arthrosc Tech. 2018;8(1):e7–e10.
26. Li J, Kong F, Gao X, Shen Y, Gao S. Prospective randomized comparison of knee stability and proprioception for posterior cruciate ligament reconstruction with autograft, hybrid graft, and γ-irradiated allograft. Arthroscopy. 2016;32(12):2548–55.
27. Wajsfisz A, Christel P, Djian P. Does reconstruction of isolated chronic posterior cruciate ligament injuries restore normal knee function? Orthop Traumatol Surg Res. 2010;96(4):388–93.
28. Shelbourne KD, Clark M, Gray T. Minimum 10-year follow-up of patients after an acute, isolated posterior cruciate ligament injury treated nonoperatively. Am J Sports Med. 2013;41(7):1526–33.
29. Torg JS, Barton TM, Pavlov H, Stine R. Natural history of the posterior cruciate ligament-deficient knee. Clin Orthop Relat Res. 1989;246:208–16.
30. Wang SH, Chien WC, Chung CH, Wang YC, Lin LC, Pan RY. Long-term results of posterior cruciate ligament tear with or without reconstruction: A nationwide, population-based cohort study. PLoS One. 2018;13(10):e0205118. https://doi.org/10.1371/journal.pone.0205118.
31. Gwinner C, Weiler A, Denecke T, Rogasch JMM, Boeth H, GTM. Degenerative changes after posterior cruciate ligament reconstruction are irrespective of posterior knee stability: MRI-based long-term results. Arch Orthop Trauma Surg. 2018;138(3):377–85.
32. Gill TJ, DeFrate LE, Wang C, Carey CT, Zayontz S, Zarins B, Li G. The effect of posterior cruciate ligament reconstruction on patellofemoral contact pressures in the knee joint under simulated muscle loads. Am J Sports Med. 2004;32(1):109–15.
33. Wang D, Graziano J, Williams RJ 3rd, Jones KJ. Nonoperative treatment of PCL injuries: goals of rehabilitation and the natural history of conservative care. Curr Rev Musculoskelet Med. 2018;11(2):290–7.
34. Bernhardson AS, Aman ZS, DePhillipo NN, Dornan GJ, Storaci HW, Brady AW, Nakama G, LaPrade RF. Tibial slope and its effect on graft force in posterior cruciate ligament reconstructions. Am J Sports Med. 2019;47(5):1168–74.
35. Novaretti JV, Sheean AJ, Lian J, De Groot J, Musahl V. The role of osteotomy for the treatment of PCL injuries. Curr Rev Musculoskelet Med. 2018;11(2):298–306.
36. Nha KW, Kim HJ, Ahn HS, Lee DH. Change in posterior Tibial slope after open-wedge and closed-wedge high Tibial osteotomy: a meta-analysis. Am J Sports Med. 2016;44(11):3006–13.
37. Savarese E, Bisicchia S, Romeo R, Amendola A. Role of high tibial osteotomy in chronic injuries of posterior cruciate ligament and posterolateral corner. J Orthop Traumatol. 2011;12(1):1–17.
38. Agolley D, Gabr A, Benjamin-Laing H, Haddad FS. Successful return to sports in athletes following non-operative management of acute isolated posterior cruciate ligament injuries: medium-term follow-up. Bone Joint J. 2017;99-B(6):774–8.
39. Lee DW, Kim JG, Yang SJ, Cho SI. Return to sports and clinical outcomes after arthroscopic anatomic posterior cruciate ligament reconstruction with remnant preservation. Arthroscopy. 2019;35(9):2658–68.
40. Devitt BM, Dissanayake R, Clair J, Napier RJ, Porter TJ, Feller JA, Webster KE. Isolated Posterior Cruciate Reconstruction Results in Improved Functional Outcome but Low Rates of Return to Preinjury Level of Sport: A Systematic Review and Meta-analysis. Orthop J Sports Med. 2018;6(10):2325967118804478. https://doi.org/10.1177/2325967118804478.
41. Yoon KH, Kim EJ, Kwon YB, Kim SG. Minimum 10-year results of single- versus double-bundle posterior cruciate ligament reconstruction: clinical, radiologic, and survivorship outcomes. Am J Sports Med. 2019;47(4):822–7.
42. Lee YS, Lee SH, Lee OS. Graft sources do not affect to the outcome of transtibial posterior cruciate ligament reconstruction: a systematic review. Arch Orthop Trauma Surg. 2018;138(8):1103–16. https://doi.org/10.1007/s00402-018-2946-5.

Chapter 58
Medial Collateral Ligament Knee Instability

This is a condition whereby there is symptomatic instability of the tibiofemoral articulation due to dysfunction of the medial collateral ligament (MCL) of the knee.

58.1 Causes of Medial Collateral Ligament Instability [1–7]

Disruption of the MCL may be:

- Acquired
  - Acute substantial trauma

  Disruption of the MCL may be:

- Isolated, single ligament
- Associated with other ligamentous dysfunction/injuries
- Associated with bony abnormalities—developmental, traumatic, degenerative

Although MCL instability may be part of multiligament instability, isolated post-traumatic anterior instability is considered in this chapter.

Traumatic MCL disruption may be described:

According to the Ligaments Disrupted

- Superficial MCL
- Deep MCL
- Posterior oblique ligament (POL)
- Combinations of the above

C. Panayiotou Charalambous, *The Knee Made Easy*,
https://doi.org/10.1007/978-3-030-54506-2_58

According to the Extent of Disruption of Each Ligament

- Partial (proportion of ligament fibres disrupted)
- Complete (all ligament fibres disrupted)

According to the Type of Disruption

- Avulsion of the MCL ligaments from their femoral origin
  - Soft tissue avulsion
  - Bony avulsion
- Avulsion of the MCL ligaments from their tibial insertion
  - Soft tissue avulsion
  - Bony avulsion
- Intra-substance tear

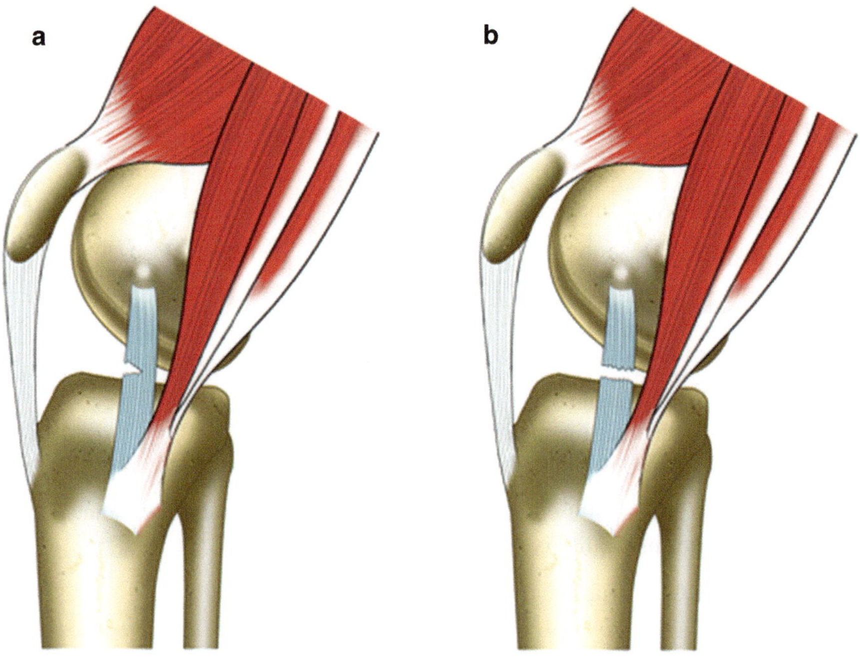

Partial (**a**) and complete (**b**) MCL tear

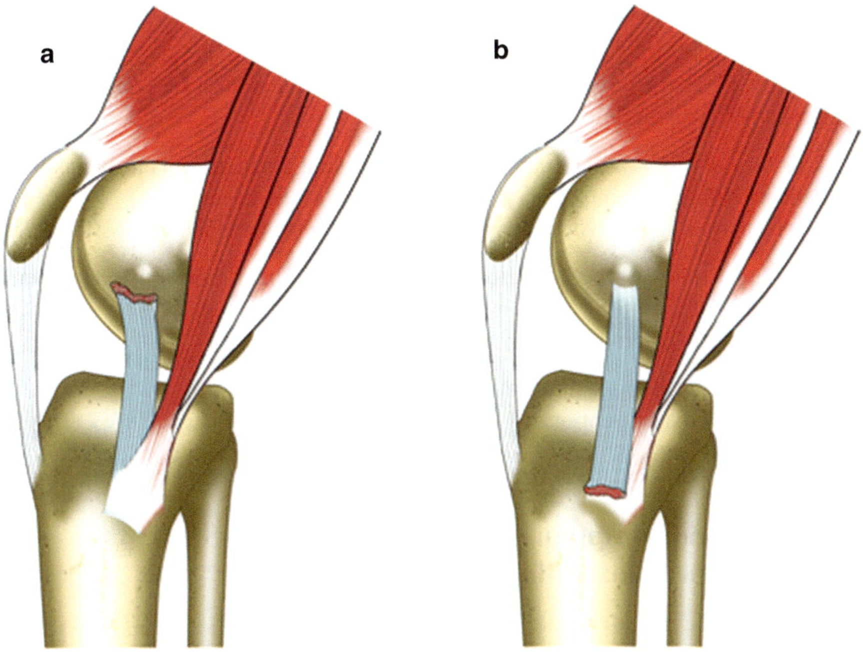

MCL avulsion from its femoral origin (**a**). MCL avulsion from its tibial insertion with interposition of the pes anserinus tendons (**b**)

According to the Mechanism of Injury Leading to Disruption

- Contact—with another player or a surface/object (more common)
- Non-contact

58.2 Effects of Medial Collateral Ligament Disruption

A ligament is taut only when it is firmly attached at its two ends, analogous to hanging from a rope. The rope may lose part of its substance (partial tear) but still provide support, but if completely torn then one may fall down. Similarly, if the MCL is disrupted it may compromise its ability to maintain the position of the tibia relative to the femur. With MCL dysfunction the following exaggerated displacements of the tibia in relation to the femur (subluxations of the tibiofemoral articulation) may occur:

- Lateral (valgus) displacement of the tibia relative to the femur
- External rotation of the tibia relative to the femur

58.3 Clinical History of a Traumatic Event

The following characteristics of the injury that led to the onset of symptoms may suggest a MCL disruption:

- A history of a substantial traumatic event (an event a patient can easily recall)
- Patient felt/heard snap/pop on the medial aspect of the knee
- Mechanism of injury whereby an elongating force was applied to the MCL:
  - Contact (blow to the lateral part of the knee-football, rugby) or non-contact (skiing)
  - Valgus +/– external rotation mechanism
- Difficulty in walking/standing after injury
- Required medical attention

58.4 Clinical Symptoms of Medial Collateral Ligament Instability

- Acute presentation
  - Painful, swollen knee, tenderness on the medial aspect of the knee (need to palpate MCL origin, insertion and mid-substance and distinguish it from posteromedial tibiofemoral tenderness that may be seen in meniscal tears)
  - Bruising medial aspect of the knee
- Chronic presentation
  - Medial pain
  - Clicking, clunking due to abnormal translation of the knee
  - Feeling of abnormal displacement—"giving way", feeling "wobbly"
  - Side to side instability—valgus
  - Rotational instability—instability upon turning
  - Dead leg syndrome, heavy leg, paraesthesia
  - Locking—possible associated meniscal injury

Following the acute injury, the acute pain may improve, knee motion restored and the patient is left with feeling of instability or other symptoms.

58.5 Clinical Signs of Medial Collateral Ligament Instability

- Swelling and bruising medial side of the knee—if acute
- Increased valgus laxity—it is important to determine:

- Amount of medial joint opening on valgus loading
- If there is a firm end point
- If there is increased valgus laxity in:
  - 20–30° knee flexion —superficial MCL disruption
  - Knee in extension—signifies a more severe injury (superficial MCL + POL+/− anterior cruciate ligament (ACL))
- Valgus thrust
- Increased external rotation—dial test positive in 30° and 90°
- Anterior drawer test—with foot in external rotation—suggestive of POL tear (or associated ACL tear)

58.6 Investigations for MCL Instability

Investigations for MCL instability aim to:

1. Confirm the MCL disruption
2. Determine:
   (a) The site of MCL disruption
   (b) The type of MCL disruption (partial/complete)
3. In cases of tibial avulsion injuries, it is vital to determine whether the pes anserinus tendon is superimposed between the detached MCL and its tibial insertion site, which may stop the MCL from healing down with non-surgical management
4. Identify any associated structural lesions (ligamentous, bony, meniscal, chondral)

   These investigations include:

- Radiological [2, 7, 8]
  - Plain radiographs—may demonstrate avulsion fracture, assess alignment
  - MRI Scan
  - CT scan—assess alignment if planning corrective surgery for chronic injuries
  - Stress views—If diagnostic uncertainty persists an anteroposterior plain radiograph whilst applying a valgus load may help determine the amount of medial joint opening and compare it to the opposite knee (stress radiograph). It has been shown [8] that:
    - An increase >3.2 mm gapping at 20° flexion compared to opposite side—suggests a complete superficial MCL tear
    - An increase >6.5 mm gapping at 0° flexion or 9.8 mm at 20° knee flexion compared to the opposite side—suggests a complete medial knee injury (superficial, deep and POL)

- Examination under general anaesthesia—joint translation and laxity is assessed with the patient under general anaesthesia to abolish pain and allow muscle relaxation
- Arthroscopic evaluation—distraction of the medial compartment, look for associated injuries, distinguish between medial meniscal tears and injuries of the deep MCL which may cause similar clinical findings

58.7 Management of MCL Instability [8–29]

Initial management aims at:

- Reducing the acute inflammation of the knee using the Rest, Ice, Compression, Elevation (RICE) principles
- Restore motion (tibiofemoral/patellofemoral)
- Quadriceps/hamstring activation
- Proprioception training
- Activity specific mobilisation
- External devices—knee bracing 6–8 weeks to limit valgus but allowing free range of motion and weightbearing
  - Partial disruptions—limit valgus forces on the MCL and thus improve pain and allow early mobilisation (but bracing not essential)
  - Complete disruptions—limit valgus forces on the MCL and thus encourage MCL healing in a near normal length position

Further management aims at improving ongoing symptoms of instability and hence improve a patient's function. This depends on:

- Underlying disruption—partial/complete

58.7.1 Non-surgical

Non-surgical management is preferable in partial injuries, with minimal associated laxity, or in low functionally demand patients.

- Leave alone
- Activity modification, avoiding unstable positions
  - Incomplete—mobilise FWB guided by pain.
  - Complete tears:

- Mobilise full weight bearing in knee brace with vertical posts that allows range of motion (to limit valgus loading of the MCL and limit extension to 30°)—utilised in complete disruptions for 6 weeks
- Physiotherapy to address:
  - Core imbalance—core strengthening
  - Hip muscle weakness —strengthening of hip muscles
  - Proprioception—proprioceptive training
  - Medial hamstring strengthening—dynamic medial stabilisers

It should be noted that non-surgical management does not specifically address the MCL disruption but aims to improve stability by enhancing the function of dynamic stabilisers (through strengthening, better control and coordination).

58.7.2 Surgical

MCL disruptions have a good healing potential hence most isolated MCL disruptions are treated non-surgically initially. Surgical intervention is preferable in:

1. Acute injuries:
   (a) Where there is complete MCL avulsion from its tibial insertion with superimposed pes anserinus tendons' insertion (equivalent to the "Stener-lesion" in tears of the ulnar collateral ligament of the metacarpophalangeal joint of the thumb)
   (b) Where the torn ligament displaces and is caught in the medial compartment of the knee
2. Chronic injuries—patients who continue with substantial symptoms of instability

Surgical options include:

- Reattachment of disrupted structures +/− augmentation with graft
  - Avulsion fracture fixation
  - Soft tissue avulsion
- Reconstruction—using a graft that is secured to the femur and tibia
  - Anatomical or non-anatomical
  - Isolated superficial MCL or combined with POL reconstruction
  - Grafts
    - Autograft—hamstring tendons (the hamstring tendons may be left attached to their tibial insertion, divided proximally and inserted onto the distal femur)
    - Allograft
    - Synthetic graft

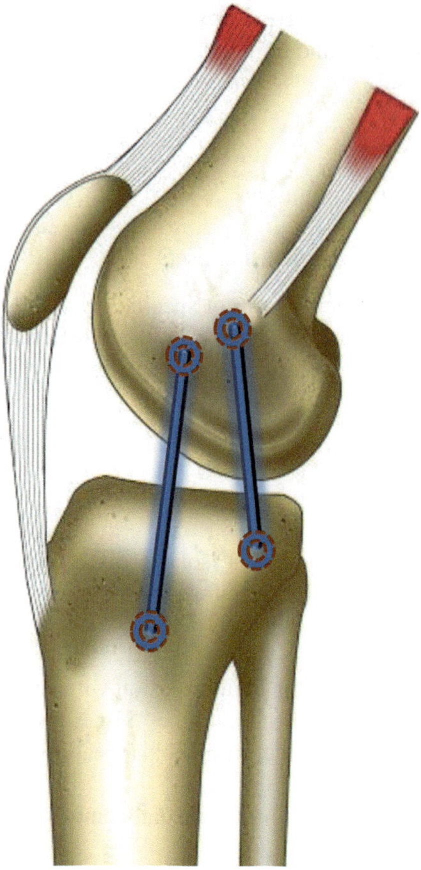

MCL reconstruction (anatomic reconstruction of the superficial MCL and posterior oblique ligament components)

58.8 Considerations in the Management of Post-Traumatic MCL Deficiency

In considering the definitive management of MCL disruption several considerations must be taken into account some of which are described below.

58.8.1 Natural History

It is recognised that:

- MCL disruption may be treated non-surgically in most cases even when there is complete disruption. Hence, it is important not to miss a MCL injury in the acutely injured knee.

- Reider B et al.[19] reported 5-year outcomes of the treatment of isolated grade III sprains of the MCL with early functional rehabilitation in 35 athletes. Following MCL injury, patients were placed in lateral hinged braces (to provide valgus support) with free flexion and extension of the knee. Range of motion exercises were performed in a whirlpool or swimming pool. Patients were then started on quadriceps setting and leg raises. Resistive exercises were added when 90° of flexion was restored. At recovery patients were allowed to return to unrestricted sports. Assessment was done with a 50-point Hospital for Special Surgery scale. At a mean follow-up of 5.3 years (range, 2.5 to 8) the mean Hospital for Special Surgery knee rating score was 45.9 points (range, 41 to 50). The authors concluded that their outcomes were comparable with those achieved with surgery or immobilization by earlier investigators.
- Mok DW and Good C[20] evaluated prospectively the non-surgical management of MCL injury in 25 patients who had acute complete tear of the MCL with associated ACL injury. They were treated by cast bracing and physiotherapy. Their average age was 27.6 years (range 15–53 years) and the average follow-up was 24.2 months (range 12–48 months). All 25 patients had good or excellent results, with return to the pre-injury level of sports by 1 year and with restoration of medial stability. The authors concluded that non-surgical treatment can restore stability to the medial side of the knee, even in the presence of ACL disruption.

58.8.2 Timing of Encountering the Patient

The patient may present at different stages following MCL disruption to the clinician:

- Acute—just after the injury
- Chronic—after the patient returned to normal activities but has experienced further instability

Hence, the approach on how to deal with the underlying MCL disruption may differ according to the above.

58.8.3 MCL Disruption Associated with Malalignemnt [30, 31]

Malalignment may put excessive forces on a MCL reconstruction graft, leading to dysfunction of the reconstruction. Hence, in cases of chronic MCL instability, combination of MCL reconstruction with a distal femoral osteotomy (single stage or two-stage procedure) may be considered:

- Valgus malalignment—opening/closing wedge distal femoral osteotomy
-

Learning Pearls

- In the acute scenario:
  - Complete MCL tears may be associated with less pain than partial tears (as the torn ligament is not under tension as it has completely torn)
  - Joint effusion may be seen in partial MCL tears but may be absent in complete tears (as in complete tears the associated torn capsule allows the effusion to escape into the surrounding subcutaneous tissues)
- The dial test may be easily performed in the acute scenario, and may be positive in the presence of an MCL tear
- MCL disruption may be treated non-surgically even if there are other associated ligamentous injuries (such as ACL tear)
- It may be difficult to quantify clinically the degree of medial tibiofemoral joint opening upon valgus loading. The presence or absence of an end point may be a more reliable sign.
- Early knee motion may facilitate healing through collagen re-organisation and may minimise stiffness. It is thus preferable in non-surgically treated MCL tears.
- Isolated injury to the deepMCL femoral origin has been described, as a cause of ongoing pain in high level football players. Chronic pain due to the femoral origin not healing may need exploration and repair.

References

1. Lundblad M, Hägglund M, Thomeé C, Hamrin Senorski E, Ekstrand J, Karlsson J, Waldén M. Medial collateral ligament injuries of the knee in male professional football players: a prospective three-season study of 130 cases from the UEFA elite Club injury study. Knee Surg Sports Traumatol Arthrosc. 2019;27(11):3692–8.
2. Wijdicks CA, Griffith CJ, Johansen S, Engebretsen L, LaPrade RF. Injuries to the medial collateral ligament and associated medial structures of the knee. J Bone Joint Surg Am. 2010;92(5):1266–80.
3. Corten K, Hoser C, Fink C, Bellemans J. Case reports: a Stener-like lesion of the medial collateral ligament of the knee. Clin Orthop Relat Res. 2010;468(1):289–93.
4. Nandi S, Parker R. Deep medial collateral ligament tear during knee arthroscopy. J Knee Surg. 2012;25(1):79–81.
5. Jung KH, Youm YS, Cho SD, Jin WY, Kwon SH. Iatrogenic medial collateral ligament injury by Valgus stress during arthroscopic surgery of the knee. Arthroscopy. 2019;35(5):1520–4.
6. Robinson JR, Bull AM, Thomas RR, Amis AA. The role of the medial collateral ligament and posteromedial capsule in controlling knee laxity. Am J Sports Med. 2006;34(11):1815–23.
7. Alaia EF, Rosenberg ZS, Alaia MJ. Stener-like lesions of the superficial medial collateral ligament of the knee: MRI features. AJR Am J Roentgenol. 2019;213(6):W272–6. https://doi.org/10.2214/AJR.19.21535.
8. Laprade RF, Bernhardson AS, Griffith CJ, Macalena JA, Wijdicks CA. Correlation of valgus stress radiographs with medial knee ligament injuries: an in vitro biomechanical study. Am J Sports Med. 2010;38(2):330–8.

9. Walsh S, Frank C, Shrive N, Hart D. Knee immobilization inhibits biomechanical maturation of the rabbit medial collateral ligament. Clin Orthop Relat Res. 1993;297:253–61.
10. Georgiev GP, Kotov G, Iliev A, Kinov P, Angelova J, Landzhov B. Comparison between operative and non-operative treatment of the medial collateral ligament: histological and Ultrastructural findings during early healing in the Epiligament tissue in a rat knee model. Cells Tissues Organs. 2018;206(3):165–82.
11. Inoue M, Woo SL, Gomez MA, Amiel D, Ohland KJ, Kitabayashi LR. Effects of surgical treatment and immobilization on the healing of the medial collateral ligament: a long-term multidisciplinary study. Connect Tissue Res. 1990;25(1):13–26.
12. Goldstein WM, Barmada R. Early mobilization of rabbit medial collateral ligament repairs: biomechanic and histologic study. Arch Phys Med Rehabil. 1984;65(5):239–42.
13. Padgett LR, Dahners LE. Rigid immobilization alters matrix organization in the injured rat medial collateral ligament. J Orthop Res. 1992;10(6):895–900.
14. Petermann J, von Garrel T, Gotzen L. Non-operative treatment of acute medial collateral ligament lesions of the knee joint. Knee Surg Sports Traumatol Arthrosc. 1993;1(2):93–6.
15. Indelicato PA, Hermansdorfer J, Huegel M. Nonoperative management of complete tears of the medial collateral ligament of the knee in intercollegiate football players. Clin Orthop Relat Res. 1990;256:174–7.
16. Mok DW, Good C. Non-operative management of acute grade III medial collateral ligament injury of the knee: a prospective study. Injury. 1989;20(5):277–80.
17. Ballmer PM, Jakob RP. The non operative treatment of isolated complete tears of the medial collateral ligament of the knee. A prospective study. Arch Orthop Trauma Surg. 1988;107(5):273–6.
18. Holden DL, Eggert AW, Butler JE. The nonoperative treatment of grade I and II medial collateral ligament injuries to the knee. Am J Sports Med. 1983;11(5):340–4.
19. Reider B, Sathy MR, Talkington J, Blyznak N, Kollias S. Treatment of isolated medial collateral ligament injuries in athletes with early functional rehabilitation. A five-year follow-up study. Am J Sports Med. 1994;22(4):470–7.
20. Woo SL, Inoue M, McGurk-Burleson E, Gomez MA. Treatment of the medial collateral ligament injury. II: Structure and function of canine knees in response to differing treatment regimens. Am J Sports Med. 1987;15(1):22–9.
21. DeLong JM, Waterman BR. Surgical Repair of Medial Collateral Ligament and Posteromedial Corner Injuries of the Knee: A Systematic Review. Arthroscopy. 2015;31(11):2249–55.e5. https://doi.org/10.1016/j.arthro.2015.05.010.
22. Malinowski K, Hermanowicz K, Góralczyk A, LaPrade RF. Medial collateral ligament reconstruction with anteromedial reinforcement for medial and anteromedial rotatory instability of the knee. Arthrosc Tech. 2019;8(8):e807–14. https://doi.org/10.1016/j.eats.2019.03.019.
23. Kim MS, Koh IJ, In Y. Superficial and deep medial collateral ligament reconstruction for chronic medial instability of the knee. Arthrosc Tech. 2019;8(6):e549–54. https://doi.org/10.1016/j.eats.2019.01.016.
24. Lind M, Jacobsen K, Nielsen T. Medial collateral ligament (MCL) reconstruction results in improved medial stability: results from the Danish knee ligament reconstruction registry (DKRR). Knee Surg Sports Traumatol Arthrosc. 2020;28(3):881–7.
25. Trofa DP, Sonnenfeld JJ, Song DJ, Lynch TS. Distal Knee Medial Collateral Ligament Repair With Suturementation. Arthrosc Tech. 2018;7(9):e921–6.
26. Varelas AN, Erickson BJ, Cvetanovich GL, Bach BR Jr. Medial Collateral Ligament Reconstruction in Patients With Medial Knee Instability: A Systematic Review. Orthop J Sports Med. 2017;5(5):2325967117703920.
27. DeLong JM, Waterman BR. Surgical Techniques for the Reconstruction of Medial Collateral Ligament and Posteromedial Corner Injuries of the Knee: A Systematic Review. Arthroscopy. 2015;31(11):2258–72.e1. https://doi.org/10.1016/j.arthro.2015.05.011.
28. Lubowitz JH, MacKay G, Gilmer B. Knee medial collateral ligament and posteromedial corner anatomic repair with internal bracing. Arthrosc Tech. 2014;3(4):e505–8.

29. Lind M, Jakobsen BW, Lund B, Hansen MS, Abdallah O, Christiansen SE. Anatomical reconstruction of the medial collateral ligament and posteromedial corner of the knee in patients with chronic medial collateral ligament instability. Am J Sports Med. 2009;37(6):1116–22.
30. Encinas-Ullán CA, Rodríguez-Merchán EC. Isolated medial collateral ligament tears: An update on management. EFORT Open Rev. 2018;3(7):398–407.
31. Phisitkul P, Wolf BR, Amendola A. Role of high tibial and distal femoral osteotomies in the treatment of lateral-posterolateral and medial instabilities of the knee. Sports Med Arthrosc Rev. 2006;14(2):96–104.

Chapter 59
Posterolateral Corner Ligament Knee Instability

This is a condition whereby there is symptomatic instability of the tibiofemoral articulation due to dysfunction of the ligaments of the posterolateral corner (PLC) of the knee.

59.1 Causes of Posterolateral Corner Ligament Instability [1–4]

Disruption of the PLC may be:

- Congenital—as part of multiligament deficiency
- Acquired
  - Acute substantial trauma

Disruption of the PLC may be:

- Isolated, single ligament
- Associated with other ligamentous dysfunction/injuries
- Associated with bony abnormalities—developmental, traumatic, degenerative

Although PLC instability is usually part of multiligament instability, isolated post-traumatic PLC instability is considered in this chapter. It has been shown [1] that in acute knee injuries presenting with a haemarthrosis:

- Isolated PLC injuries comprise about 2% of cases of ligament tears.
- 87% of PLC injuries have multiple ligament injuries. The most common ligament injured with the PLC is the posterior cruciate ligament (PCL) followed by the anterior cruciate ligament (ACL).

Traumatic PLC disruption may be described:

C. Panayiotou Charalambous, *The Knee Made Easy*,
https://doi.org/10.1007/978-3-030-54506-2_59

According to the Ligaments Disrupted

- Lateral collateral ligament (LCL)
- Popliteus tendon
- Popliteofibular ligament
- Biceps femoris tendon
- Combinations of the above

According to the Extent of Disruption of Each Ligament

- Partial (proportion of ligament fibres disrupted)
- Complete (all ligament fibres disrupted)

According to the Type of Disruption

- Avulsion of the PLC structures from their origin:
  - Soft tissue avulsion
  - Bony avulsion
- Avulsion of the PLC structures from their fibular or tibial insertion:
  - Soft tissue avulsion
  - Bony avulsion (fibular head, tibia-Gerdy's tubercle)
- Intra-substance tear

According to the mechanism of injury leading to disruption

- Contact—with another player or a surface/object
- Non-contact

59.2 Classification of Posterolateral Corner Ligament Instability

The Hughston [5] classification is based on the assessment of varus instability or rotational instability under varus stress force with the knee in full extension. Grade III injuries are associated with a PCL tear.

Hughston classification of posterolateral instability based on the assessment of varus or rotational laxity upon varus loading with the knee in full extension

Grade	Varus or rotational instability	Associated PCL injury
I	0–5 mm or 0°–5°	Intact
II	5–10 mm or 6°–10°	Intact
III	>10 mm or > 10° (soft endpoint)	PCL tear

59.3 Effects of Posterolateral Ligament Disruption

A ligament is taut only when it is firmly attached at its two ends. This is analogous to hanging from a rope. The rope may lose part of its substance (partial tear) but still provide support, but if completely gone then one may fall down. Similarly, if the PLC is disrupted it may compromise its ability to maintain the position of the tibia relative to the femur. With PLC dysfunction the following exaggerated displacements of the tibia in relation to the femur (subluxations of the tibiofemoral articulation) may occur:

- Varus displacement of the tibia relative to the femur
- External rotation of the tibia relative to the femur

59.4 Clinical History of Trauma in Posterolateral Corner Ligament Instability

The following characteristics of the injury that led to the onset of symptoms may suggest a PLC disruption:

- A history of a substantial traumatic event (an event a patient can easily recall):
- Patient felt/heard pop in the knee
- Mechanism of injury:
  - Tibial external rotation with the knee in flexion
  - Hyperextension-(isolated knee hyperextension has been shown to cause a PLC injury and partial ACL injury but not PCL injury)
  - Blow to the anteromedial thigh
  - Varus injury
  - Pivoting activities
- Patient unable/difficult to get up and stand/ walk
- Required medical attention

59.5 Clinical Symptoms of Posterolateral Corner Ligament Instability

- Acute presentation
  - Painful, swollen knee, tenderness posterolateral part of the knee
- Chronic presentation

- Clicking, clunking due to abnormal translation of the knee
- Feeling of abnormal displacement—"giving way", feeling "wobbly"
- Instability upon:
  - Walking downstairs
  - Pivoting
  - Walking on uneven ground
- Dead leg syndrome, heavy leg, paraesthesia
- Nerve dysfunction symptoms if associated common peroneal nerve dysfunction

Following the acute injury, the acute pain, may improve, knee motion restored and the patient is left with feeling of instability or other symptoms.

59.6 Clinical Signs of Posterolateral Corner Ligament Instability [6]

- Increased varus laxity
- Dial test
- Reverse pivot shift test
- Varus thrust
- Neurological dysfunction—peroneal nerve

59.7 Investigations for Posterolateral Corner Ligament Instability

Investigations for PLC instability aim to confirm the PLC disruption, determine the type of PLC disruption, identify any associated structural lesions (ligamentous, bony, meniscal, chondral). These include:

- Radiological
  - Plain radiographs—may demonstrate avulsion fracture, assess malalignment
  - MRI Scan
    - Discontinuity of the PLC structures
    - MRI has a low sensitivity especially in chronic cases, hence its results must be interpreted with caution. It has been reported that MRI may only diagnose 26% of cases when performed at more than 12 weeks post injury [7].
  - CT scan
    - Assess comminution of bony avulsion injuries

    - Assess alignment if planning surgery for chronic injuries

- Examination under general anaesthesia—joint translation and laxity are assessed with the patient under general anaesthesia to abolish pain and allow muscle relaxation. It has been shown [8] that with the knee in 20° flexion:
  - Increased varus opening of > = 2.7 mm was suggestive of a LCL complete tear
  - > = 4 mm was suggestive of a grade III PLC injury
- Arthroscopic evaluation—distraction of lateral compartment (drive through sign), look for associated injuries

59.8 Management of PLC Instability

Initial management aims at:

- Reducing the acute inflammation of the knee using the Rest, Ice, Compression, Elevation (RICE) principles
- Restore motion (tibiofemoral/patellofemoral)
- Quadriceps/hamstring activation
- Proprioception training
- Activity specific mobilisation
- External devices—bracing

Further management aims at improving ongoing symptoms of instability and hence improve a patient's function or reducing the risk of further instability. This depends on:

- Underlying disruption—partial/complete

59.8.1 Non-surgical [9–11]

Non-surgical management is preferable in partial injuries with minimal associated laxity, or in functionally low-demand patients.

- Leave alone
- Activity modification, avoiding unstable positions
- Physiotherapy to address:
- Core imbalance—core strengthening
- Hip muscle weakness —strengthening of hip muscles
- Proprioception—proprioceptive training
- Hamstring (biceps femoris) strengthening
- External devices—bracing

It should be noted that non-surgical management does not specifically address the PLC disruption but aims to improve stability by enhancing the function of dynamic stabilisers (through strengthening, better control and coordination).

Non-surgical management has been shown to confer good outcomes in grade II but not grade III injuries.

59.8.2 *Surgical* [12–22]

Surgical intervention is preferable in:

1. Acute injuries—complete/displaced injuries
2. Chronic injuries—patients who continue with substantial symptoms of instability

Surgical options include:

- Reattachment of disrupted structures ± augmentation with graft
  - Avulsion fracture fixation
  - Soft tissue avulsion
- Reconstruction—using a graft that is secured in bone tunnels in the femur and fibula. Several grafts and techniques may be used:
  - Autograft—hamstring tendons
  - Allograft
  - Synthetic graft
  - Anatomical versus non-anatomical reconstruction

Reconstruction techniques may be described as anatomical or non-anatomical.

- *Non-anatomical*—these attempt to tighten the non-injured PLC structures and include:
  - Extracapsular Iliotibial band sling, biceps femoris tenodesis
- *Anatomical*—these aim to reconstruct the injured structures and include:
  - Larsen reconstruction [17]—aims to reconstruct the LCL and popliteus using a graft sling passing through the fibula.

Early surgical intervention (3 weeks from injury) is preferable as there is a higher probability of being able to reattach the disrupted structures rather than having to use a graft. Hence, it is important not to miss a PLC injury in the acutely injured knee.

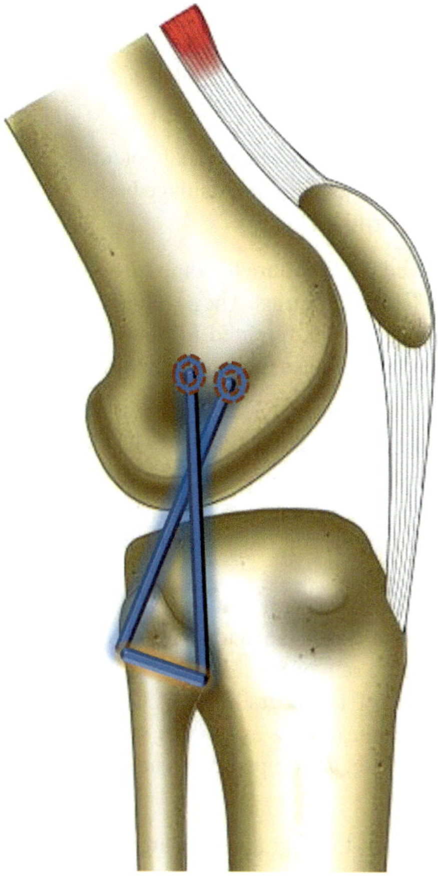

PLC reconstruction

59.9 Considerations in the Management of Post-Traumatic Posterolateral Corner Deficiency

In considering the definitive management of PLC disruption several considerations must be taken into account some of which are described below.

59.9.1 *Natural History* [17–20]

It is recognised that:

- PLC disruption is associated with poor functional outcomes if left untreated
- However, it is also recognised that PLC surgery outcomes are limited.
- Persistent instability may:
  - Limit ability of an individual to achieve high level functional potential
  - Predispose to further meniscal tears or further chondral damage both of which are related to the development of knee arthritis
- Geeslin AG et al.[18] systematically reviewed the literature to compare clinical outcomes of the treatment for acute grade III PLC injuries. They included 8 studies with 134 patients. The mean time to surgery was reported in 5 studies (range, 15–24 days). Surgery was performed within 3 weeks in the other 3 studies. They reported that:
  - An overall success rate of 81% and failure rate of 19% based on objective evaluation with varus stress examinations or radiographs
  - In 2 studies, the LCL and popliteus tendon were repaired and staged cruciate reconstruction was subsequently performed for most cases—these had 17 failures out of 45 patients (38%).
  - In the remaining studies, patients were treated with acutely local tissue transfer, hybrid repair or reconstruction for mid-substance tears, or reconstruction of all torn structures—these had a failure rate of 9%.
  - The authors concluded that the repair of acute grade III PLC injuries and staged treatment of combined cruciate injuries was associated with a substantially higher postoperative PLC failure rate, as compared to a more aggressive acute approach.
- Moulton SG et al.[20] systematically reviewed the literature of surgical treatment strategies for chronic grade III PLC injuries. Fifteen studies with a total of 456 patients were included in this study. More than half of the patients had a combined posterior cruciate ligament-PLC injury. The mean age of the patients in each study ranged from 25 to 40 years and the mean time to surgery ranged from 5.5 to 53 months. They reported that:
  - Based on objective stability, there was an overall success rate of 90% and a 10% failure rate of PLC reconstruction according to the individual investigators' examination or stress radiographic assessment of objective outcomes.

59.9.2 *Timing of Encountering the Patient*

The patient may present at different stages following PLC disruption to the clinician:

- Acute—just after the injury

- Chronic—after the patient returned to normal activities but has experienced further instability

Hence, the approach on how to deal with the underlying PLC disruption may differ according to the above. With chronicity, reconstruction rather repair of most structures is more appropriate. Furthermore, in chronic cases associated malalignment may need to be addressed along with soft tissue surgery.

59.9.3 PLC Disruption Associated with Malalignment [21, 22]

Malalignment may put excessive forces on a PLC reconstruction, leading to dysfunction of the reconstruction. Hence, in cases of chronic PLC instability, combination of PLC reconstruction with a proximal tibial osteotomy may be considered:

Varus malalignment—opening wedge high tibial osteotomy

Learning Pearls

- The dial test may be easily performed in the acute scenario
- A thorough clinical history is essential in order to determine the exact symptoms of the patient with a disrupted PLC
- There is no strong clinical evidence supporting one reconstruction technique over another

References

1. LaPrade RF, Wentorf FA, Fritts H, Gundry C, Hightower CD. A prospective magnetic resonance imaging study of the incidence of posterolateral and multiple ligament injuries in acute knee injuries presenting with a hemarthrosis. Arthroscopy. 2007;23(12):1341–7.
2. Yoo JH, Lee JH, Chang CB. Pure Varus injury to the knee joint. Clin Orthop Surg. 2015;7(2):269–74.
3. Davanzo D, Fornaciari P, Barbier G, Maniglio M, Petek D. Review and long-term outcomes of cruciate ligament reconstruction versus conservative treatment in siblings with congenital anterior cruciate ligament aplasia. Case Rep Orthop. 2017:1636578–8. https://doi.org/10.1155/2017/1636578.
4. Kupczik F, Schiavon MEG, Vieira LA, Tenius DP, Fávaro RC. Knee Dislocation: Descriptive Study of Injuries. Rev Bras Ortop. 2013;48(2):145–51.
5. Hughston JC, Andrews JR, Cross MJ, Moschi A. Classification of knee ligament instabilities. Part II. The lateral compartment. J Bone Joint Surg Am. 1976;58(2):173–9.
6. Clinical examination of the knee.
7. Pacheco RJ, Ayre CA, Bollen SR. Posterolateral corner injuries of the knee: a serious injury commonly missed. J Bone Joint Surg Br. 2011;93(2):194–7.
8. LaPrade RF, Heikes C, Bakker AJ, Jakobsen RB. The reproducibility and repeatability of varus stress radiographs in the assessment of isolated fibular collateral ligament and grade-III posterolateral knee injuries: an in vitro biomechanical study. J Bone Joint Surg Am. 2008;90:2069–76.

9. Davenport D, Arora A, Edwards MR. Non-operative management of an isolated lateral collateral ligament injury in an adolescent patient and review of the literature. BMJ Case Rep. 2018;2018. pii: bcr-2017-223478 https://doi.org/10.1136/bcr-2017-223478.
10. Haddad MA, Budich JM, Eckenrode BJ. Conservative management of an isolated grade III lateral collateral ligament injury in an adolescent multi-sport athlete: a case. Int J Sports Phys Ther. 2016;11(4):596–606.
11. Kannus P. Nonoperative treatment of grade II and III sprains of the lateral ligament compartment of the knee. Am J Sports Med. 1989;17(1):83–8.
12. Hopper GP, Heusdens CHW, Dossche L, Mackay GM. Posterolateral Corner Repair With Suture Tapementation. Arthrosc Tech. 2018;7(12):e1299–303.
13. Gilmer BB. Double-Row Suture Anchor Repair of Posterolateral Corner Avulsion Fractures. Arthrosc Tech. 2017;6(4):e997–e1001. https://doi.org/10.1016/j.eats.2017.03.011.
14. Kandeel AA. Biceps femoris tenodesis revisited a prospective cohort study of concurrent anterior cruciate and postero-lateral corner reconstruction. Injury. 2020;51(2):483–9.
15. Sanders TL, Johnson NR, Pareek A, Krych AJ, XRG, Stuart MJ, Levy BA. Satisfactory knee function after single-stage posterolateral corner reconstruction in the multi-ligament injured/dislocated knee using the anatomic single-graft technique. Knee Surg Sports Traumatol Arthrosc. 2018;26(4):1258–65.
16. Yoon KH, Lee SH, Park SY, Park SE, Tak DH. Comparison of anatomic Posterolateral knee reconstruction using 2 different Popliteofibular ligament techniques. Am J Sports Med. 2016;44(4):916–21.
17. Larsen MW, Moinfar AR, Moorman CT 3rd. Posterolateral corner reconstruction: fibular-based technique. J Knee Surg. 2005;18(2):163–6.
18. Geeslin AG, Moulton SG, LaPrade RF. A systematic review of the outcomes of Posterolateral corner knee injuries, part 1: surgical treatment of acute injuries. Am J Sports Med. 2016;44(5):1336–42.
19. Laprade RF, Griffith CJ, Coobs BR, Geeslin AG, Johansen S, Engebretsen L. Improving outcomes for posterolateral knee injuries. J Orthop Res. 2014;32(4):485–91.
20. Moulton SG, Geeslin AG, LaPrade RF. A systematic review of the outcomes of Posterolateral corner knee injuries, part 2: surgical treatment of chronic injuries. Am J Sports Med. 2016;44(6):1616–23.
21. Helito CP, Sobrado MF, Giglio PN, Bonadio MB, Demange MK, Pécora JR, Camanho GL, Angelini FJ. Posterolateral reconstruction combined with one-stage tibial valgus osteotomy: technical considerations and functional results. Knee. 2019;26(2):500–7.
22. Tischer T, Paul J, Pape D, Hirschmann MT, Imhoff AB, Hinterwimmer S, Feucht MJ. The impact of osseous malalignment and realignment procedures in knee ligament surgery: a systematic review of the clinical evidence. Orthop J Sports Med. 2017;5(3):2325967117697287. https://doi.org/10.1177/2325967117697287.

Chapter 60
Multiligament Knee Instability

This is a condition whereby there is symptomatic instability of the tibiofemoral articulation due to disruption of two or more ligaments of the knee. This may involve the anterior cruciate ligament (ACL), posterior cruciate ligament (PCL), medial collateral ligament (MCL) or the ligaments of the posterolateral corner (PLC).

60.1 Causes of Multiligament Knee Instability [1–6]

Disruption of multiple knee ligaments may be:

- Congenital—as part of multiligamentous deficiency
- Acquired
  - Acute substantial trauma (most common)

  Disruption of multiple knee ligaments may be:

- Associated with bony abnormalities—developmental, traumatic, degenerative

Although multiple ligament disruption may be seen in some congenital/developmental conditions, post-traumatic multiligament disruption is considered in this chapter.

Traumatic multiligament disruption may be described:

According to the Ligaments Disrupted
The Anatomic classification [7] describes multiligament disruption as:

C. Panayiotou Charalambous, *The Knee Made Easy*,
https://doi.org/10.1007/978-3-030-54506-2_60

KD I	Injury to single cruciate + collaterals
KD II	Injury to ACL and PCL with intact collaterals
KD III M	Injury to ACL, PCL, MCL
KD III L	Injury to ACL, PCL, PLC
KD IV	Injury to ACL, PCL, MCL, PLC
KD V	Dislocation + fracture

"C" and "N" are utilized for associated injuries:
"C" indicates an arterial injury.
"N" indicates a neural injury.

Moatshe G et al. [8] reported the ligament injury patterns in 303 patients with knee dislocations treated at a single level 1 trauma centre. The mean age at injury was 38 ± 15 years, 65% male and 35% female. There was an equal distribution of high-energy and low-energy injuries. The combination of soft ligament injuries encountered were:

- ACL + PCL + medial ligaments—52%
- ACL + PCL + PLC—28%
- All ligaments—12%
- ACL + PCL, intact collateral ligaments –5%

Associated injuries included:

- Meniscal injuries in 37%
- Cartilage injuries in 28%
- Patients with acute injuries had significantly lower odds of a cartilage injury than those with chronic injuries (odds ratio [OR] 0.28; 95% CI 0.15–0.50)
- Peroneal nerve injuries were recorded in 19% of patients (11% partial, 8% complete deficit)
- Vascular injuries in 5%
- The odds of having a common peroneal nerve injury were 42 times greater in those with PLC injury than those without
- The odds for popliteal artery injury were 9 times greater in those with KD III-L injuries than other ligament injury types

According to Extent of Disruption of Each Ligament

- Partial (proportion of ligament fibres disrupted)
- Complete (all ligament fibres disrupted)

According to the Type of Disruption

- Avulsion of the involved ligaments from their origin
  - Soft tissue avulsion
  - Bony avulsion

- Avulsion of the involved ligaments from their tibial insertion
  - Soft tissue avulsion
  - Bony avulsion
- Intra-substance tear

According to the Mechanism of Injury Leading to Disruption

- Contact—with another player or a surface/object
- Non-contact

Multiligament disruption is usually the result a very high energy injury to the knee. It may be associated with a knee subluxation or dislocation:

- Subluxation—displaced but part of the articular surfaces of the femur and tibia remaining in contact
- Dislocation—with loss of all articular contact

Knee dislocations are most often due to road traffic accidents, with sports injuries and falls accounting for a smaller proportion. Some dislocations may spontaneously reduce.

60.2 Effects of Multiligament Disruption

A ligament is taut only when it is firmly attached at its two ends. This is analogous to hanging from a rope. The rope may lose part of its substance (partial tear) but still provide support, but if completely gone then one may fall down. In multiligament disruption exaggerated displacements of the tibia in relation to the femur may occur in multiple directions (multiligament knee instability).

60.3 Timing of Encountering the Patient

The patient may present at different stages following multiligament disruption to the clinician:

- Acute—just after the injury
- Chronic—after the patient returned to normal activities but has experienced further instability. This may be due to a missed injury or an initial attempt to manage the condition non-surgically

Hence, the approach on how to deal with the underlying multiligament disruption disruption may differ according to the above.

60.4 Clinical History of a Traumatic Event in Multiligament Knee Instability

A detailed history of the traumatic event is essential even if the patient is first encountered in the chronic stage, as it will help determine the extent of injury that the knee sustained.

The following characteristics of the injury that led to the onset of symptoms may suggest multiple ligament disruption:

- A history of a substantial traumatic event (an event a patient can easily recall):
- Patient felt/heard snap/pop in the knee
- Mechanism of injury—usually high energy, contact/non-contact
- Patient not able to stand up/walk after injury
- Required medical attention
  - Knee may have dislocated and required medical reduction
  - Knee may have felt dislocating and spontaneously relocating

60.5 Clinical Symptoms of Multiligament Knee Instability

- Acute presentation
  - Painful, swollen, tender knee, limited range of motion, reduced ability to weightbear
- Chronic presentation
  - Knee pain
  - Clicking, clunking due to abnormal translation of the knee
  - Feeling of abnormal displacement—“giving way”, feeling “wobbly”
  - Abnormal displacement in multiple directions
  - Varus/valgus thrust
  - Dead leg syndrome, heavy leg, paraesthesia
  - Symptoms of neurological or vascular dysfunction

Following the acute injury, the acute pain may improve, knee motion restored and the patient is left with feeling of instability or other symptoms.

60.6 Clinical Signs of Multiligament Knee Instability

- Acute presentation
  - Swollen, tender knee, limitation of motion, limitation of weightbearing
  - Vascular/neurological dysfunction [9–12]

  - Increased knee laxity in multiple directions/ need to determine if there is firm end point

- Chronic presentation

  - Knee effusion/synovitis
  - Knee tenderness
  - Stiffness
  - Peri-articular muscle wasting
  - Neurological dysfunction
  - Increased knee laxity in multiple directions

    Determine if there is a firm end point

  - Valgus/varus thrust
  - Signs of neurological dysfunction

60.7 Investigations for Multiligament Knee Instability

Investigations for multiligament knee instability aim to:

1. Confirm the presence and pattern of multiligament disruption
2. For each disrupted ligament determine the site and extent of disruption
3. Identify any associated structural lesions (ligamentous, bony, meniscal, chondral)
4. Assess associated vascular/neurological dysfunction
5. Assess lower limb alignment if chronic reconstruction is indicated

   These include:

- Radiological

  - Plain radiographs—may demonstrate avulsion fracture, assess alignment
  - MRI Scan [13]
  - Vascular Doppler studies/CT angiogram—in the acute scenario to determine an associated vascular injury
  - CT scan—assess alignment if planning surgery for chronic injuries
  - Nerve conduction studies/electromyography—if associated nerve injury

- Examination under general anaesthesia—joint translation and laxity is assessed with the patient under general anaesthesia to abolish pain and allow muscle relaxation
- Arthroscopic evaluation—direct visualisation—distraction of lateral/medial compartment, look for associated injuries

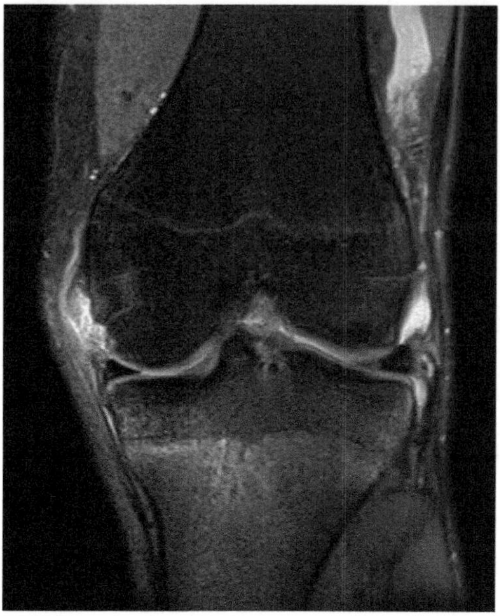

Medial collateral ligament and anterior cruciate ligament disruption

60.8 Management of Multiligament Knee Instability

Management of multiligament knee instability is influenced by several factors including the patient's extent of injury, symptoms, and timing of presentation [14–20].

60.8.1 Acute Presentation

Initial management aims at:

- Reducing the acute inflammation of the knee using the Rest, Ice, Compression, Elevation (RICE) principles
- If knee is dislocated—reduce
- If knee is in situ or post-reduction—maintain reduction by:
  - Temporary stabilisation
    - Bracing/casting
    - External-fixator (if bracing/casting not sufficient to provide stability)
  - Definitive stabilisation
    - Ligament surgery

- Restore motion (tibiofemoral/patellofemoral)
- Quadriceps/hamstring activation
- Proprioception training

60.8.2 Chronic Presentation

In chronic presentation the knee is usually in situ, and the patient presents with recurrent episodes of instability or instability related limitation of function.

In dealing with multiple ligament disruptions the options are:

1. Manage each disruption surgically
2. Manage all disruptions non-surgically (low demand/medically unfit individuals)
3. Manage some ligaments non-surgically and some surgically

60.8.3 Non-surgical

Non-surgical management is preferable in partial injuries, with minimal associated laxity, or in low functionally demand patients.

- Leave alone
- Activity modification, avoiding unstable positions
- External devices—chronic knee bracing
- Physiotherapy to address:
  - Core imbalance—core strengthening
  - Hip muscle weakness —strengthening of hip muscles
  - Proprioception—proprioceptive training
  - Quadriceps and Hamstring strengthening- dynamic stabilisers

It should be noted that non-surgical management does not specifically address the multiligament disruption but aims to improve stability by enhancing the function of dynamic stabilisers (through strengthening, better control and coordination).

60.8.4 Surgical

Surgical intervention is preferable in:

1. Acute injuries—preferable in most cases
2. Chronic injuries—patients who continue with substantial symptoms of residual instability

Surgical options for each disrupted ligament include:

- Reattachment of disrupted structures +/– augmentation with graft
  - Avulsion fracture fixation
  - Soft tissue avulsion
- Reconstruction—using a graft
  - Autograft—hamstring tendons (the hamstring tendons may be left attached to their tibial insertion, divided proximally and inserted onto the distal femur)
  - Allograft
  - Synthetic graft
- Re-alignment procedures for chronic injuries

In acute injuries—reattachment +/–augmentation+/–reconstruction may be utilised:

- Intra-substance tears—require reconstruction
- Avulsion tears—may be reattached

In chronic injuries—reconstruction is utilised.

60.9 Considerations in the Management of Multiligament Knee Instability

In considering the definitive management of multiligament knee instability several considerations must be taken into account some of which are described below.

60.9.1 Surgical Management for All vs. Some of the Ligaments

It is recognised that:

- It is possible to treat only some of the ligaments surgically and allow others to heal with non-surgical intervention, hence a selective surgery approach may be used
- An all surgical approach may be utilised

Disruption of the PLC increases substantially the forces on both ACL (varus, internal rotation) and PCL (varus) reconstruction grafts, predisposing to their failure. Hence, addressing PLC injuries is essential.

60.9.2 Multiligament Knee Instability Associated with Malalignment

Malalignment may put excessive forces on a multiligament reconstruction graft, leading to dysfunction of the reconstruction. Hence, in cases of chronic multiligament instability, combination of ligament reconstruction with a distal femoral osteotomy or tibial osteotomy (single stage or two-stage procedure) may be considered.

60.10 Prognosis of Multiligament Knee Instability

Hatch GFR et al. [21] evaluated the quality of life in 31 patients (33 knees) at a minimum of 12 months (12–111 months) post multiligament knee reconstruction surgery. They reported that patients with a history of knee ligament surgery had a significantly worse quality of life relative to those with no history of knee ligament surgery.

Everhart JS et al. [22] systematically reviewed studies which looked at rates of return to work or sport after multiligament knee injury. They analysed 524 patients (in 21 studies) and reported:

- Return to high-level sport in 22%–33%
- Return to any level of sport —54%
  - In studies with all surgical patients –59% (114/193 patients)
  - In studies with mixed surgical and non-surgical treatment —46% (64/139 patients)
- Rate of return to work with little or no modifications—62% (146/200)
- Return to any work—88% (190/215)
- They concluded that:
  - Return to sport after multi-ligament knee injury occurs in about 60% of surgically treated patients, but return to high-level sport is lower
  - Return to work is often possible but may require workplace or job duty modifications.
  - Obesity, non-surgical treatment, higher injury severity and vascular injury are associated with poorer functional outcomes

Hanley J et al. [23] looked at the factors associated with knee stiffness following surgical management of multiligament knee Injuries. They reported that knee dislocation and surgical intervention on 3 or more ligaments was significantly associated with knee stiffness.

Learning Pearls

- It is vital to recognise a PLC injury in acute multiligament knee instability presentations. The dial test may be easily performed in the acute scenario.

References

1. Sobrado MF. State of the art in multiligament knee injuries: from diagnosis to treatment. Ann Transl Med. 2019;7(Suppl 3):S97. https://doi.org/10.21037/atm.2019.04.55.
2. Levy BA, Freychet B. Knee multiligament injury. Clin Sports Med. 2019;38(2):xv–xvi. https://doi.org/10.1016/j.csm.2019.01.001.
3. Neri T, Myat D, Beach A, Parker DA. Multiligament knee injury: injury patterns, outcomes, and gait analysis. Clin Sports Med. 2019;38(2):235–46.
4. Burrus MT, Werner BC, Griffin JW, Gwathmey FW, Miller MD. Diagnostic and Management Strategies for Multiligament Knee Injuries: A Critical Analysis Review. JBJS Rev. 2016;4(2) https://doi.org/10.2106/JBJS.RVW.O.00020.
5. Stannard JP, Bauer KL. Current concepts in knee dislocations: PCL, ACL, and medial sided injuries. J Knee Surg. 2012;25(4):287–94.
6. Fanelli GC, Edson CJ, Reinheimer KN. Evaluation and treatment of the multiligament-injured knee. Instr Course Lect. 2009;58:389–95.
7. Schenck RC Jr, Richter DL, Wascher DC. Knee Dislocations: Lessons Learned From 20-Year Follow-up. Orthop J Sports Med. 2014;2(5):2325967114534387. https://doi.org/10.1177/2325967114534387.
8. Moatshe G, Dornan GJ, Løken S, Ludvigsen TC, LaPrade RF, Engebretsen L. Demographics and Injuries Associated With Knee Dislocation: A Prospective Review of 303 Patients. Orthop J Sports Med. 2017;5(5):2325967117706521. https://doi.org/10.1177/2325967117706521.
9. Matthewson G, Kwapisz A, Sasyniuk T, MacDonald P. Vascular injury in the multiligament injured knee. Clin Sports Med. 2019;38(2):199–213.
10. Worley JR, Brimmo O, Nuelle CW, Cook JL, Stannard JP. Incidence of concurrent peroneal nerve injury in multiligament knee injuries and outcomes after knee reconstruction. J Knee Surg. 2019;32(6):560–4.
11. O'Malley MP, Pareek A, Reardon P, Krych A, Stuart MJ, Levy BA. Treatment of peroneal nerve injuries in the multiligament injured/dislocated knee. J Knee Surg. 2016;29(4):287–92.
12. Mook WR, Ligh CA, Moorman CT 3rd, Leversedge FJ. Nerve injury complicating multi-ligament knee injury: current concepts and treatment algorithm. J Am Acad Orthop Surg. 2013;21(6):343–54.
13. Porrino J, Wang A, Kani K, Kweon CY, Gee A. Preoperative MRI for the Multiligament Knee Injury: What the Surgeon Needs to Know. Curr Probl Diagn Radiol. 2019; https://doi.org/10.1067/j.cpradiol.2019.02.004.
14. Gella S, Whelan DB, Stannard JP, MacDonald PB. Acute management and surgical timing of the multiligament-injured knee. Instr Course Lect. 2015;64:521–30.
15. Cook S, Ridley TJ, McCarthy MA, Gao Y, Wolf BR, Amendola A, Bollier MJ. Surgical treatment of multiligament knee injuries. Knee Surg Sports Traumatol Arthrosc. 2015;23(10):2983–91.
16. Levy BA, Stuart MJ. Treatment of PCL, ACL, and lateral-side knee injuries: acute and chronic. J Knee Surg. 2012;25(4):295–305.
17. Levy BA, Fanelli GC, Whelan DB, Stannard JP, MacDonald PA, Boyd JL, XRG, Stuart MJ, Knee Dislocation Study Group. Controversies in the treatment of knee dislocations and multi-ligament reconstruction. J Am Acad Orthop Surg. 2009;17(4):197–206.
18. Bagherifard A, Jabalameli M, Ghaffari S, Rezazadeh J, Abedi M, Mirkazemi M, Aghamohamadi J, Hesabi A, Mohammadpour M. Short to mid-term outcomes of single-stage reconstruction of multiligament knee injury. Arch Bone Jt Surg. 2019;7(4):346–53.

19. Hantes M, Fyllos A, Papageorgiou F, Alexiou K, Antoniou I. Long-term clinical and radiological outcomes after multiligament knee injury using a delayed ligament reconstruction approach: a single-center experience. Knee. 2019;26(6):1271–7.
20. Buyukdogan K, Laidlaw MS, Miller MD. Surgical Management of the Multiple-Ligament Knee Injury. Arthrosc Tech. 2018;7(2):e147–64.
21. Hatch GFR 3rd, Villacis D, Damodar D, Dacey M, Yi A. Quality of life and functional outcomes after multiligament knee reconstruction. J Knee Surg. 2018;31(10):970–8.
22. Everhart JS, Du A, Chalasani R, Kirven JC, Magnussen RA, Flanigan DC. Return to work or sport after multiligament knee injury: a systematic review of 21 studies and 524 patients. Arthroscopy. 2018;34(5):1708–16.
23. Hanley J, Westermann R, Cook S, Glass N, Amendola N, Wolf BR, Bollier M. Factors associated with knee stiffness following surgical Management of Multiligament Knee Injuries. J Knee Surg. 2017;30(6):549–54.

Chapter 61
Patellofemoral Instability

Patellofemoral (PF) instability is a condition whereby there is abnormal displacement of the patella in relation to the femoral trochlea. In most cases the patella displaces laterally in relation to the trochlea, and in a small proportion medially [1–11]. Hence, this chapter refers mainly to lateral patellar instability, but a consideration of medial patellar instability is also made.

61.1 Spectrum of Patellofemoral Instability

PF instability may be described according to:

Timing of Onset
- Congenital
- Acquired

Degree of Displacement
- Partial displacement (subluxation)
- Complete displacement (dislocation)

C. Panayiotou Charalambous, *The Knee Made Easy*,
https://doi.org/10.1007/978-3-030-54506-2_61

Frequency of Instability

- Static—the patella is fixed in the displaced position
- Dynamic—the patella displaces intermittently
  - Habitual—occurring every time the knee flexes/extends
  - Occasional

Number of Instability Episodes

- First time instability—refers to the first episode of instability
- Recurrent instability—more than one episode of instability

According to the Presence of Volition

- Voluntary—the patient may sublux/dislocate the patella at will, by influencing muscular contraction or by placing the knee in a particular position—flex the knee to tighten the quadriceps and selectively contract vastus lateralis
- Involuntary—the patient cannot achieve the above

Reducibility

- Spontaneously reducible
- Spontaneously irreducible—needs medical intervention to achieve reduction

Upon dislocation the patella may either spontaneously relocate or be locked in a dislocated position and need to be reduced medically (by closed or open means).

According to the Direction of Translation of the Patella in Relation to the Trochlea

- Lateral (most common)
- Medial

The direction of instability can be determined by:

- Clinical history—identifying the position that causes instability symptoms
- Clinical examination

  - Visual inspection
  - Palpation
  - Instability provocation tests
- If the patient is seen between dislocations, there may be a need to review:
  - Any radiological investigations obtained at the time of dislocation prior to reduction
  - Any available report of the clinical findings obtained at the time of patellar dislocation prior to reduction. Usually the diagnosis of patellar dislocation is made clinically, and the patella is reduced prior to radiographs obtained.
  - Any photograph images taken by the patient or clinicians when the patella was dislocated, prior to reduction

61.2 Causes of Patellofemoral Instability

PF instability may be caused by disruption of the stabilising ligaments due to:

- Substantial trauma
  - Contact injury—external impact on the knee, direct fall on the knee
  - Non-contact injury—twisting injury, valgus injury
  - Iatrogenic—during knee or femoral surgey [7]
- Non-traumatic—secondary to underlying soft tissue or bony derangements
- Static stabilisers
  - Imbalance between medial and lateral patellofemoral ligaments—hyperlaxity/tightness
  - Bony dysplasia—trochlea/patella
  - Rotational malalignment

    Excessive internal femoral torsion
    Tibial external torsion
  - Coronal malalignment

    Tibiofemoral joint valgus
  - Sagittal malalignment

    Patella alta—a patella that rides abnormally high in relation to the femoral trochlea

Trochlear and patellar dysplasia may be classified as below:

Dejour's Classification of Trochlear Dysplasia [12]

- Type A—shallow
- Type B—flat or convex trochlea
- Type C—asymmetry of the trochlear facets with hypoplasia of the medial condyle, and a flat or convex lateral condyle
- Type D—asymmetry of the trochlear facets and supratrochlear spur

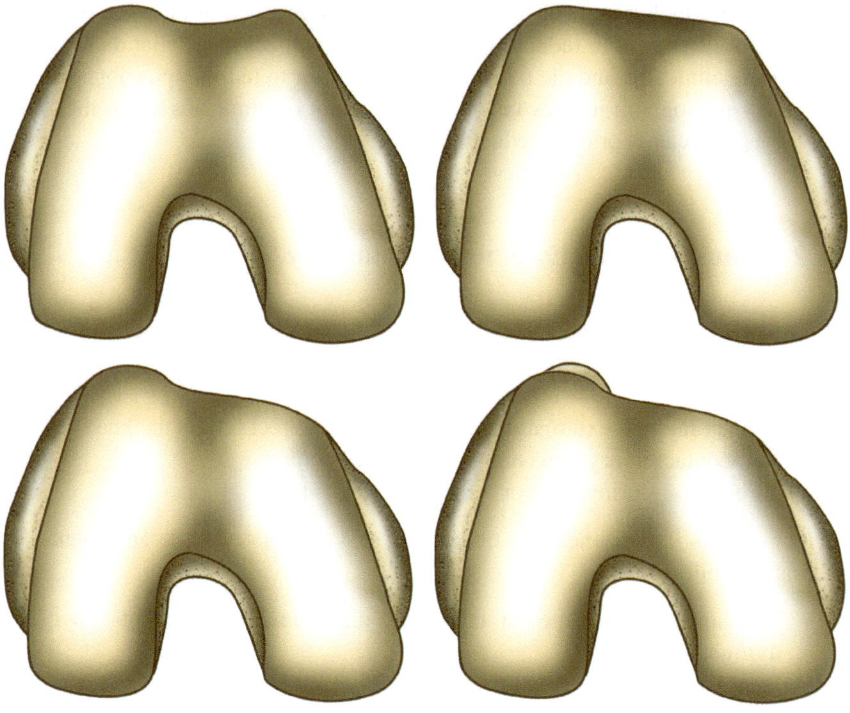

Dejour's classification of trochlear dysplasia

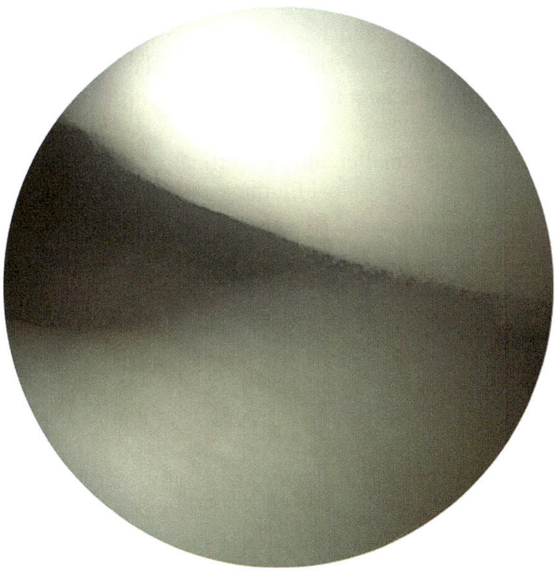

U shaped trochlea

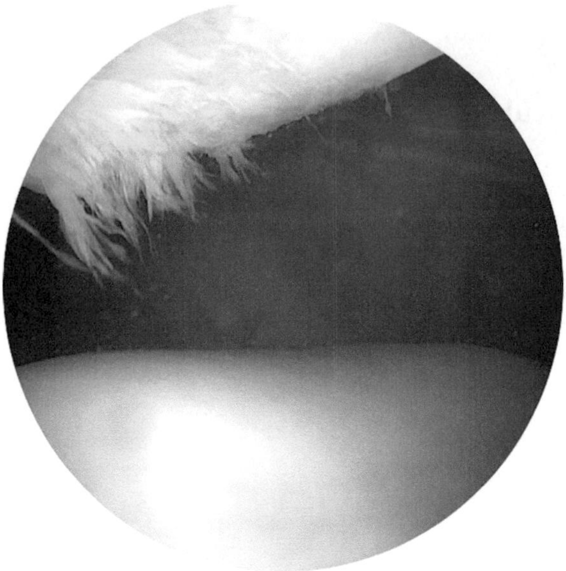

Flat trochlea

Wiberg Classification of Patellar Dysplasia [13]

- Type I—medial facet has concave shape and has almost the same size as the lateral facet which is also concave- 16.1% —symmetrical patella
- Type II—medial facet is smaller than the lateral facet, lateral facet is concave but medial facet is flat or slightly convex 80%
- Type III—medial facet is substantially smaller, almost vertical 12.9%

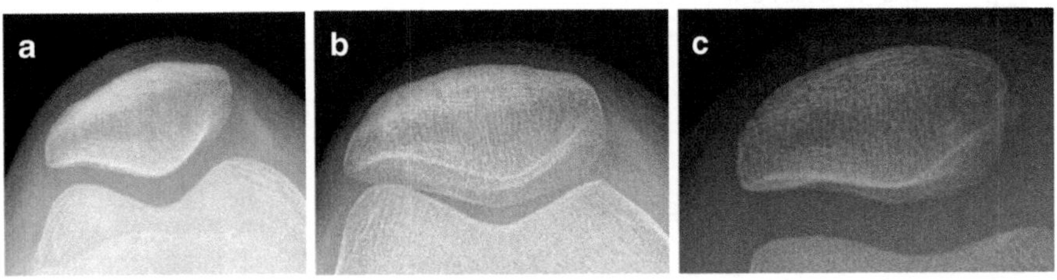

Patellar morphology may be classified according to the Wiberg classification—(a) Similar lateral and medial facets (b) Larger lateral facet (c) Vertical medial facet

Flat or concave patellae (with no separation between lateral and medial facets) also occur and are associated with PF instability.

- Dynamic stabilisers—(core, hip, knee, ankle/foot)
  - Weak
  - Discoordinated
  - Lack of stable platform to act upon
- Combination of the above
  - Trauma occurring in the background of pre-existing derangements

The most common cause of PF instability encountered in clinical practise is non-traumatic, or traumatic occurring in the background of pre-existing derangements.

61.3 Clinical Symptoms of Patellofemoral Instability

- Pain over the PF joint
  - Chronic due to:
    - Maltracking
    - PF overload
    - Chondral damage
  - Acute due to:
    - Sudden subluxation or dislocation
- Clicking/clunking of the PF joint
- Feeling of exaggerated mobility of the PF joint
- Feeling of knee instability—knee gives way, buckles
- Clinical deformity with the patella visibly displacing lateral or medially in relation to the femur
- Limitation of knee motion when the patella is dislocated

61.4 Clinical Signs of Patellofemoral Instability

- Visible and palpable displacement of the patella in relation to the femur:
  - Static
  - Dynamic—patellar maltracking with knee flexion/extension, prominent inverse J sign
- Malalignment of the knee and lower limb:
  - Coronal—valgus knee, planovalgus feet
  - Rotational—increased femoral anteversion, femoral intorsion, external tibial torsion
  - Sagittal—patella alta
- Increased ligament tightness—lateral patellar retinaculum, iliotibial band
- Hyperlaxity
  - Medial patellar retinaculum
  - Generalised

61.5 Investigations for Patellofemoral Instability [14–22]

- Plain radiographs:
  - AP, lateral and skyline views can demonstrate the position of the patella in relation to the trochlea, long leg film to assess coronal alignment when clinically indicated
- CT
  - Rotational profile of the lower limb—to provide an accurate evaluation of the rotational relation of the femur and tibia
  - Trochlear dysplasia
- MRI
  - Rotational profile of the lower limb
  - Evaluate lateralization of the tibial tubercle—Tibial Tubercle-Trochlear Groove(TT-TG) distance
  - Trochlear dysplasia
  - Demonstrate concomitant soft tissue injuries—Medial PF ligament (MPFL) disruption

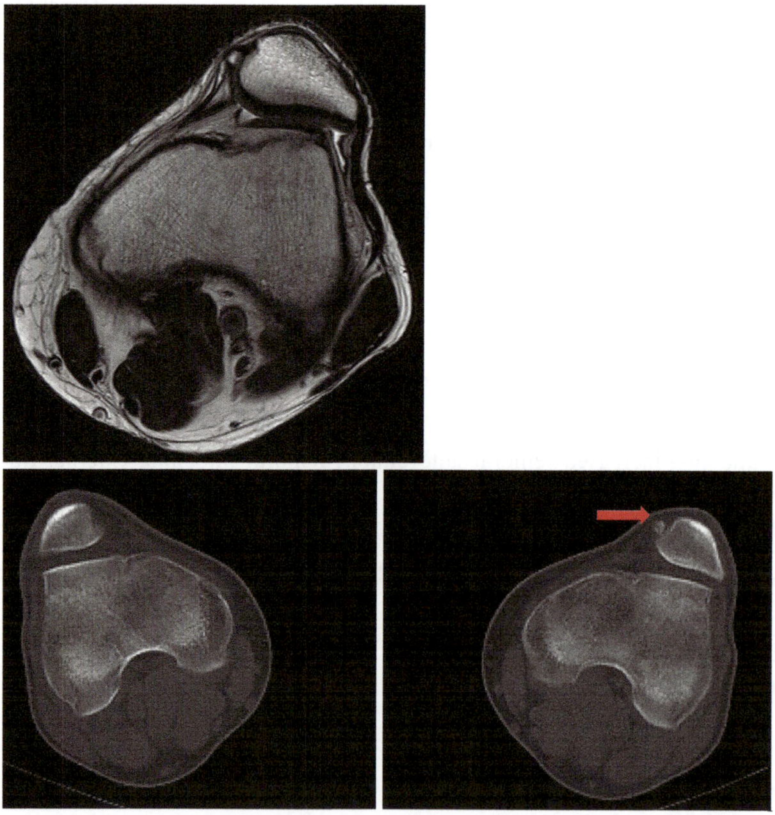

Trochlear dysplasia, lateral subluxation of the patella, and medial ossicle (red arrow) consistent with MPFL avulsion injury

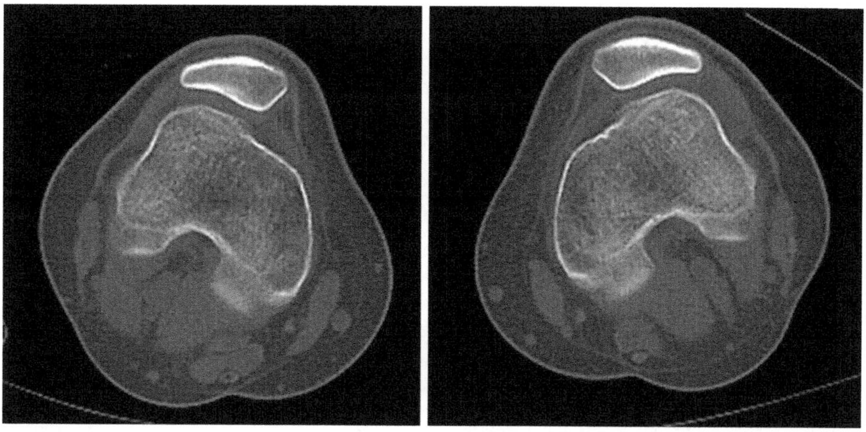

Bilateral lateral patellar subluxation, associated with femoral anteversion and trochlear dysplasia (convex trochlea, medial condyle hypoplasia)

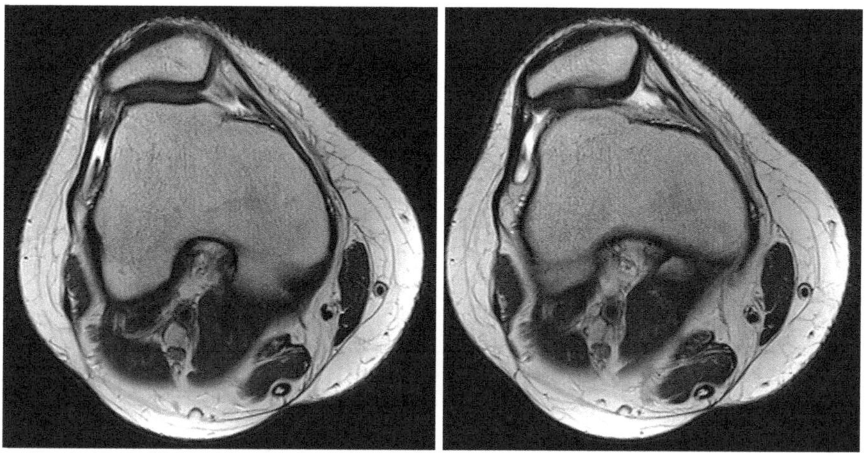

Lateral patellar subluxation, associated with trochlear dysplasia (convex trochlea, medial condyle hypoplasia)

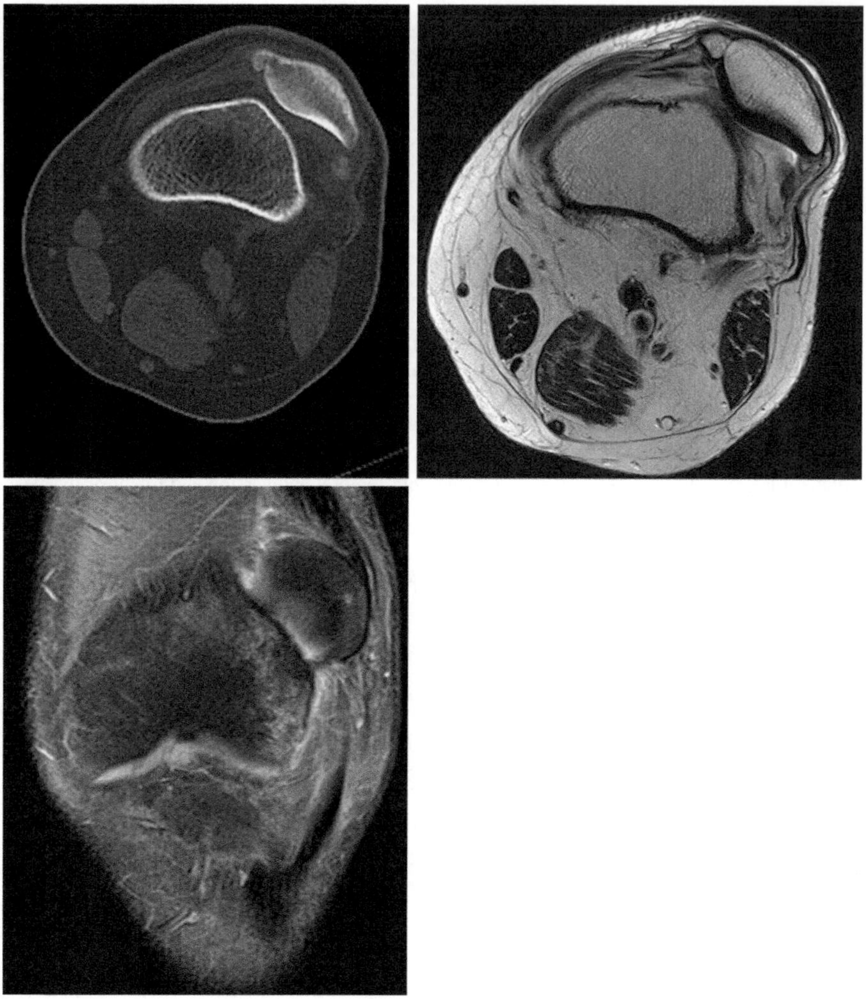

Lateral patellar dislocation, associated with convex trochlea and evidence of MPFL bony avulsion. The patella remains dislocated throughout the flexion cycle

Several radiological indices have been described to assess anatomical variants that have been related to instability. These include:

61.5.1 Sagittal Evaluation

1. Caton-Deschamps ratio—assessed on lateral plain radiographs. It measures the distance between the inferior edge of the patellar joint surface and the antero-superior angle of the tibia on sagittal X-rays and is normally equal to 1.

- A ratio equal or superior to 1.2 is defined as patella alta
- A ratio less than or equal to 0.6 is defined as patella infera (patella baja)

2. Patellar articular overlap—on sagittal MRI the patellar articular length is measured. The length of the patellar cartilage that overlaps the trochlear cartilage is also measured. The overlap may be expressed as absolute value (with <6 mm considered indicative of patella alta) or as a percentage of the total patellar articular cartilage.

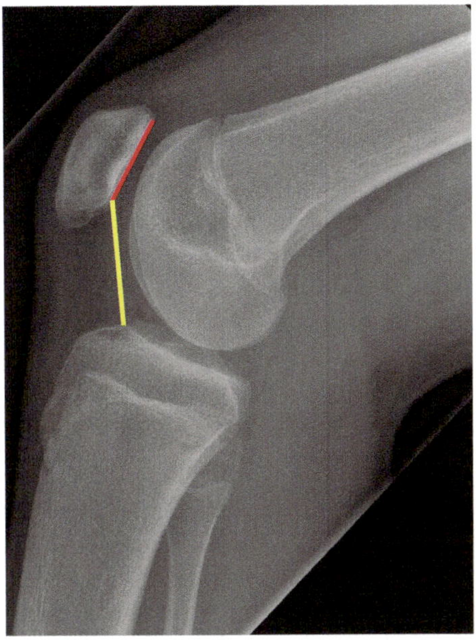

Caton-Deschamps index: The distance from the inferior border of the patellar articular surface to the superior/anterior border of the tibial plateau (length of the yellow line) is divided by the length of the patellar articular surface (red line)

61.5.2 Coronal Evaluation

1. Femoral-tibial anatomical axis—to look for valgus deformity at the knee

61.5.3 Axial Evaluation

1. TT-TG distance—assesses the position (lateralisation) of the tibial tubercle in relation to the trochlear groove. Reported values in non-symptomatic knees are: 15.5+/−1.5 mm on CT, 12.5+/−2 mm on MRI

2. Trochlear sulcus angle—this is the angle between a line drawn from the centre of the deepest part of the trochlea along the medial trochlear facet and a similar line drawn along the lateral trochlear facet. It may be assessed on plain radiographs (skyline view), axial CT (bony sulcus angle) or axial MRI (cartilaginous sulcus angle) scans. Tan SHS [15] systematically assessed the values reported for the sulcus angle in asymptomatic knees and knees with PF instability. They reported that in all studies examined the cartilaginous sulcus angle was greater than the bony sulcus angle. They showed that:
   - The mean cartilaginous sulcus angle for the non-symptomatic group was 142° (95% CI:140°-144°) and for the PF instability group 156° (95% CI: 154–159).
   - The mean bony sulcus angle for the non-symptomatic group was 134° (95% CI:131°-136°) and for the PF instability group 148° (95% CI: 144°-153°).
3. Femoral neck version angle—the angle between a line passing along the long axis of the femoral neck (midpoint between the anterior and posterior femoral neck cortices to the centre of the femoral head) in relation to a line passing across the posterior condyles of the distal femur. Assessed on axial CT or MRI scans. 15+/− 7° of femoral anteversion has been reported as normal range.
4. Tibial torsion—the angle between a line passing along the posterior condyles of the proximal tibia and a line passing across the centre of the ankle joint (through the transmalleolar axis). Values of 25+/−7° of tibial external rotation have been reported as normal range.

In assessing radiological indices it is important to appreciate their limitations as explained in the investigations chapter. Furthermore, it is vital to recognise that there may be a relation between the various radiological indices, hence they shouldn't be looked at in isolation. A high positioned patella has been shown to be associated with trochlear dysplasia. Similarly, a substantial correlation may exist between femoral and tibial torsion, trochlear dysplasia, TT-TG distance, and coronal mechanical axis.

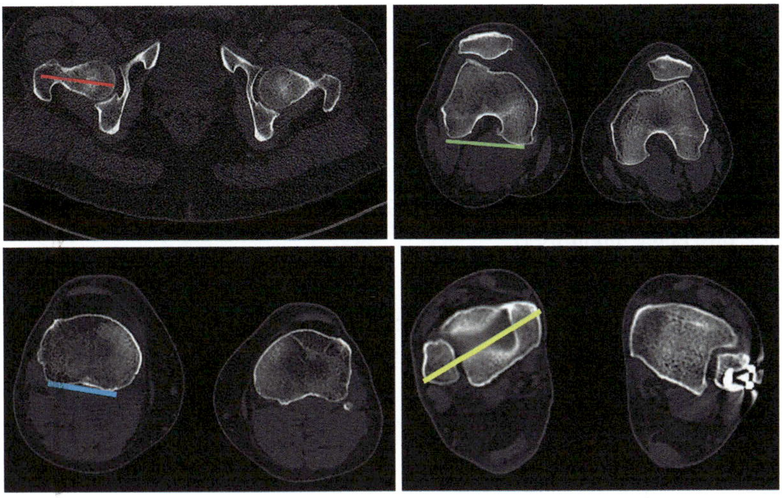

CT assessment of rotational profile. The lines passing through the middle of the femoral neck (red line), along the posterior tibial condyles (green line), posterior condyles of the widest part of the proximal tibia (blue line) and transmalleolar axis (yellow line) are determined and the angle between them is measured

61.6 Management of Patellofemoral Instability [22–56]

In those presenting with an acute traumatic dislocation the initial aim is to reduce the dislocation. This is usually done:

- Under sedation or general anaesthetic
- The patella is pushed medially whilst the knee is extended

In those patients presenting with chronic symptoms of patellar instability, further management depends on the patient's symptoms, functional demands, extent of patellar instability, and frequency of patellar instability as well as underlying cause.

Chronic symptoms may be those of:

1. Instability
2. Instability and pain

61.6.1 *Non-surgical*

- Leave alone
- Analgesia
- Activity modification
- Physiotherapy
  - Core, hip, knee, ankle/foot
    - Strengthening—core, hip abductors/external rotators, quadriceps
    - Stretching—iliotibial band, lateral patellar retinaculum
- External devices
  - Knee bracing
    - Correct coronal malalignment
    - Patellar taping, bracing
  - Foot orthotics
    - Medial arch support, heel cups

61.6.2 *Surgical*

If symptoms do not improve with non-surgical intervention and patient has structural lesions that are amenable to surgery, surgery may be considered.

Surgical interventions for stability may be described according to the structures addressed as:

- Soft tissue procedure
- Bony procedure
- Combined soft-tissue/bony procedure

It is important to recognise that:

- Surgery addresses only structural defects, hence, other contributors to instability may still need to be dealt with non-surgical measures
- Correcting structural defects may facilitate the subsequent improvement of:
  - Muscle strengthening, balancing
  - Proprioception

Several procedures have been described which aim to address the underlying derangement including:

- MPFL tear—MPFL reconstruction

- Trochlear dysplasia—trochleoplasty to deepen the trochlear groove
- Patella alta—tibial tubercle transfer distally (distalisation)
- Lateralised tibial tubercle in relation to the trochlear groove—tibial tubercle medialization
- Knee valgus—distal femoral varus osteotomy (closing wedge or opening wedge). Opening wedge may also decrease the patellar height (whereas closing wedge may not influence patellar height) which is of value if associated patella alta
- Increased femoral internal rotation—femoral external rotation osteotomy
- Increased tibial external rotation—tibial internal rotation osteotomy
- Patellar dysplasia—patellar osteotomy
- Tight iliotibial band/lateral patellar retinaculum—release of tight structures

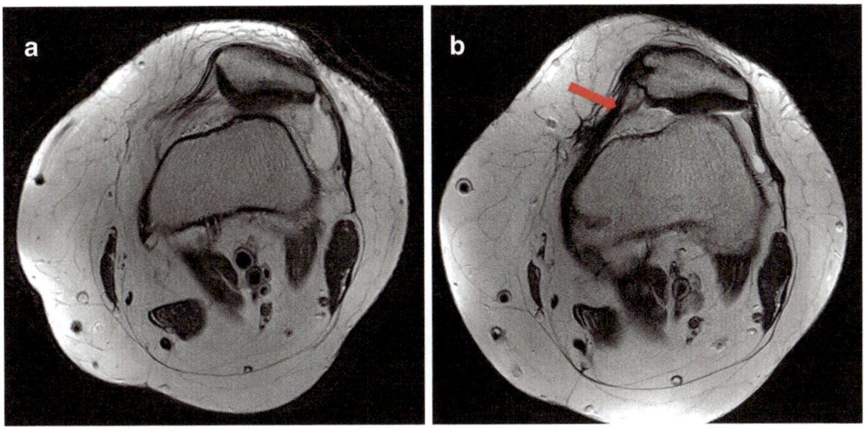

Patellar instability with MPFL tear (a), treated with MPFL reconstruction red arrow (b)

It may be suggested (even though this is not an absolute rule) [3] that:

- Intermittent, infrequent, non-substantially troublesome instability is treated non-surgically
- Frequent, troublesome instability, that fails to respond to non-surgical treatment is treated surgically

Various techniques for MPFL reconstruction have been described. These include:

- Using an autograft, allograft, or synthetic ligament
- Using a slip of quadriceps tendon

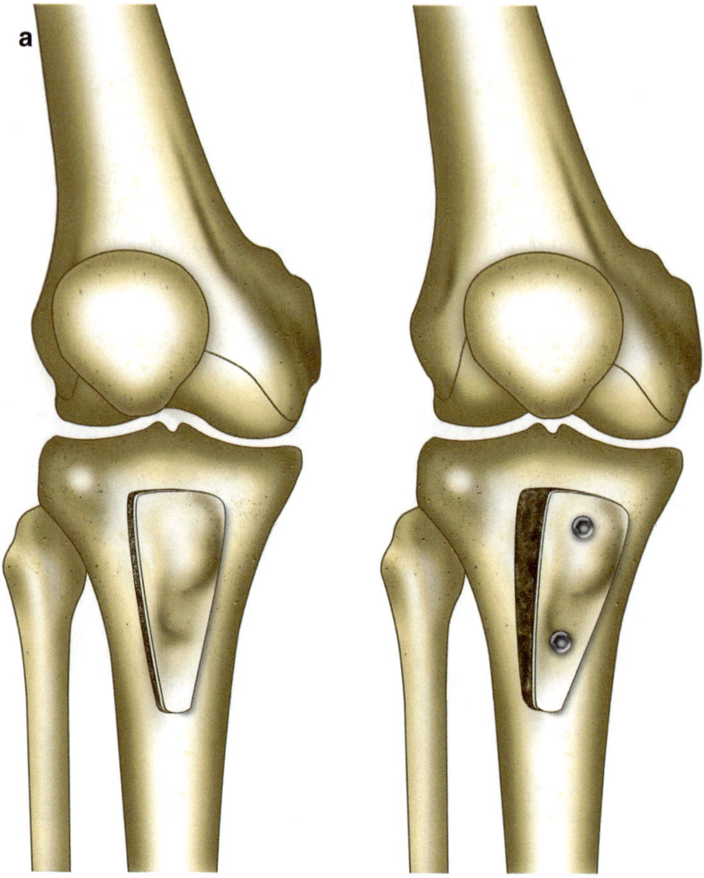

Tibial tubercle medialization

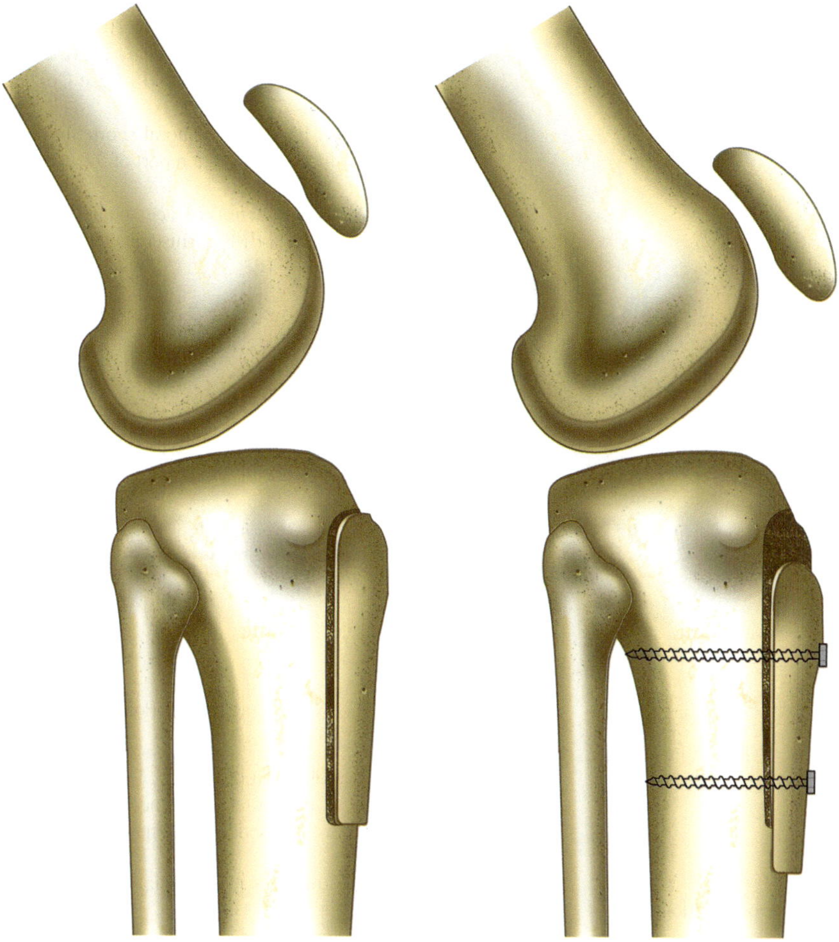

Tibial tubercle distalization

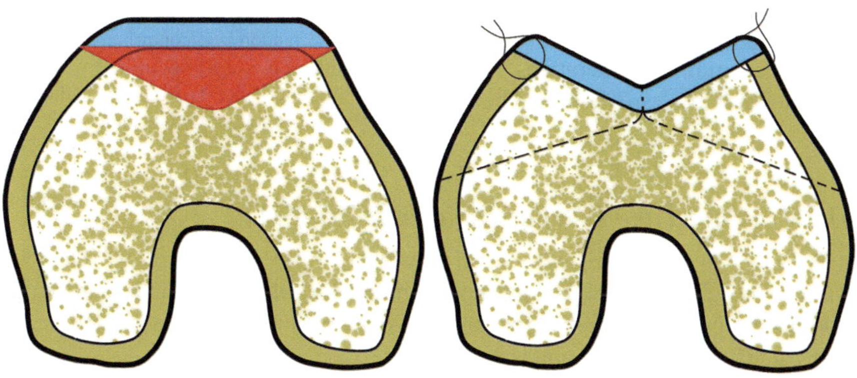

Trochleoplasty

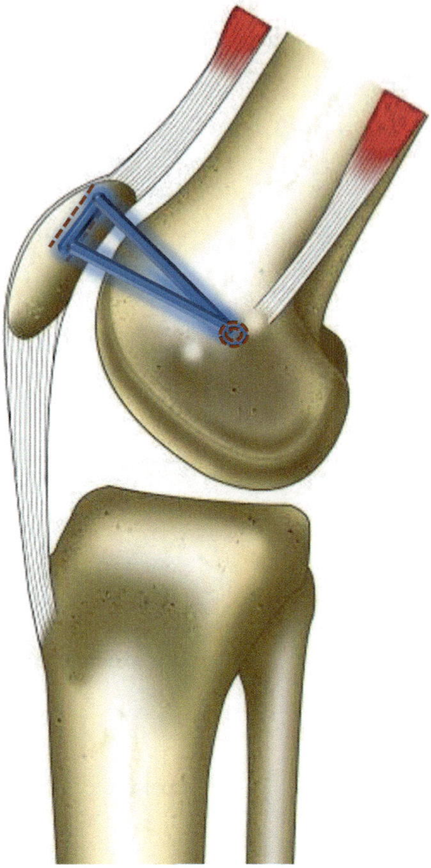

MPFL reconstruction

61.7 Special Situations of Patellofemoral Instability

There are certain considerations that must be made for some specific instability scenarios and these are described below:

61.7.1 First Time Patellar Dislocator [57–62]

It is recognised that an initial dislocation of the patella is associated with an increased risk of subsequent instability, especially in young patients. When faced with a first time patellar dislocator the aim is to either:

- Reduce the patella but also intervene surgically to stabilise the patella to minimise the risk of subsequent dislocations (such as with MPFL repair or reconstruction). This may be applied to:
  - All first time patellar dislocators
  - Those at high risk of developing recurrent instability
- Reduce the patella, observe and rehabilitate, and only consider intervening if recurrent dislocations occur

At the moment there is no high quality evidence supporting one approach over the other, hence the second option is favoured by the author as that is the least invasive approach.

Several scoring systems have looked at prognostic factors for developing recurrent patellar instability:

- The Recurrent Instability of the Patella score (RIP) [61] provides information on the risk of instability recurrence based on patient's age, skeletal maturity, trochlear dysplasia and tibial tubercle to trochlear groove distance over the patellar length ratio. It stratifies cases into low, intermediate and high risk categories with 0%, 31% and 79% 10 year recurrent instability rates respectively.
- The "Patellar Instability Severity Score" described by Balcarek et al. [62] included 6 risk factors: age (<16), bilateral instability, trochlear dysplasia, patellar height, TT-TG distance and patellar tilt. Each risk factor scored up to 1 or 2 points, with the Odds Ratio for recurrence being 5 times higher when the total score was greater than 4 points.
- A recent meta-analysis by Huntington LS et al. [57] reported that the overall rate of recurrent dislocation after a first time patellar lateral dislocation was 33.6%. An increased risk of recurrence was reported in:
  - Younger patients
  - Open physes
  - Trochlear dysplasia
  - Elevated TT-TG distance
  - Patella alta
- In studies that reported multiple risk factors, recurrence rate was about 8%–14%, but increased to 30%–60% when 2 risk factors were present and 70%–79% when 3 risk factors were present.

However, although such systems may guide as to the risk of recurrence, they cannot predict at an individual level what exactly will happen, hence cannot fully guide management.

61.7.2 Instability vs. Hyperlaxity

Laxity is a physiological condition that is different to instability but may predispose to the development of patellar instability.

Lax joints have longer and more stretchable ligaments which allow greater translation of the articular surfaces, and a higher range of motion. Most hyperlaxity patients do not have instability and can maintain their joints in situ (through dynamic muscle control). Hence, they do not exhibit symptoms of abnormal joint translation.

Excessive joint translation does not equate to instability. Similarly, it is possible to have patellar instability without hyperlaxity. Hyperlaxity, however, may increase the risk of patellar instability and may be associated with inferior results following surgery to improve patellar stability [63, 64].

Causes of hyper-laxity include:
Congenital

- Benign joint hyper-mobility syndrome (may affect up to 20% of the population, more common in women, Asians and Africans) [65, 66]
- Connective tissue disorders
  - Ehlers-Danlos syndrome
  - Marfan's syndrome
  - Osteogenesis imperfecta

Acquired

- Repetitive micro-trauma causing stretching of ligaments

Generalized joint laxity per se does not require treatment and is usually asymptomatic.

61.8 Medial Patellofemoral Instability

This is a condition whereby there is abnormal displacement of the patella medially in relation to the femoral trochlea [67–73].

61.8.1 Causes

These include:

- Iatrogenic
  - Lateral retinacular release
  - Tibial tubercle medialisation
  - MPFL reconstruction with tight graft positioning
- Hyperlaxity (connective tissue disorders)
- Deficient vastus lateralis

In most cases of medial patellar instability the patient has had previous surgery, which overtightened the medial PF structures or disrupted the lateral patellar stabilisers. Spontaneous medial PF instability may be encountered but is very rare.

61.8.2 Clinical Symptoms

- Patients may report a sudden lateral movement of the patella upon flexion—this however is not a displacement out of joint but the relocation of an already medially subluxed patella (in extension).
- Pain
- Popping
- Instability
- Clinical deformity
- Limited knee motion

61.8.3 Clinical Signs

- Medial subluxation of the patella with the knee in extension, lateral translation and reduction as the knee flexes
- Increased passive medial patellar translation
- Reduced passive lateral patellar translation
- Medial apprehension test—flexing the knee from full extension whilst applying a medial force to the patella—causes pain and apprehension

61.8.4 Management

61.8.4.1 Non-surgical

- Physiotherapy
  - Strengthen vastus lateralis
  - Address core or hip muscle weakness

61.8.4.2 Surgical

- Direct repair of the lateral retinaculum
- Lateral retinaculum reconstruction (using local iliotibial band, patellar tendon, or other natural or synthetic graft)
- Medial retinacular release
- Revision or release of MPFL reconstruction if overtight

Learning Pearls

- There is a need to distinguish between pain and instability symptoms in the presence of patellar dislocation or subluxation—the former may improve with less extensive interventions and avoid the need for a stabilisation procedure. Furthermore, stabilisation surgery and resultant stiffening of the PF joint may exacerbate pain
- In dealing with recurrent patellar instability one of two approaches may be utilised:
  - Multiple surgical procedures may be undertaken according to the underlying pathology (ala carte approach). This may involve a combination of soft tissue and more extensive bony procedures. Supporting factors for this approach include:

    Reported successful results
    Definite procedure utilised
  - A step wise approach, in which less extensive surgery is undertaken with more invasive procedures performed if less extensive surgery fails. MPFL reconstruction may be undertaken in isolation and if it fails then revision surgery addresses any other anatomical deficiencies. Supporting factors for this approach include:

    Avoids more extensive bony procedures
    Reported successful results—isolated MPFL reconstruction has shown to be effective even in the presence of substantial trochlear dysplasia, tibial tubercle lateralization or patella alta
    Recognition that patients with anatomical deficiencies related to patellar instability never develop instability symptoms
    Patients who develop patellar instability and have associated anatomical deficiencies, have often been asymptomatic for many years prior to their first instability event
- Early surgery in patellar dislocation may be necessary to address osteochondral fractures (that require fixation, or excision if causing mechanical symptoms such as locking)
- Deepening trochleoplasty may be associated with a high rate of osteoarthritis (OA), hence it needs to be used with caution. Von Knoch F et al. [74] reported 30% rate of OA after a mean of 8.3 years following a trochlear deepening procedure.
- The role of lateral release in patella instability is controversial with biomechanical studies suggesting that it may hinder rather than improve patellar stability, due to a reduction in patellar compression forces. However, a

recent meta-analysis of lateral release has shown it to be effective as an isolated procedure in decreasing the rate of PF dislocation [34].

- Nomura E et al. [63] showed that although a hypermobile patella and generalized joint laxity were encountered more commonly in cases of recurrent patellar dislocation as compared to controls, a hypermobile patella was more significant than generalised joint laxity as the predisposing factor of patellar dislocation.

References

1. Koh JL, Stewart C. Patellar instability. Orthop Clin North Am. 2015;46(1):147–57.
2. Clark D, Metcalfe A, Wogan C, Mandalia V, Eldridge J. Adolescent patellar instability: current concepts review. Bone Joint J. 2017;99-B(2):159–70.
3. Zaffagnini S, Grassi A, Zocco G, Rosa MA, Signorelli C, Muccioli GMM. The patellofemoral joint: from dysplasia to dislocation. EFORT Open Rev. 2017;2(5):204–14.
4. Arendt EA, Dahm DL, Dejour D, Fithian DC. Patellofemoral joint: from instability to arthritis. Instr Course Lect. 2014;63:355–68.
5. Dewan V, Webb MSL, Prakash D, Malik A, Gella S, Kipps C. When does the patella dislocate? A systematic review of biomechanical & kinematic studies. J Orthop. 2019;20:70–7.
6. Maia Rosa J, Carvalho AD, Coutinho LL, Esteves J, Pereira P, Vilaça A. Surgical treatment for congenital dislocation of the Patella in a young adult: a case report. JBJS Case Connect. 2019;9(4):e0196. https://doi.org/10.2106/JBJS.CC.18.00196.
7. Cvetanovich GL, Ukwuani G, Kuhns B, Weber AE, Beck E, Nho SJ. Antegrade Femoral Nail Distal Interlocking Screw Causing Rupture of the Medial Patellofemoral Ligament and Patellar Instability. Am J Orthop (Belle Mead NJ). 2018;47(7) https://doi.org/10.12788/ajo.2018.0054.
8. Maine ST, O'Gorman P, Barzan M, Stockton CA, Lloyd D, Carty CP. Rotational Malalignment of the Knee Extensor Mechanism: Defining Rotation of the Quadriceps and Its Role in the Spectrum of Patellofemoral Joint Instability. JB JS Open Access. 2019;4(4) https://doi.org/10.2106/JBJS.OA.19.00020.
9. Keshmiri A, Schöttle P, Peter C. Trochlear dysplasia relates to medial femoral condyle hypoplasia: an MRI-based study. Arch Orthop Trauma Surg. 2020;140(2):155–60.
10. Hochreiter B, Hess S, Moser L, Hirschmann MT, Amsler F, Behrend H. Healthy knees have a highly variable patellofemoral alignment: a systematic review. Knee Surg Sports Traumatol Arthrosc. 2020;28(2):398–406.
11. Parikh SN. Patellar Instability. Orthop Clin North Am. 2016;47(1):xxiii. https://doi.org/10.1016/j.ocl.2015.10.006.
12. Dejour H, Walch G, e-Josserand L, Guier C. Factors of patellar instability: an anatomic radiographic study. Knee Surg Sports Traumatol Arthrosc. 1994;2(1):19–26.
13. Wibeeg G. Roentgenographs and anatomic studies on the Femoropatellar joint: with special reference to chondromalacia patellae. Acta Orthop Scand. 1941;12(1–4):319–410.
14. Vairo GL, Moya-Angeler J, Siorta MA, Anderson AH, Sherbondy PS. Tibial tubercle-trochlear groove distance is a reliable and accurate Indicator of patellofemoral instability. Clin Orthop Relat Res. 2019;477(6):1450–8.
15. Tan SHS, Chng KSJ, Lim BY, Wong KL, Doshi C, Lim AKS, Hui JH. The difference between cartilaginous and bony sulcus angles for patients with or without patellofemoral instability: a systematic review and meta-analysis. J Knee Surg. 2020;33(3):235–41.
16. Tan SHS, Lim BY, Chng KSJ, Doshi C, Wong FKL, Lim AKS, Hui JH. The difference between computed tomography and magnetic resonance imaging measurements of Tibial tubercle-trochlear groove distance for patients with or without patellofemoral instability: a

systematic review and meta-analysis. J Knee Surg. 2019;7:768–76. https://doi.org/10.1055/s-0039-1688563.
17. Tanaka MJ, Cosgarea AJ. Measuring Malalignment on Imaging in the Treatment of Patellofemoral Instability. Am J Orthop (Belle Mead NJ). 2017;46(3):148–51.
18. Xiong R, Chen C, Yin L, Gong X, Luo J, Wang F, Yang L, Guo L. How do axial scan orientation deviations affect the measurements of knee anatomical parameters associated with patellofemoral instability? A simulated computed tomography study. J Knee Surg. 2018;31(5):425–32.
19. Caton J, Deschamp G, Chambat P, Lerat JL, Dejour H. Les rotules basses (patellae inferae)—a propos de 128 observations. Rev Chir Orthop. 1982;68:317–25.
20. Caton J. Méthode de mesure de la hauteur de la rotule. Acta Orthop Belg. 1989;55:385–6.
21. Galland O, Walch G, Dejour H, Carret JP. An anatomical and radiological study of the femoropatellar articulation. Surg Radiol Anat. 1990;12(2):119–25.
22. Munch JL, Sullivan JP, Nguyen JT, et al. Patellar articular overlap on MRI is a simple alternative to conventional measurements of patellar height. Orthop J Sports Med. 2016;4(7):2325967116656328.
23. Moiz M, Smith N, Smith TO, Chawla A, Thompson P, Metcalfe A. Clinical Outcomes After the Nonoperative Management of Lateral Patellar Dislocations: A Systematic Review. Orthop J Sports Med. 2018;6(6):2325967118766275. https://doi.org/10.1177/2325967118766275.
24. Gruskay JA, Strickland SM, Casey E, Chiaia TA, Green DW, Gomoll AH. Team approach: patellofemoral instability in the skeletally immature. JBJS Rev. 2019;7(7):e10. https://doi.org/10.2106/JBJS.RVW.18.00159.
25. Luceri F, Roger J, Randelli PS, Lustig S, Servien E. How does isolated medial patellofemoral ligament reconstruction influence patellar height? Am J Sports Med. 2020;14:363546520902132.
26. Gruskay JA, Gomoll AH, Arendt EA, Dejour DH, Strickland SM. Patellar instability and dislocation: optimizing surgical treatment and how to avoid complications. Instr Course Lect. 2020;69:671–92.
27. Puzzitiello RN, Waterman B, Agarwalla A, Zuke W, Cole BJ, Verma NN, Yanke AB, Forsythe B. Primary medial patellofemoral ligament repair versus reconstruction: rates and risk factors for instability recurrence in a young. Active Patient Population Arthroscopy. 2019;35(10):2909–15.
28. Sappey-Marinier E, Sonnery-Cottet B, O'Loughlin P, Ouanezar H, Reina Fernandes L, Kouevidjin B, Thaunat M. Clinical outcomes and predictive factors for failure with isolated MPFL reconstruction for recurrent patellar instability: a series of 211 reconstructions with a minimum follow-up of 3 years. Am J Sports Med. 2019;47(6):1323–30.
29. Gupta SK. Surgical Management of Patellofemoral Instability in the Skeletally Immature Patient. J Am Acad Orthop Surg. 2019;27(21):e954. https://doi.org/10.5435/JAAOS-D-18-00654.
30. Redler LH, Wright ML. Surgical Management of Patellofemoral Instability in the Skeletally Immature Patient. J Am Acad Orthop Surg. 2018;26(19):e405–15.
31. Erickson BJ, Nguyen J, Gasik K, Gruber S, Brady J, Shubin Stein BE. Isolated medial patellofemoral ligament reconstruction for patellar instability regardless of Tibial tubercle-trochlear groove distance and patellar height: outcomes at 1 and 2 years. Am J Sports Med. 2019;47(6):1331–7.
32. Hiemstra LA, Kerslake S, Kupfer N, Lafave MR. Generalized joint hypermobility does not influence clinical outcomes following isolated MPFL reconstruction for patellofemoral instability. Knee Surg Sports Traumatol Arthrosc. 2019;27(11):3660–7.
33. Ellis HB Jr, Dennis G, Wilson PL. Patellofemoral Instability in the Skeletally Immature Patient: A Review and Technical Description of Medial Patellofemoral Ligament Reconstruction in Patients with Open Physes. Am J Orthop (Belle Mead NJ). 2018;47(12) https://doi.org/10.12788/ajo.2018.0110.
34. Tan SHS, Chua CXK, Doshi C, Wong KL, Lim AKS, Hui JH. The outcomes of isolated lateral release in patellofemoral instability: a systematic review and meta-analysis. J Knee Surg. 2019;25 https://doi.org/10.1055/s-0039-1688961.
35. Zhang Z, Zhang H, Song G, Zheng T, Ni Q, Feng H. Increased femoral anteversion is associated with inferior clinical outcomes after MPFL reconstruction and combined tibial tubercle

osteotomy for the treatment of recurrent patellar instability. Knee Surg Sports Traumatol Arthrosc. 2019;4:2261–9. https://doi.org/10.1007/s00167-019-05818-3.
36. Rush J, Diduch D. When is Trochleoplasty a rational addition? Sports Med Arthrosc Rev. 2019;27(4):161–8.
37. Ren B, Zhang X, Zhang L, Zhang M, Liu Y, Tian B, Zhang B, Zheng J. Isolated trochleoplasty for recurrent patellar dislocation has lower outcome and higher residual instability compared with combined MPFL and trochleoplasty: a systematic review. Arch Orthop Trauma Surg. 2019;139(11):1617–24.
38. Kaiser P, Schmoelz W, Schöttle PB, Heinrichs C, Zwierzina M, Attal R. Isolated medial patellofemoral ligament reconstruction for patella instability is insufficient for higher degrees of internal femoral torsion. Knee Surg Sports Traumatol Arthrosc. 2019;27(3):758–65.
39. Imhoff FB, Cotic M, Liska F, Dyrna FGE, Beitzel K, Imhoff AB, Herbst E. Derotational osteotomy at the distal femur is effective to treat patients with patellar instability. Knee Surg Sports Traumatol Arthrosc. 2019;27(2):652–8.
40. Nelitz M. Femoral Derotational osteotomies. Curr Rev Musculoskelet Med. 2018;11(2):272–9.
41. Dickschas J, Tassika A, Lutter C, Harrer J, Strecker W. Torsional osteotomies of the tibia in patellofemoral dysbalance. Arch Orthop Trauma Surg. 2017;137(2):179–85.
42. Tan SHS, Lim SY, Wong KL, Doshi C, Lim AKS, Hui JH. The outcomes of isolated distal realignment procedures in patellofemoral instability: a systematic review and meta-analysis. J Knee Surg. 2019;1:547–52. https://doi.org/10.1055/s-0039-1681052.
43. Tan SHS, Hui SJ, Doshi C, Wong KL, Lim AKS, Hui JH. The outcomes of distal femoral Varus osteotomy in patellofemoral instability: a systematic review and meta-analysis. J Knee Surg. 2019;1:504–12. https://doi.org/10.1055/s-0039-1681043.
44. Parikh SN, Redman C, Gopinathan NR. Simultaneous treatment for patellar instability and genu valgum in skeletally immature patients: a preliminary study. J Pediatr Orthop B. 2019;28(2):132–8.
45. Frings J, Krause M, Akoto R, Wohlmuth P, Frosch KH. Combined distal femoral osteotomy (DFO) in genu valgum leads to reliable patellar stabilization and an improvement in knee function. Knee Surg Sports Traumatol Arthrosc. 2018;26(12):3572–81.
46. Nha KW, Ha Y, Oh S, Nikumbha VP, Kwon SK, Shin WJ, Lee BH, Hong KB. Surgical treatment with closing-wedge distal femoral osteotomy for recurrent patellar dislocation with genu Valgum. Am J Sports Med. 2018;46(7):1632–40.
47. Tan SHS, Tan LYH, Lim AKS, Hui JH. Hemiepiphysiodesis is a potentially effective surgical management for skeletally immature patients with patellofemoral instability associated with isolated genu valgum. Knee Surg Sports Traumatol Arthrosc. 2019;27(3):845–9.
48. Enea D, Canè PP, Fravisini M, Gigante A, Dei GL. Distalization and Medialization of Tibial Tuberosity for the Treatment of Potential Patellar Instability with Patella Alta. Joints. 2018;6(2):80–4.
49. Bartsch A, Lubberts B, Mumme M, Egloff C, Pagenstert G. Does patella Alta lead to worse clinical outcome in patients who undergo isolated medial patellofemoral ligament reconstruction? A systematic review. Arch Orthop Trauma Surg. 2018;138(11):1563–73.
50. Grimm NL, Lazarides AL, Amendola A. Tibial tubercle osteotomies: a review of a treatment for recurrent patellar instability. Curr Rev Musculoskelet Med. 2018;11(2):266–71.
51. Batailler C, Neyret P. Trochlear dysplasia: imaging and treatment options. EFORT Open Rev. 2018;3(5):240–7.
52. Dejour D, Le Coultre B. Osteotomies in Patello-femoral instabilities. Sports Med Arthrosc Rev. 2018;26(1):8–15.
53. Dejour D, Saggin P. The sulcus deepening trochleoplasty-the Lyon's procedure. Int Orthop. 2010;34(2):311–6.
54. Nelitz M, Dreyhaupt J, Williams SRM. No growth disturbance after Trochleoplasty for recurrent patellar dislocation in adolescents with open growth plates. Am J Sports Med. 2018;46(13):3209–16.
55. Fulkerson JP. Editorial commentary: medial patellofemoral ligament reconstruction alone works well when the patient has Normal alignment, but Don't forget to move the Tibial tubercle when necessary! Arthroscopy. 2018;34(4):1355–7.

56. Singhal R, Rogers S, Charalambous CP. Double-bundle medial patellofemoral ligament reconstruction with hamstring tendon autograft and mediolateral patellar tunnel fixation: a meta-analysis of outcomes and complications. Bone Joint J. 2013;95-B(7):900–5.
57. Huntington LS, Webster KE, Devitt BM, Scanlon JP, Feller JA. Factors associated with an increased risk of recurrence after a first-time patellar dislocation: a systematic review and meta-analysis. Am J Sports Med. 2019;11:363546519888467. https://doi.org/10.1177/0363546519888467.
58. Parikh SN, Lykissas MG, Gkiatas I. Predicting risk of recurrent patellar dislocation. Curr Rev Musculoskelet Med. 2018;11(2):253–60.
59. Migliorini F, Driessen A, Quack V, Gatz M, Tingart M, Eschweiler J. Surgical versus conservative treatment for first patellofemoral dislocations: a meta-analysis of clinical trials. Eur J Orthop Surg Traumatol. 2020;11:771–80. https://doi.org/10.1007/s00590-020-02638-x.
60. Askenberger M, Bengtsson Moström E, Ekström W, Arendt EA, Hellsten A, Mikkelsen C. Arv PM. Operative repair of medial patellofemoral ligament injury versus knee brace in children with an acute first-time traumatic patellar dislocation: a randomized controlled trial. Am J Sports Med. 2018;46(10):2328–40.
61. Hevesi M, Heidenreich MJ, Camp CL, Hewett TE, Stuart MJ, Dahm DL, Krych AJ. The recurrent instability of the Patella score: a statistically based model for prediction of long-term recurrence risk after first-time dislocation. Arthroscopy. 2019;35(2):537–43.
62. Balcarek P, Oberthür S, Hopfensitz S, et al. Which patellae are likely to redislocate? Knee Surg Sports Traumatol Arthrosc. 2014;22(10):2308–14.
63. Nomura E, Inoue M, Kobayashi S. Generalized joint laxity and contralateral patellar hypermobility in unilateral recurrent patellar dislocators. Arthroscopy. 2006;22(8):861–5.
64. Howells NR, Eldridge JD. Medial patellofemoral ligament reconstruction for patellar instability in patients with hypermobility: a case control study. J Bone Joint Surg Br. 2012;94(12):1655–9.
65. Hakim A, Grahame R. Joint hypermobility. Best Pract Res Clin Rheumatol. 2003;17(6):989–1004.
66. Jessee EF, Owen DS Jr, Sagar KB. The benign hypermobile joint syndrome. Arthritis Rheum. 1980;23(9):1053–6.
67. Saper MG, Shneider DA. Medial patellar subluxation: diagnosis and treatment. Am J Orthop (Belle Mead NJ). 2015;44(11):499–504.
68. McCarthy MA, Bollier MJ. Medial Patella subluxation: diagnosis and treatment. Iowa Orthop J. 2015;35:26–33.
69. Bollier M, Fulkerson J, Cosgarea A, Tanaka M. Technical failure of medial patellofemoral ligament reconstruction. Arthroscopy. 2011;27(8):1153–9.
70. Hughston JC, Deese M. Medial subluxation of the patella as a complication of lateral retinacular release. Am J Sports Med. 1988;16(4):383–8.
71. Nonweiler DE, DeLee JC. The diagnosis and treatment of medial subluxation of the patella after lateral retinacular release. Am J Sports Med. 1994;22(5):680–6.
72. Fulkerson JP. A clinical test for medial patella tracking. Tech Orthop. 1997;12:144.
73. Hughston JC, Flandry F, Brinker MR, Terry GC, Mills JC. 3rd surgical correction of medial subluxation of the patella. Am J Sports Med. 1996;24(4):486–91.
74. von Knoch F, Böhm T, Bürgi ML, von Knoch M, Bereiter H. Trochleaplasty for recurrent patellar dislocation in association with trochlear dysplasia. A 4- to 14-year follow-up study. J Bone Joint Surg Br. 2006;88(10):1331–5.

Chapter 62
Proximal Tibiofibular Joint Instability

Proximal tibiofibular joint instability is a condition where there is abnormal displacement of the protimal fibula in relation to the tibia.

62.1 Causes of Proximal Tibiofibular Joint Instability [1–8]

Disruption of the proximal tibiofibular joint may be:

- Congenital/developmental
- Acquired
  - Spontaneous—associated with generalised ligamentous laxity
  - Acute substantial trauma

  Disruption of the proximal tibiofibular joint may be due to:

- Ligamentous dysfunction/injuries
- Associated with bony abnormalities—developmental, traumatic, degenerative

Proximal tibiofibular joint instability may be described:

According to the Degree of Instability
- Subluxation
- Dislocation

C. Panayiotou Charalambous, *The Knee Made Easy*,
https://doi.org/10.1007/978-3-030-54506-2_62

According to the Direction of instability [1]
- Anterolateral dislocation
- Posteromedial dislocation
- Superior dislocation

According to the Mechanism of Injury Leading to Disruption
- Contact—direct trauma
- Non-contact—twisting injury of the lower limb with the knee in flexion

62.2 Clinical History of a Traumatic Event

The following injury characteristics may suggest a proximal tibiofibular joint disruption:

- A history of substantial trauma
- Patient felt/heard pop in the knee
- Mechanism of injury:
  - Anterolateral dislocation—knee hyperflexed and foot dorsiflexed and inverted (activities including skiing, rugby, soccer, roller skating, wrestling, parachute landing, football, basketball, volleyball)
  - Posteromedial dislocation—landing on minimal flexed knee

62.3 Clinical Symptoms of Proximal Tibiofibular Joint Instability

- Acute presentation
  - Lateral knee pain, swelling, clinical deformity (prominence of fibular head)
  - Symptoms of common peroneal nerve dysfunction
- Chronic presentation
  - Lateral knee pain aggravated by ankle/foot motion
  - Prominence of the fibular head—visual, palpable
  - Clicking/clunking due to abnormal translation of the fibula aggravated by ankle/foot motion

- Fibular head tenderness
- Symptoms of common peroneal nerve dysfunction

62.4 Clinical Signs of Proximal Tibiofibular Joint Instability

- Displacement of the fibular head in relation to the tibia—visible or palpable deformity
- Tenderness over the proximal tibiofibular joint
- With the knee flexed 90° the fibular head may be subluxed/dislocated by gentle pressure in an anterior or posterior direction
- Signs of common peroneal nerve dysfunction

62.5 Investigations for Proximal Tibiofibular Joint Instability [9–12]

- Radiological—comparison with opposite knee may improve diagnostic accuracy
  - Plain radiographs—anteroposterior, lateral
    - May demonstrate avulsion fracture
    - Assess position of the fibular head in relation to the tibia
  - MRI Scan—allows assessment of ligamentous disruption
  - CT scan—axial—investigation of choice to determine presence of fibular head dislocation/subluxation
- Examination under general anaesthesia

62.6 Management of Proximal Tibiofibular Joint Instability [13–20]

Initial management aims to:

- Reduce a dislocated joint—by closed or open means
  - Closed reduction—anterolateral dislocation—flex the knee and apply posterior force on the fibular head
  - If closed reduction cannot be achieved then open reduction is performed

- Maintain reduction by:
  - Immobilisation for 4 weeks in an above knee brace or cylinder cast
  - Temporary fixation with k-wires or screw between fibula and tibia

Further management aims at improving chronic ongoing symptoms of instability or pain and hence improve a patient's function. This depends on:

- Symptoms—severity, frequency
- Underlying cause
- Functional demand of the patient

62.6.1 Non-surgical

- Leave alone
- Activity modification, avoiding unstable positions
- Physiotherapy to address:
  - Gastrocnemius and hamstring (biceps femoris) strengthening

62.6.2 Surgical

- Fusion arthroplasty of the proximal tibiofibular joint
- Fibular head resection (if associated pressure symptoms on the common peroneal nerve)
- Ligamentous reconstruction to stabilise the joint

Learning Pearls

- Examination of the distal syndesmosis and interosseous membrane should be performed in acute injuries, as they may coexist and need addressing
- Spontaneous reduction due to the posterior pull of the biceps femoris in knee flexion may occur following an injury, and the patient thus present some time later with chronic residual symptoms

References

1. Ogden JA. Subluxation and dislocation of the proximal tibiofibular joint. J Bone Joint Surg Am. 1974;56:145–54.
2. Van Seymortier P, Ryckaert A, Verdonk P, Almqvist KF, Verdonk R. Traumatic proximal tibiofibular dislocation. Am J Sports Med. 2008;36(4):793–8.
3. Sekiya JK, Kuhn JE. Instability of the proximal tibiofibular joint. J Am Acad Orthop Surg. 2003;11(2):120–8.

4. Reynolds AW, Bhat SB, Stull JD, Krieg JC. Case report of an isolated proximal tibiofibular joint dislocation in a professional ice hockey player. J Orthop Case Rep. 2018;8(1):93–5.
5. O'Reilly OC, Carruthers KH, Siparsky PN. Bilateral, Atraumatic Proximal Tibiofibular Joint Instability Treated With Suspensory Button Fixation. Orthopedics. 2017;40(6):e1107–11.
6. Morrison TD, Shaer JA, Little JE. Bilateral, atraumatic, proximal tibiofibular joint instability. Orthopedics. 2011;34(2):133.
7. Haupt S, Frima H, Sommer C. Proximal tibiofibular joint dislocation associated with tibial shaft fractures - 7 cases. Injury. 2016;47(4):950–3.
8. Jabara M, Bradley J, Merrick M. Is stability of the proximal tibiofibular joint important in the multiligament-injured knee? Clin Orthop Relat Res. 2014;472(9):2691–7.
9. Burke CJ, Grimm LJ, Boyle MJ, Moorman CT 3rd, Hash TW 2nd. Imaging of Proximal Tibiofibular Joint Instability: A 10 year retrospective case series. Clin Imaging. 2016;40(3):470–6.
10. Forster BB, Lee JS, Kelly S, O'Dowd M, Munk PL, Andrews G, Chinkow L. Proximal tibiofibular joint: an often-forgotten cause of lateral knee pain. AJR Am J Roentgenol. 2007;188(4):W359–66.
11. Voglino JA, Denton JR. Acute traumatic proximal tibiofibular joint dislocation confirmed by computed tomography. Orthopedics. 1999;22(2):255–8.
12. Keogh P, Masterson E, Murphy B, McCoy CT, Gibney RG, Kelly E. The role of radiography and computed tomography in the diagnosis of acute dislocation of the proximal tibiofibular joint. Br J Radiol. 1993;66(782):108–11.
13. Halbrecht JL, Jackson DW. Recurrent dislocation of the proximal tibiofibular joint. Orthop Rev. 1991;20(11):957–60.
14. Kruckeberg BM, Cinque ME, Moatshe G, Chetti D, NN DP, Chahla J, RF LP. Proximal Tibiofibular Joint Instability and Treatment Approaches: A Systematic Review of the Literature. Arthroscopy. 2017;33(9):1743–51.
15. Dekker TJ, DePhillipo NN, Kennedy MI, Aman ZS, Schairer WW, LaPrade RF. Clinical Characteristics and Outcomes Following Isolated Anatomic Reconstruction of the Proximal Tibiofibular Joint. Arthroscopy. 2020. pii: S0749-8063(20)30141-9
16. Oksum M, Randsborg PH. Treatment of Instability of the Proximal Tibiofibular Joint by Dynamic Internal Fixation with a Suture Button. Arthrosc Tech. 2018;7(10):e1057–61.
17. Goljan P, Pierce TP, Scillia AJ, Festa A. Soft Tissue Reconstruction of the Proximal Tibiofibular Joint by Using Split Biceps Femoris Graft with 5-Year Clinical Follow-up. Am J Orthop (Belle Mead NJ). 2018;47(5) https://doi.org/10.12788/ajo.2018.0029.
18. Bédard M, Corriveau-Durand S. Instability of the proximal tibiofibular joint associated with total knee arthroplasty. Arthroplast Today. 2016;2(3):93–6.
19. Cazeneuve JF, Bracq H, Meeseman M. Weinert and Giachino ligament arthroplasty for the surgical treatment of chronic superior tibiofibular joint instability. Knee Surg Sports Traumatol Arthrosc. 1997;5(1):36–7.
20. Falkenberg P, Nygaard H. Isolated anterior dislocation of the proximal tibiofibular joint. J Bone Joint Surg Br. 1983;65(3):310–1.

Chapter 63
Knee Hyperextension: Recurvatum

This is a condition whereby there is excessive knee extension (greater than 10° or 15°) [1–21]. Knee extension is influenced by static and dynamic factors, which under normal conditions work in a coordinated and balanced way to ensure the knee straightens but not excessively. Disruption of any of these factors may lead to knee hyperextension. Knee recurvatum may cause local troublesome knee symptoms. Furthermore, its presence may be of clinical significance in the management of other knee conditions.

Knee recurvatum may be described according to:

The Timing of its Development:

- Congenital–congenital knee dislocation
- Acquired
  - Idiopathic
  - Post-traumatic
  - Post-surgical (skeletal traction distal femur or proximal tibia)

The Structures Involved in its Genesis:

- Soft tissue factors
  - Ligamentous
  - Muscle
- Bony factors
  - Femur
  - Tibia
- Combination of soft tissue and bony components

C. Panayiotou Charalambous, *The Knee Made Easy*,
https://doi.org/10.1007/978-3-030-54506-2_63

According to the Underlying Process:

- Ligamentous
  - Benign ligamentous hyperlaxity
  - Connective tissue disorders
  - Ligamentous disruption
    - Posterior capsule
    - Posterior oblique ligament (POL)—This has been shown by cadaveric studies to be the main ligamentous restraint to knee hyperextension
    - Posterolateral corner (PLC)
  - Ligamentous tightness

    Iliotibial band in valgus tibiofemoral degeneration. In valus deformity the iliotibial band may be tight in knee extension, pulling the tibia (and the knee) into hyperextension.
- Muscle
  - This may be due to imbalance between the activity of quadriceps and the hamstrings, or it may be compensatory in response to other muscle changes in the lower limb.
    - Knee extensor spasticity (quadriceps over activity) pulling the tibia into hyperextension
    - Weakness of knee flexors, elongated hamstring tendons
    - Quadriceps weakness—patient may hyperextend to lock the knee to compensate for muscle weakness
    - Limited ankle dorsiflexion, equinus deformity
    - Weakness of the hip extensors, excessive hip flexion
  - Muscle dysfunction may be due to:
    - Myopathy
    - Neurological cause
      - Upper motor neurone lesion—stroke, cerebral palsy, multiple sclerosis
      - Lower motor neurone lesion—poliomyelitis
- Bony
  - Posterior tibial overgrowth in relation to the anterior tibia
    - Due to asymmetric closure of the proximal tibial physis
    - Reduced posterior tibial slope
  - Posterior femoral overgrowth in relation to the anterior femur
- Inflammatory arthropathy

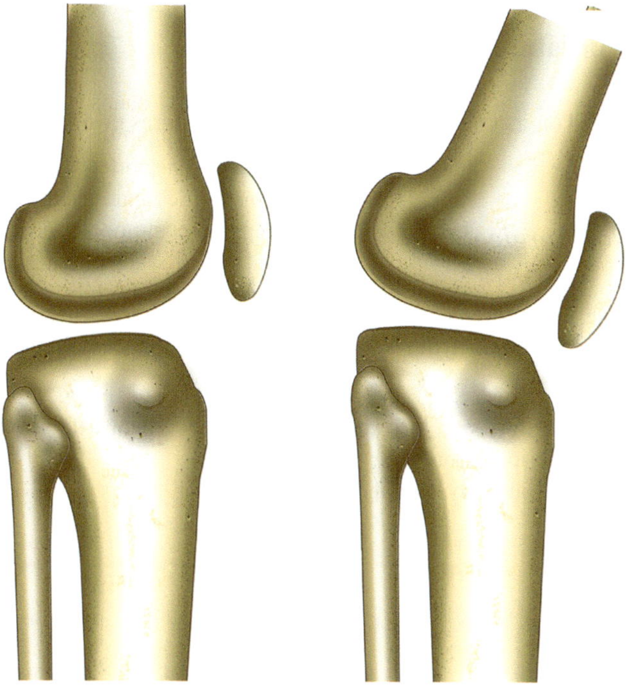

Recurvatum due to increased anterior tibial slope

63.1 Clinical Symptoms of Knee Hyperextension—Recurvatum

- Anterior knee pain—due to increased pressure and irritation/impingement of anterior knee structures—tibiofemoral, fat pad, patellofemoral articulation
- Posterior knee pain—due to tension on posterior knee structures
- Symptoms of instability

63.2 Clinical Signs of Knee Hyperextension—Recurvatum

- Recurvatum
- Accompanied valgus deformity in many cases
- Ligamentous instability
- Muscle weakness/wasting
- Muscle tightness
- Poor proprioception
- Tender anterior joint line and infrapatellar fat pad

63.3 Management of Knee Hyperextension—Recurvatum [22–47]

This will depend on its underlying cause and the structures involved.

63.3.1 Non-surgical

- Leave alone
- External devices—anti-hyperextension bracing, ankle/foot orthotics
- Physiotherapy
  - Muscle strength—core, hip, knee (quadriceps and hamstrings rebalancing)
  - Enhance proprioception
  - Biofeedback (auditory, visual)

63.3.2 Surgical

- Proximal tibial osteotomy—anterior opening wedge to increase posterior slope of tibia
- Distal femoral osteotomy
- Posterior capsule plication/advancement to tighten the posterior capsule

Anti-hyperextension bracing may help to predict improvement following osteotomy.

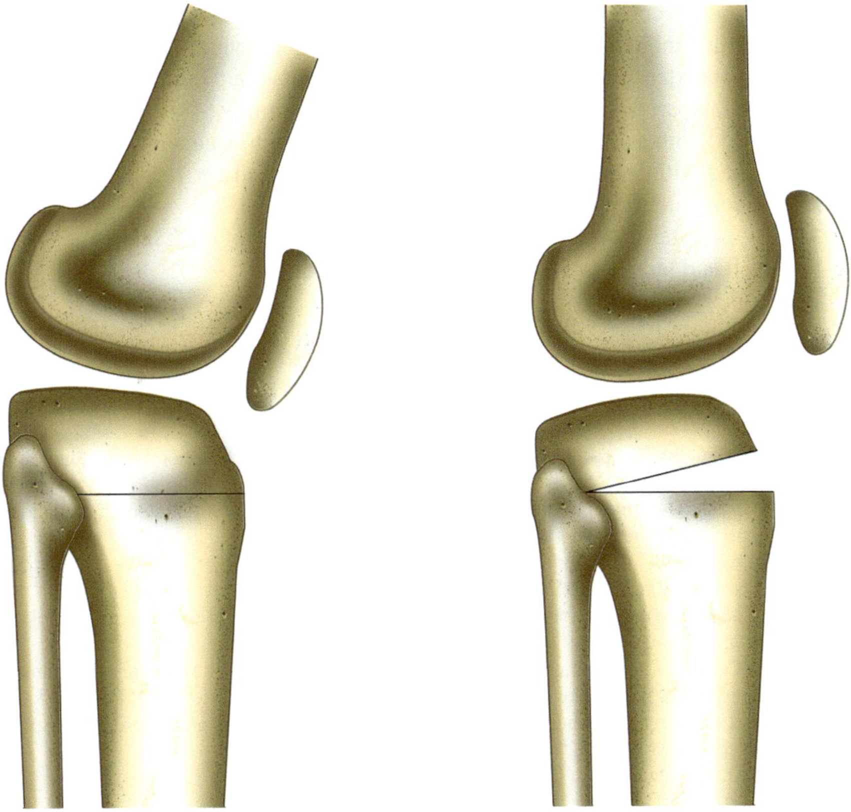

Anterior opening wedge osteotomy of the proximal tibia to reduce knee hyperextension

63.4 Clinical Significance of Knee Hyperextension—Recurvatum

In addition to the above described symptoms, the presence of knee recurvatum may influence several other knee conditions including:

- Its presence may warrant constrained implants in total knee replacement arthroplasty (TKR) to ensure stability
- Cruciate retaining TKR in the presence of recurvatum (5°–20°) and in the absence of any major ligamentous instability, neuromuscular disease, or inflammatory arthropathy has been shown to confer good outcomes at an average follow up of 4.5 years [46]

- Preoperative recurvatum has been shown to be a predictor of poor clinical outcomes following unicompartmental knee replacement arthroplasty (UKR) [43]
- Knee hyperextension has been associated with worse outcomes at 2 years post TKR as compared with those with fixed flexion deformity [48].
- Associated with an increased risk of anterior cruciate ligament (ACL) injury
- Associated with a higher risk of graft failure and need for revision following ACL reconstruction surgery
- Knee hyperextension has been related to increased risk of graft impingement on the notch and failure following ACL reconstruction [49].

References

1. Loudon JK, Goist HL, Loudon KL. Genu recurvatum syndrome. J Orthop Sports Phys Ther. 1998;27(5):361–7.
2. Knight JL. Genu recurvatum deformity secondary to partial proximal tibial epiphyseal arrest: case report. Am J Knee Surg. 1998 Spring;11(2):111–5.
3. Howard AC, Redden JF. Neglected bilateral congenital recurvatum of the knee. Clin Orthop Relat Res. 1994;303:198–202.
4. Ooishi T, Sugioka Y, Matsumoto S, Fujii T. Congenital dislocation of the knee. Its pathologic features and treatment. Clin Orthop Relat Res. 1993;287:187–92.
5. Takai R, Grant AD, Atar D, Lehman WB. Minor knee trauma as a possible cause of asymmetrical proximal tibial physis closure. A case report. Clin Orthop Relat Res. 1994;307:142–5.
6. Moorhead JF. Cervical myelopathy presenting as a genu recurvatum gait disorder. Arch Phys Med Rehabil. 1993;74(3):320–3.
7. Gupta AD, Mahalanabis D. Genu recurvatum in hemophilia: a case report. Arch Phys Med Rehabil. 2007;88(6):791–3.
8. Kerrigan DC, Deming LC, Holden MK. Knee recurvatum in gait: a study of associated knee biomechanics. Arch Phys Med Rehabil. 1996;77(7):645–50.
9. Bauer J, Patrick Do K, Feng J, Pierce R, Aiona M. Knee Recurvatum in children with spastic Diplegic cerebral palsy. J Pediatr Orthop. 2019;39(9):472–8.
10. Segev E, Hendel D, Wientroub S. Genu recurvatum in an adolescent girl: hypothetical etiology and treatment considerations. A case report. J Pediatr Orthop B. 2002;11(3):260–4.
11. Feczko P, Emans P. Hereditary bilateral genu recurvatum: case report of a family. Knee. 2017;24(1):137–43.
12. Saito N, Tensyo K, Horiuchi H, Aoki K, Kobayashi S, Kato H, Kosho T. Brothers with genu recurvatum. Knee. 2007;14(6):500–1.
13. Domzalski M, Mackenzie W. Growth arrest of the proximal tibial physis with recurvatum and valgus deformity of the knee. Knee. 2009;16(5):412–6.
14. Ishikawa H, Abrahan LM Jr, Hirohata K. Genu recurvatum: a complication of prolonged femoral skeletal traction. Arch Orthop Trauma Surg. 1984;103(3):215–8.
15. Van Meter JW, Branick RI. Bilateral genu recurvatum after skeletal traction. A case report. J Bone Joint Surg Am. 1980;62(5):837–9.
16. Llario S, Brandon ML, Bonamo JR, Flynn MI, Sherman MF. Genu recurvatum presenting as PCL insufficiency. J Knee Surg. 2004;17(4):214–7.
17. Gross R, Delporte L, Arsenault L, Revol P, Lefevre M, Clevenot D, Boisson D, Mertens P, Rossetti Y, Luauté J. Does the rectus femoris nerve block improve knee recurvatum in adult stroke patients? A kinematic and electromyographic study. Gait Posture. 2014;39(2):761–6.

18. Klotz MC, Wolf SI, Heitzmann D, Gantz S, Braatz F, Dreher T. The influence of botulinum toxin a injections into the calf muscles on genu recurvatum in children with cerebral palsy. Clin Orthop Relat Res. 2013;471(7):2327–32.
19. Zwick EB, Svehlík M, Steinwender G, Saraph V, Linhart WE. Genu recurvatum in cerebral palsy--part B: hamstrings are abnormally long in children with cerebral palsy showing knee recurvatum. J Pediatr Orthop B. 2010;19(4):373–8.
20. Shultz SJ, Levine BJ, Nguyen AD, Kim H, Montgomery MM, Perrin DH. A comparison of cyclic variations in anterior knee laxity, genu recurvatum, and general joint laxity across the menstrual cycle. J Orthop Res. 2010;28(11):1411–7.
21. Morgan PM, LaPrade RF, Wentorf FA, Cook JW, Bianco A. The role of the oblique popliteal ligament and other structures in preventing knee hyperextension. Am J Sports Med. 2010;38(3):550–7.
22. Bleyenheuft C, Bleyenheuft Y, Hanson P, Deltombe T. Treatment of genu recurvatum in hemiparetic adult patients: a systematic literature review. Ann Phys Rehabil Med. 2010;53(3):189–99.
23. Requier B, Bensoussan L, Mancini J, Delarque A, Viton JM, Kerzoncuf M. Knee-ankle-foot orthoses for treating posterior knee pain resulting from genu recurvatum: Efficiency, patients' tolerance and satisfaction. J Rehabil Med. 2018;50(5):451–6.
24. Portnoy S, Frechtel A, Raveh E, Schwartz I. Prevention of genu Recurvatum in Poststroke patients using a hinged soft knee Orthosis. PM R. 2015;7(10):1042–51.
25. Appasamy M, De Witt ME, Patel N, Yeh N, Bloom O, Oreste A. Treatment strategies for genu recurvatum in adult patients with hemiparesis: a case series. PM R. 2015;7(2):105–12.
26. Basaglia N, Mazzini N, Boldrini P, Bacciglieri P, Contenti E, Ferraresi G. Biofeedback treatment of genu-recurvatum using an electrogoniometric device with an acoustic signal. One-year follow-up. Scand J Rehabil Med. 1989;21(3):125–30.
27. Hogue RE, McCandless S. Genu recurvatum: auditory biofeedback treatment for adult patients with stroke or head injuries. Arch Phys Med Rehabil. 1983;64(8):368–70.
28. Laurà G, Berruto M, Bianchi M. Genu recurvatum following distal epiphysiodesis of the femur: X-ray evaluation and therapeutical approach. Ital J Orthop Traumatol. 1992;18(4):505–14.
29. Moroni A, Pezzuto V, Pompili M, Zinghi G. Proximal osteotomy of the tibia for the treatment of genu recurvatum in adults. J Bone Joint Surg Am. 1992;74(4):577–86.
30. Jung YB, Lee YS, GHJ, Nam CH, Yang JJ. Correction of bony genu recurvatum combined with ligamentous instability of the knee: three case reports. Knee Surg Sports Traumatol Arthrosc. 2008;16(2):185–7.
31. Mehta SN, Mukherjee AK. Flexion osteotomy of the femur for genu recurvatum after poliomyelitis. J Bone Joint Surg Br. 1991;73(2):200–2.
32. Flandry F, Sinco SM. Surgical treatment of chronic posterolateral rotatory instability of the knee using capsular procedures. Sports Med Arthrosc Rev. 2006;14(1):44–50.
33. Piriou P, Garreau C, Combelles F, Judet T. Original technique for the treatment of ligament-related genu recurvatum: preliminary results. Knee Surg Sports Traumatol Arthrosc. 2002;10(4):260–4.
34. Bellicini C, Khoury JG. Correction of genu recurvatum secondary to Osgood-Schlatter disease: a case report. Iowa Orthop J. 2006;26:130–3.
35. Choi IH, Chung CY, Cho TJ, Park SS. Correction of genu recurvatum by the Ilizarov method. J Bone Joint Surg Br. 1999;81(5):769–74.
36. van Raaij TM, de Waal Malefijt J. Anterior opening wedge osteotomy of the proximal tibia for anterior knee pain in idiopathic hyperextension knees. Int Orthop. 2006;30(4):248–52.
37. Gasbarrini A, Fravisini M, Pascarella R, Boriani S. Severe genu recurvatum treated with arthrodesis and external fixation: case report. J Knee Surg. 2005;18(3):209–11.
38. Cheng CC, Ko JY. Early reduction for congenital dislocation of the knee within twenty-four hours of birth. Chang Gung Med J. 2010;33(3):266–73.
39. Beslikas T, Christodoulou A, Chytas A, Gigis I, Christoforidis J. Genu Recurvatum deformity in a child due to salter Harris type V fracture of the proximal Tibial Physis treated

with high Tibial dome osteotomy. Case Rep Orthop. 2012;2012:219231–6. https://doi.org/10.1155/2012/219231.
40. Manohar Babu KV, Fassier F, Rendon JS, Saran N, Hamdy RC. Correction of proximal tibial recurvatum using the Ilizarov technique. J Pediatr Orthop. 2012;32(1):35–41.
41. Brooks JT, Bernholt DL, Tran KV, Ain MC. The Tibial slope in patients with Achondroplasia: its characterization and possible role in genu Recurvatum development. J Pediatr Orthop. 2016;36(4):349–54.
42. Kim TW, Lee S, Yoon JR, Han HS, Lee MC. Proximal tibial anterior open-wedge oblique osteotomy: Ael technique to correct genu recurvatum. Knee. 2017;24(2):345–53.
43. Jiang L, Chen JY, Chong HC, Chia SL, Lo NN, Yeo SJ. Early outcomes of Unicompartmental knee Arthroplasty in patients with preoperative genu Recurvatum of non-neurological origin. J Arthroplast. 2016;31(6):1204–7.
44. Nishitani K, Nakagawa Y, Suzuki T, Koike K, Nakamura T. Rotating-hinge total knee arthroplasty in a patient with genu recurvatum after osteomyelitis of the distal femur. J Arthroplast. 2007;22(4):630–3.
45. Seo SS, Kim CW, Lee CR, Seo JH, Kim DH, Kim OG. Outcomes of total knee arthroplasty in degenerative osteoarthritic knee with genu recurvatum. Knee. 2018;25(1):167–76.
46. Meding JB, Keating EM, Ritter MA, Faris PM, Berend ME. Total knee replacement in patients with genu recurvatum. Clin Orthop Relat Res. 2001;393:244–9.
47. Prasad A, Donovan R, Ramachandran M, Dawson-Bowling S, Millington S, Bhumbra R, Achan P, Hanna SA. Outcome of total knee arthroplasty in patients with poliomyelitis: A systematic review. EFORT Open Rev. 2018;3(6):358–62.
48. Koo K, Silva A, Chong HC, Chin PL, Chia SL, Lo NN, Yeo SJ. Genu Recurvatum versus fixed flexion after Total knee Arthroplasty. Clin Orthop Surg. 2016;8(3):249–53.
49. Owens BD. Recurvatum. Am J Sports Med. 2018;46(12):2833–5.

Chapter 64
Post-Traumatic Knee Stiffness

This is a condition where the knee loses movement. This may occur following a specific and usually substantial knee injury. It is often seen following a fracture of the distal femur, proximal tibia or patella. Patients may have had surgery to stabilise their fracture, but still develop stiffness. It may also be encountered following a soft tissue injury such as quadriceps tear, cruciate ligament tear, meniscal tear [1–9].

Post-traumatic knee stiffness may have a pure soft tissue component, a bony component or a combination of both.

The mechanical block to motion accounting for the loss of motion may be secondary to several causes including:

- Contracture of the capsule, ligaments or tendons. This may be due to:
  - Sprain of these tissues by the injury force, leading to their inflammation and contracture
  - Surgical repair of torn tendons which may lead to tendon shortening
  - Immobilisation of the knee in a position where tendons or ligaments are shortened—to protect a healing fracture or a soft tissue repair
  - Infrapatellar contracture syndrome
- Intra-articular adhesions (adhesions between the articulating surfaces) or adhesions between the peri-articular muscles/tendons and the knee bones
- Displaced bony fragments which lead to impingement on surrounding parts of the joint or soft tissues limiting motion, or reduce conformity between the articulating surfaces (such as depressed tibial plateau fracture)
- Displaced torn meniscal fragments

64.1 Clinical Symptoms of Post-Traumatic Stiffness

- Loss of knee motion
- Pain

C. Panayiotou Charalambous, *The Knee Made Easy*,
https://doi.org/10.1007/978-3-030-54506-2_64

64.2 Clinical Signs of Post-Traumatic Stiffness

- Loss or reduction of knee motion in one or more directions
- Both active and passive movements are affected

64.3 Investigations for Post-Traumatic Stiffness

- Plain radiographs (knee anteroposterior and lateral views) to assess the bony morphology and relation of articulating surfaces
- CT scan with 3D reconstruction to assess the bony morphology and look for displaced/mal-united fragments
- MRI to look for associated soft tissue injuries (meniscal, ligamentous)
- Inflammatory markers—ESR, CRP, white cell count—to exclude underlying infection

64.4 Differential Diagnosis of Post-Traumatic Stiffness

- Apparent stiffness—mediated by pain
- Knee arthritis

64.5 Management of Post-Traumatic stiffness [10–17]

64.5.1 Non-surgical

Treatment is guided by symptoms:

Pain

- o Oral analgesia, non-steroidal anti-inflammatories (oral, topical)
- Physiotherapy (localised ultrasound, mega-pulse, acupuncture)
- Knee steroid injection

Stiffness

- Physiotherapy—stretching exercises that aim to elongate the contracted, shrunk capsule and ligaments, break down adhesions

Adequate pain control is essential for stretching exercises to be performed. Even in cases where there is obvious displacement of bony fragments, stretching the soft tissues may improve joint motion, by compensating for the bony block.

64.5.2 Surgical

Persistent stiffness may be treated with surgery:

- o Manipulation—under general anaesthesia the knee is moved by the surgeon and stretched, to tear the contracted tissue and regain movement. This is performed once union of the fracture is confirmed. Loss of knee flexion may be easier to improve with manipulation as compared to loss of extension.
- Arthroscopic release:
  - Remove intra-articular adhesions
  - Remove obstructing loose bodies or meniscal tears or other intra-articular lesions
  - Capsular release
- Open arthrolysis:
  - Division/lengthening of contracted soft tissue (capsular release)
  - Excision of adhesions
  - Removal of impinging hardware
    - o Loss of flexion—may be improved by quadriceps release
    - o Loss of extension—may be improved by posterior capsular release
- Osteotomy and realignment of displaced bony fragments—to address mechanical block due to bony components
- Knee replacement arthroplasty to improve conformity of the articulating surfaces

References

1. Predictive factors for knee stiffness after periarticular fracture: a case-control study. J Bone Joint Surg Am. 2012;94(20):1833–8.
2. Kugelman DN, Qatu AM, Strauss EJ, Konda SR, Egol KA. Knee stiffness after tibial plateau fractures: predictors and outcomes (OTA-41). J Orthop Trauma. 2018;32(11):e421–7.
3. Hanley J, Westermann R, Cook S, Glass N, Amendola N, Wolf BR, Bollier M. Factors associated with knee stiffness following surgical management of multiligament knee injuries. J Knee Surg. 2017;30(6):549–54.
4. Reahl GB, Inos D, NN OH, Howe A, Degani Y, Wise B, Maceroli M, RV OT. Risk factors for knee stiffness surgery after tibial plateau fracture fixation. J Orthop Trauma. 2018;32(9):e339–43.
5. Paulos LE, Wnorowski DC, Greenwald AE. Infrapatellar contracture syndrome. Diagnosis, treatment, and long-term followup. Am J Sports Med. 1994;22(4):440–9.
6. Bishop J, Agel J, Dunbar R, Ludvig D, Perreault EJ. The dynamic effect of muscle activation on knee stiffness. Conf Proc IEEE Eng Med Biol Soc. 2014;2014:1599–602.
7. Gage A, Kluczynski MA, Bisson LJ, Zo JM. Factors associated with a delay in achieving full knee extension before anterior cruciate ligament reconstruction. Orthop J Sports Med. 2019;7(3):2325967119829547. https://doi.org/10.1177/2325967119829547.

8. Huang GS, Lee CH, Chan WP, Lee HS, Chen CY, Yu JS. Acute anterior cruciate ligament stump entrapment in anterior cruciate ligament tears: MR imaging appearance. Radiology. 2002;225(2):537–40.
9. Tonin M, Saciri V, Veselko M, Rotter A. Progressive loss of knee extension after injury. Cyclops syndrome due to a lesion of the anterior cruciate ligament. Am J Sports Med. 2001;29(5):545–9.
10. Bonutti PM, McGrath MS, Ulrich SD, McKenzie SA, Seyler TM, Mont MA. Static progressive stretch for the treatment of knee stiffness. Knee. 2008;15(4):272–6.
11. Bhave A, Sodhi N, Anis HK, Ehiorobo JO, Mont MA. Static progressive stretch orthosis-consensus modality to treat knee stiffness-rationale and literature review. Ann Transl Med. 2019;7(Suppl 7):S256. https://doi.org/10.21037/atm.2019.06.55.
12. Kukreja M, Kang J, Curry EJ, Li X. Arthroscopic lysis of adhesions and anterior interval release with manipulation under anesthesia for severe post-traumatic knee stiffness: a simple and reproducible step-by-step guide. Arthrosc Tech. 2019;8(5):e429–35.
13. Xing W, Sun L, Sun L, Liu C, Kong Z, Cui J, Zhang Z. Comparison of minimally invasive arthrolysis vs. conventional arthrolysis for post-traumatic knee stiffness. J Orthop Sci. 2018;23(1):112–6.
14. Mousavi H, Mir B, Safaei A. Evaluation of Thompson's quadricepsplasty results in patients with knee stiffness resulted from femoral fracture. J Res Med Sci. 2017;22:50.
15. Pujol N, Boisrenoult P, Beaufils P. Post-traumatic knee stiffness: surgical techniques. Orthop Traumatol Surg Res. 2015;101(1 Suppl):S179–86.
16. Liu KM, Liu S, Cui Z, Han X, Tang T, Wang A. A less invasive procedure for posttraumatic knee stiffness. Arch Orthop Trauma Surg. 2011;131(6):797–802.
17. Bassi G, Zaffarana VG, Roberto F, Braito W. Arthroscopic arthrolysis of intra-articular knee stiffness. Chir Organi Mov. 1992;77(3):271–4.

Chapter 65
Common Peroneal Nerve Dysfunction

This is a condition where there is impairment in the function of the common peroneal nerve (CPN), involving its motor, sensory component or both. This may be complete involving the main nerve trunk, or partial involving one or more of its branches (superficial/deep). Recognition of the anatomy of the CPN is essential in explaining the clinical findings in nerve dysfunction, as well as in minimising the risk of damage to the nerve during surgical interventions of the knee.

65.1 Causes of Common Peroneal Nerve Dysfunction

Lesions of the CPN may be defined as intrinsic or extrinsic [1–51]:

- Intrinsic
  - Neuritis
  - Systemic disorders (e.g. diabetes, alcohol abuse)
  - Neurological (Charcot Marie Tooth disease)
  - Neoplastic (schwannoma, intraneural cyst)
- Extrinsic
  - Compression
  - Traction
  - Laceration

Causes of extrinsic lesions include:

C. Panayiotou Charalambous, *The Knee Made Easy*,
https://doi.org/10.1007/978-3-030-54506-2_65

Compression
- Fabellar compression syndrome
- Displaced knee fractures
- Mass lesions—bony, soft tissue, vascular
- External compression—thromboprophylaxis stockings, lower limb plaster casts, positioning during surgery, sudden weight loss

Traction
- By a dislocated tibiofemoral joint or proximal tibiofibular joint

Laceration
- Penetrating trauma—stab wounds
- Displaced knee fractures
- Surgery:
  - Open knee surgery—posterolateral corner ligamentous surgery, knee arthroplasty
  - Hip surgery—in sciatic disruption the CPN component of the sciatic nerve is most commonly affected
  - Arthroscopic knee surgery (meniscal repairs)

65.2 Clinical Symptoms of CPN Dysfunction

- Foot drop
- Neurogenic pain in the knee area
- Leg weakness
- Sensory disturbance (reduced/altered/absent) —over the anterior and lateral aspects of the leg and foot

65.3 Clinical Signs of CPN Nerve Dysfunction

- Weakness of lower leg muscles ankle and foot extensors—foot drop
- Weakness of the peroneal muscles—foot eversion
- Muscle wasting
- Sensory disturbance around the lower leg

65.4 Investigations for CPN Dysfunction [52–54]

- Plain radiographs—look for bony disruptions, bony mass lesions
- Ultrasound
- MRI
  - Look for compressive cause of the nerve due to a space occupying lesion
  - Evaluate other causes of leg weakness such as nerve root compromise at the lumbosacral spine
- Electromyography looking for muscle denervation
- Nerve Conduction studies

65.5 Management of CPN Dysfunction [55–66]

- Expectant, await recovery
- Control pain and maintain passive motion
- Surgical exploration if recovery does not occur within about 3 months:
  - Nerve decompression
  - Nerve repair, cable grafting, nerve transfer
  - Tendon transfers

References

1. Pattyn R, Loder R, Mullis BH. Iatrogenic peroneal nerve palsy rates secondary to open reduction internal fixation for tibial plateau fractures using an intraoperative distractor. J Orthop Trauma. 2020;31:359–62. https://doi.org/10.1097/BOT.0000000000001748.
2. Pendleton C, Broski SM, Spinner RJ. Concurrent schwannoma and intraneural ganglion cyst involving branches of the common peroneal nerve. World Neurosurg. 2019;135:171–2. https://doi.org/10.1016/j.wneu.2019.12.078.
3. Asadollahi S, Bucknill A, Robertson PL. Oblique proximal locking screw in tibial fracture intramedullary nailing: a clinical imaging study of proximity to common peroneal nerve. Eur J Orthop Surg Traumatol. 2019;28:523–7. https://doi.org/10.1007/s00590-019-02599-w.
4. Simske NM, Krebs JC, Heimke IM, Scarcella NR, Vallier HA. Nerve injury with acetabulum fractures: incidence and factors affecting recovery. J Orthop Trauma. 2019;33(12):628–34.
5. van Zantvoort A, Setz M, Hoogeveen A, van Eerten P, Scheltinga M. Chronic lower leg pain: entrapment of common peroneal nerve or tibial nerve. Unfallchirurg. 2020;123(Suppl 1):20–4.
6. Mckenna J, Ibrahim A. Isolated common peroneal nerve palsy in sarcoidosis. Ir Med J. 2008;101(10):313–4.
7. Zeng X, Xie L, Qiu Z, Sun K. Compression neuropathy of common peroneal nerve caused by a popliteal cyst: a case report. Medicine (Baltimore). 2018;97(16):e9922. https://doi.org/10.1097/MD.0000000000009922.
8. Margulis M, Ben Zvi L, Bernfeld B. Bilateral common peroneal nerve entrapment after excessive weight loss: case report and review of the literature. J Foot Ankle Surg. 2018;57(3):632–4.

9. Souter J, Swong K, McCoyd M, Balasubramanian N, Nielsen M, Prabhu VC. Surgical results of common peroneal nerve neuroplasty at lateral fibular neck. World Neurosurg. 2018;112:e465–72. https://doi.org/10.1016/j.wneu.2018.01.061.
10. Kara A, Yalçın S, Çelik H, Kuyucu E, Şeker A. Compression neuropathy of the common peroneal nerve caused by an intraosseous ganglion cyst of fibula. Int J Surg Case Rep. 2017;40:10–2.
11. Kitamura T, Kim K, Morimoto D, Kokubo R, Iwamoto N, Isu T, Morita A. Dynamic factors involved in common peroneal nerve entrapment neuropathy. Acta Neurochir. 2017;159(9):1777–81.
12. Ferris S, Maciburko SJ. Partial tibial nerve transfer to tibialis anterior for traumatic peroneal nerve palsy. Microsurgery. 2017;37(6):596–602.
13. Öz TT, Aktaş B, Özkan K, Özturan B, Kilic B, Demiroğlu M. A Case of Schwannoma of the Common Peroneal Nerve in the Knee. Orthop Rev (Pavia). 2017;9(1):6825. https://doi.org/10.4081/or.2017.6825.
14. Fukuda A, Nishimura A, Nakazora S, Kato K, Sudo A. Entrapment of common peroneal nerve by surgical suture following distal biceps femoris tendon repair. Case Rep Orthop. 2016;2016:7909805.
15. Jenkins MJ, Farhat M, Hwang P, Kanawati AJ, Graham E. The distance of the common peroneal nerve to the posterolateral structures of the knee. J Arthroplast. 2016;31(12):2907–11.
16. Emamhadi M, Bakhshayesh B, Andalib S. Surgical outcome of foot drop caused by common peroneal nerve injuries; is the glass half full or half empty? Acta Neurochir. 2016;158(6):1133–8.
17. Poloni TE, Alimehmeti R, Galli A, Gambini S, Mangieri M, Ceroni M. "malignant" foot drop: Enzinger epithelioid sarcoma of the common fibular nerve. Muscle Nerve. 2016;54(4):805–6.
18. O'Malley MP, Pareek A, Reardon P, Krych A, Stuart MJ, Levy BA. Treatment of peroneal nerve injuries in the multiligament injured/dislocated knee. J Knee Surg. 2016;29(4):287–92.
19. Myers RJ, Murdock EE, Farooqi M, Van Ness G, Crawford DC. A Unique Case of Common Peroneal Nerve Entrapment. Orthopedics. 2015;38(7):e644–6.
20. Ghazala CG, Elsaid TA, Mudawi A. Popliteal Artery Pseudoaneurysm with Secondary Chronic Common Peroneal Nerve Neuropathy and Foot Drop after Total Knee Replacement. Ann Vasc Surg. 2015;29(7):1453.e5–8.
21. Woodmass JM, Romatowski NP, Esposito JG, Mohtadi NG, Longino PD. A systematic review of peroneal nerve palsy and recovery following traumatic knee dislocation. Knee Surg Sports Traumatol Arthrosc. 2015;23(10):2992–3002.
22. Sobol GL, Lipschultz TM. Successful surgical treatment of an intraneural ganglion of the common peroneal nerve. Am J Orthop (Belle Mead NJ). 2015;44(4):E123–6.
23. Güzelküçük Ü, Skempes D, Kumnerddee W. Common peroneal nerve palsy caused by compression stockings after surgery. Am J Phys Med Rehabil. 2014;93(7):609–11.
24. Wendt MC, Spinner RJ, Shin AY. Iatrogenic transection of the peroneal and partial transection of the tibial nerve during arthroscopic lateral meniscal debridement and removal of osteochondral fragment. Am J Orthop (Belle Mead NJ). 2014;43(4):182–5.
25. Patel A, Singh R, Johnson B, Smith A. Compression neuropathy of the common peroneal nerve by the fabella. BMJ Case Rep. 2013;2013. pii: bcr2013202154 https://doi.org/10.1136/bcr-2013-202154.
26. Mook WR, Ligh CA, Moorman CT 3rd, Leversedge FJ. Nerve injury complicating multiligament knee injury: current concepts and treatment algorithm. J Am Acad Orthop Surg. 2013;21(6):343–54.
27. Ozden R, Uruc V, Kalacı A, Dogramacı Y. Compression of common peroneal nerve caused by an extraneural ganglion cyst mimicking intermittent claudication. J Brachial Plex Peripher Nerve Inj. 2013;8(1):5. https://doi.org/10.1186/1749-7221-8-5.
28. Park JH, Hozack B, Kim P, Norton R, Mandel S, Restrepo C, Parvizi J. Common peroneal nerve palsy following total hip arthroplasty: prognostic factors for recovery. J Bone Joint Surg Am. 2013;95(9):e55. https://doi.org/10.2106/JBJS.L.00160.
29. Thompson AT, Gallacher PD, Rees R. Lateral meniscal cyst causing irreversible peroneal nerve palsy. J Foot Ankle Surg. 2013;52(4):505–7.

30. Manoharan A, Suresh SS, Sankaranarayanan L. Proximal fibular Osteochondroma producing common peroneal nerve palsy in a post-cesarean section patient. Oman Med J. 2013;28(3):e047. https://doi.org/10.5001/omj.2013.63.
31. Park JH, Restrepo C, Norton R, Mandel S, Sharkey PF, Parvizi J. Common peroneal nerve palsy following total knee arthroplasty: prognostic factors and course of recovery. J Arthroplast. 2013;28(9):1538–42.
32. Mitsiokapa EA, Mavrogenis AF, Antonopoulos D, Tzanos G, Papagelopoulos PJ. Common peroneal nerve palsy after grade I inversion ankle sprain. J Surg Orthop Adv. 2012;21(4):261–5.
33. Girolami M, Galletti S, Montanari G, Mignani G, Schuh R, Ellis S, Di Motta D, D'Apote G, Bevoni R. Common peroneal nerve palsy due to hematoma at the fibular neck. J Knee Surg. 2013;26(Suppl 1):S132–5.
34. Shariq O, Radha S, Konan S. Common peroneal nerve schwannoma: an unusual differential for a symptomatic knee lump. BMJ Case Rep. 2012;2012. pii: bcr2012007346 https://doi.org/10.1136/bcr-2012-007346.
35. Spinner RJ, Binaghi D, Socolovsky M, Amrami KK. Torsional injury to the ankle resulting in fibular neuropathy affects the common fibular nerve as well as its terminal branches, specifically, the articular branch. Clin Anat. 2012;25(4):515–7.
36. Agrawal M, Bhardwaj V, Wangchuk T, Sural S, Dhal A. Common peroneal nerve palsy secondary to peroneus longus abscess: case report. J Foot Ankle Surg. 2012;51(4):479–81.
37. Harvie P, Torres-Grau J, Beaver RJ. Common peroneal nerve palsy associated with pseudotumour after total knee arthroplasty. Knee. 2012;19(2):148–50.
38. Babwah T. Common peroneal neuropathy related to cryotherapy and compression in a footballer. Res Sports Med. 2011;19(1):66–71.
39. Park SE, Lee JU, Ji JH. Intraneural chondroid lipoma on the common peroneal nerve. Knee Surg Sports Traumatol Arthrosc. 2011;19(5):832–4.
40. Jang SH, Lee H, Han SH. Common peroneal nerve compression by a popliteal venous aneurysm. Am J Phys Med Rehabil. 2009;88(11):947–50.
41. Mnif H, Koubaa M, Zrig M, Zammel N, Abid A. Peroneal nerve palsy resulting from fibular head osteochondroma. Orthopedics. 2009;32(7):528–30.
42. Anderson AW, LaPrade RF. Common peroneal nerve neuropraxia after arthroscopic inside-out lateral meniscus repair. J Knee Surg. 2009;22(1):27–9.
43. Bruzzone M, Ranawat A, Castoldi F, Dettoni F, Rossi P, Rossi R. The risk of direct peroneal nerve injury using the Ranawat "inside-out" lateral release technique in valgus total knee arthroplasty. J Arthroplast. 2010;25(1):161–5.
44. Blakey CM, Biant LC. Transection of the common peroneal nerve during harvesting of tendons for anterior cruciate ligament reconstruction. A case report. J Bone Joint Surg Am. 2008;90(7):1567–9.
45. Jowett AJ, Johnston JF, Gaillard F, Anderson SE. Lateral meniscal cyst causing common peroneal palsy. Skelet Radiol. 2008;37(4):351–5.
46. O'Brien CM, Eltigani T. Common peroneal nerve palsy as a possible sequelae of poorly fitting below-knee thromboembolic deterrent stockings (TEDS). Ann Plast Surg. 2006;57(3):356–7.
47. Nonthasoot B, Sirichindakul B, Nivatvongs S, Sangsubhan C. Common peroneal nerve palsy: an unexpected complication of liver surgery. Transplant Proc. 2006;38(5):1396–7.
48. Yamamoto N, Koyano K. Neurovascular compression of the common peroneal nerve by varicose veins. Eur J Vasc Endovasc Surg. 2004;28(3):335–8.
49. Giannas J, Bayat A, Watson SJ. Common peroneal nerve injury during varicose vein operation. Eur J Vasc Endovasc Surg. 2006;31(4):443–5.
50. Bottomley N, Williams A, Birch R, Noorani A, Lewis A, Lavelle J. Displacement of the common peroneal nerve in posterolateral corner injuries of the knee. J Bone Joint Surg Br. 2005;87(9):1225–6.
51. Gray KV, Robinson J, Bernstein RM, Otsuka NY. Splitting of the common peroneal nerve by an osteochondroma: two case reports. J Pediatr Orthop B. 2004;13(4):281–3.

52. Visser LH, Hens V, Soethout M, De Deugd-Maria V, Pijnenburg J, Brekelmans GJ. Diagnostic value of high-resolution sonography in common fibular neuropathy at the fibular head. Muscle Nerve. 2013;48(2):171–8.
53. Van den Bergh FR, Vanhoenacker FM, De Smet E, Huysse W, Verstraete KL. Peroneal nerve: Normal anatomy and pathologic findings on routine MRI of the knee. Insights Imaging. 2013;4(3):287–99.
54. Vasudevan JM, Freedman MK, Beredjiklian PK, Deluca PF, Nazarian LN. Common peroneal entrapment neuropathy secondary to a popliteal lipoma: ultrasound superior to magnetic resonance imaging for diagnosis. PM R. 2011;3(3):274–9.
55. Prabhala T, Hellman A, Walling I, Maietta T, Qian J, Burdette C, Neubauer P, Shao M, Stapleton A, Thibodeau J, Pilitsis JG. External focused ultrasound treatment for neuropathic pain induced by common peroneal nerve injury. Neurosci Lett. 2018;684:145–51.
56. Liang T, Panu A, Crowther S, Low G, Lambert R. Ultrasound-guided aspiration and injection of an intraneural ganglion cyst of the common peroneal nerve. HSS J. 2013;9(3):270–4.
57. Maalla R, Youssef M, Ben Lassoued N, Sebai MA, Essadam H. Peroneal nerve entrapment at the fibular head: outcomes of neurolysis. Orthop Traumatol Surg Res. 2013;99(6):719–22.
58. Reichl H, Ensat F, Dellon AL, Wechselberger G. Successful delayed reconstruction of common peroneal neuroma-in-continuity using sural nerve graft. Microsurgery. 2013;33(2):160–3.
59. Giuffre JL, Bishop AT, Spinner RJ, Shin AY. Surgical technique of a partial tibial nerve transfer to the tibialis anterior motor branch for the treatment of peroneal nerve injury. Ann Plast Surg. 2012;69(1):48–53. https://doi.org/10.1097/SAP.0b013e31824c94e5.
60. Titolo P, Panero B, Ciclamini D, Battiston B, Tos P. New tendon transfer for correction of drop-foot in common peroneal nerve palsy. Clin Orthop Relat Res. 2013;471(10):3382. https://doi.org/10.1007/s11999-013-3175-4.
61. Tarabay B, Abdallah Y, Kobaiter-Maarrawi S, Yammine P, Maarrawi J. Outcome and prognosis of Microsurgicalompression in idiopathic severe common fibular nerve entrapment: prospective clinical study. World Neurosurg. 2019;126:e281–7.
62. Terzis JK, Kostas I. Outcomes with microsurgery of common peroneal nerve lesions. J Plast Reconstr Aesthet Surg. 2020;73(1):72–80. https://doi.org/10.1016/j.bjps.2019.02.031.
63. Horteur C, Forli A, Corcella D, Pailhé R, Lateur G, Saragaglia D. Short- and long-term results of common peroneal nerve injuries treated by neurolysis, direct suture or nerve graft. Eur J Orthop Surg Traumatol. 2019;29(4):893–8.
64. Garozzo D, Ferraresi S, Buffatti P. Surgical treatment of common peroneal nerve injuries: indications and results. A series of 62 cases. J Neurosurg Sci. 2004;48(3):105–12.
65. Ferraresi S, Garozzo D, Buffatti P. Common peroneal nerve injuries: results with one-stage nerve repair and tendon transfer. Neurosurg Rev. 2003;26(3):175–9.
66. Irgit KS, Cush G. Tendon transfers for peroneal nerve injuries in the multiple ligament injured knee. J Knee Surg. 2012;25(4):327–33.

Chapter 66
Superficial Peroneal Nerve Dysfunction

This is a condition where there is impairment in the function of the superficial peroneal nerve (SPN), involving its motor, sensory component or both. Recognition of the anatomy of the SPN is essential in explaining the clinical findings in nerve dysfunction, as well as in minimising the risk of damage to the nerve during surgical interventions of the knee and lower leg.

66.1 Causes of Superficial Peroneal Nerve Dysfunction

Lesions of the SPN may be defined as intrinsic or extrinsic [1–23]:

- Intrinsic
  - Neuritis
  - Systemic disorders (e.g. diabetes, alcohol abuse)
  - Neurological (Charcot Marie Tooth disease)
- Extrinsic
  - Compression
  - Traction
  - Laceration

Causes of extrinsic lesions include:

C. Panayiotou Charalambous, *The Knee Made Easy*,
https://doi.org/10.1007/978-3-030-54506-2_66

Compression

- Mass lesions (ganglia arising from the proximal tibiofibular joint)
- Displaced knee fractures (tibia, fibula)
- At emergence through lower limb deep fascia, muscle herniations
- Ankle fractures

Traction

- By a dislocated tibiofemoral or proximal tibiofibular joint

Laceration

- Penetrating trauma—stab wounds
- Displaced knee fractures (tibia/fibula)
- Surgery:
  - Open (posterolateral corner ligamentous surgery, tibial fracture fixation, fasciotomy) [24]
  - Arthroscopic (meniscal repairs)
  - Ankle surgery (fixation of distal fibular fractures, ankle joint surgery-open or arthroscopic)

66.2 Clinical Symptoms of SPN Dysfunction

- Neurogenic pain in the lower leg and dorsum of foot
- Foot weakness
- Sensory disturbance (reduced/altered/absent) —over the dorsum of the foot excluding dorsum of first web space

66.3 Clinical Signs of SPN Dysfunction

- Weakness of the peroneal muscles—foot eversion
- Muscle wasting
- Sensory disturbance around the lower leg and foot (over the dorsum of the foot excluding dorsum of first web space)

66.4 Investigations for Superficial Peroneal Nerve Dysfunction [25, 26]

- Plain radiographs
- Ultrasound
- MRI
  - Look for compressive cause of the nerve due to a space occupying lesion, peroneal muscle wasting/fatty infiltration
  - Evaluate other causes of leg weakness such as nerve root compromise at the lumbosacral spine, common peroneal nerve or sciatic nerve
- Electromyography looking for muscle denervation
- Nerve conduction studies

66.5 Management of Superficial Peroneal Nerve Dysfunction [27–29]

- Expectant, await recovery
- Control pain and maintain passive motion
- Surgical exploration if recovery does not occur within about 3 months:
  - Nerve decompression
  - Nerve repair, cable grafting, nerve transfer

References

1. Haddad SF, Harrington M, Adams C, Arain A, Czajka C. Acute superficial Peroneal nerve entrapment mimicking compartment syndrome: a case report. JBJS Case Connect. 2019;9(4):e0137. https://doi.org/10.2106/JBJS.CC.19.00137.
2. Malagelada F, Vega J, Guelfi M, Kerkhoffs G, Karlsson J, Dalmau-Pastor M. Anatomic lectures on structures at risk prior to cadaveric courses reduce injury to the superficial peroneal nerve, the commonest complication in ankle arthroscopy. Knee Surg Sports Traumatol Arthrosc. 2020;28(1):79–85.
3. Maselli F, Testa M. Superficial peroneal nerve schwannoma presenting as lumbar radicular syndrome in a non-competitive runner. J Back Musculoskelet Rehabil. 2019;32(2):361–5.
4. de Bruijn JA, van Zantvoort APM, Hundscheid HPH, Hoogeveen AR, Teijink JAW, Scheltinga MR. Superficial Peroneal nerve injury risk during a semiblind fasciotomy for anterior chronic exertional compartment syndrome of the leg: an anatomical and clinical study. Foot Ankle Int. 2019;40(3):343–51.
5. Paolasso I, Cambise C, Coraci D, Del Tedesco FM, Erra C, Fernandez E, Padua L. Tibialis anterior muscle herniation with superficial peroneal nerve involvement: ultrasound role for diagnosis and treatment. Clin Neurol Neurosurg. 2016;151:6–8.
6. Kang J, Yang P, Zang Q, He X. Traumatic neuroma of the superficial peroneal nerve in a patient: a case report and review of the literature. World J Surg Oncol. 2016;14(1):242. https://doi.org/10.1186/s12957-016-0990-6.

7. Corey RM, Salazar DH. Entrapment of the superficial Peroneal nerve following a distal fibula fracture. Foot Ankle Spec. 2017;10(1):69–71.
8. Bregman PJ, Schuenke M. Current diagnosis and treatment of superficial fibular nerve injuries and entrapment. Clin Podiatr Med Surg. 2016;33(2):243–54.
9. Ribak S, da Silva Filho PR, Tietzmann A, Hirata HH, de Mattos CA, da Gama SA. Use of superficial peroneal nerve graft for treating peripheral nerve injuries. Rev Bras Ortop. 2016;51(1):63–9.
10. McAlister JE, DeMill SL, Hyer CF, Berlet GC. Anterior Approach Total Ankle Arthroplasty: Superficial Peroneal Nerve Branches at Risk. J Foot Ankle Surg. 2016;55(3):476–9.
11. Martin D, Dowling J, Rowan F, Casey M, O'Grady P. Superficial peroneal nerve paresis in a dancer caused by a midfoot ganglion: case report. J Dance Med Sci. 2015;19(2):77–9.
12. Ellanti P, Mohamed KM, O'Shea K. Superficial Peroneal Nerve Incarceration in the Fibular Fracture Site of a Pronation External Rotation Type Ankle Fracture. Open Orthop J. 2015;9:214–7.
13. Tzika M, Paraskevas G, Natsis K. Entrapment of the superficial peroneal nerve: an anatomical insight. J Am Podiatr Med Assoc. 2015;105(2):150–9.
14. Ang CL, Foo LS. Multiple locations of nerve compression: an unusual cause of persistent lower limb paresthesia. J Foot Ankle Surg. 2014;53(6):763–7.
15. Maurya PK, Kulshreshtha D, Singh AK, Thacker AK, Malhotra KP. Isolated superficial peroneal neuropathy: a rare presentation of Hansen's disease (leprosy). QJM. 2015;108(5):419.
16. Nguyen JT, Nguyen JL, Wheatley MJ, Nguyen TA. Muscle hernias of the leg: a case report and comprehensive review of the literature. Can J Plast Surg. 2013 Winter;21(4):243–7.
17. Halm JA, Schepers T. Damage to the superficial peroneal nerve in operative treatment of fibula fractures: straight to the bone? Case report and review of the literature. J Foot Ankle Surg. 2012;51(5):684–6.
18. Anandkumar S. Physical therapy management of entrapment of the superficial peroneal nerve in the lower leg: a case report. Physiother Theory Pract. 2012;28(7):552–61.
19. Suzangar M, Rosenfeld P. Ankle arthroscopy: is preoperativeking of the superficial peroneal nerve important? J Foot Ankle Surg. 2012;51(2):179–81.
20. Ozsoy MH. Percutaneous plating of the distal tibia and fibula: risk of injury to the saphenous and superficial peroneal nerves. J Orthop Trauma. 2011;25(9):e95. author reply e95. https://doi.org/10.1097/BOT.0b013e31822c58b1.
21. Mirza A, Moriarty AM, Probe RA, Ellis TJ. Percutaneous plating of the distal tibia and fibula: risk of injury to the saphenous and superficial peroneal nerves. J Orthop Trauma. 2010;24(8):495–8.
22. Terrence Jose Jerome J. Superficial peroneal nerve lipoma. Romanian J Morphol Embryol. 2009;50(1):137–9.
23. Sevinç TT, Kalaci A, Doğramaci Y, Yanat AN. Bilateral superficial peroneal nerve entrapment secondary to anorexia nervosa: a case report. J Brachial Plex Peripher Nerve Inj. 2008;3:12. https://doi.org/10.1186/1749-7221-3-12.
24. Ogrodnik J. Superficial Peroneal Nerve Injured During Fasciotomy: A Successful Repair with Cadaveric Nerve Allograft. Am Surg. 2018;84(2):e59–60.
25. Nwawka OK, Lee S, Miller TT. Sonographic evaluation of superficial Peroneal nerve abnormalities. AJR Am J Roentgenol. 2018;211(4):872–9.
26. Tong O, Bieri P, Herskovitz S. Nerve entrapments related to muscle herniation. Muscle Nerve. 2019;60(4):428–33.
27. Daghino W, Pasquali M, Faletti C. Superficial peroneal nerve entrapment in a young athlete: the diagnostic contribution of magnetic resonance imaging. J Foot Ankle Surg. 1997;36(3):170–2.
28. Guo D, Guo D, Harrison R, McCool L, Wang H, Tonkin B, Kliot M. A cadaveric study using the ultra-minimally invasive thread transection technique toompress the superficial peroneal nerve in the lower leg. Acta Neurochir. 2019;161(10):2133–9.
29. Matsumoto J, Isu T, Kim K, Iwamoto N, Yamazaki K, Isobe M. Clinical Features and Surgical Treatment of Superficial Peroneal Nerve Entrapment Neuropathy. Neurol Med Chir (Tokyo). 2018;58(7):320–5.

Chapter 67
Deep Peroneal Nerve Dysfunction

This is a condition where there is impairment in the function of the deep peroneal nerve, involving its motor, sensory component or both. This may be complete involving the main nerve trunk, or partial involving one or more of its branches. Recognition of the anatomy of the deep peroneal nerve is essential in explaining the clinical findings in nerve dysfunction, as well as in minimising the risk of damage to the nerve during surgical interventions of the knee or lower leg and foot.

67.1 Causes of Deep Peroneal Nerve Dysfunction

Lesions of the deep peroneal nerve may be defined as intrinsic or extrinsic [1–16]:

- Intrinsic
  - Neuritis
  - Systemic disorders (e.g. diabetes, alcohol abuse)
  - Neurological (Charcot Marie Tooth disease)
- Extrinsic
  - Compression
  - Traction
  - Laceration

Causes of extrinsic lesions include:

Compression
- Mass lesions
- Displaced knee fractures

C. Panayiotou Charalambous, *The Knee Made Easy*,
https://doi.org/10.1007/978-3-030-54506-2_67

Traction
- By a dislocated tibiofemoral or proximal tibiofibular joint

Laceration
- Penetrating trauma—stab wounds
- Displaced knee fractures (tibia/fibula)
- Surgery:
  - Open (posterolateral corner ligamentous surgery)
  - Arthroscopic (meniscal repairs)
  - Tibial/foot surgery

67.2 Clinical Symptoms of Deep Peroneal Nerve Dysfunction

- Foot drop
- Neurogenic pain in the knee area
- Leg weakness
- Sensory disturbance (reduced/altered/absent) —over the dorsal first web space of the foot

67.3 Clinical Signs of Deep Peroneal Nerve Dysfunction

- Weakness of lower leg muscles ankle and foot extensors—foot drop, big toe drop, weakness of foot inversion
- Muscle wasting
- Sensory disturbance—over the dorsal first web space of the foot

67.4 Investigations for Deep Peroneal Nerve Dysfunction

- Plain radiographs
- Ultrasound
- MRI
  - Look for compressive cause of the nerve due to a space occupying lesion
  - Evaluate other causes of leg weakness such as nerve root compromise at the lumbosacral spine, common peroneal nerve or sciatic nerve

- Electromyography looking for muscle denervation
- Nerve conduction studies

67.5 Management of Deep Peroneal Nerve Dysfunction [17–21]

- Expectant, await recovery
- Control pain and maintain passive motion
- Surgical exploration if recovery does not occur within about 3 months:
  - Nerve decompression
  - Nerve repair, cable grafting, nerve transfer
  - Tendon transfers

References

1. Ciucci G, Callegarini C, Stumpo M, Poppi M. Ganglionic cyst of the deep peroneal nerve: description of a case. Ital J Neurol Sci. 1996;17(1):83–6.
2. Lu H, Chen L, Jiang S, Shen H. A rapidly progressive foot drop caused by the posttraumatic Intraneural ganglion cyst of the deep peroneal nerve. BMC Musculoskelet Disord. 2018;19(1):298. https://doi.org/10.1186/s12891-018-2229-x.
3. Demiroğlu M, Özkan K, Kılıç B, Akçal A, Akkaya M, Özkan FÜ. Deep peroneal nerve palsy due to osteochondroma arising from fibular head and proximal lateral tibia. Int J Surg Case Rep. 2017;31:200–2.
4. Nikolopoulos D, Safos G, Sergides N, Safos P. Deep peroneal nerve palsy caused by an extraneural ganglion cyst: a rare case. Case Rep Orthop. 2015;2015:861697.
5. Itoh M, Itou J, Kuwashima U, Fujieda H, Okazaki K. Deep peroneal nerve injury during plate fixation for medial open-wedge high tibial osteotomy: A case report and cadaveric study. Clin Case Rep. 2019;7(11):2225–30.
6. Genç B, Solak A, Kalaycıoğlu S, Şahin N. Distal tibial osteochondroma causing fibular deformity and deep peroneal nerve entrapment neuropathy: a case report. Acta Orthop Traumatol Turc. 2014;48(4):463–6.
7. Jeong JH, Chang MC, Lee SA. Deep peroneal nerve palsy after opening wedge high tibial osteotomy: a case report. Medicine (Baltimore). 2019;98(27):e16253. https://doi.org/10.1097/MD.0000000000016253.
8. Tan ET, Tan TJ, Poon KB. Entrapment of the deep peroneal nerve and anterior tibial vessels by a spiral tibial fracture causing partial non-union: a case report. Skelet Radiol. 2016;45(4):551–4.
9. Yıldırım E, Sarıkaya İA, İnan M. Unusual entrapment of deep peroneal nerve after femoral distal extension osteotomy. J Pediatr Orthop B. 2015;24(5):440–3.
10. Erdil M, Ozkan K, Ozkan FU, Bilsel K, Turkmen I, Senol S, Sarar S. A rare cause of deep peroneal nerve palsy due to compression of synovial cyst - case report. Int J Surg Case Rep. 2013;4(5):515–7.
11. Hey HW, Tan TC, Lahiri A, Wilder-Smith EP, Kumar VP, Kagda FH, Lim AY. Deep peroneal nerve entrapment by a spiral fibular fracture: a case report. J Bone Joint Surg Am. 2011;93(19):e113(1–5).
12. Lui TH, Chan LK. Deep peroneal nerve injury following external fixation of the ankle: case report and anatomic study. Foot Ankle Int. 2011;32(5):S550–5.

13. Ahmad I, Patil S. Isolated deep peroneal (fibular) nerve palsy in association with primary total hip arthroplasty. Clin Anat. 2007;20(6):703–4.
14. Rubin DI, Nottmeier E, Blasser KE, Peterson JJ, Kennelly K. Acute onset of deep peroneal neuropathy during a golf game resulting from a ganglion cyst. J Clin Neuromuscul Dis. 2004;6(2):49–53.
15. Brestas P, Protopsaltis I, Drossos C. Role of sonography in the diagnosis and treatment of a ganglion cyst compressing the lateral branch of deep peroneal nerve. J Clin Ultrasound. 2017;45(2):108–11.
16. De Maeseneer M, Madani H, Lenchik L, Kalume Brigido M, Shahabpour M, Celis S, de Mey J, Scafoglieri A. Normal Anatomy and Compression Areas of Nerves of the Foot and Ankle: US and MR Imaging with Anatomic Correlation. Radiographics. 2015;35(5):1469–82.
17. Wood MB. Peroneal nerve repair. Surgical results. Clin Orthop Relat Res. 1991;267:206–10.
18. Giuffre JL, Bishop AT, Spinner RJ, Levy BA, Shin AY. Partial tibial nerve transfer to the tibialis anterior motor branch to treat peroneal nerve injury after knee trauma. Clin Orthop Relat Res. 2012;470(3):779–90.
19. Wu CC, Tai CL. Anterior transfer of tibialis posterior tendon for treating drop foot: technique of enforcing tendon implantation to improve success rate. Acta Orthop Belg. 2015;81(1):147–54.
20. Cohen JC, de Freitas Cabral E. Peroneus longus transfer for drop foot in Hansen disease. Foot Ankle Clin. 2012;17(3):425–36.
21. Kihm CA, Camasta CA. Review of Drop Hallux: Assessment and Surgical Repair. J Foot Ankle Surg. 2017;56(1):103–7.

Chapter 68
Tibial Nerve Dysfunction

This is a condition where there is impairment in the function of the tibial nerve, involving its motor, sensory component or both. This may be complete involving the main nerve trunk, or partial involving one or more of its branches. Recognition of the anatomy of the tibial nerve is essential in explaining the clinical findings in nerve dysfunction, as well as in minimising the risk of damage to the nerve during surgical interventions of the knee and tibia.

68.1 Causes of Tibial Nerve Dysfunction

Lesions of the tibial nerve may be defined as intrinsic or extrinsic [1–27]:

- Intrinsic
  - Neuritis
  - Systemic disorders (e.g. diabetes, alcohol abuse)
  - Neurological
- Extrinsic
  - Compression
  - Traction
  - Laceration

Causes of extrinsic lesions include:

C. Panayiotou Charalambous, *The Knee Made Easy*,
https://doi.org/10.1007/978-3-030-54506-2_68

Compression
- Popliteal aneurysm in popliteal fossa
- Displaced knee fractures/tibial fractures

Traction
- By a dislocated tibiofemoral joint

Laceration
- Penetrating trauma—stab wounds
- Displaced knee fractures
- Surgery—to posterior part of the knee, tibia, lower leg, ankle

68.2 Clinical Symptoms of Tibial Nerve Dysfunction

- Neurogenic pain in the knee or lower limb
- Leg weakness
- Sensory disturbance (reduced/altered/absent)—over the plantar aspect of the foot

68.3 Clinical Signs of Tibial Nerve Dysfunction

- Weakness of lower leg muscles ankle and toe plantar flexors
- Weakness of tibialis posterior—week foot inversion
- Muscle wasting
- Sensory disturbance on plantar aspect of the foot

68.4 Investigations for Tibial Nerve Dysfunction

- Plain radiographs
- Ultrasound
- MRI
  - Look for compressive cause for the nerve due to a space occupying lesion
  - Evaluate other causes of leg weakness such as nerve root compromise at the lumbosacral spine, or sciatic nerve
- Electromyography looking for muscle denervation
- Nerve conduction studies

68.5 Management of Tibial Nerve Dysfunction [28–32]

- Expectant, await recovery
- Control pain and maintain passive motion
- Surgical exploration if recovery does not occur within about 3 months:
  - Nerve decompression
  - Nerve repair, cable grafting, nerve transfer

References

1. Badr IT, Hassan S, Fotoh DS, Moawad MM. Extrinsic compression neuropathy of the tibial nerve secondary to accessory soleus muscle in a young teenager. J Clin Orthop Trauma. 2020;11(2):302–6.
2. Buchanan V, Rawat M. Schwannoma of the posterior Tibial nerve. J Orthop Sports Phys Ther. 2020;50(2):111.
3. Falovic R, Nambiar M, Boekel P, Lenaghan J. Varicose veins causing tibial nerve compression in the tarsal tunnel. BMJ Case Rep. 2019;12(5). pii: e230072 https://doi.org/10.1136/bcr-2019-230072.
4. Moretti E, da Silva IB, Boaviagem A, Barbosa L, de Lima AMJ, Lemos A. "posterior Tibial nerve" or "Tibial nerve"? Improving the reporting in health papers. Neurourol Urodyn. 2020;39(2):847–53.
5. Hashimoto K, Nishimura S, Fujii K, Kakinoki R, Akagi M. Intraneural synovial sarcoma of the tibial nerve. Rare Tumors. 2018;10:2036361318776495.
6. Nam SH, Kim JY, Ahn J, Park Y. Plexiform Neurofibroma of the Posterior Tibial Nerve Misdiagnosed as Proximal Tarsal Tunnel Syndrome: A Case Report. Surg J (N Y). 2018;4(1):e18–22.
7. Bernardi G, Tudisco C. Transient Common Peroneal and Tibial Nerve Palsy Following Knee Arthroscopy for the Treatment of Discoid Lateral Meniscus. Joints. 2017;5(2):118–20.
8. Moussa A, Chakhachiro Z, Sawaya RA. Posterior Tibial Nerve Lymphoma Presenting as Tarsal Tunnel Syndrome: A Case Report. J Foot Ankle Surg. 2018;57(1):167–9.
9. Silveira CRS, Vieira CGM, Pereira BM, Pinto Neto LH, Chhabra A. Cystic degeneration of the tibial nerve: magnetic resonance neurography and sonography appearances of an intraneural ganglion cyst. Skelet Radiol. 2017;46(12):1763–7.
10. Scacchi P, Gousopoulos L, Juon B, Ahmed S, Krause FG. Tibial nerve palsy by a crossing posterior Tibial artery branch after lateral sliding calcaneal osteotomy. Foot Ankle Int. 2017;38(5):580–3.
11. Shin YS, Sim HB, Yoon JR. Tibial nerve neuropathy following medial opening-wedge high tibial osteotomy-case report of a rare technical complication. Eur J Orthop Surg Traumatol. 2017;27(4):563–7.
12. Murphy AD, Chan M, Fairbank SM. Tibial nerve palsy as the presenting feature of posterior tibial artery pseudoaneurysm. ANZ J Surg. 2018;88(11):1206–8.
13. Krzywosinski TB, Bingham AL, Fallat LM. Intraneural lipoma of the tibial nerve: a case report. J Foot Ankle Surg. 2017;56(1):125–8.
14. Reddy CG, Amrami KK, Howe BM, Spinner RJ. Combined common peroneal and tibial nerve injury after knee dislocation: one injury or two? An MRI-clinical correlation. Neurosurg Focus. 2015;39(3):E8. https://doi.org/10.3171/2015.6.FOCUS15125.

15. Palit V, Paddle A, Rozen WM, Fairbank S, McCombe D. Case of knee pain in a child: intraneural ganglion of the tibial nerve. J Paediatr Child Health. 2015;51(7):727–30. https://doi.org/10.1111/jpc.12851.
16. Ladak A, Spinner RJ, Amrami KK, Howe BM. MRI findings in patients with tibial nerve compression near the knee. Skelet Radiol. 2013;42(4):553–9.
17. Milnes HL, Pavier JC. Schwannoma of the tibial nerve sheath as a cause of tarsal tunnel syndrome--a case study. Foot (Edinb). 2012;22(3):243–6.
18. Williams EH, Rosson GD, Hagan RR, Hashemi SS, Dellon AL. Soleal sling syndrome (proximal tibial nerve compression): results of surgicalompression. Plast Reconstr Surg. 2012;129(2):454–62.
19. Cugat R, Ares O, Cuscó X, Garcia M, Samitier G, Seijas R. Posterior tibial nerve lesions in ankle arthroscopy. Arch Orthop Trauma Surg. 2008;128(5):485–7.
20. Ji JH, Shafi M, Kim WY, Park SH, Cheon JO. Compressive neuropathy of the tibial nerve and peroneal nerve by a Baker's cyst: case report. Knee. 2007;14(3):249–52.
21. Adn M, Hamlat A, Morandi X, Guegan Y. Intraneural ganglion cyst of the tibial nerve. Acta Neurochir. 2006;148(8):885–9.
22. Tseng KF, Hsu HC, Wang FC, Fong YC. Nerve sheath ganglion of the tibial nerve presenting as a Baker's cyst: a case report. Knee Surg Sports Traumatol Arthrosc. 2006;14(9):880–4.
23. Sansone V, Sosio C, da Gama MM, de Ponti A. Two cases of tibial nerve compression caused by uncommon popliteal cysts. Arthroscopy. 2002;18(2):E8.
24. Leblebicioglu G, Atay A, Doral MN, Dogan R, Yilmaz M. Neurilemoma of the tibial nerve causing intermittent claudication. Case report. Am J Knee Surg. 2001 Summer;14(3):181–3.
25. Mastaglia FL. Tibial nerve entrapment in the popliteal fossa. Muscle Nerve. 2000;23(12):1883–6.
26. Oh SJ, Meyer RD. Entrapment neuropathies of the tibial (posterior tibial) nerve. Neurol Clin. 1999;17(3):593–615.
27. Whiteley MS, Smith JJ, Galland RB. Tibial nerve damage during subfascial endoscopic perforator vein surgery. Br J Surg. 1997;84(4):512.
28. Higgins TF, DeLuca PA, Ariyan S. Salvage of open tibial fracture with segmental loss of tibial nerve: case report and review of the literature. J Orthop Trauma. 1999;13(5):380–5.
29. Ducic I, Felder JM 3rd. Tibial nerveompression: reliable exposure using shorter incisions. Microsurgery. 2012;32(7):533–8.
30. De Maeseneer M, Madani H, Lenchik L, Kalume Brigido M, Shahabpour M, Celis S, de Mey J, Scafoglieri A. Normal anatomy and compression areas of nerves of the foot and ankle: US and MR imaging with anatomic correlation. Radiographics. 2015;35(5):1469–82.
31. Murovic JA. Lower-extremity peripheral nerve injuries: a Louisiana State University health sciences center literature review with comparison of the operative outcomes of 806 Louisiana State University health sciences center sciatic, common peroneal, and tibial nerve lesions. Neurosurgery. 2009;65(4 Suppl):A18–23.
32. Kim DH, Ryu S, Tiel RL, Kline DG. Surgical management and results of 135 tibial nerve lesions at the Louisiana State University health sciences center. Neurosurgery. 2003;53(5):1114–24.

Chapter 69
Saphenous Nerve Dysfunction

This is a condition where there is impairment in the function of the saphenous nerve, which is a pure sensory nerve. This may be complete involving the main nerve trunk, or partial involving one or more of its branches. Recognition of the anatomy of the saphenous nerve is essential in explaining the clinical findings in nerve dysfunction, as well as in minimising the risk of damage to the nerve during surgical interventions of the knee and lower leg.

69.1 Causes of Saphenous Nerve Dysfunction

Lesions of the saphenous nerve may be defined as intrinsic or extrinsic [1–21]:

- Intrinsic
  - Neuritis
  - Systemic disorders (e.g. diabetes, alcohol abuse)
  - Neurological
- Extrinsic
  - Compression
  - Traction
  - Laceration

Causes of extrinsic lesions include:

C. Panayiotou Charalambous, *The Knee Made Easy*,
https://doi.org/10.1007/978-3-030-54506-2_69

Compression
- By the femoral vessels (aberrant branches, aneurysms)
- Adductor canal entrapment—mass lesion
- As the nerve pierces the fascia between vastus medialis and adductor magnus (knee valgus or tibial internal rotation predisposing to this)
- External compression (knee braces, splints, surf board in surfers)
- Trapped in scar tissue as a result of surgery or trauma
- Trapped by suture material in meniscal repairs (posteromedial branches)
- Direct acute blunt trauma

Traction
- During knee surgery
- Displaced knee fractures/tibial fractures

Laceration
- Penetrating trauma—stab wounds
- Displaced knee/lower leg fractures
- Surgery—femoral artery surgery or catheterisation, saphenous vein harvesting, saphenous vein cut down, saphenous vein stripping or laser ablation, hamstring tendon harvesting, arthroscopic surgery, meniscal repair surgery

69.2 Clinical Symptoms of Saphenous Nerve Dysfunction

- May walk "stiff legged" to limit pain due to knee flexion
- Neurogenic pain in the knee and/or lower limb (medial aspect)
- Sensory disturbance (reduced/altered/absent/hyperalgesia) —over the medial aspect of the thigh, lower leg and anterior knee

69.3 Clinical Signs of Saphenous Nerve Dysfunction

- Light palpation along the course of the nerve causing
  - Tenderness
  - Sensory symptoms

- Tender adductor canal on palpation
- Altered sensation over the medial aspect of the thigh, lower leg and anterior knee, medial ankle, dorsum of foot (but not toes)
- Tinel's test positive at or distal to the site of dysfunction
- Palpable neuroma
- Complex regional pain syndrome (CRPS) signs—tenderness on light touch, skin discolouration
- Pain and sensory symptoms may radiate proximally to the groin
- Symptoms aggravated by hyperextension and abduction with the knee in flexion

69.4 Investigations for Saphenous Nerve Dysfunction [22, 23]

- Plain radiographs
- Ultrasound
- MRI
  - Look for compressive cause of the nerve due to a space occupying lesion
  - Evaluate other causes of nerve dysfunction such as nerve root compromise at the lumbosacral spine, or femoral nerve
- Ultrasound—evaluate nerve and guide diagnostic local anaesthetic injections
- Nerve conduction studies
- Electromyography to confirm no motor involvement
- Diagnostic local anaesthetic nerve block to determine if improvement in symptoms

69.5 Management of Saphenous Nerve Dysfunction [17–21, 24–26]

- Expectant, await recovery
- Control pain
- Physiotherapy
  - Maintain joint motion
  - Nerve mobilisation (gliding, stretching)
  - Myofascial release
  - Acupuncture
- Perineural injections
  - Steroid
  - Normal saline (hydrodissection)

- Neuro-ablation
  - Cryo-ablation
  - Pulsed radiofrequency
- Nerve blocks
- Surgical exploration if non-surgical measures fail and symptoms troublesome:
  - Nerve decompression
  - Neurolysis
  - Neuroma resection
  - Neurectomy

Learning Pearls

- The nerve is more susceptible to entrapment in the adductor canal or at the point of exit from the canal

References

1. Wisbech Vange S, Tranum-Jensen J, Krogsgaard MR. Gracilis tendon harvest may lead to both incisional and non-incisional saphenous nerve injuries. Knee Surg Sports Traumatol Arthrosc. 2020;28(3):969–74.
2. Cubas Farinha N, Livraghi S. Saphenous nerve schwannoma as a cause of vascular claudication - case report and review of the literature. Br J Neurosurg. 2018;13:1–4.
3. Bugelli G, Dell'Osso G, Bottai V, Celli F, Loggini B, Guido G, Giannotti S. Giant Schwannoma of the saphenous nerve in the distal thigh: a case report. Surg Technol Int. 2016;28:285–8.
4. de Padua VB, Nascimento PE, Silva SC, de Gusmão Canuto SM, Zuppi GN, de Carvalho SM. Saphenous nerve injury during harvesting of one or two hamstring tendons for anterior cruciate ligament reconstruction. Rev Bras Ortop. 2015;50(5):546–9.
5. Tertemiz O, Akçalı D, Köseoğlu BF, Ordu Gökkaya NK, Uçar M, Esen E, Babacan A, Özçakar L. Chronic unexplained thigh pain from saphenous nerve entrapment due to a leiomyoma. Pain Med. 2015;16(2):408–10.
6. Jaworucka-Kaczorowska A, Oszkinis G, Huber J, Wiertel-Krawczuk A, Gabor E, Kaczorowski P. Saphenous vein stripping surgical technique and frequency of saphenous nerve injury. Phlebology. 2015;30(3):210–6.
7. Henningsen MH, Jaeger P, Hilsted KL, Dahl JB. Prevalence of saphenous nerve injury after adductor-canal-blockade in patients receiving total knee arthroplasty. Acta Anaesthesiol Scand. 2013;57(1):112–7.
8. Flu HC, Breslau PJ, Hamming JF, Lardenoye JW. A prospective study of incidence of saphenous nerve injury after total great saphenous vein stripping. Dermatol Surg. 2008;34(10):1333–9.
9. Iizuka M, Yao R, Wainapel S. Saphenous nerve injury following medial knee joint injection: a case report. Arch Phys Med Rehabil. 2005;86(10):2062–5.
10. Pyne D, Jawad AS, Padhiar N. Saphenous nerve injury after fasciotomy for compartment syndrome. Br J Sports Med. 2003;37(6):541–2.
11. Kornbluth ID, Freedman MK, Sher L, Frederick RW. Femoral, saphenous nerve palsy after tourniquet use: a case report. Arch Phys Med Rehabil. 2003;84(6):909–11.
12. Widmer F, Gerster JC. Medial meniscal cyst imitating a tumor, with compression of the saphenous nerve. Rev Rhum Engl Ed. 1998;65(2):149–52.

13. Abram LJ, Froimson AI. Saphenous nerve injury. An unusual arthroscopic complication. Am J Sports Med. 1991;19(6):668–9.
14. Murayama K, Takeuchi T, Yuyama T. Entrapment of the saphenous nerve by branches of the femoral vessels. A report of two cases. J Bone Joint Surg Am. 1991;73(5):770–2.
15. Hemler DE, Ward WK, Karstetter KW, Bryant PM. Saphenous nerve entrapment caused by pes anserine bursitis mimicking stress fracture of the tibia. Arch Phys Med Rehabil. 1991;72(5):336–7.
16. Holme JB, Skajaa K, Holme K. Incidence of lesions of the saphenous nerve after partial or complete stripping of the long saphenous vein. Acta Chir Scand. 1990;156(2):145–8.
17. Worth RM, Kettelkamp DB, Defalque RJ, Duane KU. Saphenous nerve entrapment. A cause of medial knee pain. Am J Sports Med. 1984;12(1):80–1.
18. Romanoff ME, Cory PC Jr, Kalenak A, Keyser GC, Shall WK. Saphenous nerve entrapment at the adductor canal. Am J Sports Med. 1989;17(4):478–81.
19. Porr J, Chrobak K, Muir B. Entrapment of the saphenous nerve at the adductor canal affecting the infrapatellar branch - a report on two cases. J Can Chiropr Assoc. 2013;57(4):341–9.
20. Pendergrass TL, Moore JH. Saphenous neuropathy following medial knee trauma. J Orthop Sports Phys Ther. 2004;34(6):328–34.
21. Settergren R. Conservative management of a saphenous nerve entrapment in a female ultramarathon runner. J Bodyw Mov Ther. 2013;17(3):297–301.
22. Mumenthaler M, Schlaick H. Peripheral nerve lesions, diagnosis and therapy. New York, NY: Thieme Medical Publishers; 1991.
23. Tranier S, Durey A, Chevallier B, Liot F. Value of somatosensory evoked potentials in saphenous entrapment neuropathy. J Neurol Neurosurg Psychiatry. 1992;55(6):461–5.
24. Batistaki C, Saranteas T, Chloros G, Savvidou O. Ultrasound-guided Saphenous Nerve Block for Saphenous Neuralgia after Knee Surgery: Two Case Reports and Review of Literature. Indian J Orthop. 2019;53(1):208–12.
25. Watanabe K, Tokumine J, Lefor AK, Moriyama K, Yorozu T. Ultrasound-Guided Hydrodissection of an Entrapped Saphenous Nerve After Lower Extremity Varicose Vein Stripping: A Case Report. A A Pract. 2020;14(1):28–30.
26. Ulloa M, Coronel BM. Scar Tissue Causing Saphenous Nerve Entrapment: Percutaneous Scar Release and Fat Grafting. Plast Reconstr Surg Glob Open. 2017;5(9):e1495. https://doi.org/10.1097/GOX.0000000000001495.

Chapter 70
Infrapatellar Nerve Dysfunction

This is a condition where there is impairment in the function of the infrapatellar nerve (IPN), which is a pure sensory nerve. This may be complete involving the nerve, or partial involving one or more of its branches. Recognition of the anatomy of the IPN is essential in explaining the clinical findings in nerve dysfunction, as well as in minimising the risk of damage to the nerve during surgical interventions of the knee.

70.1 Causes of Infrapatellar Nerve Dysfunction

Lesions of the IPN nerve may be defined as intrinsic or extrinsic [1–14]:

- Intrinsic
  - Neuritis/idiopathic
  - Systemic disorders (e.g. diabetes, alcohol abuse)
  - Neurological
- Extrinsic
  - Compression
  - Traction
  - Laceration

Causes of extrinsic lesions include:

C. Panayiotou Charalambous, *The Knee Made Easy*,
https://doi.org/10.1007/978-3-030-54506-2_70

Compression

- Between sartorius and the medial femoral condyle
- Displaced knee fractures/tibial fractures
- Blunt trauma to the knee
- Compression by scar tissue following surgery

Traction

- By a dislocated tibiofemoral joint

Laceration

- Penetrating trauma—stab wounds
- Displaced knee fractures
- Surgery—knee arthroscopy, anterior approach to the knee (knee arthroplasty, pes anserinus tendon harvesting)

70.2 Clinical Symptoms of Infrapatellar Nerve Dysfunction

- Light palpation along the course of the nerve causing
  - Tenderness
  - Sensory symptoms
- Neurogenic pain around the anterior aspect of the knee
- Sensory disturbance (reduced/altered/absent) —over the anterior aspect of the knee

70.3 Clinical Signs of Infrapatellar Nerve Dysfunction

- Sensory disturbance on the anterior aspect of the knee
- Tinel's test positive at or distal to the site of dysfunction
- Palpable neuroma
- Complex regional pain syndrome (CRPS) signs—tenderness on light touch, skin discolouration

70.4 Investigations for Infrapatellar Nerve Dysfunction [15, 16]

- Plain radiographs
- Ultrasound
- MRI
  - Look for compressive cause of the nerve due to a space occupying lesion
  - Evaluate other causes of sensory disturbance, such as nerve root compromise at the lumbosacral spine, femoral or saphenous nerve
- Nerve conduction studies
- Electromyography to confirm no motor involvement

70.5 Management of Infrapatellar Nerve Dysfunction [17–20]

- Expectant, await recovery
- Control pain and maintain passive motion
- Physiotherapy
  - Maintain joint motion
  - Nerve mobilisation (gliding, stretching)
  - Myofascial release
  - Acupuncture
- Perineural injections
  - Steroid
  - Normal saline (hydrodissection)
- Neuro-ablation
  - Cryo-ablation
  - Pulsed radiofrequency
- Surgical exploration if non-surgical measures fail and symptoms troublesome:
  - Nerve decompression
  - Neurolysis
  - Neuroma resection
  - Nerve ablation

Learning Pearls

- Diagnosis is usually clinical, based on clinical findings and relevant medical history
- The nerve is susceptible to entrapment between sartorius and the medial femoral condyle
- Sensory changes due to IPN damage during total knee joint replacement arthroplasty (TKR) is a common occurrence and can interfere with patient satisfaction.
- A medial parapatellar incision may confer higher risk of injuring the nerve as compared to a midline or more laterally placed incision.
- James NF et al. [2] looked for the IPN in 76 knees having primary TKR using a standard midline skin incision with a medial parapatellar arthrotomy. The IPN was encountered in all knees with a mean distance of 2.82 cm (95% CI 2.58–3.06) distal to the inferior pole of the patella during the arthrotomy. They concluded that the IPN is routinely encountered by the general orthopaedic surgeon during a standard TKR medial parapatellar approach and hence is at risk of injury.
- Subramanian S et al. [21] reported that following TKR 81% of their patients had lateral skin flap numbness with only 19% having normal skin sensation around their scar. The size of the numb area was large in 73% of cases. Only 50% fully recovered from skin numbness at a two year follow up suggesting that in a large proportion the numbness is permanent.

References

1. van Dijk W, van Eerten P, Scheltinga M. Infrapatellar nerve damage: a neglected cause of severe localized leg pain. Unfallchirurg. 2020;123(Suppl 1):25–8.
2. James NF, Kumar AR, Wilke BK, Shi GG. Incidence of encountering the infrapatellar nerve branch of the saphenous nerve during a midline approach for total knee arthroplasty. J Am Acad Orthop Surg Glob Res Rev. 2019;3(12). pii: e19.00160 https://doi.org/10.5435/JAAOSGlobal-D-19-00160.
3. Mistry D, O'Meeghan C. Fate of the infrapatellar branch of the saphenous nerve post total knee arthroplasty. ANZ J Surg. 2005;75(9):822–4.
4. Xiang Y, Li Z, Yu P, Zheng Z, Feng B, Weng X. Neuroma of the Infrapatellar branch of the saphenous nerve following Total knee Arthroplasty: a case report. BMC Musculoskelet Disord. 2019;20(1):536. https://doi.org/10.1186/s12891-019-2934-0.
5. Kartus J, Movin T, Karlsson J. Donor-site morbidity and anterior knee problems after anterior cruciate ligament reconstruction using autografts. Arthroscopy. 2001;17(9):971–80.
6. Mochida H, Kikuchi S. Injury to infrapatellar branch of saphenous nerve in arthroscopic knee surgery. Clin Orthop Relat Res. 1995;320:88–94.
7. House JH, Ahmed K. Entrapment neuropathy of the infrapatellar branch of the saphenous nerve. Am J Sports Med. 1977;5(5):217–24.
8. Natsis K, Konstantinidis G, Geropoulos G, Totlis T, Lazaridis N, Tegos T. Transtendinous course of the infrapatellar branch of saphenous nerve. A contribution to the aetiology of entrapment neuropathy and modification of the existing classification. Folia Morphol (Warsz). 2016;75(4):481–5.

9. Grabowski R, Gobbi A, Zabierek S, Domzalski ME. Nonspecific Chronic Anteromedial Knee Pain Neuroma as a Cause of Infrapatellar Pain Syndrome: Case Study and Literature Review. Orthop J Sports Med. 2018;6(1):2325967117751042. https://doi.org/10.1177/2325967117751042.
10. Grassi A, Perdisa F, Samuelsson K, Svantesson E, Romagnoli M, Raggi F, Gaziano T, Mosca M, Ayeni O, Zaffagnini S. Association between incision technique for hamstring tendon harvest in anterior cruciate ligament reconstruction and the risk of injury to the infra-patellar branch of the saphenous nerve: a meta-analysis. Knee Surg Sports Traumatol Arthrosc. 2018;26(8):2410–23.
11. Koch G, Kling A, Ramamurthy N, Edalat F, Cazzato RL, Kahn JL, Garnon J, Clavert P. Anatomical risk evaluation of iatrogenic injury to the infrapatellar branch of the saphenous nerve during medial meniscus arthroscopic surgery. Surg Radiol Anat. 2017;39(6):611–8.
12. Leliveld MS, Kamphuis SJM, Verhofstad MHJ. An infrapatellar nerve block reduces knee pain in patients with chronic anterior knee pain after tibial nailing: a randomized, placebo-controlled trial in 34 patients. Acta Orthop. 2019;90(4):377–82.
13. Kim KT, Kim YK, Yoon JR, Ko Y, Chung ME. Reference value for infrapatellar branch of saphenous nerve conduction study: cadaveric and clinical study. Ann Rehabil Med. 2018;42(2):321–8.
14. Blazina ME, Cracchiolo A 3rd. Neurilemoma of the infrapatellar branch of the saphenous nerve. A case report. Clin Orthop Relat Res. 1968;60:213–5.
15. Bademkiran F, Obay B, Aydogdu I, Ertekin C. Sensory conduction study of the infrapatellar branch of the saphenous nerve. Muscle Nerve. 2007;35(2):224–7.
16. Ackmann T, Von Düring M, Teske W, Ackermann O, Muller P, Von Schulze Pellengahr C. Anatomy of the infrapatellar branch in relation to skin incisions and as the basis to treat neuropathic pain by cryodenervation. Pain Physician. 2014;17(3):E339–48.
17. Clendenen S, Greengrass R, Whalen J, O'Connor MI. Infrapatellar saphenous neuralgia after TKA can be improved with ultrasound-guided local treatments. Clin Orthop Relat Res. 2015;473(1):119–25.
18. Trescot AM, Brown MN, Karl HW. Infrapatellar saphenous neuralgia - diagnosis and treatment. Pain Physician. 2013;16(3):E315–24.
19. Hosahalli G, Sierakowski A, Venkatramani H, Sabapathy SR. Entrapment Neuropathy of the Infrapatellar Branch of the Saphenous Nerve: Treated by Partial Division of Sartorius. Indian J Orthop. 2017;51(4):474–6.
20. Harris JD, Fazalare JJ, Griesser MJ, Flanigan DC. Infrapatellar branch of saphenous neurectomy for painful neuroma: a case report. Am J Orthop (Belle Mead NJ). 2012;41(1):37–40.
21. Subramanian S, Lateef H, Massraf A. Cutaneous sensory loss following primary total knee arthroplasty. A two years follow-up study. Acta Orthop Belg. 2009;75(5):649–53.

Chapter 71
Sciatic Nerve Dysfunction

This is a condition where there is impairment in the function of the sciatic nerve, involving its motor, sensory component or both. This may be complete involving the main nerve trunk, or partial involving part of its components (most often the common peroneal component). Recognition of the anatomy of the sciatic nerve is essential in explaining the clinical findings in nerve dysfunction, as well as in minimising the risk of damage to the nerve during surgical interventions of the lower limb.

71.1 Causes of Sciatic Nerve Dysfunction

Lesions of the sciatic nerve may be defined as intrinsic or extrinsic [1–36]:

- Intrinsic
  - Neuritis/idiopathic
  - Systemic disorders (e.g. diabetes, alcohol abuse)
  - Neurological
- Extrinsic
  - Compression
  - Traction
  - Laceration

Causes of extrinsic lesions include:

Compression
- Piriformis syndrome
- Displaced fractures—knee/tibial, hip/femoral

C. Panayiotou Charalambous, *The Knee Made Easy*,
https://doi.org/10.1007/978-3-030-54506-2_71

- Blunt trauma to the knee
- Compression by scar tissue following surgery

Traction
- By a dislocated hip joint
- Hip or proximal femoral surgery

Laceration
- Penetrating trauma—stab wounds, injections into the gluteal region (avoid the lower medial quadrant)
- Displaced proximal femoral fractures
- Surgery—to the hip or femur

71.2 Clinical Symptoms of Sciatic Nerve Dysfunction

- Light palpation along the course of the nerve causing
  - Tenderness
  - Sensory symptoms
- Neurogenic pain
- Sensory disturbance (reduced/altered/absent)

71.3 Clinical Signs of Sciatic Nerve Dysfunction

- Sensory disturbance
- Tinel's test positive at or distal to the site of dysfunction

71.4 Investigations for Sciatic Nerve Dysfunction

- Plain radiographs
- Ultrasound
- MRI

- Look for compressive cause of the nerve due to a space occupying lesion (such as haematoma)
- Evaluate other causes of nerve dysfunction, such as nerve root compromise at the lumbosacral spine, lumbosacral plexus dysfunction

- Nerve conduction studies
- Electromyography to distinguish between a sciatic nerve, or more proximal or distal lesion

71.5 Management of Sciatic Nerve Dysfunction

- Expectant, await recovery
- Control pain and maintain passive motion
- Physiotherapy
  - Maintain joint motion
  - Nerve mobilisation (gliding, stretching)
  - Myofascial release
  - Acupuncture
- Surgical exploration if non-surgical measures fail and symptoms troublesome:
  - Nerve decompression
  - Neurolysis
  - Neuroma resection
  - Tendon transfers

References

1. Godkin O, Ellanti P, O'Toole G. Large schwannoma of the sciatic nerve. BMJ Case Rep. 2016;2016. pii: bcr2016217717 https://doi.org/10.1136/bcr-2016-217717.
2. Mezian K, Záhora R, Vacek J, Kozák J, Navrátil L. Sciatic nerve schwannoma in the gluteal region mimicking sciatica. Am J Phys Med Rehabil. 2017;96(7):e139–40.
3. Balaji G, Sriharsha Y, Sharma D. Delayed onset sciatic nerve palsy secondary to wound hematoma following anticoagulant therapy post-bipolar hemiarthroplasty - an uncommon complication: a case report. Malays Orthop J. 2019;13(2):49–51.
4. Macdonald J, McMahon SE, O'Longain D, Acton JD. Delayed sciatic nerve compression following hamstring injury. Eur J Orthop Surg Traumatol. 2018;28(2):305–8.
5. Kadioglu HH. Sciatic nerve injuries from gluteal intramuscular injection according to Records of the High Health Council. Turk Neurosurg. 2018;28(3):474–8.
6. Monteleone G, Stevanato G. Entrapment of the sciatic nerve at the linea aspera: A case report and literature review. Surg Neurol Int. 2016;7:89.
7. Burks SS, Levi DJ, Hayes S, Levi AD. Challenges in sciatic nerve repair: anatomical considerations. J Neurosurg. 2014;121(1):210–8.

8. Ditino A, Papapietro N, Denaro V. Sciatic nerve compression by a gluteal vein varicosity. Spine J. 2014;14(8):1797. https://doi.org/10.1016/j.spinee.2014.03.008.
9. Shim HY, Lim OK, Bae KH, Park SM, Lee JK, Park KD. Sciatic nerve injury caused by a stretching exercise in a trained dancer. Ann Rehabil Med. 2013;37(6):886–90.
10. Mert M, Oztürkmen Y, Unkar EA, Erdoğan S, Uzümcügil O. Sciatic nerve compression by an extrapelvic cyst secondary to wear debris after a cementless total hip arthroplasty: a case report and literature review. Int J Surg Case Rep. 2013;4(10):805–8.
11. Howe BM, Amrami KK, Nathan MA, Garcia JJ, Spinner RJ. Perineural spread of cervical cancer to the sciatic nerve. Skelet Radiol. 2013;42(11):1627–31.
12. Kayani B, Rahman J, Hanna SA, Cannon SR, Aston WJ, Miles J. Delayed sciatic nerve palsy following resurfacing hip arthroplasty caused by metal debris. BMJ Case Rep. 2012;2012. pii: bcr2012006856 https://doi.org/10.1136/bcr-2012-006856.
13. Telleria JJ, Safran MR, Harris AH, Gardi JN, Glick JM. Risk of sciatic nerve traction injury during hip arthroscopy—is it the amount or duration? An intraoperative nerve monitoring study. J Bone Joint Surg Am. 2012;94(22):2025–32.
14. Justice PE, Katirji B, Preston DC, Grossman GE. Piriformis syndrome surgery causing severe sciatic nerve injury. J Clin Neuromuscul Dis. 2012;14(1):45–7.
15. Yacoubian SV, Sah AP, Estok DM 2nd. Incidence of sciatic nerve palsy after revision hip arthroplasty through a posterior approach. J Arthroplast. 2010;25(1):31–4.
16. Beksaç BP, Della Valle AG, Salvati EA. Acute sciatic nerve palsy as a delayed complication of low-molecular-weight heparin prophylaxis after total hip arthroplasty. Am J Orthop (Belle Mead NJ). 2009;38(2):E28–30.
17. Turan Ilica A, Yasar E, Tuba Sanal H, Duran C, Guvenc I. Sciatic nerve compression due to femoral neck osteochondroma: MDCT and MR findings. Clin Rheumatol. 2008;27(3):403–4.
18. Weil Y, Mattan Y, Goldman V, Liebergall M. Sciatic nerve palsy due to hematoma after thrombolysis therapy for acute pulmonary embolism after total hip arthroplasty. J Arthroplast. 2006;21(3):456–9.
19. Sosna A, Pokorny D, Jahoda D. Sciatic nerve palsy after total hip replacement. J Bone Joint Surg Br. 2005;87(8):1140–1.
20. Austin MS, Klein GR, Sharkey PF, Hozack WJ, Rothman RH. Late sciatic nerve palsy caused by hematoma after primary total hip arthroplasty. J Arthroplast. 2004;19(6):790–2.
21. Vardi G. Sciatic nerve injury following hamstring harvest. Knee. 2004;11(1):37–9.
22. Crawford JR, Van Rensburg L, XC. Compression of the sciatic nerve by wear debris following total hip replacement: a report of three cases. J Bone Joint Surg Br. 2003;85(8):1178–80.
23. Pego-Reigosa R, Brañas-Fernández F, Garcia-Porrua C, Gonzalez-Gay MA. Sciatic nerve palsy as presenting sign of a perianal abscess. Joint Bone Spine. 2003;70(1):85–6.
24. Cai C, Kamath A, Nesathurai S. Traumatic sciatic nerve contusion. J Back Musculoskelet Rehabil. 2000;15(2):89–92.
25. Kim DH, Murovic JA, Tiel R, Kline DG. Management and outcomes in 353 surgically treated sciatic nerve lesions. J Neurosurg. 2004;101(1):8–17.
26. Robertson CM, Robertson RF, Strazerri JC. Proximal dissection of a popliteal cyst with sciatic nerve compression. Orthopedics. 2003;26(12):1231–2.
27. Tomaino MM. Complete sciatic nerve palsy after open femur fracture: successful treatment with neurolysis 6 months after injury. Am J Orthop (Belle Mead NJ). 2002;31(10):585–8.
28. Lee WY, Hwang DS, Kang C, Zheng L. Entrapment neuropathy of the sciatic nerve caused by a paralabral cyst: three cases treated arthroscopically: a case report. JBJS Case Connect. 2016;6(4):e82. https://doi.org/10.2106/JBJS.CC.16.00064.
29. Puliero B, Blakeney WG, Beaulieu Y, Roy A, Vendittoli PA. Distal femoral shortening osteotomy for treatment of sciatic nerve palsy after total hip arthroplasty - a report of 3 cases. Acta Orthop. 2018;89(6):696–8.
30. Yoon SJ, Park MS, Matsuda DK, Choi YH. Endoscopic resection of acetabular screw tip toompress sciatic nerve following total hip arthroplasty. BMC Musculoskelet Disord. 2018;19(1):184.

31. Aguilera-Bohorquez B, Cardozo O, Brugiatti M, Cantor E, Valdivia N. Endoscopic treatment of sciatic nerve entrapment in deep gluteal syndrome: clinical results. Rev Esp Cir Ortop Traumatol. 2018;62(5):322–7.
32. Kay J, de Sa D, Morrison L, Fejtek E, Simunovic N, Tin HD, Ayeni OR. Surgical Management of Deep Gluteal Syndrome Causing Sciatic Nerve Entrapment: a systematic review. Arthroscopy. 2017;33(12):2263–78.
33. Xu LW, Veeravagu A, Azad TD, Harraher C, Ratliff JK. Delayed presentation of sciatic nerve injury after total hip arthroplasty: neurosurgical considerations, diagnosis, and management. J Neurol Surg Rep. 2016;77(3):e134–8.
34. Park MS, Yoon SJ, GSY, Kim SH. Clinical results of endoscopic sciatic nerveompression for deep gluteal syndrome: mean 2-year follow-up. BMC Musculoskelet Disord. 2016;17:218.
35. Son BC, Kim DR, Jeun SS, Lee SW. Ompression of the sciatic nerve entrapment caused by post-inflammatory scarring. J Korean Neurosurg Soc. 2015;57(2):123–6.
36. Martin HD, Shears SA, Johnson JC, Smathers AM, Palmer IJ. The endoscopic treatment of sciatic nerve entrapment/deep gluteal syndrome. Arthroscopy. 2011;27(2):172–81.

Chapter 72
Myofascial Trigger Points of the Knee

A condition whereby there are areas of discreet bands of taut skeletal muscle or fascia that may give rise to pain and other clinical symptoms and which are tender on palpation. Tender spots may also reflect areas within the muscle which are hypersensitive secondary to muscle overload (abnormal posture, overuse, trauma) [1–3].

72.1 Clinical Symptoms of Myofasial Trigger Points

- Localised muscle or fascial pain, exacerbated by movements of the knee
- Common areas around the knee [4–10] are:
  - Quadriceps
  - Hamstrings
  - Gastrocnemius heads
  - Iliotibial band
- Referred pain distant to the tender spot (may thus mimic neuropathic pain, radiculopathies)—however, the distribution of pain referred from a trigger spot does not follow a specific nerve pattern
- Apparent stiffness or weakness of the lower limb
- Autonomic phenomena—sweating, erythema
- Altered sensation, increased sensitivity to pain (hyperalgesia), pain on light touch

72.2 Clinical Signs of Myofascial Trigger Points

- Tender muscular or fascial spots that on palpation cause pain reproducing the clinical symptoms (including any referred pain)
- Apparent muscle weakness or knee stiffness due to pain
- Pain worsened by stretching the involved muscle or fascia

C. Panayiotou Charalambous, *The Knee Made Easy*,
https://doi.org/10.1007/978-3-030-54506-2_72

72.3 Investigations for Myofasial Trigger Points

- These aim to exclude other causes:
  - Plain radiographs, ultrasound, MRI
  - Nerve conduction studies

72.4 Management of Myofascial Trigger Points [11–20]

- Leave alone
- Inactivate tender points
- Eliminate any causative factors
- Physiotherapy:
  - Manual techniques (compression on the trigger point or massage)
  - Gradual stretching of the involved muscle
  - Postural correction
  - Relaxation of tense muscles
  - Core strengthening
- Injection
  - Dry needling acupuncture
  - Normal saline
  - Local anaesthetic
  - Steroid
  - Botulinum toxin
- Ultrasound
- TENS
- Skin cooling
- Local heat treatment

Learning Pearls

- The diagnosis of myofascial trigger points is clinical and must be considered when dealing with the painful knee, especially in the presence of normal radiological findings
- Referred pain may have a neurological source but may also originate from trigger points
- It has been shown that a substantial number of patients with knee osteoarthritis (OA) have trigger points and that treatment of these may result in a substantial improvement in pain

- Henry R et al. [10] studied the presence of myofascial pain in 25 arthritis patients placed on the waiting list for total knee arthroplasty (TKR) and the response to their pain to trigger point injections. Myofascial trigger points were found in all cases mainly in the medial muscles (gastrocnemius). Trigger point injections significantly reduced pain and improved mobility immediately and this effect persisted during the 8 weeks of their follow up period.

References

1. Lavelle ED, Lavelle W, Smith HS. Myofascial trigger points. Med Clin North Am. 2007;91(2):229–39.
2. Fernández-de-Las-Peñas C, Dommerholt J. International consensus on diagnostic criteria and clinical considerations of myofascial trigger points: a delphi study. Pain Med. 2018;19(1):142–50.
3. Money S. Pathophysiology of trigger points in Myofascial pain syndrome. J Pain Palliat Care Pharmacother. 2017;31(2):158–9.
4. Moraska AF, Schmiege SJ, Mann JD, Butryn N, Krutsch JP. Responsiveness of myofascial trigger points to single and multiple trigger point release massages: a randomized, placebo controlled trial. Am J Phys Med Rehabil. 2017;96(9):639–45.
5. Rozenfeld E, Finestone AS, Moran U, Damri E, Kalichman L. The prevalence of myofascial trigger points in hip and thigh areas in anterior knee pain patients. J Bodyw Mov Ther. 2020;24(1):31–8.
6. Sánchez-Romero EA, Pecos-Martín D, Calvo-Lobo C, García-Jiménez D, Ochoa-Sáez V, Burgos-Caballero V, Fernández-Carnero J. Clinical features and myofascial pain syndrome in older adults with knee osteoarthritis by sex and age distribution: a cross-sectional study. Knee. 2019;26(1):165–73.
7. Dor A, Kalichman L. A myofascial component of pain in knee osteoarthritis. J Bodyw Mov Ther. 2017;21(3):642–7.
8. Alburquerque-García A, Rodrigues-de-Souza DP, Fernández-de-las-Peñas C, Alburquerque-Sendín F. Association between muscle trigger points, ongoing pain, function, and sleep quality in elderly women with bilateral painful knee osteoarthritis. J Manip Physiol Ther. 2015;38(4):262–8.
9. Torres-Chica B, Núñez-Samper-Pizarroso C, Ortega-Santiago R, Cleland JA, Salom-Moreno J, Laguarta-Val S, Fernández-de-las-Peñas C. Trigger points and pressure pain hypersensitivity in people with postmeniscectomy pain. Clin J Pain. 2015;31(3):265–72.
10. Henry R, Cahill CM, Wood G, Hroch J, Wilson R, Cupido T, Vandenkerkhof E. Myofascial pain in patients waitlisted for total knee arthroplasty. Pain Res Manag. 2012;17(5):321–7.
11. Velázquez-Saornil J, Ruíz-Ruíz B, Rodríguez-Sanz D, Romero-Morales C, López-López D, Calvo-Lobo C. Efficacy of quadriceps vastus medialis dry needling in a rehabilitation protocol after surgical reconstruction of complete anterior cruciate ligament rupture. Medicine (Baltimore). 2017;96(17):e6726.
12. Núñez-Cortés R, Cruz-Montecinos C, Vásquez-Rosel Á, Paredes-Molina O, Cuesta-Vargas A. Dry needling combined with physical therapy in patients with chronic postsurgical pain following total knee arthroplasty: a case series. J Orthop Sports Phys Ther. 2017;47(3):209–16.

13. Mayoral O, Salvat I, Tín MT, Tín S, Santiago J, Cotarelo J, Rodríguez C. Efficacy of myofascial trigger point dry needling in the prevention of pain after total knee arthroplasty: a randomized, double-blinded, placebo-controlled trial. Evid Based Complement Alternat Med. 2013;2013:694941.
14. Fredericson M, Guillet M, Debenedictis L. Innovative solutions for iliotibial band syndrome. Phys Sportsmed. 2000;28(2):53–68.
15. Kalichman L, Ben DC. Effect of self-myofascial release on myofascial pain, muscle flexibility, and strength: a narrative review. J Bodyw Mov Ther. 2017;21(2):446–51.
16. Vernon H, Schneider M. Chiropractic management of myofascial trigger points and myofascial pain syndrome: a systematic review of the literature. J Manip Physiol Ther. 2009;32(1):14–24.
17. Li X, Wang R, Xing X, Shi X, Tian J, Zhang J, Ge L, Zhang J, Li L, Yang K. Acupuncture for Myofascial pain syndrome: a network meta-analysis of 33 randomized controlled trials. Pain Physician. 2017;20(6):E883–902.
18. Sánchez-Romero EA, Pecos-Martín D, Calvo-Lobo C, Ochoa-Sáez V, Burgos-Caballero V, Fernández-Carnero J. Effects of dry needling in an exercise program for older adults with knee osteoarthritis: a pilot clinical trial. Medicine (Baltimore). 2018;97(26):e11255.
19. Espejo-Antúnez L, Tejeda JF, Albornoz-Cabello M, Rodríguez-Mansilla J, de la Cruz-Torres B, Ribeiro F, Silva AG. Dry needling in the management of myofascial trigger points: a systematic review of randomized controlled trials. Complement Ther Med. 2017;33:46–57.
20. Borg-Stein J, Iaccarino MA. Myofascial pain syndrome treatments. Phys Med Rehabil Clin N Am. 2014;25(2):357–74.

GPSR Compliance

The European Union's (EU) General Product Safety Regulation (GPSR) is a set of rules that requires consumer products to be safe and our obligations to ensure this.

If you have any concerns about our products, you can contact us on ProductSafety@springernature.com

In case Publisher is established outside the EU, the EU authorized representative is:

Springer Nature Customer Service Center GmbH
Europaplatz 3
69115 Heidelberg, Germany

Batch number: 10732021

Printed by Printforce, the Netherlands